The

Dental Assistant

This book is dedicated to my husband Larry for his understanding through-out this project, to my son Greg for his helpful contribution, and to my daughter Julie who devoted countless hours to this project by lending her support, artistic ability, and innovative ideas.

Alice Pendleton

The Dental Assistant

7th Edition

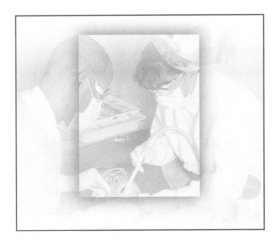

Pauline C. Anderson, CDA, MA

Alice E. Pendleton, CDA, RDAEF, MA

DELMAR
CENGAGE Learning

Australia • Brazil • Japan • Korea • Mexico • Singapore • Spain • United Kingdom • United States

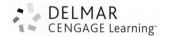

The Dental Assistant, Seventh Edition
Pauline C. Anderson, Alice E. Pendleton

Health Care Publishing Director: William Brottmiller

Executive Editor: Cathy L. Esperti

Acquisitions Editor: Maureen Muncaster

Senior Developmental Editor: Elisabeth F. Williams

Channel Manager: Tara Carter

Executive Production Manager: Karen Leet

Production Editor: James Zayicek

Project Editor: Patricia Gillivan

Executive Marketing Manager: Dawn F. Gerrain

Cover Design: Timothy J. Conners

Senior Art/Design Coordinator: Timothy J. Conners

For product information and technology assistance, contact us at
Cengage Learning Customer & Sales Support, 1-800-354-9706
For permission to use material from this text or product,
submit all requests online at **www.cengage.com/permissions**
Further permissions questions can be emailed to
permissionrequest@cengage.com

Library of Congress Control Number: 00-050846

ISBN-13: 978-0-7668-1113-3

ISBN-10: 0-7668-1113-1

Delmar
Executive Woods
5 Maxwell Drive
Clifton Park, NY 12065
USA

Cengage Learning is a leading provider of customized learning solutions with office locations around the globe, including Singapore, the United Kingdom, Australia, Mexico, Brazil, and Japan. Locate your local office at **international.cengage.com/region**

Cengage Learning products are represented in Canada by Nelson Education, Ltd.

For your lifelong learning solutions, visit **www.cengage.com/delmar**

Visit our corporate website at **www.cengage.com**

Notice to the Reader

Publisher does not warrant or guarantee any of the products described herein or perform any independent analysis in connection with any of the product information contained herein. Publisher does not assume, and expressly disclaims, any obligation to obtain and include information other than that provided to it by the manufacturer. The reader is expressly warned to consider and adopt all safety precautions that might be indicated by the activities described herein and to avoid all potential hazards. By following the instructions contained herein, the reader willingly assumes all risks in connection with such instructions. The publisher makes no representations or warranties of any kind, including but not limited to, the warranties of fitness for particular purpose or merchantability, nor are any such representations implied with respect to the material set forth herein, and the publisher takes no responsibility with respect to such material. The publisher shall not be liable for any special, consequential, or exemplary damages resulting, in whole or part, from the readers' use of, or reliance upon, this material.

Printed in the United States of America
12 13 14 15 16   19 18 17 16 15

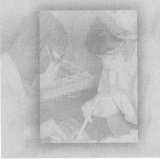

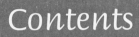

Contents

SECTION 6 Dental Histology

SECTION 7 Odontology

SECTION 8 Oral Exam and Dental Charting

SECTION 9 Dental Instruments

SECTION 10 Chairside Assisting

SECTION 11 Dental Materials

SECTION 12 Pharmacology and Anesthesia

SECTION 13 Dental Specialties

SECTION 14 Dental Radiography

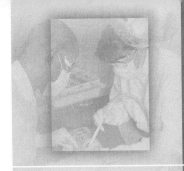

The philosophy and objectives of *The Dental Assistant*, seventh edition, are to prepare students with a lifelong career that will enable them to contribute their values, skills, and knowledge to the profession of dental assisting.

The first priority is to present a comprehensive text that will provide students with information to qualify as entry-level dental assistants. Emphasis continues to be placed on the *what, why,* and *how* in the development of manipulative skills using critical thinking values, based on the selection and application of theoretical knowledge.

The second priority is to present the material in understandable terms as applied to the practice of dentistry. The reader is introduced to terminology in sequence, as the subject matter is presented. New terms are boldfaced within chapters and included in the master text glossary. The text material is kept within the knowledge required in a basic, yet scientific, approach to dentistry. The student is encouraged to use additional sources of information and to seek continuing education in the quest for professional growth.

The facts, techniques, and methods, as they apply to clinical or laboratory procedures, are provided for the student. Review exercises and suggested activities are included. The format for review questions is matching and multiple choice to prepare students for successful completion of upcoming national and state board examinations.

New chapters in the seventh edition include Dental Ethics and Legal Issues, Using the Computer in the Dental Office, Basic Microbiology, Coronal Polishing, Oral Exam, Pharmacology, Anesthesia and Anxiety Control, Digital Imaging Systems in Oral Radiography, and Radiographic Interpretation.

Coverage of dental specialties, including Public Health, Pediatric Dentistry, Orthodontics, Endodontics, Prosthodontics, Periodontics, Oral and Maxillofacial Surgery, and Oral Pathology has been expanded.

New illustrations, photographs, line drawings, and tables have been included to facilitate interpretation of the subject matter.

The authors believe the text is one that can be effectively used by beginning dental assistant students as well as by dental assistants who are trained on-the-job, whether in a private dental office or clinic setting. It also provides current information to those dental assistants who wish to upgrade their skills and increase knowledge.

About the Authors

Pauline C. Anderson, CDA, MA—Professor Emerita and former Chairperson, Department of Allied Health, Pasadena City College, Pasadena, California

Life Member, American Dental Assistants Association

Co-founder and Honorary Member, California Association of Dental Assisting Teachers (CADAT)

Alice E. Pendleton, CDA, RDAEF, MA—Associate professor and former Program Director of Dental Assisting Program, Pasadena City College, Pasadena, California

Over 30 years in dental assisting, including 23 years in education

Life Member, American Dental Assistants Association

ADAA representative to the Commission on Dental Accreditation Appeal Board from 1994 to 1998

State director, California Dental Assistants Association (CDAA) from 1991 to 1995

Member and past secretary and treasurer, California Association of Dental Assisting Teachers (CADAT)

Active member and past president (1997) of the local component dental assistants society

Visiting instructor at University of Southern California, Los Angeles, California

Member, Organization for Safety & Asepsis Procedures (OSAP)

Acknowledgments

Many people contributed their talents and gave invaluable assistance in preparing this text. They took unexpected time and effort to ensure that each chapter fit the format, theme, and objectives of the book. It is our pleasure to express thanks and appreciation to the dental auxiliary staff at Pasadena City College:

Linda K. Teilhet, CDA, RDAEF for continued assistance in chairside procedures.

Joan K. Brandlin, RDH, BS for her guidance in the anesthesia and anxiety control chapter.

Lori Gagliardi, CDA, RDA, RDH, MEd for continued assistance in providing resource materials.

Claudia Pohl, RDA, BA for her assistance in the periodontics chapter.

Anita Bobich, CDT for assistance in dental laboratory technology avenues of education.

Jeanne Porush, RDH, MA for assistance in the education of dental hygienists.

Kathy Talaro, BA for her contribution to Chapter 5 on Microbiology.

Our grateful thanks to our friends at the University of Southern California School of Dentistry for their expertise, guidance, and support:

Robert Danforth, DDS who spent many hours providing invaluable assistance in the dental radiology section.

Terry E. Donovan, DDS who provided up-to-date resource material based on his research of dental materials.

Gayle Macdonald, RDH, PhD, a recognized authority on infection control, who provided direction on current bloodborne pathogen standards.

It is also our desire to thank key people involved in the development of this text:

Julie C. Scoon, CDA, RDA, RDH for the tremendous task and untiring efforts in coordinating the figure control sheets and illustrations.

Gregory D. Yost, computer programmer/analyst, for his invaluable contribution and expertise in the chapter related to computers.

Julie C. Scoon, CDA, RDA, RDH and Nicole Campanaro, RDA, RDH who served as models for various photographs.

Roger W. Lindner, DDS and staff who provided the dental office photographic setting and who served as models for various photographs.

Oscar Chavez, official Pasadena City College photographer, for his specialized advice and artistic contributions.

Nancy White, artist, for designing selected artistic renderings in this book.

Larry E. Pendleton, husband, for his understanding, patience, support, and assistance.

Delmar/Thomson Learning Staff:

Developmental Editor—Elisabeth F. Williams for her continual expert advice and support in formulating this text.

Acquisitions Editor—Maureen Muncaster for her contributions to this text.

Project Editor—Pat Gillivan for her support.

Art Coordinator—Timothy J. Conners for his artistic contributions.

The Dental Health Care Team and Its Responsibilities

CHAPTER 1

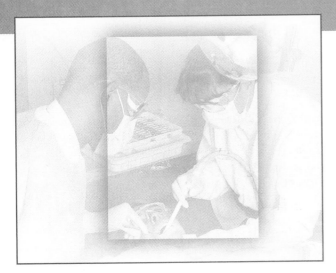

OBJECTIVES

After studying this chapter, the student will be able to:

- Identify the members of the dental health team.
- Discuss the basic qualifications and requirements for all members of the dental health team.
- Discuss the acceptable personal appearance of a well-groomed dental assistant.
- State the shared goal of the dental health care team.
- State the responsibilities of the chairside assistant.
- State the responsibilities of the business office assistant.
- Discuss how to achieve the status of a Certified Dental Assistant (CDA).
- Discuss the requirements for the registration and licensure of the dental hygienist.
- Determine the educational requirements for the dental laboratory technician.
- Describe the manner in which a visitor/colleague of the dentist should be received.
- Discuss the housekeeping procedures for maintaining an attractive dental office.
- Describe the daily function of handling the mail.
- Discuss the methods used for maintaining dental supplies.

Introduction

Given the ever-increasing demand for dental care, the modern dental office is designed with a dental team approach for the delivery of dental care. Although this chapter deals with **dental health care workers (DHCWs)**, their requirements, and their functions, it seems appropriate first to introduce the dental health team.

The first individual a prospective patient meets in the dental office may be the **dental assistant**. Many people base their first impression of the dental practice on the dental assistant's personal appearance. It is at this first meeting that the dental assistant has the opportunity to build patient confidence and a pleasing atmosphere. Both are necessary for proper patient and practice rapport. Rapport can be defined as having a relationship of mutual trust and confidence between persons.

The Dental Health Care Team

The dental team is composed of dentist(s), dental assistant(s), dental hygienist(s), and dental laboratory technician(s). Although the composition of the team may vary from office to office, it is the dentist(s) who always supervises the delivery of services to the patient.

Basic Qualifications and Requirements

The first requirement for any member of a dental health team is to maintain good physical and mental health. A dental practice cannot afford to have an employee who is not physically well, has less-than-average ability to reason, or is unable to adjust to the dental environment. Failure to care for his or her own person cannot be tolerated.

Second, each team member must know and practice the rules of professional **ethics** (dealing with moral conduct, judgment, and the ability to apply these capacities) and conduct. Each team member must exhibit social and professional self-assurance. Such proper behavior invites the confidence of the patient, and that confidence and trust must be treated with sincerity.

Third, a friendly approach is highly desirable and is shown by a smile and a pleasant, calm, and patient attitude. Friendliness, rather than familiarity, indicates to the dental patient that the team members are courteous representatives of dentistry. Courtesy is capable of attracting many persons to a dental practice. Patients tend to come back to a dental office for help, empathy (feelings, thoughts, and motives that can be understood by another), and assurance. In contrast, patients will not tolerate a disinterested or egotistical dental team. Patients need to know they have a team that is honest and interested in their welfare.

Fourth, a neat, well-groomed team member who exhibits good personal hygiene is an asset to any dental practice. In many offices the dental assistant wears a uniform that must be kept immaculate. Dental uniforms vary from the traditional dress-type to pants and a top and may be in white or a color. The hair should be attractively styled and easy to control. Long hair, for either male or female team members, should be pulled back and secured. Males should be clean-shaven on a daily basis. Comfortable duty shoes of standard design must be kept clean and polished. Nails must be clean, short, and with smooth cuticles. Nail polish is discouraged; colored nails have proven offensive and nonprofessional in the eyes of patients and doctors. Using a chamois buffer to give sheen to the nails is recommended. If the female dental assistant uses cosmetics, any makeup should be applied in good taste and not readily noticeable.

Good grooming and personal cleanliness are vital to the success of a dental team member. Spending a few minutes each day will ensure that the dental team member's appearance is orderly.

All members of the dental team have specific duties and responsibilities. As a team, they are working together with the shared goal of providing the best possible dental care. The success of such a team depends on the attitudes and cooperation of all team members. The efficiency of the team depends on the ability of each member to contribute those particular talents and capabilities required in providing quality dentistry to patients.

The Dentist

In the practice of dentistry, the licensed **dentist** is the individual who sets up practice to provide dental care to persons who need such services. Dentists may limit their practices to general dentistry or may specialize in pediatric dentistry, periodontics, prosthodontics, oral and maxillofacial surgery, orthodontics, oral pathology, endodontics, or dental public health. If a dentist specializes in one of the specialties, additional postgraduate education is required that could take from two to three years or more. The duties include:

- Diagnosis of dental diseases and lesions and the correction of malpositioned teeth, bony structures, soft tissues, and associated structures

- Management of drugs and medicaments used in dentistry

- Providing patients with advice on their dental health

- Utilizing skills for patient treatment in all necessary related procedures, including operative or surgical procedures

To be able to practice dentistry, an individual must be a graduate of a dental school accredited by the **American Dental Association (ADA)**, Commission on Dental Accreditation, and pass both the written and clinical exams in the state. Dentists are awarded one of the following degrees depending on the school granting it: DDS (Doctor of Dental Surgery) or DMD (Doctor of Medical Dentistry).

The Dental Assistant

With the modernization of dental equipment and improved operating techniques, such as sit-down, fourhanded dentistry, qualified dental assistants are required.

Whether the office is a private (solo) or group practice, more than one dental assistant is needed. The delegation of responsibilities may be divided into separate areas.

Chairside Dental Assistant

Dental assistants who work directly with the dentist in the operatory (treatment room) are the chairside dental assistants (Figure 1-1). The duties include:

- Seating and dismissing the patient

- Infection control procedures

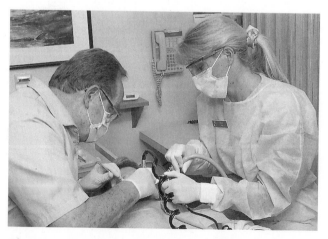

Figure 1-1 The chairside dental assistant.

- Sterilization procedures
- Assisting in chairside procedures
- Preparing restorative materials
- Exposing, processing, and mounting radiographs
- Caring for and maintaining dental equipment
- Inventory and ordering supplies
- Performing selected laboratory procedures
- Other delegated tasks permitted under the state's Dental Practice Act

Extended Functions Dental Assistant

The **extended functions dental assistant (EFDA)** or the **registered dental assistant in extended functions (RDAEF)** performs duties that are beyond the scope of what dental assistants are required to do. Thus, additional education is required for licensure in this category. The duties delegated to EFDAs, in addition to all dental assisting duties, are generally performed within the patient's mouth. However, duties vary between EFDAs and RDAEFs depending on what is delineated in the Dental Practice Act for each level. Duties may include:

- Taking final impressions for cast restorations
- Taking impressions for appliance construction
- Acid etching the teeth for bonding
- Cord retraction of gingiva for impression procedures
- Coronal polishing
- Applying pit and fissure sealants
- Fitting of trial endodontic points
- Placing, carving, and finishing amalgam and composite restorations (not RDAEF)

Business Office Assistant

A business office assistant, sometimes known as the secretarial assistant or receptionist, handles all business procedures and is responsible for the smooth operation of the front or business office (Figure 1-2). The duties include:

- Office management
- Telephone management
- Controlling the appointment book (scheduling all appointments)
- Making financial arrangements for patient fees
- Using computer skills
- Banking
- Bookkeeping
- Managing office correspondence and mail
- Dental insurance billing
- Regular monthly billing

Rover

Some offices may employ a third assistant. A rover, also referred to as the coordinating assistant, may have specific duties or assist wherever needed, at chairside or the front office. A rover assistant may perform in situations where certain procedures require six-handed dentistry. Duties delegated to the rover assistant would be dependent on where the immediate need might be.

Certification

For those dental assistants who meet the eligibility and examination requirements, certification may be earned in one or more areas. To earn any of the available certifications, a dental assistant must first meet one of the eligibility pathways for the certification being sought; generally, graduation from a dental assisting program accredited by the ADA Commission on Dental Accreditation or two years of full-time work experience (3500 hours) as a dental assistant. Second, the dental assistant must pass the certification examination directly related to the area of certification. Documentation for each of the requirements in the eligibility pathway sought must be submitted to the **Dental Assisting National Board (DANB)**.

The **Certified Dental Assistant (CDA)** credentials will include certification in general chairside, radiation health and safety, and infection control. All pathways require verification of current Health Care Provider cardiopulmonary resuscitation (CPR) certification from the American Heart Association or the American Red Cross. The following certifications are available:

- Certified Dental Assistant, which includes the General Chairside (GC), Radiation Health & Safety Examination (RHS), and Infection Control Examination (ICE)

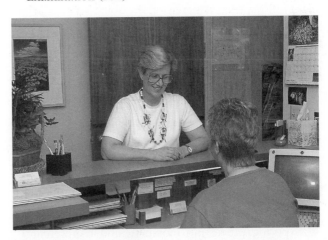

Figure 1-2 The business office dental assistant.

- Certified Dental Practice Management Assistant (CDPMA)

- Certified Orthodontic Assistant (COA), which includes the ICE

Certification is in no sense a degree, nor does it hold any legal status. However, it does carry with it knowledge in the dental field and the ability to apply it.

Some states require the dental assistant to pass a written and/or clinical examination to become *registered* or *licensed*. Rather than requiring a second exam, some states will accept the DANB examination and grant registration to those dental assistants. Having met the requirements, the dental assistant is known as a **registered dental assistant,** extended functions dental assistant, or registered dental assistant in extended functions (RDA, EFDA or RDAEF). Most registration or licensure requires periodic renewal.

Many states require certification, registration, or licensure for all dental personnel who expose dental radiographs.

Areas of Service

Dental assistants currently serve the profession in dental offices, in federal agencies, or in facilities of the armed services. Dentists employ the majority of dental assistants in private (solo) practice. Both general practitioners and specialists maintain these offices in the dental profession.

Other dental assistants are employed by the rapidly growing group-practice system. In the group-practice setting, several general-practice dentists or specialists join and share one receptionist, one business office, and one dental laboratory. Federal agencies, including clinics and hospitals of the Veterans Administration and the U.S. Public Health Service, also employ dental assistants.

The national organization for dental assistants is the **American Dental Assistants Association (ADAA)** with state and local components.

The Registered Dental Hygienist

The dental hygienist is the auxiliary member employed specifically to perform oral hygiene care (Figure 1-3). The duties include:

- Recording health histories

- Scaling and polishing teeth

- Applying topical fluoride treatment

- Applying pit and fissure sealants

- Placing and removing periodontal dressings

- Exposing, processing, mounting, and interpreting radiographs

- Oral health education

- Preventive oral care, including plaque control

- Providing oral hygiene instruction

- Diet and nutrition counseling

- Maintaining an active recall system. Such a system is used to inform patients, either by postcard or telephone, of their next prophylaxis (teeth cleaning) appointment. In many offices, the business office assistant assumes this responsibility. The recall system is most vital in that it affords the patient an opportunity to be involved in his or her own preventive dental care program.

Although the dental hygienist is licensed and sees patients on an independent basis within the dental office, clinic, or hospital, the responsibilities remain under the supervision of the dentist in some states. However, in recent times within certain states, there has been a change in which dental hygienists are allowed to practice independently in alternative settings without the supervision of dentists. This allows qualified dental hygienists to perform in such alternative settings as retirement homes and hospitals for easy patient access to care. Dental hygienists are licensed and must comply with the regulations within the state Dental Practice Act. In certain states the hygienist is permitted to perform some expanded functions such as soft tissue curettage, administering local anesthesia and nitrous oxide-oxygen, and assuming some dental assisting chairside duties when necessary.

Requirements for licensure of a dental hygienist are as follows:

- Graduation from a dental hygiene program accredited by the ADA Commission on Dental Accreditation

- Current CPR certification

- Successful completion of the National Board in Dental Hygiene (NBDH) written examination

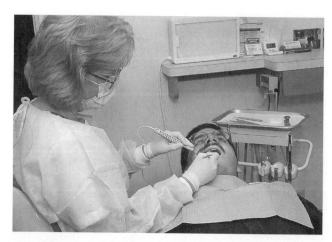

Figure 1-3 The registered dental hygienist.

● Successful completion of the state dental hygiene licensure practical examination *or* completion of a state regional practical board examination (for participating states). For a fee, applicants may be licensed in more than one state; applicants may complete a state regional board examination in more than one state.

Results of the examination will be sent to member state boards in which the person holds state licensure.

A hygienist uses the title of **registered dental hygienist (RDH)** and is licensed and governed by the Dental Practice Act of the state in which he or she practices.

The national organization for dental hygienists is the **American Dental Hygienists Association (ADHA)** with state and local components.

The Dental Laboratory Technician

Unlike other auxiliary members of the dental team (dental assistants and hygienists), dental technicians do not perform work directly on the patient, but in a laboratory.

A **dental laboratory technician (DLT)** is educated to perform the mechanical and technical tasks necessary to prepare dental restorations and appliances, such as fabrication of gold and porcelain restorations, partials, or full dentures. However, the dental technician is under the guidance and supervision of the dentist and must have a written prescription from the dentist to complete the required laboratory procedures. Generally, the dental technician is not a member of the dentist's immediate staff but either is self-employed or works in a commercial laboratory. The procedures that dental technicians perform are many. There are five subspecialties, each requiring certification:

1. Ceramics: constructing porcelain restorations
2. Crown and bridge: constructing gold restorations
3. Dentures: constructing removable teeth
4. Partials: constructing removable teeth with metal substructures
5. Orthodontics: constructing appliances for the purpose of tooth movement

Dental laboratory technicians may complete programs approved by the ADA Commission on Dental Accreditation. Programs approved by the ADA are two years in length and are usually conducted in a two- or four-year college or post–high school institution. Upon successful completion of an ADA-approved program and successfully passing the written and practical parts of the **Certified Dental Technicians (CDT)** examination given by the **National Board for Certification (NBC)**, the technician receives the Certified Dental Technician certificate.

Dental laboratory technicians may also receive their education through apprenticeship (by agreement, the learner agrees to work for a specific amount of time for instruction in the area of concern). Commercial dental laboratories offer apprenticeships leading to employment. In some states a dental laboratory may use the title of **Certified Dental Laboratory (CDL)** if the owner is a CDT and the laboratory is an approved facility; otherwise, that title is not applicable.

Front-Office Routine and Management

The responsibility for the care and management of the front office and reception room is usually delegated to the business office assistant, who is in close proximity to them.

The Reception Room

When greeting a dental patient, the business office assistant should always check the appointment book to know the correct name of the patient. The patient should be greeted by name, promptly, upon arrival. The business office assistant should enter the reception room to greet each patient rather than just peeking around the door. A business-like, dignified, courteous manner should be maintained at all times.

Conversation in the reception room between patients and the dental assistant should be kept to a minimum. Personal comments are in order only when the patient and dental assistant are well acquainted. Lengthy conversations are time consuming and do not contribute to the atmosphere of the office. Idle chatter cannot reduce the fears of apprehensive patients.

An efficient dental assistant is considerate and concerned about the patient's welfare but does not talk too much. The dental assistant makes certain the patient is as comfortable as possible and offers special help when necessary. In dismissing the patient, the chairside dental assistant will accompany the patient to see the business office assistant for any necessary appointments, then thank the patient for coming in. The dental assistant should also have a special good-bye for children, praise them for being good patients, and, if it is the dentist's routine, reward them with a small token.

Should an individual enter the reception room and introduce herself or himself as a doctor (colleague) or personal friend of the dentist, the business office assistant should offer a seat in the reception room. The dentist should be notified as soon as it is convenient to do so. Professional colleagues of the dentist who are not members of the office staff should not be allowed into the dental treatment room unless the patient and dentist have given permission.

Reception Room Reading Material. A variety of magazines with different subject matter should be provided for patients in the reception room. It is suggested that several areas of interest be included in the magazine selection:

- Sports
- Homemaking
- Business
- Pictorials
- Children's books
- Children's coloring books with colored pencils or crayons situated at a child-size table with chairs (Figure 1-4)

Reading material must be updated and kept orderly at all times. The business office assistant should sort the magazines and discard all except the last two editions of each periodical. Current issues, if damaged, should be repaired or discarded.

Housekeeping

The dental office should be completely and periodically cleaned professionally. Woodwork, tables, and table lamps must be checked daily for finger marks and kept clean. Furniture should be free of dust and soil. When the reception room is carpeted, the carpeting should be inspected daily for tread marks left by foot traffic and soil. Routine vacuuming and spot cleaning should keep maintenance at a minimum.

Proper lighting and ventilation in the dental office with midmorning and a midafternoon temperature check will ensure comfort for the patients and staff.

Business Office Assistant's Desk. Because the business office assistant's desk is usually in view of the

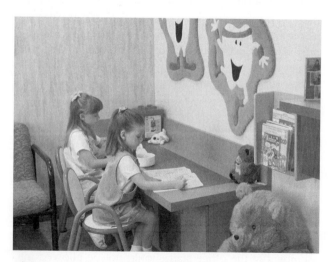

Figure 1-4 Children's table in the reception room.

patients in the reception room, it is essential that the desk be kept free of clutter. Everything should have its place—and be kept in its place. When an item is efficiently filed, it should not be difficult to find it later. Personal belongings must be kept out of sight. Papers, patient records, dental radiographs, and like items must not be allowed to pile up on the business office assistant's desk. Tiered desk trays will help greatly in keeping order.

Doctor's Office and Treatment Rooms. Good housekeeping in the inner office provides the dental staff with the proper environment for conducting dental treatment. As each patient is dismissed, the dental assistant should quickly clean and disinfect the treatment room before the next patient is seated. Any evidence of the preceding patient must be removed.

Administrative Duties

An important function of the dental staff is the handling of mail. The mail includes display advertisements, personal letters, bills, checks, professional announcements, magazines, laboratory reports, samples from drug houses, and so forth. Most often, it is the business office assistant who opens the mail.

As a general rule, every doctor has a preference for the way the office mail is handled. For instance, the dentist may prefer to open certain mail and delegate the rest of the responsibility to the dental assistant. There are certain classes of mail separated according to their importance:

- Special-delivery letters
- Express mail
- Payment envelopes
- Personal letters
- Facsimile correspondence
- Advertising material
- Magazines and newspapers
- Other routine mail

Handling the Mail. Once the routine has been established, the business office assistant can direct special-delivery letters, express mail, and personal mail to the doctor's office without opening them. Occasionally there is some doubt in the dental assistant's mind regarding a particular piece of mail. A good rule to follow in such cases is this: If one is uncertain about opening a letter or parcel, *don't*. Discretion in handling the mail is very important, and it is essential that communications containing personal items for the doctor be routed unopened to the doctor's desk.

The business office assistant will then group the mail into the mentioned categories and handle as necessary. Magazines, for example, should be placed in the reception room in exchange for dated magazines. Payment envelopes from patients can be separated and recorded immediately in the day's receipts. Other items may need to be filed, shown to the doctor, or thrown away. The more accomplished the dental assistant becomes with this routine, the more time the dentist can devote to professional duties.

There are fewer problems involved in handling outgoing mail than there are with incoming mail. Letters, for example, that are sent from the doctor's office should always be checked for correct spelling and punctuation. Care must be taken that the correct letter goes into the right envelope. A copy of all outgoing correspondence is maintained and filed in the office. However, copies of letters should not be filed until the doctor has signed the original letter. Should a particular letter be one the doctor prefers not to sign (because of an inaccuracy), both letter and copy can be destroyed without having to remove the copy from the file.

When mailing letters, local mail should be separated from out-of-town and foreign mail that may require special postage. Such letters or parcels should be taken directly to the post office for mailing. Group the mail together, and schedule a time each day to send it on its way.

In the event that the doctor is not at the office and cannot be contacted when important mail arrives, the dental assistant should try to get in touch with the sender immediately, explain the reasons for the delay, and ask for the sender's cooperation. It is wise when forwarding mail to the doctor to inform the sender that the mail has been forwarded and that there will be some delay. In some cases, the doctor will respond directly to the sender. In other cases, the doctor will dictate a message to the dental assistant for forwarding to the sender. Other mail not requiring special handling that arrives during the doctor's absence can be placed in a folder and held until the doctor returns.

Ordering Supplies. Ordering supplies is performed by the chairside dental assistant, the business office dental assistant, or both. The task of ordering supplies is delegated to the individual(s) who is (are) in close contact with their use.

To keep the supply area well stocked, it is necessary to have a record, or inventory, of supplies to be ordered. Accurate records, systematically kept, will enable the dentist and office staff to devote more time to patient care.

Surveys of various manufacturers of dental products indicate that the dental assistant is in charge of ordering and maintaining supplies.

It is important to set up a method of inventory control and to maintain a well-balanced stock. A spiral notebook may be used as an inventory logbook, with additional information retained on file cards or maintained in the computer. A complete inventory should be conducted on a monthly basis.

The inventory log should include the following:

- Date order is placed
- Name of supplier
- Reference or ID number for each order
- Name and quantity of product
- Projected cost of each item
- Items on back order and approximate shipping date
- Name of the supply house and individual taking order
- Check-off column for items received

When ordering by mail or phone, the name, address, and telephone number of the doctor's office should be included with the ordering information. These orders should also be indicated in the log.

Keeping a separate index of file cards on which product name, price of item, supplier name, address, and telephone number are recorded provides easy reference when ordering.

A complete inventory once a month (in addition to the daily routine checking of supplies) before an order is placed is highly recommended.

Storing Supplies. After the supplies have been ordered and received, it is necessary to have a storage plan. A neat, well-arranged supply cupboard will aid in better and more efficient dental assisting. As a rule, supplies should be stored according to accessibility, temperature, light, and effects of moisture on each item. When an article is removed from its place, care should be taken that it is returned to the same place. Expiration dates of chemicals and other supplies that deteriorate during storage must be checked periodically and replaced as a routine part of ordering.

SUGGESTED ACTIVITIES

- Do some role playing whereby another student plays the part of a patient. Practice greeting and welcoming the patient to the office. Also, practice dismissing the patient and make a hypothetical appointment.
- Take inventory of supplies and calculate how much is needed of each item for one month. Based on the inventory, list needed supplies with projected amounts as if they were to be ordered at this time.

REVIEW

1. The shared goal of the whole dental team is to:
   a. Recruit as many patients as possible.
   b. Have increased production by serving more patients.
   c. Allow team members to practice their skills.
   d. Provide the best possible dental care.

2. One of the responsibilities of the chairside dental assistant is to:
   a. Confirm patients for the next day.
   b. Possess computer skills.
   c. Take inventory and order supplies.
   d. Make financial arrangements while the patient is seated at the chair.

3. All eligibility pathways for dental assistant certification (CDA) require:
   a. Hepatitis B vaccination
   b. Current CPR certification
   c. High school diploma
   d. Current radiation certification

4. Indicate which two of the following factors are of greatest importance to ensure comfort for patients and office staff: (1) proper lighting, (2) proper décor, (3) proper filing system, or (4) proper ventilation.
   a. 1, 2
   b. 2, 3
   c. 3, 4
   d. 1, 4

5. Indicate which of the following type of mail should be directed to the doctor's office: (1) payment envelopes, (2) special delivery, (3) personal mail, and/or (4) express mail.
   a. 1, 2, 3
   b. 2, 3, 4
   c. 1, 3, 4
   d. 1, 4

Dental Ethics and Legal Issues

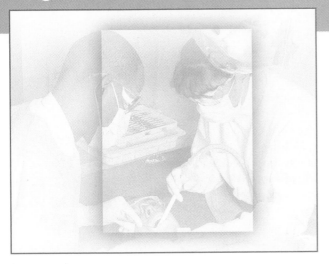

Legal issues are addressed that should cause the dental professional to be aware of laws that govern issues in the delivery of dental care. Dental auxiliaries need to know their boundaries within which they perform duties legally. It is wise to know the duties that are listed in the state Dental Practice Act for each member of the dental health team. These duties are developed through legislative action, which regulates the scope of practice in dentistry. Dental professionals also need to have an understanding of basic law and apply this knowledge when maintaining records and carrying out routine tasks in the dental office.

OBJECTIVES

After studying this chapter, the student will be able to:

- Define the concept of ethics.
- Discuss the purpose for the state Dental Practice Act.
- Discuss the role of the Board of Dental Examiners and who serves on it.
- Explain the difference between criminal and civil law.
- Explain what the term "negligence" means.
- Explain the difference between direct supervision and general supervision.
- Identify whom the Americans with Disabilities Act protects.
- Discuss what is involved in the duty of care for which the dentist is responsible.
- Explain the two types of consent.

Introduction

Dental health care workers (DHCWs) have ethical and moral responsibilities to patients. It is their obligation to provide patients with quality dental care. Their moral concerns together with technical skills must be acceptable and they should have a clear understanding of pertinent issues of the law that deal with the practice of dentistry when providing desired patient care. The principles of the **golden rule** ("Do unto others as you would have them do unto you") as well as the code of ethics for each group should be used as basic guidelines when dealing with patients as well as other health care professionals and the public domain. The dental team must work harmoniously in the delivery of care and take responsibility to promote the well-being of everyone concerned.

Ethics

Ethics may be defined as that part of philosophy (love of learning) that deals with moral conduct (knowing right from wrong), judgment (the mental capacity to make reasonable decisions), and being able to apply these capacities. As a result, one is able to feel a sense of duty (moral obligation).

A **code of ethics** is the standard of moral principles and practices that a profession closely follows. Although they are voluntary controls, rather than laws, they serve as a method of self-policing within a profession. In dentistry, a code of ethics is the standard of professional rules by which DHCWs are guided. Each group within the dental team has a code of ethics, specifically, the American Dental Association (ADA) for dentists, the American Dental Hygienists Association (ADHA) for dental hygienists and the American Dental Assistants Association (ADAA) for dental assistants (Figure 2-1).

The dental professional must maintain ethical standards that reflect the responsibilities established for the primary purpose of providing quality care to the patient. In dentistry and medicine, the Hippocratic oath is a standard that serves as a guide to protect the rights of the patient and to "above all, do no harm." The principles of the golden rule should also be practiced. There are standards for dental care set forth in each state. These are known as the state Dental Practice Act.

The State Dental Practice Act

Each state imposes legal rules and regulations of professional standards for dental practice upon every DHCW

AMERICAN DENTAL ASSISTANTS ASSOCIATION
PRINCIPLES OF ETHICS AND CODE
OF PROFESSIONAL CONDUCT

Each individual involved in the practice of dentistry assumes the obligation of maintaining and enriching the profession. Each member shall choose to meet this obligation according to the dictates of personal conscience based on the needs of the general public the profession of dentistry is committed to serve.

The member shall refrain from performing any professional service which is prohibited by state law and has the obligation to prove competence prior to providing services to any patient. The member shall constantly strive to upgrade and expand technical skills for the benefit of the employer and consumer public. The member should additionally seek to sustain and improve the local organization, state association, and the American Dental Assistants Association through active participation and personal commitment.

As a member of the American Dental Assistants Association, I pledge to:

• Abide by the Bylaws of the Association
• Maintain loyalty to the Association
• Pursue the objectives of the Association
• Hold in confidence the information entrusted to me by the Association
• Maintain respect for the members and employees of the Association
• Serve all members of the Association in an impartial manner
• Recognize and follow all laws and regulations relating to activities of the Association
• Exercise and insist on sound business principles in the conduct of the affairs of the Association
• Use legal and ethical means to influence legislation or regulation affecting members of the Association
• Issue no false or misleading statements to fellow members or to the public
• Refrain from disseminating malicious information concerning the Association or any member or employee of the Association
• Maintain high standards of personal conduct and integrity
• Not imply Association endorsement of personal options or positions
• Cooperate in a reasonable and proper manner with staff and members
• Accept no personal compensation from fellow members, except as approved by the Association
• Promote and maintain the highest standards of performance in service to the Association
• Assure public confidence in the integrity and service of the Association

Figure 2-1 American Dental Assistants Association Principles of Ethics and Code of Professional Conduct (Courtesy of American Dental Assistants Association).

through its state **Dental Practice Act**. It contains the legal restrictions and controls for the dentist, the dental auxiliaries, and the practice of dentistry. It defines regulations in all areas of dentistry developed for the protection of society and, most importantly, the dental consumer (patient).

The requirements listed in the Dental Practice Act have been developed through legislative action and, therefore, are legal. It lists all the rules and regulations affecting each dental professional and thereby describes the types of supervision under which **dental auxiliaries** (dental assistants and hygienists) may perform. For example, it specifies whether a function/duty may be performed under direct supervision or general supervision.

Under **direct supervision**, the auxiliary may perform a procedure/duty while the dentist is physically present in the dental office and who will evaluate the procedure upon completion.

Under **general supervision**, the auxiliary may perform a procedure/duty with the dentist's permission but without the physical presence of the dentist.

The state Board of Dental Examiners, created by the act and designated as an administrative board, usually interprets and provides a definite procedure to ensure that regulations are fulfilled.

The State Board of Dental Examiners. The **state Board of Dental Examiners** is the body responsible for the administration of examinations for licensure, enforcement of **statutes** (laws), rules, and regulations, and the establishment of standards for quality continuing education for license renewal.

The board adopts rules and regulations that define, interpret, and provide a plan that follows the intent of the Dental Practice Act. The state Board of Dental Examiners supervises and regulates the practice of dentistry within the state.

The Board of Dental Examiners is usually comprised of dentists, public members, and in some states dental auxiliaries. This body of representatives meets several times a year in different locations of the state for the purpose of addressing concerns on the board's agenda. These concerns are usually related to dental educational changes, developing and implementing **mandates** (something the board imposes as a moral obligation) for the improvement of dental care delivery, suspending and revoking licenses when there has been a violation or criminal act, or regulating the practice of dentistry. The main purpose of this body is the protection of the patient.

Legal Issues

The legal system is composed to two types of law, criminal law and civil law. **Criminal law** can be defined as a law that deals with a person who has committed an act or crime that threatens society and may be subject to **punitive** (punishment) action. **Civil law** is a law that generally deals with a situation between two persons where there was damage or injury or where there was a binding agreement. There are two branches under civil law, contract law and tort law. Contract law can be considered to have a binding agreement involving compensation, whereas tort law basically involves injury to a person or property, as in a "malpractice action," and is considered a civil wrongdoing.

Negligence

If a practitioner is careless about the manner in which the patient is treated, thus causing mental and physical harm, this action could be labeled as negligent. Therefore, **negligence** is defined as an act that a reasonable person would not do under the same or similar circumstance (act of commission) or, on the other hand, failure to act as a reasonable person would under the same or similar circumstance (act of omission). A **malpractice** action usually would fall under negligence committed by a professional. When a patient brings a malpractice action, it could involve the dentist, dental hygienist, or dental assistant and it could be due to the professional's conduct, performing a duty illegally, or evil doing.

It is imperative that each member of the dental team carries liability insurance. Dentists and dental hygienists usually do; however, many dental assistants assume that the dentist has a policy that covers them. As dental assistants assume more responsibilities in providing direct clinical care to the patient, they have an obligation to themselves to carry their own liability insurance. The ADAA provides members with its own professional liability insurance, naming the member in the policy. Where there is no other affordable alternative, such a policy should be given careful consideration.

Consent

Consent is defined as the authorization for proposed treatment performed by an adult. To minimize problems in a dental office, it is imperative that the patient give the practitioner his or her consent to perform dental treatment; otherwise, the practitioner may be liable for committing battery (unauthorized touching). When a patient comes in for treatment, the patient, being an adult and of sound mind, must give consent for himself, for his children who are under legal age, or for someone who is mentally incompetent. This consent could be either informed consent or implied consent.

Informed Consent. **Informed consent** is the written authorization given by an adult who agrees to proposed treatment. It is the doctor's responsibility to give an adequate explanation of the proposed treatment in terms that the patient will fully understand, the manner in which it will be performed, the outcome of such treatment, alternative plans for treatment, and the estimated cost of the proposed treatment. The patient must not be pressured into making a hasty decision, should be given an opportunity to ask questions with satisfactory answers, and have ample time to make a reasonable decision about proceeding with the treatment.

It may be the practice of a dentist to have a form for the patient to sign to affirm that consent has been given. This may be viewed as a contractual agreement (Figure 2-2).

Implied Consent. **Implied consent** is a verbal authorization given by an adult who agrees to proposed treatment. Most of the time it may be a general oral agreement between the dentist and the patient, in which case an implied consent would result. It is wise to have a written statement giving authorization for proposed treatment. In an emergency, and lacking either informed or implied consent prior to treatment, the practitioner performs dental treatment without it; however, there must be evidence of urgency and gravity of the emergency.

INFORMED CONSENT

Patient's name _____ Date _____
Dentist's name _____

Proposed treatment _____
_____
_____

Benefits and alternative treatments _____
_____
_____

Common risks _____
_____
_____

Consequences of not performing treatment _____
_____
_____
_____
_____

Every reasonable effort will be made to ensure that your condition is treated properly, although it is not possible to guarantee perfect results. By signing below, you acknowledge that you have received adequate information about the proposed treatment, that you understand this information, and that all of your questions have been answered fully.

☐ I give my consent for the proposed treatment as described above.

☐ I refuse to give my consent for the proposed treatment as described above.

☐ I have been informed of the potential consequences of my decision to refuse treatment.

_____
Patient's signature   Date

_____
Dentist's signature   Date

_____
Witness's signature   Date

Figure 2-2 Informed consent (Courtesy of Roger W. Lindner, DDS).

Duty of Care

Duty of care is the ethical responsibility owed by one individual to another. When a dentist accepts the responsibility of treating a patient, the duty of care owed to the patient is as follows.

- Possess proper credentials (licenses) to be able to practice dentistry.
- Possess proper knowledge and skills in providing treatment.
- Obtain informed consent prior to initiating treatment.
- Make a record of the patient's medical history to provide proper care.
- Inform the patient of his or her findings or diagnosis using proper diagnostic aids.
- Refer patients to specialists or other practitioners who offer expertise, when indicated.
- Use approved materials and medicaments.
- Provide dental care that meets ethical and professional standards.
- Complete treatment once initiated in a given period of time and not abandon the patient.
- Charge fees that are in accordance with other similar offices in the community.
- Give clear and understandable instructions to patients.
- Practice using infection control measures on all patients.

When the patient agrees to receive dental care, there are certain responsibilities owed to the dentist as follows:

- Provide the dentist with an accurate health history.
- Cooperate in following the dentist's special instructions dealing with medication or care.

- Show good faith in keeping appointments.
- Pay fees for services rendered in a timely manner.

Termination or Abandonment

In situations where dental care is discontinued for unforeseen circumstances, such as relocation of the dental office or terminal illness of a practitioner, patients should be informed of the subsequent change. Dental care should continue for at least 30 more days until such time when other arrangements can be made; otherwise this act may be viewed as **abandonment** (wrongful cessation of dentist-patient relationship where the patient is still undergoing treatment). On the other hand, if a patient becomes undesirable, the dentist should notify the patient by correspondence using a return-receipt registered letter, informing the patient that the dentist-patient relationship is being terminated. The letter should indicate that the local dental society is able to provide information regarding referrals to other dentists. A copy of the letter and receipt should be filed in the patient's chart (see Chapter 3).

Documentation of Patient Records

Accurate record keeping is one of most important tasks a dental assistant and other dental team members can accomplish. The information must be dated and clearly written in complete form, and the person responsible for entering the data should sign his or her name for each entry made. If an error in entering data is made, the assistant *cannot* use an eraser or "white out." A simple line across the area to be deleted is acceptable in a court of law; this correction should be initialed and dated by the person making the adjustment. It is recommended that all information reflect with accuracy what was performed. Using abbreviations or ambiguity is not recommended.

With increased attention given by the media on the exposure to radiation for the purpose of making radiographs, patients are becoming more apprehensive in subjecting themselves to its effects. If patients refuse to comply with having current radiographs made, this statement should be clearly dated, documented, and signed by the patient.

Radiographs. Many times patients think that radiographs made on the recommendation of a dentist are theirs to keep and carry around from dentist to dentist, but in reality they are the property of the dentist who ordered them. Radiographs are considered to be part of the patient's record, used as an aid in diagnosis, and not simply for legal documentation. Should a situation arise where it is necessary for the patient to access his or her radiographs to make them available to the succeeding dentist, it is customary to make a copy and forward the copy of the radiographs. It should be noted that when this transaction takes place, the patient needs to give written consent for the transfer of any radiographs or records. There may be a fee charged to the patient for duplication and mailing costs.

Confidentiality

Confidentiality is defined as the nondisclosure of certain patient information except to another authorized person. The Americans with Disabilities Act protects individuals who are afflicted by an illness, such as a communicable disease that could cause embarrassment or harm to the patient, if the nature of the disease is divulged to others. In the dental office, a patient may communicate such information to the dentist. It is of utmost importance that this type of information be kept confidential except in cases where it is obligatory for the dentist to report certain health hazards to appropriate authorities. Otherwise, it is possible that the patient be entitled to file a lawsuit for "invasion of privacy" and be compensated monetarily for damages incurred.

SUGGESTED ACTIVITIES

- Record services rendered on a simulated patient's chart. Realizing that the wrong entry was made, make the proper correction based on information from this chapter.
- Prepare a set of radiographs to forward to another dental office to include all necessary documentation.

REVIEW

1. Standards for dental care in each state, which impose legal rules and regulations, are found in:
   a. The Centers for Disease Control and Prevention (CDC) reports
   b. Board of Dental Examiners reports
   c. OSHA guidelines
   d. State Dental Practice Act

2. Name the administrative board responsible for enforcement of laws, rules, and regulations for dentistry within each state.
   a. Board of Consumer Affairs
   b. State Board of Dental Examiners
   c. Committee on Dental Auxiliaries
   d. OSHA

3. A malpractice action committed by a professional would be known as:
   a. Negligence
   b. Criminal act
   c. Civil act
   d. Punitive act

4. The written authorization given by an adult for proposed dental treatment is known as:
   a. Confidentiality
   b. Informed consent
   c. Duty of care
   d. Implied consent

5. The nondisclosure of certain patient information, except to another authorized person, is known as:
   a. The golden rule
   b. Implied consent
   c. Statute
   d. Confidentiality

Dental Patient Management and Communication

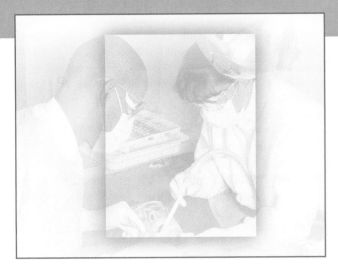

CHAPTER 3

OBJECTIVES

After studying this chapter, the student will be able to:

- Discuss human relationships as they apply to the practice of dentistry.
- Determine the skills necessary to establish a sound professional relationship.
- Discuss the need for dental patient questions.
- Determine the role of dental staff when verbally communicating with a patient.
- Discuss time management.
- Define the term patient's advocate.
- Determine the influence of office environment on the patient.
- Discuss the method used for emergency coverage of dental patients.
- Determine the meaning of division of responsibilities as it applies to dental patients.
- Define proper distance from patients.
- Determine what information should be included when taking a telephone message.
- Discuss making appointments.
- Evaluate the need for keeping good dental records.
- Understand the necessity of sound financial management.
- Discuss how a dentist-patient relationship is terminated.

Introduction

Dentistry is both a technical- and person-oriented profession. The success of a dental practice and the satisfaction enjoyed by the dentist, the staff, and the patients largely depend on how well needs and expectations can be shared and adjusted. Patients find dentistry more rewarding when they understand the importance of sound personal oral hygiene and appreciate the value of the technical work performed. When the dental staff shares a common system of values and goals, only then can the needs of the patient be met. These goals are all more likely to be achieved when there is good communication.

Communication

What is communication? **Communication** is an exchange of information, ideas, views, meanings, and understanding, be it **verbal** (spoken, written) or **nonverbal** (actions, attitudes, gestures).

Patients look for competence, commitment, and caring. Dental professionals must be able to communicate through words and actions that the dentist knows what he or she is doing and the team is committed to the patient's health and care about him or her as a person, as well as about his or her overall health. Communicating these values to the patient will improve patient satisfaction.

Communication can also be seen as a way to involve others in the problems faced in the practice of dentistry. Good interpersonal (between-people) communication skills are essential for getting better control of what goes on in the dental office. Control involves the capacity to predict and adequately influence the present environment with the task at hand. Control implies fewer hassles, fewer surprises, and a greater sense of accomplishment. Consequently, control benefits all concerned. The dental professional who is at ease, effective, and predictable, because he or she communicates well, helps the dentist, patients, and co-workers gain control.

Human Relationships

Rather than stressing the technical aspects of dentistry when speaking with patients, the focus should be on human relationships. Dental health care professionals can find great satisfaction in their work when they make a conscious and continuous effort to study human behavior—both their own and that of other people. **Behavior** is the manner in which a person conducts him- or herself under specified circumstances.

With some patients, it will be easy to establish a pleasant relationship, one in which the patient believes that he or she is understood and that everyone in the dental office is concerned. This relationship is termed **rapport**.

Good rapport may be more difficult to establish with other patients. Perhaps, the patient's behavior arouses unfavorable feelings in the staff. Perhaps, the patient is not found to be "interesting" to staff. It is easy to project blame or label the patient "difficult."

The patient who has been labeled difficult is probably most in need of special attention from the dental team. The behavior that causes the patient to appear difficult may actually be signals that the patient's needs are not being met. On the other hand, the pleasant, agreeable patient may be covering up true feelings and may have just as much need for concern and understanding. In other words, providers of dental care will need to apply interpersonal skills, to establish rapport with each patient on an individual basis. Some patients will present more of a challenge than others, but all need to be shown understanding and a sincere interest in making a positive contribution to their health care.

During the first visit, the patient and dentist establish a rapport that will assist them in their future professional relationship. As a result, all dental staff will want to make this initial visit as successful as possible. The following are suggested ways in which dentist and staff can let patients know that they will be taken care of, that their questions will be answered, and that their concerns will be addressed.

Listening Skills

Three things that dentists and staff can do to make patient relationships stronger are (1) listen, (2) listen, and (3) listen. Listening takes work and it takes time. Changes in the office scheduling procedures may need to be made to allow time for adequate listening.

Eye Contact. When listening, good eye contact should be maintained with the patient. Good eye contact is recognized by the public as representing honesty, cooperativeness, regard for others, and self-confidence. These are characteristics the dental team seeks to have associated with it. When dentist and staff have developed a comfortable and effective eye contact with the patient, the doctor-patient-staff relationship will increase in value.

Avoiding Distracters. When patients are talking, every effort should be made to avoid shuffling papers, viewing radiographs, or doing anything that would indicate to patients they do not have the full individual attention of the listener.

Sitting with the Patient. Another technique that helps the patient feel that he or she has been given ample time for discussion is the simple act of sitting down in the patient's presence. It is customary for this to occur during a prophylactic appointment with the

hygienist, but less likely when the dentist enters the treatment room to check the patient's chart and mouth after the prophylactic exam is completed.

Allowing the patient to sit upright and at a level where the dentist and patient have good eye contact will help the communication process. The patient who receives information of extreme importance regarding dental care, while staring at the acoustical tiles of the ceiling or the nose of the dentist, will gain little from this sort of communication and may, in fact, resent such inconsiderate behavior.

Body Posture. Keeping a body posture that is open and relaxed is also important when listening to a patient. Slouched or closed posture habits, such as sitting or standing with only one side facing the patient rather than full-face, could suggest a disinterest in the patient's problems and concerns.

Patient Questions. Dental professionals should avoid becoming defensive about questions asked by the patient. Questions are opportunities for better patient satisfaction and should be encouraged. Often, the patient is looking for a way to better understand, to remove doubt, or for various reasons to feel comfortable with treatment recommendations. Patient questions are often opportunities for the dental personnel to help rid the patient of perceived notions about dental care.

Patients who leave the dental office with unanswered questions may be dissatisfied with the recommendations, which can lead to discontent with completed treatment. The patient can be encouraged to ask questions simply by being asked for them.

Careful listening to patient's questions and concerns can often enable the dentist and staff to recognize a problem, or realize the patient is unhappy at a very early stage of treatment. Before the patient leaves the office, every effort should be made to determine any questions the patient might have and to mutually agree on the appropriate solutions.

Speaking Skills

Adjusting language and terminology to a level the patient understands will assist both the dentist and the staff in communicating with the patient. While some patients understand technical terminology, others will need **lay terms** (adjusting technical terms into ones that will be understood by the average person) for complete comprehension. Patients should be asked if they are following the explanation being offered. Answering questions or clearing up information will help patients recognize that they have a part to play in their health care. Patients need to understand their role in the treatment process.

Staff Communication. The dentist will set the tone for the communication style of the office and direct the interaction with the patients. However, all dental personnel are responsible for good communications with the patients. Staff should check on the patient on a regular basis, making certain the patient is not left alone for long periods of time. They can also help to reassure the patient even when the doctor is present. Often, the patient is more willing to seek support from the staff member (assistant) rather than from the dentist. Thus, the assistant becomes the *patient's advocate*, one who will speak on the patient's behalf.

Time Management

Time management is another technique for making the patient feel comfortable. A patient should not have to wait for lengthy periods of time in the reception room or be kept waiting in a treatment or consultation room. Likewise, the patient should not be detained at the front desk to make future appointments or settle an account.

When an emergency alters an orderly schedule, the scheduled patient should be informed immediately and be offered the opportunity to reschedule. Tardiness reflects an uncaring attitude, and such timely explanations will go far in soothing ruffled feelings.

Nonverbal Communication

Office Design and Decorative Style. The office environment will often influence how the patient feels about the treatment offered by a particular dental practice. Is the office kept clean? Has it been decorated in a manner that is suitable to the clientele? Are the furnishings updated or decades old?

Since patients do not have the technical expertise to judge the clinical competence of the dentist, they will use other unspoken clues to assess his or her abilities. If the dental office has the appearance of being a bit untidy or dirty, patients may suspect that sterilization techniques are not thorough.

Matching the office décor to patients' taste will assist in reducing the pressure or strain felt by many patients. The mere fact that they have a dental appointment produces stress-related disturbances. If the office is decorated like one in Beverly Hills, when the practice is predominantly suburban and where patients come directly to the office from varied types of employment, some patients may feel uncomfortable in such surroundings. On the other hand, if the furnishings are not up to the acceptable modern standards, patients might think the dental practice is not keeping up with current trends and techniques in dentistry.

Personal Hygiene. All dental personnel must have a commitment to personal hygiene. Patients will be offended by poor hygiene habits of health care providers. If they think that the dental professional does not take health care recommendations seriously, they may not accept any treatment recommendations. Consider the example of working with the patient on improving daily oral health care while the dentist or staff member explaining these procedures has bad breath!

The message is clear; many factors contribute to the way patients perceive the dental office, the dentist personally, and the staff. These thoughts affect the patient's attitude about treatment success, coupled with how comfortable the patient feels within the environment.

Written Communications. Written communication to the patient will emphasize the dentist's concern for the patient's health. Follow-up letters after a treatment consultation summarizing the discussion and agreements made during the appointment serve to assure the patient that his or her needs are being met. The business office assistant will play an important role in all correspondence to the patient.

Telephone Communications. A telephone call at the end of the day to check on patients after a long or difficult procedure or treatment will reflect the concern for total patient care.

Emergency Coverage. In the event the doctor is unavailable to the patient (such as during vacation or illness), arrangements should be made by the office for another dentist to see patients on an emergency basis. When patients realize their dentist is arranging for their health care in his or her absence, they will feel reassured.

Patient Education

The patient must understand the division of responsibilities of care. The dentist's responsibility is to make a diagnosis, establish an acceptable treatment plan, and provide adequate dental care. The patient's responsibilities include making and keeping timely appointments, caring for his or her oral health before, during, and after care, and meeting the financial obligations associated with the treatment. Patients should also realize they must promptly report to the dentist any problems they might experience.

Interpersonal Distance

There are distances that are appropriate for certain relations between people and for certain activities. Any departure from these socially expected distances may cause tension and contribute to misunderstanding (Table 3-1).

Table 3-1 Interpersonal Distance

Type	Distance	Relationship
Intimate	1–18 in.	Close friends, family
Personal	18 in.–4 ft.	Friends, peers
Social	4–12 ft.	Acquaintances
Public	12 ft. or more	Strangers

Touching

Touching is an important part of dental care. Positioning the patient's head, assisting the patient in and out of the chair, and unexpected contact at the front desk are examples.

Telephone Management

Telephone communications are of utmost importance because they set the stage, in the patient's mind, about the type of dental office it is. Portraying a professional demeanor is, without question, what patients will look for and remember when forming an opinion about a dental office. The business office assistant must always maintain an attitude of professionalism and warmth. The tone of voice should be loud enough to be easily heard but not so loud that it would be uncomfortable to the listener. One should speak in a clear, easily understood, and calm but enthusiastic manner.

Things to avoid would be mumbling, holding the receiver at a distance, chewing gum, interrupting the patient, using slang terms such as "yeah" in place of "yes", not listening carefully, and making assumptions about what the patient said instead of asking the patient to repeat the statement.

Taking and Relaying Messages

When patients call the dental office, they expect a prompt reply. The business office assistant should be attentive and respond after the first ring, identifying the office and herself, then inquire how the caller can be helped. An example of the greeting may be as follows: "Good morning, this is Dr. Martin's office, Susan speaking. How may I help you?" The caller realizes that he or she has reached the correct office and is speaking with Susan. By the tone of voice used, the caller formulates an opinion instantly about the office and the business office assistant. Did she sound friendly and caring or unfriendly and uncaring?

The caller who wishes to speak with the dentist needs to be informed that the dentist is with a patient and cannot be disturbed at the moment. The business office assistant should offer to take a message, indicating that it will be relayed to the dentist as soon as possible.

When the message is taken, it should contain the following information:

- The date and time of the call
- The first and last name of the caller
- A clear message
- The name or initials of the business office assistant if there is more than one person taking calls

Screening Calls

It is important not to disturb the dentist while attending a patient so as not to interrupt productivity and create a delay in the schedule. Policies should be established to determine which calls would take precedence. Calls from immediate family members or from other dentists who need to confer would be exempt from screening. Screening others should be done in a tactful manner. Emphasis should be placed on the fact that when the dentist is with a patient, interruptions are kept to a minimum to provide continual patient care.

Keeping a Telephone Log

Keeping a log on every incoming call may be the policy in some dental practices. It is used to track persons whose call may be of value for the dentist to review at the end of the day. When entering information in the log, the following data should be recorded: the date and time of the call, the person's full name and telephone number, if they are a representative of a business company, and the purpose of the call.

Voice Mail

If the telephone will remain unattended for a period of time, a message on the voice mail should identify the dentist's name, office hours, the number to call in an emergency, the importance of their call, and instructions on how to leave a message for follow-up. The business office assistant should be prompt in the follow-up of such calls.

Appointment Control

Service to dental patients is at its best when there is complete mutual understanding and cooperation. When a series of treatments is provided to the patient, the business office assistant can expect complete cooperation in making and keeping appointments. Generally, a customary sequence of procedures is followed in making appointments for new patients, recall patients, emergency cases, and special cases. To keep a dental practice running smoothly, appointments and the handling of the appointment book are usually assigned to the business office assistant. If appointments are made systematically and efficiently, there will be more available productive time. The dentist will be able to handle emergencies, often resulting in more new patients. There will also be sufficient time allowed for each operation. A more evenly spaced day for both the dentist and chairside dental assistant is the outcome.

Initial Appointments

When scheduling an initial appointment for the new patient, enough time should be allowed for a complete dental and medical history to be completed. Adequate time should be allotted for the dentist to make a thorough examination of the patient's mouth and teeth. It is preferable to allow an additional 15 minutes to complete the patient history card, which includes health information. The dental assistant should also determine who referred the patient to the office and the reason for the appointment.

The dental hygienist may first see the patient for prophylaxis (teeth cleaning) and radiographs. Many offices will routinely take impressions for study models prior to a second diagnostic appointment. Findings from radiographs, diagnostic models, and clinical findings obtained during the first appointment are studied and diagnosed prior to the second appointment. The conditions present and the recommended proper treatment are discussed with the patient at the time of the diagnostic appointment. If more than one method of treatment warrants consideration, the alternatives are thoroughly discussed, and the patient is informed of what can be expected from each type of service. The exact fee for the services is discussed at that time. When the method of treatment has been decided, additional time is then set aside for the most efficient and the earliest possible completion of the case. In addition, a definite arrangement for the payment of fees is made by the patient. The business office assistant is usually given the responsibility for this agreement.

Emergency Appointments

Emergency appointments are frequently made by patients who are suffering from some dental discomfort or pain. It is the duty of the dental assistant to determine the extent of the dental problem and to do the utmost to arrange for an appointment. If certain hours of each day are allotted for emergency appointments, the emergency patient should be scheduled at that time. It is recommended that one-half hour of each day be scheduled for such emergencies. In nonindustrial areas, 11:30–12:00 a.m. or 1:00–1:30 p.m. may be set aside. If the day is fully appointed, the patient should be so advised. The patient should also be told there is a scheduled emergency time when the doctor will be available. As with

all cases, the dental assistant should never indicate to the patient that the office staff and the dentist are in a hurry because of a full schedule.

Confirming Appointments

Generally, it is a good idea to notify all patients 24 hours in advance of an appointment. However, if a patient has a tendency to break appointments, the following suggestions may help in keeping such broken appointments to a minimum:

1. The patient should always be notified 24 hours in advance of each appointment.
2. The patient should be impressed with the fact that a broken appointment results in considerable inconvenience to the dental routine.
3. The patient should be reminded that the doctor works on a schedule.
4. If the doctor has such a policy, the patient should be informed that there will be a charge for broken appointments.
5. The patient should be encouraged not to make any more appointments until he or she feels the appointments can be kept.

Should a patient cancel an appointment, the business office assistant should remain courteous. The patient should be thanked for calling, and another appointment should be scheduled. In the event the patient does not wish to make another appointment at the time of cancellation, the business office assistant should ask if it is agreeable to call the patient in a week or two to reschedule the appointment. If the patient desires this service, the business office assistant should note this and be certain to call the patient at that time to reschedule the appointment.

Management of Patient Records

It is essential to keep accurate patient records. Several entries are necessary to have these records complete:

1. Correct name, address, home telephone number
2. Place of employment and telephone number
3. Dental insurance carrier (if applicable)
4. Birthdate (month, day, and year)
5. Dental and health histories
6. Mold and shade of teeth used in denture and bridgework; shade of synthetics and plastics

Such records should be posted on the patient's record and kept up-to-date.

Current trends in record keeping involve use of the computer, thus enabling rapid retrieval of patient records (Figure 3-1).

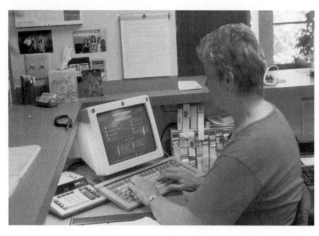

Figure 3-1 Using a computer to store dental records.

Indexing and Filing

Accurate indexing and filing in a dental office are both a convenience and a necessity and are the bulk of most dental office procedures. All dental offices, whether large or small, should keep all letters received and make copies of all letters that are mailed. In addition to correspondence, much other important information is carefully kept, such as receipts, canceled checks, purchase orders, duplicate sales slips, invoices, statements, and catalogs. There is always a chance that such items will be needed for quick reference. They must be properly indexed and filed if they are to be located quickly.

Many offices keep separate folders or sections in file drawers for correspondence, auditor information (income tax returns, bank statements, and social security information), invoices, paid statements, unpaid statements, and catalogs. All such papers should be filed properly and promptly to ensure that they can be located quickly when needed.

Financial Management

Successful financial management is the key to a successful dental practice. Such management is based on establishing a practical arrangement with each patient and includes diagnosis, case presentation, and an estimate of work to be done. A definite understanding of what is expected of both doctor and patient is essential to financial management. Even though the patient has selected a dental program and the method of payment, certain unforeseen situations may arise, causing the account to become delinquent. The business office assistant, in many instances, has the responsibility of collecting the delinquent accounts.

Delinquent accounts are usually caused by one or more factors:

● Dissatisfaction with service

● Misunderstanding of fees and work to be done

● Poor money management by the patient

● Poverty

● Dishonesty

Delinquent accounts may be collected by phone or mail solicitations. Generally, contact is made each month following the last payment of the overdue account. The method should be persuasive and the communication simple. The purpose is to have the patient willing to pay the account.

Collection Problems

Satisfying the patient can minimize collection problems. If the estimate is correct and the payment schedule is realistic, patients are appreciative and more apt to pay their accounts promptly. The paying habits of new patients should be investigated to determine their occupations, earning power, and credit histories. If a doctor is a member of a credit union, this information is readily available.

The Case Presentation

The case presentation is the responsibility of the dentist. The staff should prepare and gather all materials needed for the meeting. These include patient charts, radiographs, study models (if any), visual aids, booklets, brochures applicable to the case, schedule of fees, and "consent" form for the patient's acceptance of the treatment plan.

A treatment plan will include proposed treatment with options to that plan, if options exist. The fees associated with each treatment option should be presented during the treatment discussion.

Once the plan has been agreed upon and accepted by the patient, the payment schedule of fees will be discussed by doctor and patient. Long-term patient benefits rather than the financial aspects of the treatment should be stressed.

Documentation of Records

Good record keeping is imperative, to support not only the clinical aspect of the treatment but the dentist-patient-staff relationship as well. The doctor's notations on the patient chart should include patient questions, how a mutually agreed-upon solution was achieved or determined, and any satisfactory comments made by the patient. Such entries in the chart must be made accurately and without personal prejudice.

Staff entries can be beneficial to the patient's entire record. Staff can note on the chart additional information or comments made by the patient directly to them. Any questions concerning appointments, follow-up visits, and other nontreatment concerns the patient expressed should be noted and signed by the person making them. Staff notations should be reviewed by the dentist, signed, and dated. Once an entry is made in the patient record, it becomes documented evidence of what has transpired.

Terminating Patient Relationship

Sometimes the dentist-patient relationship must be terminated. Termination of the relationship involves three considerations:

1. The health of the patient must not be jeopardized by the termination of care.

2. There must be written notification to the patient that treatment is to be discontinued.

3. The patient must be given ample time to secure the services of another dentist.

It is recommended that this written notification be sent by registered mail, with a return receipt to be permanently filed in the patient's chart.

Ways to find another dentist should be offered to the patient. The local dental society may maintain a referral service or have a list of dentists' names within the same geographic area. The patient should be notified that copies of dental records, radiographs, and other materials that would be helpful and beneficial to future care would be forwarded to the new dental practice.

SUGGESTED ACTIVITIES

Using a videotape recorder, do some role playing in which one student acts as the office assistant and a fellow student acts as the patient. Later on view the tape and evaluate communication effectiveness and problem solving. Discuss the following hypothetical topics:

● Confirm an appointment with a patient who is known to break appointments. What should be communicated?

● Dental work has just been completed and the fee needs to be collected. The patient was previously informed that the fee would be collected at the end of the appointment time, but came unprepared to pay. What is the best option?

● A colleague of the dentist walks in the office and wishes to speak with him right away; however, the dentist is treating a difficult case. What is the best way of handling this situation?

REVIEW

1. Describe a key to building positive doctor-staff-patient relationship.
   a. Having good eye contact
   b. Improving behavior patterns
   c. Improving communication
   d. Using technical terms to impress others

2. How can the dental assistant improve speaking skills with patients?
   a. Adjust language and terminology to the patient's level.
   b. Refer all patients' questions to the dentist.
   c. Avoid telephone interruptions.
   d. Record everything that was communicated on paper.

3. What four elements should the telephone log include?
   a. Date, time, caller's name, purpose of call
   b. Date, caller's name, when available for a return call, purpose of call
   c. Date and time, caller's name and phone number, company representative, purpose of call
   d. Time, caller's name, purpose of call, relation to dentist

4. How many hours in advance should patients be notified of their appointment?
   a. 48
   b. 2
   c. 8
   d. 24

5. Indicate which of the following factors usually cause delinquent accounts: (1) misunderstanding of fees and work to be done, (2) dissatisfaction with service, (3) having to wait for an appointment, and/or (4) not being able to schedule a weekend appointment.
   a. 1, 2
   b. 2, 3
   c. 3, 4
   d. 1, 4

CHAPTER 4

Using the Computer in the Dental Office

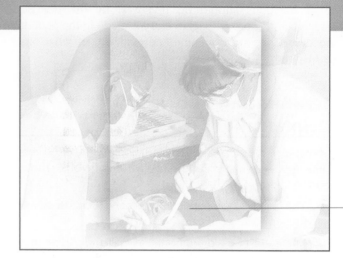

OBJECTIVES

After studying this chapter, the student will be able to:

● Explain the difference between the three types of computers.

● Explain the basic principles of how a computer operates.

● Describe the four functions of the computer.

● Explain where data is processed.

● List the components of computer hardware.

● Explain the purpose for having a diskette/floppy disk.

● Discuss the role of software in the computer system.

● Explain how dental software fits into the computer environment.

● Discuss how a database is acquired.

Introduction

Use of computers in the dental practice has revolutionized the business office. Beginning with the purchase of new computer equipment and the acquisition of new computer vocabulary, the transition from manual record keeping to sophisticated electronic entries has had a significant impact on today's dentistry. Efficiency has increased by promoting organization throughout the office. Computer use has benefited operations such as appointment scheduling, treatment plan presentation, patient tracking, accounts management, payment agreement program, insurance processing, recall system, clinical charting, marketing assistance by generating correspondence for all purposes, intraoral camera integration (see Chapter 34), and digitized radiograph (filmless x-ray system; see Chapter 68) integration.

Computer Principles

The computer originated as a large calculator that was housed in a big room. It consisted of numerous vacuum tubes acting as switches. Thus, in principle, a computer is only a large number of switches. A single computer chip may contain thousands of microscopic switches that perform mathematical calculations.

It is of great importance that all personnel in a dental office be familiar with the operation of the computer

system. There is new vocabulary to learn along with understanding the type of software being used that will be at the heart of knowing how to input **data** or information. This learning period may take place during an orientation session conducted by a software sales representative, by using resources such as a computer manual to continually improve skills in computer performance, and a lot of practice. It is no longer the case that only business office personnel will be operating the computer. Workstations using the computer are being placed in treatment rooms where chairside dental assistants or dental hygienists will be responsible for data input. Therefore, it is wise to become computer literate and contribute to the overall office productivity.

Looking into the Computer

The computer system is capable of operating in several aspects:

● gathering information by data input

● processing the data

● outputting information, also called data output

● storing information

Data Input. The most common way data input is achieved is by manually "typing" in the information using the keyboard. A person who assumes this position should have typing skills and understand key commands. There are other devices used to input data: a scanner, computer graphics, voice recognition, touch recognition screens, and a compact disk read-only memory (CD-ROM). The term "read only" refers to the fact that the information on the compact disk may be viewed as a soft copy on the monitor or be printed out as a hard copy; the user cannot "write," or change, its information but can only use it as resource material. Graphics may be purchased in this manner and incorporated in the production of a document.

Data Processing. Data is processed in the **central processing unit (CPU)**, which is referred to as the inner workings, or "brain," of the computer. It is here where all activities of the computer are controlled and where the memory capacity is located. Computers are equipped with a hard disk/drive that may have enough memory to take care of all the patients' records and their applications in one office.

Data Output. The data output takes place when information is produced by printing a copy of the document known as **hard copy** or by displaying information on the monitor making it visible, referred to as **soft copy**. A printer is used to print out a hard copy.

Data Storage. Data may be *stored* in the hard disk/drive, on a floppy disk also called a diskette, or on a tape cartridge. The **hard disk/drive** is located within the CPU. It has ample memory capacity and it is called the hard disk because it consists of a rigid metal disk that is coated with magnetic material.

The **floppy disk/diskette** is a portable unit that may be transferred from one computer to another. It consists of a thin plastic disk within a protective cover. The 3.5" double-density disk is capable of holding 720 kilobytes (kB) and the high-density disk is capable of holding 1.44 megabytes (MB). Depending on the diskette disk drive (a device designed to read and write information and programs on a diskette) options the computer unit has, a diskette may be used to record the same data that was saved on the hard drive and may be retained as **backup** (a copy made of a file usually on a diskette or tape cartridge in the event the original is lost or damaged) for future reference. A *tape cartridge* may also be used for the same purpose. At the end of the business day, all data that was entered in the computer should be backed up using one of the recording items already described.

In addition, new removable storage media continue to emerge on the marketplace. Examples would be the Zip cartridge, which holds 100 megabytes, and the Jaz/EZ-Flyer cartridge capable of holding 1–2 gigabytes of information (Table 4-1).

Computer Systems

There are three computer systems that may be used in a business setting: the mainframe, minicomputer, and microcomputer.

Table 4-1 Media Sizes and Capacity	
Media	**Capacity**
3.5" diskette	High density – 1.44 megabytes
Zip cartridge	100 megabytes
Jaz/EZ-Flyer cartridge	1-2 gigabytes
Hard drive (fixed disk)	10 megabytes – 12 gigabytes
Tape cartridge	250 megabytes – 40 gigabytes

The Mainframe. The **mainframe** is an enormous system that was designed to handle large volumes of information. All of the processing, programs, and data are located on the mainframe, not on the individual workstations. This type of system is designed for large corporations and is not normally found in dental offices.

The Minicomputer. The **minicomputer** is a medium-sized computer that provides a centralized design similar to the mainframe discussed above in that they both utilize workstations. All processing, programs, and data are located on the minicomputer, and not on the workstations. Dental software in a small- to medium-sized office may be found residing on this type of system.

The Microcomputer. The **microcomputer**, or PC (personal computer), as it is more commonly known, is the typical computer used extensively in dental offices, homes, and in most businesses. It has the capabilities of data collection, storage, and production of hard copies. Many of the more common office programs are used on this type of system (e.g., word processing, spreadsheets, database). It is capable of handling less volume of data than the minicomputer (Figure 4-1).

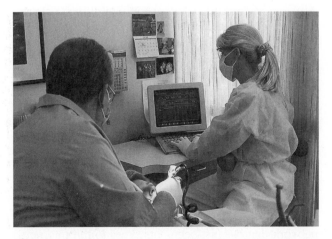

Figure 4-1 Computerized system in the dental office.

Networking

In simplest terms networking is connecting computers together so that they can communicate with each other. Computers on a network utilize a communications protocol (procedures and language used to communicate) to communicate with each other. It is important to use the same communications protocol as that of the computer with which one is attempting to communicate.

Local Area Network

A local-area network resides within a single company or department and provides communications between workstations, mainframes, minicomputers, and microcomputer servers. This gives a single workstation access to corporate information (typically found on a mainframe), departmental information (typically found on a minicomputer), and office applications (typically found on a microcomputer server). In a dental office, a minicomputer might house the dental software, whereas the microcomputer server would typically house **e-mail (electronic mail)** and other general office applications.

Wide-Area Network

A wide-area network is simply a local-area network that connects multiple local-area networks together. It is typically used to connect the local-area networks of multiple offices at different locations together to provide better communications between those offices.

Internet

The **Internet** is simply a large network similar to the wide-area network discussed above. If one were to connect a local-area network to the Internet through a **router** (a device that bridges between a local-area network and the Internet), access to resources on the Internet would be available through the local-area network. Once connected to the Internet, resources are available according to the communications protocol used. **Web sites** (a collection of viewable documents located on a computer server) utilize HTTP (hypertext transaction protocol), whereas a file download might utilize FTP (file transaction protocol). This is only an example of the many types of protocols used on the Internet and is an illustration of the fact that the Internet is simply a large network.

Once the Internet connection is made, e-mail can be sent to any of more than a thousand e-mail post offices located throughout the world, and any workstation with a web browser (e.g., Netscape Navigator, Microsoft Internet Explorer) will have access to any web site in the world. The only danger is that the local-area network that has just been connected to the Internet is also visible and potentially accessible by the millions of users on the Internet.

Hardware

The **hardware** is comprised of the computer itself, which receives, processes, and stores information; the monitor, which displays a soft copy on the screen; the keyboard, where the information is input, comprised of alphanumeric keys (keys that represent the alphabet and numbers), function keys (keys that control specific processing functions) located at the top of the keyboard, and other keys that perform specific commands (Figure 4-2); the mouse, which acts as a pointer on the screen; and a printer.

Devices that are connected to the computer but are external to the unit itself are called computer **peripherals**. They would include such things as printers, scanners, digital cameras, etc.

Software

Software is defined as a set of instructions that tells the hardware which tasks to perform. It is a very important entity in determining how the computer will be used. Software is also known as a "program" and is generally purchased separately from the hardware. However, the operating system software is usually preinstalled in the system. Software falls into several categories, such as operating system, office applications, and proprietary business software.

Operating System

The **operating system** is the software that controls the hardware directly. All other software will interact directly with the operating system rather than with the hardware directly. In this way, the operating system acts as a middleman. The operating system is responsible for all system operations but needs to be loaded from a diskette or hard drive into RAM when the computer is powered on.

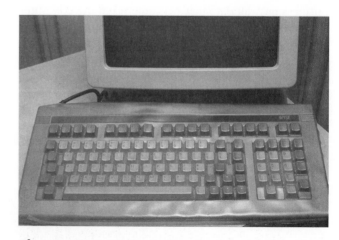

Figure 4-2 Computer keyboard.

Office Applications

Office applications are various programs or software that fall into the category of general use. In other words, they can be used for a variety of business and/or personal situations. Examples of these would be word processing (e.g., Microsoft Word, Word Perfect), **spreadsheet** used to create tables (e.g., Excel, Lotus 123), database (e.g., Access, Paradox), and presentation (e.g., PowerPoint). The most common of these is word processing, which offers the ability to enter and format text and graphics for output on a printer. When installed, one must bear in mind that it takes up a fair amount of storage capacity.

Proprietary Business Software

Proprietary business software is that software that has been developed for a specific purpose or industry. Dental software (e.g., Dentrix, Computer Age Dentist) would fall into this category and may interface with any of the office applications listed above.

Dental Applications

Dental offices that employ computerized systems (see Figure 4-1) have many advantages over ones that do not. Information is processed at high speed in a professional manner that allows for increased productivity through office automation. Increased numbers of dental office personnel are becoming computer users. The first task upon acquiring a computer system is to input a **database** (collection of data) of all patients in the practice. Once all patient data (information consisting of facts and figures that is processed to produce a final product) is recorded in the computer, it becomes a simple matter of updating it later on. For example, updating the chart is done at the time services to the patient are performed, when insurance reimbursement takes place, or when new information is received from the patient.

For security reasons, the user would enter a **password** (a meaningful number of characters used to identify a specific user) that the computer recognizes, allowing the user to gain access to its programs and also to track who posted what and when. Once it gets past this phase, it displays icons (representative recognizable figures) of all the software programs, files, or functions that have been installed. The user selects the desired icon and proceeds to enter it.

If the selected icon is the dental software program, a menu of the types of applications (e.g. appointment scheduling, patient accounts, insurance) is displayed first. Highlighting the desired application makes a selection. Once this is achieved, the operator will need to type in the patient's name.

The next step is to input data and edit it as needed. The output would take place as data were entered. A

hard copy may be made at any time whether it is for the insurance company or for patient information. All desired input data should be "saved" as a permanent document and stored on the hard drive/disk. This is done immediately after completing data input. A back-up copy should be made on a daily basis and stored safely away from magnetic environment in the event the computer is damaged or malfunctions.

Examples of Electronic Entries

Appointment Scheduling. Scheduling appointments electronically for the dentist and dental hygienist is made easy when using a color-coded module, a feature found in some software. The soft copy displayed on the monitor provides the date at the top with columns designated for each professional those patients will be scheduled to see. For example, if the dentist uses two treatment rooms, the first column may be color coded pink for the dentist's treatment room 1 schedule, the second column may be color coded yellow for the dentist's treatment room 2 schedule, and the third column may be color coded green for the dental hygienist's schedule. If the lunch hour were scheduled at the noon hour, it would be blocked out. If an appointment is canceled, all the information written for that patient, such as the name, telephone number, a code for type of work to be done, or special considerations as a medical alert, may be moved to another day electronically instead of rewriting it. It can search for open appointments, eliminating the need for time-consuming visual search (Figure 4-3).

Once appointments are scheduled, the information may be transferred automatically to a "daily schedule" sheet and a hard copy printed for the next day. This is the sheet that is posted in each treatment room to inform the dental team of the day's activities.

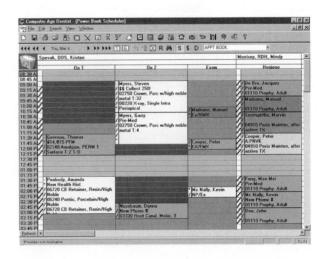

Figure 4-3 Example of computerized appointment control (Courtesy of Computer Age Dentist, Inc.).

Locating the Patient's File. Upon entering the dental computer software, a menu with a list of functions is visible on the monitor screen. If the selection for "patient information" is chosen and entered, then the patient's last name followed by first name and identification number are inserted to be able to access that patient's file. When it is brought up, data may be input (Figure 4-4).

Clinical Charting. While the patient is in the chair, electronic entries are made in the patient's file provided that the treatment room is equipped with a workstation. As the dentist examines the patient's teeth, the assistant may enter data regarding the conditions that are present. There is software that automatically enters the date, graphics, American Dental Association (ADA) diagnostic code, and proposed fee while the tooth number and involved surfaces are entered. Treatment planning and the total of proposed fees using the mathematical computation feature are done quickly, saving chairside time. Periodontal charting may be done in like manner. When the probing depth is recorded, the software program may record it graphically using distinct colors to indicate where bleeding and suppuration (discharge of pus) points are located. It is also possible to record tooth mobility, bone loss, and furcation (the space between the roots on a multirooted tooth) grades (Figure 4-5).

Patient Record Files

Although it appears that the emphasis in the modern dental office is to have a "paperless" administrative office, the need to keep patients' records in file drawers is still essential. Having the hard copy in place is necessary even though the computer is capable of storing most of the patient's information electronically. For example, radiographs are part of patients' records that need to be stored as reference material. If digitized radiographs (see Chapter 68) are integrated with the existing patient database in the computer, the need for hard copies may still be necessary to use for comparative or informational purposes. Until there is complete evolvement from the traditional business office to an absolute electronic one, there will be a need for manual filing and record keeping.

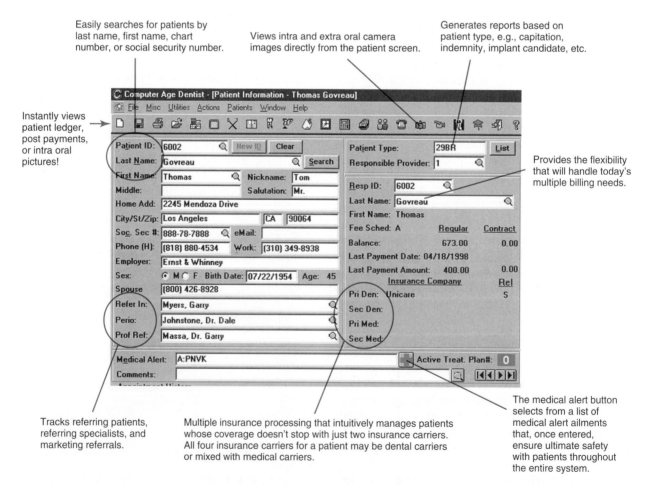

Figure 4-4 Example of a computerized patient's chart (Courtesy of Computer Age Dentist, Inc.).

Clinical and Perio Charting

Color coded, textbook charting symbols make the "clinical workstation" easy and functional. Treatment plans, procedures, dates, ADA codes, descriptions, fees, tooth numbers and surfaces are all automatically updated to the patient's chart, ledger, billing, etc. Materials used are noted along with unlimited clinical notes. Intra and extra oral camera images along with digitized x-rays are easily displayed on the chart for clinical review and patient education. X-rays may be viewed with many different effects to help diagnose difficult cases. Charting can be entered by voice, light pen, mouse, or keyboard. **Perio charting** easily charts mobility, furcations, pocket depths, bleeding, suppuration, gingival margins and attachment levels, and more! Displays and legally records perio history as well as current probings.

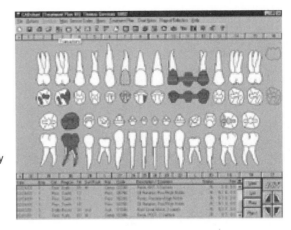

Figure 4-5 Example of computerized charting (Courtesy of Computer Age Dentist, Inc.).

SUGGESTED ACTIVITIES

- Compare the minicomputer with the microcomputer.
- Boot up the computer, following directions previously given. Enter the password. Select the desired icon for the dental software plan, and enter it. Enter the patient's name. Use the mouse to control the cursor and input data.
- Using a floppy disk, make a copy of data you entered.

REVIEW

1. Indicate which of the following are essential components of a computerized operational system: (1) mainframe, (2) data, (3) hardware, and/or (4) basic operating procedures.
   a. 1, 2, 3
   b. 2, 3, 4
   c. 1, 3, 4
   d. 1, 2, 4

2. A set of instructions that tells the hardware which task to perform is called:
   a. Software
   b. Monitor
   c. Data
   d. Memory capacity

3. The soft copy is:
   a. The software
   b. A printed copy
   c. A xeroxed copy
   d. A copy of what the screen on the monitor displays

4. When input data is saved as a permanent record, it can be stored: (1) on a diskette, (2) on the hard drive disk, (3) on a compact disk read-only memory, and/or (4) on a tape cartridge.
   a. 1, 2, 3,
   b. 2, 3, 4
   c. 1, 2, 4
   d. 1, 3, 4

5. What should take place at the end of each day when all data are entered in the computer?
   a. There is no need to do anything more.
   b. A hard copy should be made.
   c. All data should be backed up.
   d. A second copy of the hard copies should be made.

SECTION 2

Basic Microbiology

CHAPTER 5

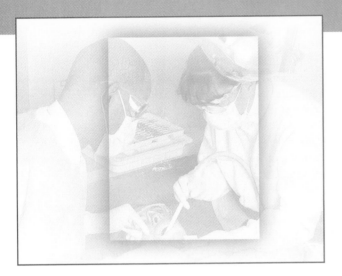

OBJECTIVES

After studying this chapter, the student will be able to:

- Define what microbiology and microorganisms are.
- Delineate several important roles of microorganisms.
- Understand the general types of cells, their basic structure, and the basic life processes they demonstrate.
- Know the general methods of classifying and naming organisms.
- Outline the general characteristics and functions of bacterial cells.
- Characterize the main groups of bacteria and know examples of nutrition, distribution, and diseases they cause.
- Describe the morphology, nutrition, and importance of fungi.
- List several major groups of fungi and types of diseases they cause.
- Describe the morphology, nutrition, and importance of protozoa.
- List several major groups of protozoa and types of diseases they cause.
- Understand several unique characteristics of viruses that make them different from other microbes, including structure and methods of multiplication.
- Discuss the major medical impact of viruses.

Introduction

Microbiology is a science devoted to studying living things that cannot readily be seen without magnification. These small **microscopic** creatures are known by several names, most commonly **microorganisms**, or microbes, and some more specific names such as **bacteria**, **viruses**, **fungi**, **protozoa**, **parasitic worms**, and **algae**. This list of microorganisms represents the major groups that microbiologists study (Figure 5-1). Sometimes they are also referred to as "germs" or "bugs" because of their role in infection and disease. This emphasis on the disagreeable reputation of microorganisms is unfortunate. It is important to recognize that most microorganisms are harmless residents of most of the habitats on earth. Here, they serve many beneficial roles such as decomposing wastes, recycling important nutrients for other organisms to use, and generally contributing to the balance of nature.

A relatively small number of microbes are **parasites**, which means that they are nourished by other living organisms, called **hosts**. Parasitic microorganisms can damage their hosts and produce an **infectious disease**. Most microbial parasites are some type of bacteria, fungi, protozoa, worm, or virus (but not algae). A few microorganisms can live either a free-living or parasitic existence. Even with modern medical technology, infectious diseases are still a serious health threat. The World Health Organization (WHO) of the United Nations estimates that more than 20 million persons die each year worldwide from preventable infectious diseases. These diseases are more common in developing countries with less access to medical care. Many new diseases such as acquired immunodeficiency syndrome (AIDS) and older diseases such as tuberculosis and cholera have increased dramatically in recent years. Another growing trend is the aging population and a higher incidence of patients with weakened immunity. These individuals are subject to infections from common environmental microorganisms that do not affect healthy people.

Microbiologists study many aspects of the biology of microorganisms, including their interactions with humans and other organisms, their morphology (structure), physiology (function), genetics (heredity), and ecology. Other subjects included in this study are food

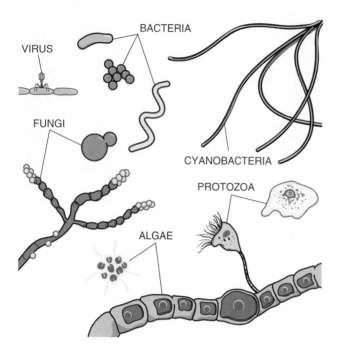

Figure 5-1 Members of the microbial world.

science, drug therapy, **epidemiology** (transmission of diseases), immunology (the systems of body defenses), genetic engineering (techniques that alter the genetic makeup of organisms), biotechnology (any process that uses microorganisms to create products), and agriculture.

The General Characteristics of Microbial Cells

The bodies of all living things consist of one or more cells, which are complex microscopic packages. Regardless of the organism, all cells share a few common characteristics. They tend to be small round or elongated compartments containing **cytoplasm**, a complex semiliquid medium where thousands of activities take place. The cytoplasm is encased in a **cell membrane**, a slender double-layered sheet composed of fats and proteins. Cells carry their genetic material in special packets called **chromosomes** and use **ribosomes** to synthesize proteins. The great diversity of life has given rise to many differences in cell structure and function. Generally, all cells fall into one of two categories: **procaryotic** cells, which are small and simple in structure, and **eucaryotic** cells, which are larger and structurally more complex.

The cytoplasm of eucaryotes is divided into a number of complex internal parts called **organelles** (little organs) that carry out a particular cell function such as transport, **synthesis** (producing a chemical or structure), energy production, and growth. Organelles are surrounded by membranes that help to separate the

eucaryotic cell into compartments. One of the most prominent of the organelles is the **nucleus**, a spherical body that contains the cells' genetic material and is surrounded by a nuclear membrane. Other organelles include the Golgi complex, endoplasmic reticulum, vacuoles, and mitochondria. Eucaryotic cells are found in protozoa, algae, fungi, animals, and plants.

Procaryotes are known by what they lack. They have no nucleus or organelles, but even though they appear simple, they are very complex in their physiology. Procaryotic cells are found only in bacteria, so all procaryotic organisms are microorganisms. Because of their role in disease and the need to use a microscope to observe their details and identify them, certain **macroscopic** (visible with the naked eye) animals such as parasitic worms and insects are included in microbiology. A number of properties that are commonly shown by living cells are summarized in Table 5-1.

Even though viruses are not cells or living organisms, they can infect cells, and so they are included in the study of microbes. Viruses are even simpler in structure than procaryotic cells, in some ways more like large, complex molecules. They could be described as a small fragment of hereditary material wrapped up in a protein covering. We will consider viruses in the last section of this chapter.

The normal size range of microbes falls somewhere within the millimeter (mm), micrometer (μm), and the nanometer (nm) scale (Figure 5-2). The largest microbes are the worms (several millimeters); protozoa and fungi (2 mm–10 μm) and the smallest microbes are bacteria (1–10 μm), and viruses (10–400 nm).

Important Concepts in Medical Microbiology

By the middle of the 1800s, microbiologists began to realize that the air and dust were full of microbes, as well as the entire surface of the earth, its waters, and all objects exposed to these elements. This discovery was especially important to medicine and health, and it led to a number of ideas and concepts that are still in use today. Early microbiologists began to suspect that not only were spoilage and decay caused by microorganisms, but so were infectious diseases. These observations led to the germ theory of disease that stated that some microbes are **pathogenic** and could be spread from one human to another. These techniques led to the use of **sterile** and aseptic techniques. Sterility means the complete absence of all life forms, and it was only made possible when it was discovered that certain microbial **spores** in dust and air have very high heat resistance and particularly vigorous treatment is required to destroy them. The surgeon Joseph Lister first introduced **aseptic techniques** (infection free) that could reduce microbes in a medical setting and prevent incision and wound

Table 5-1 Major Activities of Living Cells

Metabolism	This refers to all of the physiologic activities of cells. Protein synthesis is carried out by tiny particles called ribosomes. Chemical reactions, which produce energy, occur in the mitochondria in eucaryotes and in the cell membrane in procaryotes. Algae and certain bacteria contain a pigment for trapping light, which allows them to carry out photosynthesis and form their own nutrients.
Heredity and Reproduction	All cells contain genetic material in the form of elongated strands of DNA, packaged into compact chromosomes. In eucaryotic cells, the chromosomes are located entirely within the nucleus. Bacterial chromosomes are free in the cell, without a nuclear membrane around them. Bacteria divide mainly by binary fission, a simple process in which the cell splits in two. Many eucaryotic cells go through **mitosis**, an orderly division of chromosomes into two new cells.
Movement	The ability to move (motility) is present in many microorganisms. It is usually made possible by special locomotor appendages such as flagella (long whips), cilia (short hairs), and other structures.
Support	Many cells are supported and protected by rigid **cell walls** located directly in contact with the cell membrane. Walls prevent cells from rupturing while also providing support and shape. Cell walls occur in plants, algae, fungi, and the majority of bacteria, but not in animals or protozoa.
Obtaining Nutrients and Removing Wastes	Cells use their cell membranes to transport nutrients into the cells and to flush out waste products. They are selectively permeable, so that only certain molecules can pass through. Eucaryotes also use the Golgi complex to package materials so they can be transported from the cell.

infections. The use of disinfectants and heat sterilization as microbial control agents is still an absolutely essential part of microbiology, medicine, dentistry, and industry.

Classifying and Naming Microorganisms

The microbial world is extremely varied, with half a million known microorganisms. It has been necessary to organize this great diversity by arranging them in orderly groups and assigning unique names to these groups. The result is an orderly scheme organized into seven ranks, beginning with a kingdom, the largest and most general grouping. All the members of a kingdom share only one or a few general characteristics. For example, humans are included in the animal kingdom, but so are sponges. The final category is **species**, the smallest and most specific grouping. All members of species are the same kind of organism, that is, they share the majority of their charac-

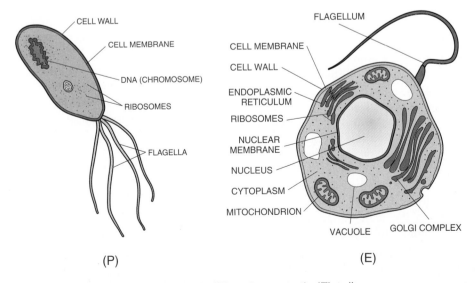

Figure 5-2A Structure of procaryotic (P) and eucaryotic (E) cells.

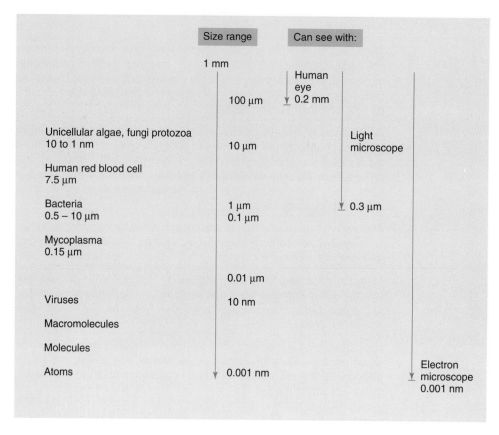

Figure 5-2B Structure and size comparisons of microorganisms.

teristics. For example, all members of the human species (*Homo sapiens*) are the same basic organism. The other taxa (taxonomic categories) between the top and bottom levels are, in order, phylum or division, class, order, family, and genus. As you move down the categories, they become less inclusive and the individual members are more closely related.

All living things are placed in one of five basic kingdoms: The simple, single-celled organisms at the base of the family tree are in the kingdom Procaryotae (also called Monera). It includes all of the microorganisms commonly known as bacteria. The other four kingdoms contain organisms composed of eucaryotic cells. The kingdom Protista contains mostly single-celled microbes that lack more complex levels of organization, such as tissues. Its members include the algae and the protozoan. Fungi belong to the kingdom Myceteae. With the exception of certain infectious worms and arthropods, the final two kingdoms, Animalia and Plantae, are generally not included in the realm of microbiology because most are large, multicellular organisms.

To aid in the organization and identification of microbes, each species is given a scientific name that is always a combination of the genus name and the species name. The following examples show the formatting.

Streptococcus Mutans

The genus part of the scientific name (*streptococus*) is capitalized, and the species part (*mutans*) begins with a lowercase letter. Both should be italicized or underlined. The source for nomenclature is usually Latin or Greek, but each organism is given a unique name. One advantage of standardized naming is that it provides a universal language, enabling free exchange of scientific information. Names are often based on characteristics of the organism such as shape, color, a location where it is found, or a disease it causes.

The next section will provide an overview of the major types of microorganisms to prepare for later chapters on dental diseases, disease transmission, and infection control.

General Characteristics of Bacteria

Bacteria are mostly single cells (unicellular), with distinct shapes called **cocci**, **bacilli**, **spirilla**, and **spirochetes** (Figure 5-3). Cocci are spherical or ovoid; bacilli (also called rods) are basically cylindrical; spirilla are thick, rigid spirals; and spirochetes are thin flexible spirals. Certain groups may assume long filaments. Cocci often

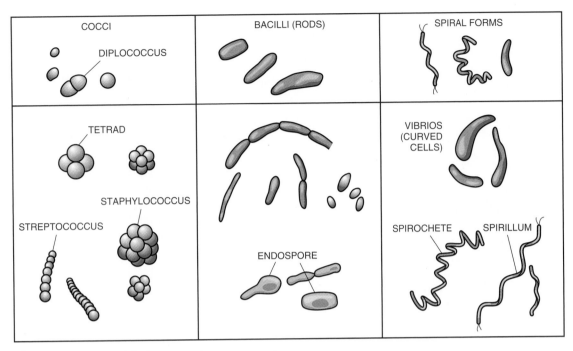

Figure 5-3 Bacterial shapes and arrangements.

exist in groupings or arrangements termed diplococci (pairs), streptococci (chains), staphylococci (clusters), and tetrads (fours). Most bacteria possess an outer covering in the form of a slime layer or capsule that helps them adhere to their surroundings.   It is this structure that helps some species adhere to the surface of the teeth and initiate dental infections.

Another special structure found in a few groups of bacteria is the **endospore** (Figure 5-3). These are highly resistant survival cells formed by only a few groups of bacteria in response to adverse conditions. They are extremely dense and can remain dormant for thousands of years. They are the most heat and chemical resistant bacterial cells in existence. Because they are common in the soil, dust, and air and are dispersed into many human habitats, endospores are the major target of infection control procedures that sterilize.

Habitat and Nutritional Requirements

Bacteria exist in nearly every habitat on earth, including water, soil, air, dust, food, plants, animals, hot springs, glaciers, deep in the ocean, in salt lakes, and in acidic swamps. Many also normally inhabit the bodies of humans and other animals. Most are adapted to temperate conditions somewhere between 10°C and 40°C. Bacteria that require oxygen in metabolism are described as **aerobic**, those that are harmed or killed by oxygen are considered **anaerobic**, and many species can grow in either condition. Most bacteria derive their nutrients by feeding on dead or living organic matter,

but only a small number of them (around 200 species) are parasites. A few are capable of deriving nutrients through photosynthesis.

Bacteria can be grown in the laboratory by inoculating them into special nutrients called **media**. A common type of medium is a solid gel (agar) that provides a substrate for them to grow into large masses of cells called **colonies** that are visible to the naked eye. These colonies can be used to isolate bacteria from samples (such as saliva) that contain many different types of bacteria, and this serves as the starting point for identification.

Classification and Identification

Bacteria are classified by their microscopic morphology. They will be identified as gram-positive and gram-negative bacteria.

Gram-positive bacteria have a thick cell wall. *Streptococcus* is typically found with skin and throat infections, dental infections, pneumonia, and serious systemic diseases (rheumatic fever); *Staphylococcus* is a major pathogen affecting the skin, wounds, and internal organs. Rod-shaped *Mycobacterium* is the agent of tuberculosis and *Clostridium* the cause of tetanus and gangrene.

Gram-negative bacteria have a thinner cell wall. *Neisseria* cocci are responsible for gonorrhea and a form of meningitis. Medically important rods include *Salmonella* and *Shigella*, which are intestinal pathogens. Other notable members of the group are *Treponema*, the spirochete of syphilis and certain dental infections.

Special groups of bacteria include the **rickettsias**, tiny gram-negative rods that are strict parasites and can only grow inside host cells. Most of them are carried by some form of arthropod (insect or tick). The most common member in the United States causes Rocky Mountain spotted fever. A similar parasitic bacterium is *Chlamydia*, the agent responsible for a very common sexually-transmitted disease.

Ecological and Economic Importance

Bacteria are the most important decomposers of organic matter. They are absolutely necessary for the cycling of elements such as nitrogen, phosphorus, sulfur, and carbon. Photosynthetic bacteria serve as an important source of nutrients for many organisms, and some of them contribute oxygen to the atmosphere through photosynthesis. Bacteria are used in a number of industries, including food technology (wine, beer, cheese, and pickled foods); production of antibiotics, vaccines, and other medicines; and making hormones, enzymes, and other proteins. On the negative side, bacteria are responsible for spoilage of food and vegetables and plant diseases. They are also very common pathogens of humans. Fortunately, most bacterial infections can be treated with antibiotics and other drugs.

Major Groups of Eucaryotic Microorganisms

Fungi

The fungi exist in both macroscopic and microscopic forms. The macroscopic fungi are large fleshy members such as mushrooms and puffballs, which are usually not considered microorganisms. The microscopic fungi include yeasts and molds (Figure 5-4).

Nutritional Mode and Distribution. All fungi feed off the organic matter from other organisms. The majority are harmless decomposers of organic matter from dead animal and plant tissues. A small number are parasites that feed on the tissues of live organisms. Such pathogenic fungi cause infections called **mycoses**. Some infections involve only superficial skin infections (athlete's foot or ringworm). A few pathogenic fungi (*Histoplasma* or *Cryptococcus*) invade deeper organs (the lung or brain). Most fungal infections can be treated with drugs; for example, *Penicillium* is the source of the drug penicillin.

Protozoa

Protozoa are unicellular animallike microorganisms that move by some form of locomotion such as flagella, cilia, or pseudopods. Like animal cells, they lack a rigid cell wall and are generally flexible, with a wide degree of variation in shape. Many protozoa alternate between two stages: a motile, feeding stage known as **trophozoite** and a dormant, resistant stage, or cyst. **Cysts** allow the protozoa to survive adverse conditions in their environment, such as drying, heat, and lack of nutrients. They may be involved in transmission of diseases.

Nutrition, Distribution, and Classification. Protozoa feed on the dead or living tissues of other organisms. Most of them are free-living in fresh or salt

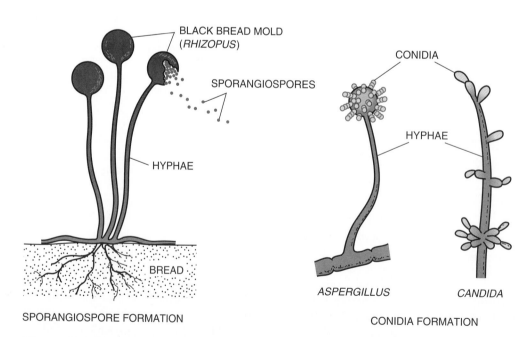

Figure 5-4 Examples of microscopic fungi and spore formation in molds.

water, where they engulf other microorganisms and organic matter. A small number are animal parasites and may be spread from host to host by insects and other carriers. They do not form spores or other special reproductive structures; they mostly divide by binary fission and mitosis.

There are several groups of protozoans, based upon mode of locomotion and type of reproduction (Figure 5-5). As a group, they are ecologically important in food chains and decomposing organic matter. Their medical significance is due to the common occurrence of **malaria** infections caused by the sporozoa *Plasmodium* restricted to certain geographic regions in the tropics where they are harbored and spread by insect vectors. A **vector** is any animal that carries a disease to humans.

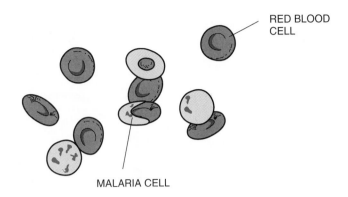

Figure 5-5 Example of the sporozoa *Plasmodium*, the malaria parasite.

Viruses: Infectious Particles

Viruses are an important group of microbes with very unusual biological characteristics. The French bacteriologist Louis Pasteur was one of the first scientists to think that some diseases were caused by microbes even smaller than bacteria. He proposed that the term virus (Latin for "poison") be used to denote this special group of infectious agents. Viruses are strict parasites that can infect every type of cell, including bacteria, algae, fungi, protozoa, plants, and animals.

Viruses have such unique structure and behavior that their connection to the rest of the microbial world has been the subject of much debate. Because they are unable to exist separately from their host cells, they cannot really be considered living. But they can also direct the activities of cells, so they are certainly more than inert and lifeless molecules. Regardless of how we view them, they are common agents of human diseases, ranging from AIDS and the common cold to influenza and cancer. Most biologists would prefer to refer to viruses as "infectious particles" (rather than organisms) and as either active or inactive (rather than alive or dead).

Major Characteristics of Viruses. Viruses are the smallest infectious agents, and they have a very specialized structure and chemical composition. They are described as **obligate intracellular parasites**, meaning that they do not display activities such as growth or metabolism unless they have been taken inside their specific host cell. It is this characteristic that causes the damage and disease to the host it invades. The major properties of viruses are summarized in Table 5-2.

Virus Size and Structure. Viruses are the smallest infectious agents. They are so tiny that it requires high magnification of 5000–10,000 times to detect them. Even higher magnification is needed to see their detailed structure. Figure 5-6 compares the sizes of several viruses.

It is important to emphasize that viruses bear no real resemblance to cells and that they lack any of the structures found in even the simplest cells. They are similar to large molecules and can even appear as crystals. Viruses contain only those parts needed to invade and control a host cell (Figure 5-7).

Table 5-2 Major Properties of Viruses

They are not cells, but very small particles.

They are not considered to be living.

They are strict parasites that can grow inside host cells.

They have a protective protein covering called a capsid that surrounds a molecule of genetic material.

The capsid carries molecules on its surface that are specific for the host cell.

They lack enzymes for producing energy and synthesizing their own proteins.

They multiply by entering the host cell and taking over its machinery.

The process of virus multiplication includes attachment of virus to host cell, penetration of genetic material, duplication of virus molecules by the host cell, assembly of viruses, and release of new viruses from host cell.

They cause disease in all living things, such as bacteria, protozoa, fungi, algae, plants, and animals.

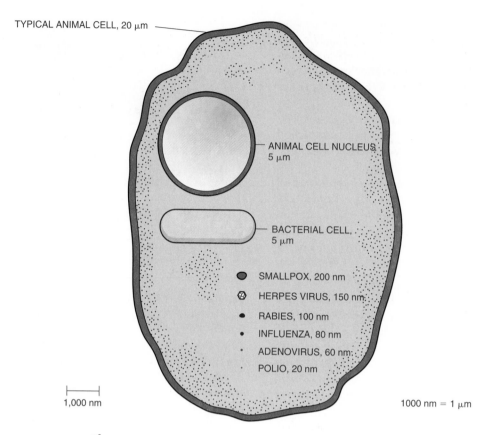

TYPICAL ANIMAL CELL, 20 μm

ANIMAL CELL NUCLEUS
5 μm

BACTERIAL CELL,
5 μm

SMALLPOX, 200 nm

HERPES VIRUS, 150 nm

RABIES, 100 nm

INFLUENZA, 80 nm

ADENOVIRUS, 60 nm

POLIO, 20 nm

1,000 nm

1000 nm = 1 μm

Figure 5-6 Comparison of relative sizes of cells and viruses.

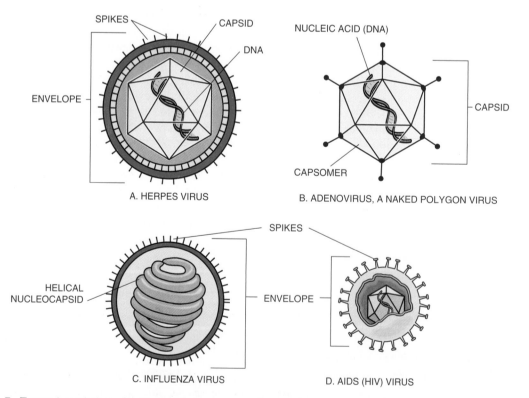

SPIKES

CAPSID

DNA

ENVELOPE

A. HERPES VIRUS

NUCLEIC ACID (DNA)

CAPSID

CAPSOMER

B. ADENOVIRUS, A NAKED POLYGON VIRUS

SPIKES

HELICAL
NUCLEOCAPSID

ENVELOPE

C. INFLUENZA VIRUS

D. AIDS (HIV) VIRUS

Figure 5-7 Examples of virus structure using common viruses that infect humans: (a) herpes virus; (b) adenovirus, a naked polygon virus; (c) Influenza virus; (d) AIDS (HIV) virus.

Table 5-3 Common Viruses That Cause Disease or Illness in Humans

Virus	Disease/Illness
Herpes simplex virus (HSV)	Cold sores, genital herpes
Herpes zoster virus	Chickenpox and shingles
Human papilloma (warts) virus	Common warts and genital warts
Poliovirus	Polio
Rhinovirus	Common cold
Hantavirus	Respiratory distress syndrome
Morbillivirus	Measles
Human immunodeficiency virus (HIV)	AIDS
Influenza virus	Influenza
Hepatitis B virus	Hepatitis B infection
Enterovirus	Hepatitis A infection
Togavirus	Rubella

How Viruses Are Classified and Named. Viruses are classified according to their host organism, the type of nucleic acid, whether they have an **envelope** (additional covering acquired from host cell membrane), the type of **capsid** (outer shell), the disease caused, and the area of the world where the virus is found. DNA viruses are subdivided into 6 families, and RNA viruses into 14 families, for a total of 20 families. Other characteristics used for placement in a particular family include overall viral size and shape and specific type of cell in which the virus multiplies. The technical names of viruses usually use some characteristic of the virus followed by "virus." For example, a rhabdovirus has a bullet-shaped envelope, an adenovirus infects adenoids (one type of tonsil), and herpesviruses are named for the spreading character of herpes rashes. In everyday usage, the common names of viruses prevail, including poliovirus, rabiesvirus, mumpsvirus all being named for the disease they cause (Table 5-3).

A Virus Multiplication Cycle. Multiplication in viruses is a fascinating process. A general knowledge of the relationship between viruses and their host cells will help in understanding how viruses cause disease, how they are transmitted, how the body develops immunity, and how virus infections are treated. The process involves a sequence of events depicted for a human virus in Figure 5-8.

- **Adsorption**, the viruses first specifically attach to the outer surface of the host cell. Most viruses are very restricted by what they can attach to. For example, hepatitis B viruses can only attach to the membranes of liver cells and HIV can only attach to cells that have special receptors.

- Penetration is the entry of the virus's genetic material into the host cell. Some viruses are totally engulfed by the host cell and pulled into the cell, and other viruses fuse with its membrane. Once the genetic material enters a host cell, the cycle may continue to the end point, which causes cell **lysis**, or destruction (the lytic cycle). In other cases, the virus can remain in an inactive, or latent, stage in which the virus does not lyse the host cell.

- During the replication phase the host cell becomes a factory to duplicate various virus components (capsid, nucleic acid) using its own machinery and resources.

- Maturation is the final assembly of individual viral parts into new finished viruses. Release is the escape of the mature viruses to the outside of the host cell. Certain naked viruses are released when the cell dies and lyses. Enveloped viruses bud off the surface of the host cell membranes. Through this process, the virus receives its envelope and spikes. Regardless of how the virus leaves, lytic viral infections are usually lethal to the cell. The number of viruses released by infected cells varies from 3000 or 4000 to over 100,000 viruses. Each of these viruses is potentially able to infect another cell.

Medical Importance of Viruses. It is thought by experts in infectious diseases that viruses are the most common cause of infections worldwide, especially when one considers widespread diseases such as colds, measles, chickenpox, influenza, herpes, and AIDS. Estimates from WHO indicate there are several billion cases per year. Most viral infections do not result in hospitalization or severe disease. Exceptions include rabies and AIDS, with very high mortality rates, and hepatitis B and C and neonatal herpes infections, which may cause permanent damage and disability. Viruses may also be

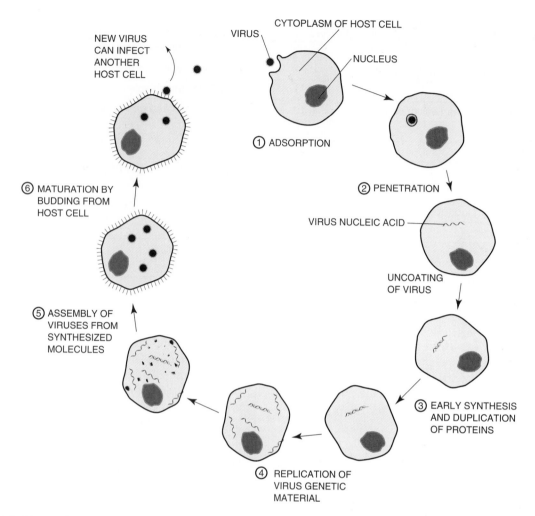

Figure 5-8 The major events in virus replication. The example here is an enveloped virus such as influenza.

connected with several chronic diseases of unknown cause, such as type I diabetes and multiple sclerosis.

Some viruses do not immediately kill the host cell but survive in a persistent state that lasts from a few weeks to life, in some cases. Some persistent viruses remain **latent** (dormant inactive phase) and can erupt to produce symptomatic infections. This is the case with herpes simplex viruses (fever blisters and genital herpes) and herpes zoster virus (chickenpox and shingles). Both viruses can persist in nerve cells and cause recurrent infections.

Some persistent viruses alter the growth of host cells, thereby causing tumors and cancers. Such viruses, which are termed oncogenic, include human papilloma virus (genital warts are associated with cervical cancer), and herpesviruses (Epstein-Barr virus causes Burkitt's lymphoma). Relatives of HIV and hepatitis B are also involved in human cancers.

Detection and Treatment of Viral Infections.
Viral diseases are usually detected and diagnosed by the overall clinical picture of the disease (specific symp-

toms). It may be necessary to examine patient's tissue or specimens to observe cytopathic effects in their cells, which are signs of changes in the cells that indicate infection. Some laboratories may scan the tissues with a high-powered microscope to directly identify the virus. A new technique that is rapidly becoming standard procedure is the polymerase chain reaction (PCR), which can identify the exact type of viral genetic material in a sample. An alternate way of determining if a patient currently has an infection or has had one in the past is to screen the blood for the presence of specific antibodies (this is the basis of the test for HIV infection).

Controlling viral infections has traditionally been difficult. This is because most drugs available to treat infections are for bacteria, and only a small number are available for treating viruses. Most of the antiviral drugs stop the virus cycle, especially at the replication and assembly stage. This is how the drugs for treating AIDS work (e.g., AZT). Some of the drugs have severe toxic side effects because they have to enter the host cell to work. Vaccines that stimulate immunity are an extremely valuable tool but are available for only a few viral diseases.

SUGGESTED ACTIVITIES

● Expose plates of agar media to various objects [fingers, lips, hair, stamps, and environmental samples (air, dust, soil, water)] around your classroom. Allow the plates to incubate for several days and observe them for colonies. Note the difference between molds and bacteria, and make an estimate of which places sampled have the greatest numbers of microorganisms.

● If microsopes are available, collect pond samples, decomposing fruit, and other food and make slides from them to observe the many different types of microorganisms that inhabit these worlds.

● Go to a web site such as *www.microworld.org* and try out several of their activities, such as "Let's Get Small," "Defend Your Surface," and Get Caught Red-Handed." Print out some of these activities to take into the classroom and share with other students in groups.

REVIEW

1. Which of the following is not a microorganism?
   a. Virus
   b. Bacteria
   c. Mushroom
   d. Protozoan

2. Most microorganisms:
   a. Are harmful germs
   b. Are able to cause disease
   c. Are beneficial and harmless
   d. Are animals

3. Which of the following is NOT a characteristic of a living cell?
   a. Metabolism
   b. Reproduction
   c. Movement
   d. Being composed of molecules

4. Aseptic techniques are:
   a. Used to prevent infection
   b. Used for growing microrganisms
   c. Used for observing microscopic organisms
   d. No longer used because they are outdated

5. Procaryotic cells lack what structure?
   a. Cell wall
   b. Cell membrane
   c. Genetic material
   d. A nucleus

6. What is an example of an organelle?
   a. Mitochondrion
   b. Ribosomes
   c. Chromosomes
   d. Capsule

7. The Kingdom is the _____ level of classification and the species is the _____.
   a. Most specific, most general
   b. Most general, most specific
   c. Smallest, largest
   d. Scientific, nonscientific

8. What part of a bacterial cell is mainly involved in supporting it and keeping it from collapsing?
   a. Cell membrane
   b. Cell wall
   c. Endospore
   d. Capsule

9. A bacterium is shaped like a spherical:
   a. Rod
   b. Spirochete
   c. Coccus
   d. Tetrad

10. An aerobic bacterium prefers to grow in
    a. Water
    b. Soil
    c. Oxygen
    d. The human body

11. Gram-positive bacteria are responsible for which disease?
    a. Rocky Mountain spotted fever
    b. Meningitis
    c. Syphilis
    d. Tuberculosis

12. An endospore is:
    a. Highly resistant to harsh environmentaL conditions
    b. Used in reproduction
    c. Produced by fungi
    d. Not alive

13. Molds are ___ composed of long filaments called ___.
    a. Bacteria, yeasts
    b. Yeasts, buds
    c. Pathogens, fibers
    d. Fungi, hyphae

14. Fungi obtain their nutrients from:
    a. The sun through photosynthesis
    b. Dead plants and animals
    c. Water and soil
    d. Bacteria

15. A protozoan goes through an inactive, survival phase during its life cycle called a:
    a. Cyst
    b. Spore
    c. Trophozoite
    d. Virus

16. Protozoans are motile by all but which organelle?
    a. Flagella
    b. Pili
    c. Cilia
    d. Pseudopods

17. The most common protozoan disease worldwide is:
    a. Amebic dysentery
    b. Ringworm
    c. Pneumonia
    d. Malaria

18. The main components found in all viruses are the:
    a. Tail and spikes
    b. Capsid and nucleic acid
    c. Envelope and capsid
    d. Spikes and nucleic acid

19. Viruses
    a. Are alive
    b. Are tiny cells
    c. Are genetic parasites
    d. Produce energy by feeding on dead cells

20. At which stage of virus multiplication does the host cell synthesize new virus parts?
    a. Replication
    b. Penetration
    c. Adsorption
    d. Release

Infectious Diseases and Disease Transmission

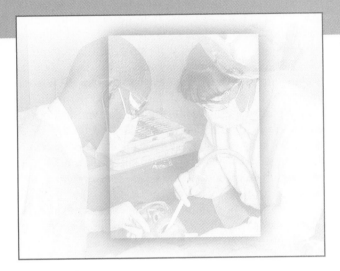

OBJECTIVES

After studying this chapter, the student will be able to:

● Define the meaning of disease.

● Discuss the etiological factors of disease.

● Identify the diseases that most often spread from person to person in the dental environment.

● Discuss the means by which indirect transmission of infectious disease may occur.

● Discuss the means by which direct transmission of infectious disease may occur.

● State the precautionary measures of control for the various infectious diseases.

Introduction

Infectious diseases that can be transmitted from one person to another have proven to spread to and from the patient in the dental environment. The patient health questionnaire, though valuable, cannot be relied upon to identify infectious patients. In fact, many patients do not realize they have been exposed and are potential disease **carriers** (individuals who harbor disease organisms without being ill with the disease); for example, only one of five persons who has had hepatitis B is aware of it.

The patient with a disease at the incubation stage may be more infectious than one with the active disease, as with hepatitis and measles. The **incubation period** of an infectious disease is measured by the time of its entry into an organism up to the time of the first appearance of signs or symptoms. Patients may not appreciate the importance of informing the dental office of their health status, past or current, because they regard the mouth as being separate from the rest of the body! Others may deliberately conceal information for fear they might be denied treatment.

Adding to public health anxiety is the emergence of acquired immunodeficiency syndrome (AIDS). This has generated a great deal of interest about the impact of viral infections on the practice of dentistry. Of major concern to all dental practitioners are tuberculosis, herpes simplex, serum hepatitis B, and AIDS. The onset and residual effects of these diseases vary greatly. They do, however, have one aspect in common: their potential to be spread in the dental office.

What is Disease?

Before entering on a discussion of the possible causes of disease, it may be well to ask ourselves, What is disease? This is a question that is a great deal easier to ask than to answer. To the patient it means dis-comfort, dis-ease, and dis-harmony with his or her environment; to a dentist or physician, it means a variety of signs and symptoms with one or more structural changes or lesions.

Disease may be defined as the pattern of response of a living organism to some form of injury. With the presence of disease, there is usually some altered or disordered cell function. Thus, disease is a response to all kinds of injury, ranging from infection with bacteria or virus to stress or depression.

The presence of **lesions** (disease-related or external injury-induced tissue damage) may bear an obvious relation to symptoms. Lesion is a broad term and includes wounds, sores, ulcers, tumors, cataracts, and other tissue damage. For disease to occur, three conditions must be present: a susceptible host, a portal of entry for the **pathogen** (germ) to enter the organism, and a pathogen of sufficient **virulence** (of sufficient strength) to cause the disease or infection.

Etiology

The relationship of cause, origin, reason for something, and effect is known as the **etiology** of a disease. It might be supposed that the relation of the etiological agent to disease, or cause to effect, was a relatively simple matter. The reverse is the case. Perhaps, we are misled into imagining that only one cause is responsible. We say that the cause of tuberculosis is the tubercle bacillus, but we know that many people may inhale these bacilli, yet only one may develop the disease. The bacilli may lurk in the body for years and only become active as a result of factors such as an existing infection, prolonged strain (stress), and starvation. In determining the cause of a disease, such elements as heredity, sex, environment, immunity, allergy, and other agents must be considered.

Infections

By far, the most common cause of disease is bacteria, which belong to the animal kingdom. Other forms of life such as molds or fungi belong to the plant life. Certain lowly forms of animal life, known as animal parasites, may live in the body and produce disease. Finally, there are *filterable* viruses, forms of living matter so minute they pass through the pores of filters fine enough to hold back bacteria, so tiny that they cannot be seen by the most powerful light microscope and are said to be *ultra-microscopic*. They can be made visible with the electron microscope. This last group has attracted a great deal of attention in recent years (see Chapter 5).

Tuberculosis

Tuberculosis (TB) was considered the number one killer in the United States at the turn of the century. Since the 1930s it has been on the decline, and by the 1980s it was no longer considered a major health threat.

In recent years, TB cases have increased in number along with the dramatic increases in HIV (human immunodeficiency virus) infected persons.

Tuberculosis is a chronic inflammation caused by human bacillus tuberculosis (*Mycobacterium tuberculosis*). There is evidence that the natural defensive power of the body against TB is sufficiently great to hold it in check in the majority of cases. This defense may be broken down by an infection such as influenza, which undermines health, by overwork, poor hygienic conditions, insufficient food, and such. This bacillus may live outside the body for six months if not exposed to sunlight and is an exceptionally resistant germ.

Transmission

Tuberculosis infection may spread from one person to another by inhalation. When an infected person coughs, the discharged droplets infect the air in the immediate area with millions of tubercle bacilli contained in tiny droplets of moisture. Transmission occurs in the dental office through handling of unclean objects and used, contaminated dental instruments, a very good reason for following the universal guidelines for infection control when treating *all patients.*

Hospital-grade disinfectants approved by the Environmental Protection Agency (EPA) and used in the

dental office *do* kill the TB bacterium. However, to be totally effective, they must be used according to the manufacturer's instructions. It is heartening to realize that in healthy persons the probability of a TB infection developing into active TB that is infectious is remote.

Besides disinfectants, there are two devices designed to intervene and interrupt the transfer of respiratory diseases. The ultra violet lamp and the high-efficiency particulate air (HEPA) filtration system, both of which are recommended by the CDC. The ultra violet device, usually mounted on the wall, is turned on while the treatment room is vacant. It kills airborne bacteria and bacteria-exposed surfaces, but does not affect hidden surfaces such as underneath a tray or inside a hollow tube. The HEPA filtration, which cleans the air, may be used continuously for environmental protection within the entire office.

Herpes Simplex

Two types of **herpes simplex** virus have been identified: HSV-1 labialis and HSV-2 genitalis. Herpes simplex virus type-1 is more common in children between one and three years of age, whereas HSV-2, also known as genital herpes, is transmitted after puberty usually through sexual contact. Both HSV-1 and HSV-2 can produce lesions around the mouth. These lesions are painful and affect the exposed pink or reddish border, called the vermillion border of the extraoral lip. Regardless of the location, the lesions begin as either a single or multiple **vesicular** (a serum-filled blister) eruption. The vesicles burst, ulcerate, and scab within 5–10 days. The lesions or herpes infections shed virus and are infective by direct contact until healing is complete.

A primary herpetic infection usually is self-limiting, and complications are rare. Unfortunately, there presently is no antiviral therapy for herpes.

Treatment

Treatment is neither specific nor very satisfactory aside from *acyclovir*, an antiviral drug used in topical ointment, oral, and tablet forms. It inhibits replication of the virus and diminishes recovery time.

Secondary or recurrent herpetic lesions may affect oral tissues as well as the human genitalia (external sex organs).

According to the Occupational Safety and Health Administration (OSHA), a splatter of herpes in saliva can cause blindness within 48 hours. Eye protection for the dental operator personnel and the patient is a must!

Herpetic whitlow exists on the fingers where a portal of entry for the herpes simplex virus takes place, affecting the area around the fingernail. Another concern is when an infected mother gives birth to her child. There is a 50% chance that the child will be infected with the virus, which may result in severe problems such as deafness, mental retardation, chronic liver disease, and possible death.

Hepatitis

The term **hepatitis** means inflammation of the liver [hepat(o) = liver, -itis = inflammation]. This inflammation can occur from a variety of injurious or harmful agents, including recognized viral forms of the disease. Individuals experiencing hepatitis infection may exhibit the following symptoms: the emotion of **malaise** (a feeling of illness or depression), nausea, vomiting, loss of appetite, fever, and **jaundice** (a yellowish appearance on the skin and eyes).

Hepatitis A (HAV) "Infectious Hepatitis"

Hepatitis A, known as *infectious hepatitis*, usually occurs in children and young adults.

Transmission. It is frequently transmitted from person to person by way of contaminated foods and liquids or by the oral-fecal route, as, for example, when someone who is carrying the virus does not wash hands after using the restroom and then handles food. Immunization is indicated for optimal protection.

Incubation. Hepatitis A is a virus that multiplies in the intestinal tract and invades the blood stream, localizing in the liver. It has an incubation period (the time between the infection of the individual by a microorganism and the first manifestation of the disease) of two to six weeks and is most infectious a week *before* the onset of any clinical symptoms. At this time, large amounts of the virus can be found in the stools and urine of the infected individual. Clinical symptoms are an acute onset accompanied by a high fever and sometimes jaundice. Most HAV infections are without severe complications and are treated with bedrest and high-protein and high-carbohydrate diets. Recovery takes six to eight weeks. Vaccine for active immunization is available. However, once exposed, a person may be immunized within the first few days after infection with the standard immune globulin for prevention or alteration of hepatitis A.

Hepatitis B (HBV) "Serum Hepatitis"

It is estimated that 600,000–1 million carriers of the **hepatitis B virus (HBV)** live in the United States. According to the Centers for Disease Control and Prevention (CDC), the number of new cases increases by approximately 200,000 each year. It is obvious that HBV,

because of its tendency to spread, is a real problem for individuals in the dental profession.

Transmission. Hepatitis B, referred to as serum hepatitis, was once thought to be transmitted only by contaminated needles during transfusion of blood or blood products. Sexual contacts, needle sharing among drug addicts, mother-to-fetus transmission, and infected blood or blood products remain the principal avenues for spreading the virus. It has been shown, however, that transmission through other body fluids besides blood exists. Saliva, semen, and vaginal fluids have been instrumental in transmitting the virus. The virus has also been found in tears, urine, menstrual blood, perspiration, and nasopharyngeal secretions.

Hepatitis B virus can be found in all body fluids, as already mentioned, and may spread from one person to another in a variety of ways, including household contact through sharing utensils, food, razors, and the like. The CDC has shown that HBV can be transmitted by a splatter of any body fluid into the eye. The CDC projects that a health care worker stands a one-third of one percent chance of contracting the disease of an AIDS patient from a splatter, but a 30% chance from an HBV patient. Hepatitis B can spread in the dental environment through patient debris on contaminated instruments, surfaces, and dental charts.

Incubation. The incubation period for HBV is from two to six months. The onset of HBV spreads in a harmful but not easily detected manner, making it difficult to diagnose. Symptoms may mimic the flu: headache, malaise, mild stomach upset, and joint pain. Infection with HBV increases the risk of developing liver cancer.

Should a needle prick (percutaneous injury) or other wound occur while a staff member is performing a procedure on a member of any high-risk group, the person should receive an injection of hepatitis B immune globulin (HBIG) as soon as possible if he or she has not been immunized against the virus already. The HBIG will provide passive immunity for two to three months.

Protection. The best protection against any disease is immunity to that disease. The American Dental Association (ADA) and OSHA recommend that all dental professionals receive the HBV vaccine. The OSHA guidelines state that the employer-dentist makes available the vaccine for his or her employees and that vaccination be kept up-to-date!

Three different vaccines used to immunize against HBV are Heptavax-B (a plasma-derived vaccine) and Recombivax-HB and Energix-B (both genetically engineered products). Energix-B has been approved for immunization against all known subtitles of hepatitis virus. Each of the vaccines requires a series of three injections and should be administered only in the deltoid muscle for adults and in the thigh muscle for infants. The vaccines have no effect on individuals who have had the disease or who are already carriers. It is not contraindicated during pregnancy.

There is one very important part of the vaccination process that many individuals do not complete. Three months after completing the last injection, a **titer** (the quantity of a substance required to cause antibody formation) for antibodies to the HBV surface antigen should be taken. The serum induced will reveal if an individual developed antibodies (protection) and what the protection level is at that time. The following should be used to determine the level of protection:

0.0–2.0	Negligible (no immunity)
2.1–9.9	Borderline
10.0+	Immunity

If the titer indicates a level below 10.0, an additional booster is recommended and the titer rechecked again. If the vaccination process was completed some time ago without ever having had a titer, one should proceed with it to determine if antibodies were ever developed. The average individual probably will need a booster vaccination somewhere between five to seven years after their initial series. However, some studies indicate that a booster requirement is based on the original titer and age of the individual and will vary from person to person.

The National AIDS Network reported that most people, including health care workers, do not consider HBV as great a threat as the AIDS virus. Furthermore, even health care workers, who should know better, have a problem taking HBV seriously. A CDC survey of hospitals with established vaccination programs found that only 30% of their health care workers were vaccinated against HBV.

Hepatitis B is a major health risk in dentistry, responsible for many lost weeks or months of work, as well as the inability to continue in dental practice, permanent disability, or death.

Hepatitis C (HCV)

Hepatitis C, previously known as hepatitis non-A, non-B, a chronic disease of the liver, is considered to be the major cause of posttransfusion hepatitis.

Transmission. Hepatitis C is transmitted through blood transfusions (although rare today due to blood screening), contaminated needles, and skin penetration. Other routes include sexual transmission and from infected mother to infant at birth.

The Food and Drug Administration (FDA) approved a test that detects antibodies to HCV. This currently used test screens blood donations and reduces the risks of transmission through transfusions. The test identifies carriers of the virus. Presently, it is effective in detecting chronic infections of six months or longer. However, it may not be as effective in detecting acute cases.

Incubation. The incubation period for HCV is from two weeks to six months with no clinical symptoms. One week before onset of symptoms, the individual is contagious but may be a chronic carrier for an indefinite period of time.

There is no effective treatment for HCV or a vaccine against it at present, and the use of postexposure prophylaxis is not recommended due to severe side effects.

Hepatitis D (HDV)

Hepatitis D, also known as the *delta* hepatitis virus, has been determined to occur simultaneously with HBV. The ability to spread rapidly and extensively among many individuals in a given area and its clinical course are similar. Fortunately immunization against HBV will provide protection against HDV.

Transmission. Transmission for HDV occurs in persons who have been exposed to HBV several times, especially hemophiliacs and intravenous drug abusers. It takes place by direct exposure to contaminated blood and serum through needles and syringes, by sexual contacts, and from infected mother to infant at birth.

Incubation. The incubation period is from 2 to 10 weeks and may be communicated at any time during that period. The disease is more severe with higher mortality rate than HBV. The symptoms are very similar to HBV.

Hepatitis E

Hepatitus E was previously known as enterically (through the intestine) transmitted non-A, non-B hepatitis. It also resembles HAV in its signs and symptoms.

Transmission. Transmission for Hepatitis E is by contaminated water or person-to-person by the fecal-oral route, affecting adults more than children, generally in areas where heavy rains caused water contamination with sewage disposal.

The best method of preventing Hepatitis E is by adopting sanitary disposal of human waste and hand washing before handling food. There is no vaccine at present.

Incubation. The incubation period is from 2 to 9 weeks (15 to 64 days).

Hepatitis G (HGV)

Not much information is presently available on Hepatitus G; however, it is known that it is found worldwide.

Transmission. Transmission occurs from the blood of an infected person, possibly from blood transfusions, intravenous injection drug users, and occupational incidences. There is no vaccine at present.

AIDS (HIV)

Acquired immunodeficiency syndrome (AIDS), now a worldwide epidemic, is one of the most serious health problems that has faced the American public. An **epidemic** may be defined as a contagious disease that spreads rapidly and extensively among many individuals in any geographic area. The hysteria created by this disease is unfounded and has resulted in misunderstanding and intolerance. Individuals have been denied access to schools, fired from jobs, harassed, evicted, and refused medical and dental treatment. It is important that everyone, regardless of whom they might be, understand this disease.

Acquired immunodeficiency syndrome is a disease caused by the **human immunodeficiency virus (HIV)**, the AIDS virus. The CDC and medical research teams in the United States have projected a sizeable increase in the number of both HIV- and AIDS-related deaths throughout the coming years.

The HIV enters the body and attaches itself to particular target cells. T-lymphocytes (helper T-cells) are the virus's main, but not exclusive, targets. As the widespread invasion continues, the virus seems to target more and more types of cells and to present itself in different ways. The HIV has been known to infect nerve cells, travel to the brain, and cause **dementia** (loss of thought processes and memory).

Transmission

Contrary to what many believe, AIDS *cannot* be transmitted by casual contact, such as sharing of household items, drinking glasses, toothbrushes, a bed or clothing, and such. The virus is not specific to any particular group of individuals. It is most important to realize that a person can be infected with HIV without showing any symptoms at all. It is possible for him or her to be infected for years, feel fine, and have no way of knowing if he or she is infected.

The AIDS virus can be transmitted from one person to another through sexual activity. Any person engaging in *unprotected* sexual intercourse with an HIV carrier is at risk. Many experts indicate that "safe sexual intercourse" can only occur between two individuals who have been in an absolutely monogamous relationship for at least seven to eight years, have both been tested, and have no other risk behavior or sexual contacts.

The second route of transmission of HIV is through blood and blood products. In many communities, sharing drug needles and syringes is the fastest route by which HIV spreads. Sharing needles, even once, is an extremely easy way to become infected with HIV. Blood from an infected person can be trapped in the needle or syringe, then injected directly into the blood stream of the next person who uses the needle.

Other behaviors involving needles increase the risk of HIV infection. Many young people pierce each other's ear lobes, using the same needle to puncture the ears of several friends. Athletes may inject themselves with steroids, then pass the needle and syringe on to others.

Testing for the HIV antibody in all donated blood has been occurring with regularity and has drastically reduced the numbers of people who contract the disease through transfusions of blood and blood products. A test developed by Abbott Laboratories can determine the presence of the virus itself and should make blood supplies safer for the transfusion recipient. Bear in mind that, although there is still a risk factor connected with transfusions, most recipients are in a life-threatening situation and may well die without the transfusion.

A third mode of transmission, and one that is increasing, is the passing on of the virus from an infected mother to her infant, either before birth or at the time of delivery.

Incubation

Since there is a long (an average of 9.8 years) incubation period between infection with HIV and the onset of AIDS symptoms, researchers believe that many young adults diagnosed with AIDS contracted the virus during their adolescent years.

Detection

The *HIV antibody test*, or so-called AIDS test, does *not* determine the presence of the AIDS disease. It *does* show if a person has been *infected* with the HIV, or AIDS virus. The test looks for changes in blood that occur after being infected. It is very reliable when testing is conducted by a reputable laboratory and the results checked by a knowledgeable physician.

When the HIV antibody test became available in 1985, most AIDS agencies remained neutral on its use. Because of complex political, ethical, and public health issues surrounding the test, it was left as a matter of personal choice. It was viewed more as an educational tool than a medical determination, and there were few treatment options to offer someone who tested positive.

It has been recommended that health care workers who are at high risk consider volunteering for anonymous testing of AIDS. The psychological stress involved in deciding to be tested is significant, and there still exists a real risk of housing, insurance, and job-related discrimination resulting from a breach of confidentiality. With new treatment options, most AIDS organizations are coming to feel the benefits of knowing antibody status outweigh the risks and burdens. They are reconsidering their attitudes on advocated testing. The gradual development of a medical model of disease management emphasizes early detection of infection and immune system monitoring.

Management

Presently, there is no vaccine and no cure for AIDS. A combination of zidovudine (2DV) and lamivudine (3TC), known as Combivir, approved by the FDA, is now used in antiviral therapy for the AIDS virus. The drug prevents the reproduction of HIV cells and has been shown in clinical studies to prolong the lives of some AIDS victims. AZT has been administered to those diagnosed with full-blown AIDS, but a few preliminary studies have indicated possible benefits from prescribing it earlier in the course of HIV infection.

The San Francisco AIDS Foundation (SFAF) notes that researchers have mixed AZT with other antiviral drugs in an attempt to find a combination of chemicals that will destroy HIV. An FDA-approved drug, didanosine (DDI), a less common medication, has been used to delay the onset of AIDS. Didanosine may be used in conjunction with AZT when AZT proves too toxic for a particular patient.

Aerosolized pentamidine, approved by the FDA in 1989, has proven effective in slowing or preventing *Pneumocystis carinii* **pneumonia (PCP)**. A diagnosis of this particular type of pneumonia depends on a laboratory culture of lung tissue. Termed an "opportunistic" disease, it occurs in people suffering from AIDS, whose natural defenses have been reduced by the AIDS disease itself. Studies indicate that in over one-half of AIDS deaths PCP was determined as the cause.

The ability to prevent, delay, or treat the complications accompanying HIV infection has lent optimism to the future of the disease. Project Inform, a San Francisco organization, provides information about therapeutic options and access to treatment.

Promising drug therapies and greater understanding of the course of HIV infection have fundamentally changed prevailing attitudes toward AIDS.

For the present, the best way to slow AIDS is through worldwide education and prevention. These efforts will fight not only the epidemic of the disease but also the "second epidemic" of fear and mistrust that AIDS often generates.

Dental Care

Like other patients with chronic diseases, AIDS patients need ongoing routine dental care. Oral findings in the AIDS patient include infections of the mucosa (mucous membranes of the mouth): **thrush**, characterized by white patches on a red, moist, inflamed surface; *recurrent herpes simplex virus*; and *progressive disease of the periodontal tissues*. Some of these disorders require treatment that can be provided in the dental office. A case in point are HIV-related periodontal problems.

Human immunodeficiency virus infections may appear in many ways, and the dental professional should become familiar with the oral evidence, because this is often the first sign of the presence of the disease. For instance, a herpes simplex ulcer that persists longer than one month is particularly significant as an indicator of AIDS. Periodontal lesions of HIV periodontitis, or *AIDS virus–associated periodontitis (AVAP)*, are marked by swelling and intense *erythema* (redness of the tissue caused by congestion of the capillaries in the lower layers of that tissue) of the free and attached gingiva. A rapidly progressive gingivitis, the symptoms of AVAP are intense pain, spontaneous bleeding, and bad breath.

Often, AIDS patients display a high incidence of **Kaposi's sarcoma** (a purplish, localized malignant cancer of the skin), which spreads from the original site to one or more sites elsewhere in the body. *Squamous* (scaly) *carcinoma* is a malignant new growth or tumor that appears on the skin surface and has a potential to infiltrate (penetrate) surrounding tissues and to spread.

If the individual with AIDS is a regular patient, a dentist must be particularly careful if he or she wishes to assist the patient in obtaining care through other sources. Referral to clinics or hospitals equipped to treat those with infectious diseases is one means of assisting these patients to receive the necessary dental care. Each patient must be evaluated individually, and in some cases referral may be the best action for that patient. The ADA recommends that local dental societies attempt to set up a referral system for patients with AIDS and other infectious diseases to enable all patients to receive quality dental care when it is needed.

Prevention of Diseases

Protection from diseases is accomplished by disinfecting contaminated surfaces; subjecting oneself to vaccines; and wearing personal protective equipment (PPE) including eyeglasses/goggles, face mask/shield, treatment/surgical gloves, utility gloves, and protective gown (see Chapter 7). Using the **Universal Precautions** protocol on all patients for every given procedure and recognizing that their blood and saliva are considered potentially infectious are steps in preventing the spread of disease (Table 6-1).

Table 6-1 Disease Transmission and Protection

Disease	Method of Transmission	Method of Protection
Tuberculosis	Inhaled airborne droplets of blood or saliva (moisture)	Personal protective equipment; Use UV light and HEPA filtration to disinfect contaminated surfaces
Herpes Simplex Labialis (HSV-1)	Direct contact with open herpetic ulcer discharge	Avoid treating patients with apparent herpetic ulcers; avoid contact with infected persons; do not drink from the same cup or use same utensils
Herpes Simplex Genitalis (HSV-2)	Sexually transmitted by direct contact with open herpetic ulcer discharge; childbirth: mother to infant	Avoid sexual contact with infected person
Hepatitis A (HAV)	Direct contact with fecal-oral route (mostly children and young adults); contaminated food or water	Vaccine currently available; personal protective equipment; disinfect contaminated surfaces; standard immune globulin after infection
Hepatitis B (HBV)	Direct contact with all body fluids; direct bloodborne contact by contaminated sharps; childbirth: mother to infant	HBV vaccine; personal protective equipment; disinfect contaminated surfaces
Hepatitis C (HCV)	Blood transfusions; contaminated sharps; infected drug needles; multiple sex partners; childbirth: mother to infant	Personal protective equipment; disinfect contaminated surfaces
Hepatitis D (HDV)	Direct bloodborne contact by contaminated sharps; sexual contact; childbirth: mother to infant	HBV vaccine; personal protective equipment; disinfect contaminated surfaces
Hepatitis E	Direct contact with fecal-oral route (mostly adults); contaminated water	Personal protective equipment; hand washing prior to food handling
Hepatitis G (HGV)	Direct bloodborne contact similar to HCV	Personal protective equipment; disinfect contaminated surfaces
AIDS/HIV	Sexual contact; blood and blood products, contaminated needles; childbirth: mother to infant	Personal protective equipment; disinfect contaminated surfaces; avoid sexual contact

SUGGESTED ACTIVITIES

- Make a list of possible ways that airborne bacteria could be created in a dental office.
- Using specific situations, explain how a DHCW could become infected and achieve the following:
  - Tuberculosis
  - Herpetic whitlow
  - Hepatitus B
  - HIV

REVIEW

1. A lesion is:
   a. A normal nonpathologic condition
   b. Disease-related or injury-induced tissue damage
   c. A symptom the patient is experiencing
   d. A congenital defect such as anodontia
2. Tuberculosis spreads by:
   a. Direct contact with fecal-oral route
   b. Sexual contact with an infected person
   c. Childbirth of an infected mother
   d. Discharged droplets of moisture from an infected person

3. The incubation stage of disease takes place:
   a. As soon as it enters the organism
   b. When signs and symptoms appear until recovery takes place
   c. At the time it enters the organism up to the time the first signs or symptoms appear
   d. Within a week of infection

4. Indicate which three of the following are ways that the AIDS virus can spread: (1) sexual activity, (2) sharing needles and syringes, (3) childbirth, or (4) discharged droplets of saliva.
   a. 1, 2, 3
   b. 1, 3, 4
   c. 2, 3, 4
   d. 1, 2, 4

5. Indicate how the hepatitis B virus (HBV) can spread in the dental environment: (1) direct contact with all body fluids, (2) childbirth, (3) needlestick injury, and/or (4) patient debris on contaminated instruments.
   a. 1, 2, 3
   b. 1, 3, 4
   c. 2, 3, 4
   d. 1, 2, 4

Principles of Personal Protection

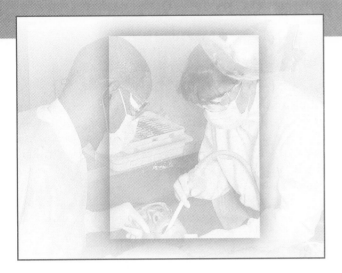

OBJECTIVES

After studying this chapter, the student will be able to:

- Discuss the principles of personal grooming for the conscientious chairside dental assistant.
- Cite the steps for disinfecting the hands and forearms.
- Demonstrate the accepted hand-washing technique.
- Compare the types of gloves used in the practice of dentistry.
- Explain the rationale for wearing gloves in dentistry.
- Demonstrate the proper method(s) for donning and removing dental treatment gloves.
- Discuss the protection provided by a face mask.
- Describe the recommended eyewear for dental operatory procedures.

Introduction

The nature of dental assisting leads to the possibility of spreading infectious organisms from patient to chairside dental assistant, and from chairside dental assistant to family and co-workers as well as to other patients. For the sake of the dental assistant, patients, co-workers, and the dental assistant's family, it is necessary to break the chain of infection wherever possible (Figure 7-1).

At least, a person should think about what is carried home to family members on clothing or being transmitted to fellow commuters. More than one spouse or child have become ill from microorganisms brought home on soiled clothing of a health care worker.

Personal Grooming

The conscientious chairside dental assistant will strictly follow several principles of good grooming in the prevention of cross-contamination:

- *Nails*–Short, clean, with smooth tips and cuticles. Long fingernails increase the possibility of puncturing a dental glove. Nail polish is not acceptable due to microscopic chips and crevices that harbor organisms.

- *Uniform*–Professional uniforms should be washable and bleachable, whether white or of a color. The uniform should be free of frills and other catchalls. Sleeves should be short to allow washing of the forearms. Uniform should be covered by a protective garment with long sleeves closed at the wrists and high neck whenever contact with spray or splashes of blood or other body fluids can be anticipated. Uniform should be removed before leaving the office at the end of the workday and laundered separately from other clothes. Studies from Centers for Disease Control and Prevention (CDC) report that professional uniforms may be laundered in a normal laundry cycle and should be given a high-temperature (140–160°F) wash cycle with normal bleach concentration followed by machine drying (212°F or more).

- *Hair*–Short, clean, off the face and neck, or tied back and firmly secured to keep loose strands from falling forward or down.

- *Jewelry*–Inappropriate items, such as rings, watches, bracelets should be removed at the beginning of the workday. It is impossible to scrub them free of organisms that are constantly working their way from deeper layers to the surface of the skin.

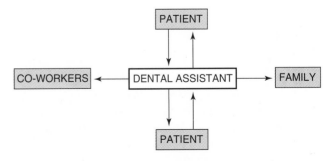

Figure 7-1 Potential chain of infection.

● *Tobacco*–Odor may be offensive to patients and fellow workers. Nicotine stains are unsightly.

Washing Hands

Assisting with or performing intraoral procedures demands that hands be as free as possible from impurities and microorganisms that contribute to infection and disease. There are no chemicals that can be depended on to kill all organisms on the skin; therefore, hand cleansing is vital. Mechanical removal (rubbing, rinsing, drying) with the use of germicidal cleaning agents helps to prevent cross-contamination.

Supplies

Germicidal Soap Preparations. Current research indicates that the antimicrobial agents proven to be most effective against a broad range of microorganisms are chlorhexidine gluconate and provisions-iodine preparations. These may be irritating to the skin of some persons; in such cases, bactericidal lotion-type cleansers containing triclosan or trilocarbon may be preferable. *Accepted Dental Therapeutics*, a publication of the American Dental Association (ADA), should be consulted for brand names.

Hand Towels. Absorbent, disposable paper hand towels for complete drying should be used. A hand towel should *never* be reused.

Procedure for Washing Hands

Effective steps must be developed for disinfection of the hands and forearms. Ideally, antimicrobial preparations should be available for use from a dispensing device and the water source operated by a foot or forearm control. Most dental offices are furnished with hand-activated water faucets. Paper hand towels should be dispensed one at a time.

It is advisable that front-office staff washes with antimicrobial soap several times during the workday to remove the number of pathogens from the hands. An ADA report, published September 1985 in the *Journal of the American Dental Association*, showed that contaminated debris on dental charts can remain active for as long as five days. Although front-office staff do not wear gloves, it seems reasonable that they should take precautions for their own protection. Hand washing is a *must* for all dental personnel prior to lunch and before leaving the office at the end of the day.

Procedure 1 Hand Washing

Materials Needed

Antimicrobial soap
Orangewood stick
Hand towel

Instructions

1 Turn on and adjust the flow of cool water. Remove rings/jewelry from hands.

2 Wet both hands, and then apply sufficient amount of antimicrobial soap to work into lather.

3 Wash hands for 15 seconds by rubbing lather over all surfaces of forearms and hands. Include the palms, knuckles, and especially tips of all fingers and under the nails. Make certain both hands are cleaned.

4 Using an orangewood stick, clean debris from under nails. Discard after use.

5 Thoroughly rinse hands in *cold* water to close pores.

6 Dry with hand towel, beginning with the fingers. Use the towel to thoroughly dry the cuticles of the nails, then run the edge of the towel under the tip of each nail. Proceed to dry hands and forearms thoroughly.

7 Turn off hand-activated faucet with hand towel. Discard towel in trash container.

8 Apply antimicrobial lotion to hands. *Note:* Keeping the hands from cracking and drying is most important. Lotion should be applied at least three to four times a day, especially before lunch and at the end of the day. Avoid lotions that are *petroleum* or *mineral oil* based as they degrade glove material.

9 Prepare to don gloves.

Personal Protective Equipment (PPE)

Personal protective equipment (PPE) consists of gloves, garments, masks, and eyewear to provide a protective barrier between the DHCW's (dental health care worker's) body and the source of contamination, thus preventing possible infection.

The procedure to apply PPE should be as follows, according to the Office Safety & Asepsis Procedures (OSAP) recommendation: Don eyewear first, then the face mask, followed by the gloves. To remove contaminated PPE, remove gloves first, then face mask by the strap, and lastly protective eyewear. Disposable items should be discarded in proper waste receptacle.

PPE Application Sequence	PPE Removal Sequence
1. Eyewear	1. Gloves
2. Face mask	2. Face mask
3. Gloves	3. Eyewear

Protective Gloves

Gloves should always be worn for protection during intraoral procedures or when handling objects that have become contaminated with saliva or blood. Bear in mind that gloves offer the best, although not perfect, barrier to organisms to and from the hands.

Gloves minimize the risk of cross-infection from patient to patient, from patient to dentist and chairside dental assistant, and from the dental operatory personnel to patient. Routine hand-washing procedures and germicidal hand-washing agents are very important, as they reduce the number of pathogens on the hands. However, these procedures alone have proved inadequate in eliminating pathogenic organisms from the hands.

In the dental situation, saliva contacted by dental personnel may become contaminated with blood. It is wise to assume that where blood and saliva are mixed, there is a potential for transmission. Dental professionals can contract infectious agents, such as herpes, human immunodeficiency virus, hepatitis B, tuberculosis, and common respiratory viruses, through microscopic cuts and skin punctures, even hangnails. (Refer to Chapter 6.) Patients may not be aware they have contracted an infectious disease and may seek dental care before diagnostic symptoms develop.

Use of Gloves. For years, dentistry personnel used gloves almost exclusively for surgical procedures. Today, they are used for every patient, under the guidelines of the CDC and the mandate of the Occupational Safety and Health Administration (OSHA). Although the CDC can only recommend the use of gloves, OSHA has the power to enforce the guidelines.

According to the CDC, Standard Precautions must be taken. This is interpreted to mean "treat every patient as though he or she has an infectious disease that is deadly."

Types of Gloves. Dentistry uses several types of gloves: vinyl, latex, or nitrile examination/treatment gloves, latex surgical gloves, cotton undergloves, plastic overgloves, and heavy utility gloves.

Examination/Treatment Gloves. Examination gloves may be made of vinyl or latex and are dispensed unsterilized. Vinyl is used in procedures where a tight fit is not absolutely necessary. Vinyl lacks the elasticity of latex and may tear when stretched. Gloves made of vinyl easily adapt to either the left or right hand. In some cases, the choice of vinyl or latex is due to skin irritations caused by the latex material (Figure 7-2).

Latex is strong, tough, and elastic, capable of stretching then returning to its molded shape to fit snugly over the hand. Latex affords an ideal sense of touch during a dental procedure. Latex gloves are designed for the left or right hand and are dispensed in sizes ranging from extra small to extra large. Nonsterile latex treatment gloves can be purchased in quantities and are adequate for most dental operatory procedures. The manufacturer may treat treatment gloves with cornstarch powder, making the process of donning them much easier.

Treatment gloves are to be worn during direct patient care. They should be worn while handling radiograph films that have been in the patient's mouth, as well as dentures, dental appliances, impressions, or other items that could contribute to disease transmission.

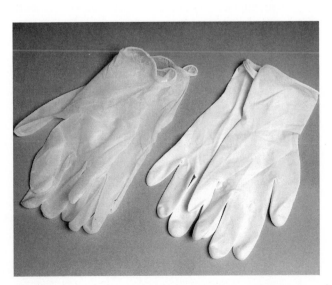

Figure 7-2 Examination/treatment gloves: (A) vinyl; (B) latex.

Surgical Gloves. Surgical gloves are made of latex, have been sterilized, and are required when dental procedures involve extensive surgical manipulation.

Note: It is not recommended that vinyl or latex gloves be washed with detergent because it can weaken stabilizers in the glove material and promote **wicking** (penetration of the glove material through inherent defects). For patient comfort, rinsing gloves to remove excess powder is preferred. If gloves become punctured, torn, or cut during treatment, they must be removed immediately, hands washed thoroughly, dried, and fresh gloves donned.

Overgloves. Plastic overgloves, also known as food-handler gloves, are very inexpensive; they are not a suitable replacement for latex or vinyl. Made of clear plastic, they are acceptable as an overglove for treatment gloves. For instance, the chairside dental assistant needs to contact a surface that cannot be covered with a barrier and cannot be disinfected. The dental assistant may dry his or her gloved hands, don the plastic gloves (for this short procedure only), then simply remove and discard the overgloves before returning to the patient. An example of such a situation might be the need to look for information on the patient chart or reach for supplies in a cabinet or drawer. Careful planning can reduce situations such as these (Figure 7-3).

Heavy Utility Gloves. Heavy utility gloves are used for treatment room disinfection and instrument clean-up. Utility gloves are made of nitrile plastic chemically bonded with rubber. These protective gloves are puncture resistant and not to be confused with household gloves sold in grocery or hardware stores. Utility gloves should be thoroughly washed and dried while still on the hands. Remove and spray with a disinfectant. Hang to dry.

Contaminated utility gloves should be washed, dried, and placed in the autoclave for sterilization, along with other disposables, before being discarded. Repeat hand washing and drying (Figure 7-4).

Allergic Reaction to Latex Gloves. There has been some misunderstanding about cornstarch powder on latex gloves being the sole cause of skin irritation for the wearer. It is a well-known fact that there are only three sources of cornstarch in the world. Most manufacturers use the same source for their cornstarch. Cornstarch powder is biodegradable and nonirritating; however, the powder absorbs latex proteins and chemical additives from the gloves and carries them into cracks and crevices on the hands that could produce irritation and adverse skin reactions.

Where the glove of one manufacturer causes irritation, that of another will not. This occurs because there are different qualities of latex material as well as variations in the manufacturing process.

Latex rubber, like maple sap, seeps from the rubber tree, *Hevea brazilienis,* according to the OSAP. Many chemical additives such as ammonia (the ammonia breaks down some of the protein into smaller fragments) are used in the latex solution before it is molded. The glove is removed from the mold and washed in water to remove the residual chemicals; otherwise, the chemicals remain in the glove. Lack of this important step, rather than the cornstarch powder, probably contributes to skin irritations.

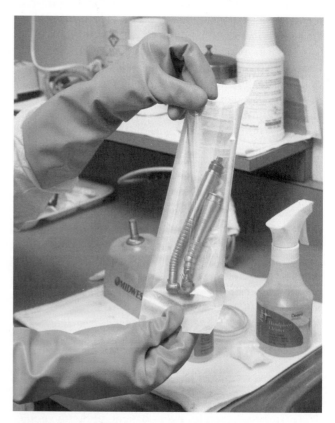

Figure 7-4 Utility gloves used for disinfection and instrument clean-up.

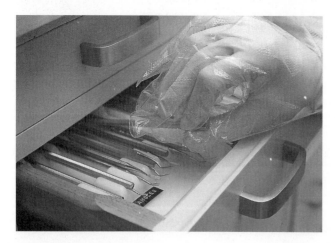

Figure 7-3 Overgloves used to reach for supplies in a cabinet or write on the patient's chart.

Powder-Free Gloves. A powder-free latex glove is chemically washed with chlorine to remove 100% of all the chemicals and the cornstarch powder. Gloves that are powder free, previously referred to as **hypoallergenic** (hypo = "below"; or below the level to cause an allergic reaction), are available. According to the Federal Drug Administration (FDA), the term *hypoallergenic* must be removed from latex glove packaging in the future. Powder-free gloves are considerably more costly than other latex gloves.

Nitrile Exam Gloves. Although more expensive than latex or vinyl, nitrile exam gloves claim to be ideal for persons sensitive to natural rubber. These gloves are made of synthetic rubber material and provide chemical and abrasion durability without compromising comfort and tactility. They are available with light powder and powder free.

Undergloves. Thin cotton undergloves are available to use under latex and vinyl gloves and help to avoid skin surface reactions. Some dental personnel are inclined to perspire under their gloves. Undergloves help in such situations without the loss of any tactile (touch) sensations. A light dusting of cornstarch on the hands prior to gloving enables the glove to slip over the hand without difficulty.

Storage of Treatment Gloves.
Latex or vinyl treatment gloves should be stored in a cool, dark place, within easy access of the dental operatory personnel. Prolonged exposure to heat and light increases the tendency to develop minute perforations. The shelf life of treatment gloves is reasonably long, but the expiration date on the container should always be checked. A variety of glove dispensers are available, either with a wall mount or countertop fitting.

Posttreatment Care of Gloves.
Upon completion of a dental procedure:

● Gloves should be removed, turned inside out, as they are pulled free of the fingers.

● One glove should be tucked inside the other. Gloves should be discarded in plastic disposal biohazard bag.

● Hands should be washed thoroughly and dried with disposable paper towels.

Protective Garments

Protective coverup gowns are available in disposable, cotton, or cotton/polyester. They are worn over a professional uniform and are required whenever contact with spray or splashes of blood or other body fluids can be reasonably anticipated to contaminate the torso, fore-

arms, or lap. Protective gowns should be changed daily and removed before leaving the dental office. They should be disposed of or laundered according to the material from which they are made.

Disposable Gowns. Disposable gowns are available in a fabric that breathes, resists absorption, and provides an effective barrier. Protective gowns should be designed with a high neck and long sleeves and be knee length for optimal protection. Change of gown should take place as soon as possible when visible soil is apparent; otherwise, they should be discarded daily. Unisex sizes range from extra small to extra large. According to OSHA regulations, traditional professional uniforms are not intended to function as protection against any hazard. Refer to Chapter 9 for stated regulations (Figure 7-5).

Reusable Gowns. An alternative to disposable gowns is the reusable cotton or cotton/polyester gown or laboratory coat. However, an employee may not launder them. In accordance with OSHA's **Bloodborne Pathogens Standard**, it is the responsibility of the employer to launder protective reusable garments whether the attire is laundered in the office, provided equipment is available and universal precautions are followed, or elsewhere. If contaminated laundry is transported away

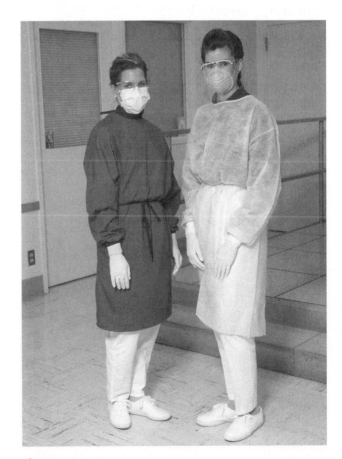

Figure 7-5 Gowns.

from the office, it must be in appropriate leak-proof bags marked with the universal symbol indicating **biohazard material** (biologically hazardous or potentially infectious material).

Face Masks, Protective Eyeware, and Face Shields

Face Masks. The choice of masks may be dictated by comfort, fit, and price. To be effective, the **FDA (Food and Drug Administration)** recommends that masks have at least 95% or greater **bacterial filtration efficiency (BFE)** of all larger particles of aerosol debris. Traditional types are the pliable pleated tie-on and the preformed dome-shaped masks. Both create a problem, because the wearer will often remove the mask from the face, then allow it to hang around the neck after treatment is completed. This action is very much discouraged due to the fact that patient blood and spatter on the outside of the mask could contaminate the skin of the DHCW. Masks are available that are pleated with slender straps that hook over the ears, making it impossible to hang around the neck! Another innovative type of mask is one that has the mask-eyewear combination with elastic strap or tie-on options.

When selecting a mask, it should fit the face well without allowing open gaps around the mask that may allow spatter to enter, transmitting it to the nose or mouth of the wearer. Should the mask become moist for any reason, its filtration efficiency will be compromised and become a "nest" for bacterial growth rather than a barrier; therefore it should be replaced. The CDC recommends that a mask be changed between patients or if it becomes moist from within or without. If masks need to be adjusted, the DHCW should refrain from handling the body of the mask, but rather should handle it only from the periphery and as little as possible, (Figure 7-6).

Protective Eyewear. The purpose of protective eyewear is to shield the DHCW from diseases such as herpes simplex or *Staphylococcus aureus* and prevent contact with caustic chemicals as well as airborne particles generated from grinding or polishing procedures.

According to OSHA, the criterion for protective eyewear is that it must have front and side protection with solid side shields (Figure 7-7). This type of eyewear offers maximum protection, resists scratching and fogging, and does not cause visual distortion. Eyewear should also be capable of being decontaminated, disinfected, or sterilized. Some manufacturers provide glasses with replaceable lenses with antifog properties that may withstand heat by autoclaving. For those who already wear corrective lens eyewear, there is eyewear that will fit over existing glasses. Each DHCW *must* wear appropriate eye protection.

Face Shields. The DHCW should be aware that face shields do not substitute for the use of masks. Therefore, if a face shield is worn, a face mask should also be worn. The face shield may be worn in place of protective eyewear but should meet the **American National Standards Institute (ANSI) Occupational and Educational Eye and Face Protection Standard (Z87.1-1989)** and be labeled as such. The criteria for face shields are that they provide protection at both the top and sides of the shield and be of chin length (Figure 7-8). There are new face shields that are specific for laser or cauterization procedures and are known as laser-plume masks.

Face shields should be washed and disinfected using the spray-wipe-spray technique before reuse, taking care not to scratch the shield.

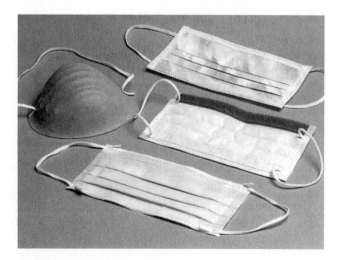

Figure 7-6 Assorted face masks.

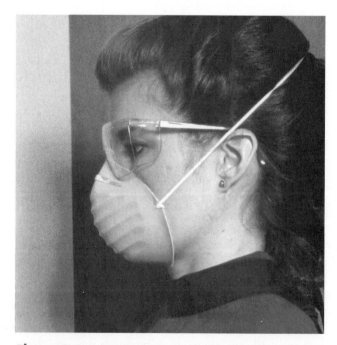

Figure 7-7 Protective eyewear with solid side shields.

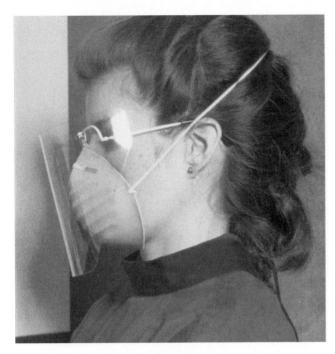

Figure 7-8 Chin length face shield.

SUGGESTED ACTIVITIES

● Using the recommended steps, practice hand washing, rinsing, and drying.

● Practice donning and removing treatment gloves.

● Orally explain the method(s) of disposal for treatment gloves.

REVIEW

1. What does PPE mean?
   a. Protective practical environment
   b. Potential protective environment
   c. Personal protective equipment
   d. Practical procedural eyewear

2. Which two principal agencies establish guidelines for glove use in dentistry?
   a. CDC, OSHA
   b. EPA, ADA
   c. FDA, ADAA
   d. ANSI, ADA

3. Indicate why plastic "food handler" overgloves are worn over treatment gloves: (1) for double protection, (2) to avoid contact with sharp instruments, (3) to avoid contact with a surface that cannot be covered with a barrier, and/or (4) to avoid contact with a surface that cannot be disinfected
   a. 1, 2
   b. 2, 3
   c. 3, 4
   d. 1, 4

4. What do disposable gowns provide when worn over professional uniforms?
   a. They don't have to be laundered.
   b. They are an effective barrier.
   c. They are disposable.
   d. They are light weight.

5. Indicate when a face mask should be changed: (1) after each patient, (2) after it was contaminated during mask adjustments, (3) after one hour of operative procedures, and/or (4) at the end of the day.
   a. 1, 2
   b. 2, 3
   c. 3, 4
   d. 1, 3

CHAPTER 8

Infection Control and Hazard Communication Management

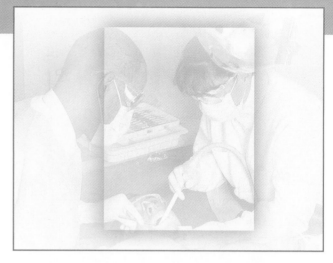

OBJECTIVES

After studying this chapter, the student will be able to:

- Determine the two best-known chemical hazards in dental practice and their routes of entry into the human body.

- Cite the most common respiratory irritants used in the dental office.

- State the prime concern of the Occupational Safety and Health Administration regarding the dental staff.

- Discuss the procedures manual and its importance in controlling the use of chemicals in dentistry.

- Discuss the Material Safety Data Sheets with regard to hazardous materials.

- Determine the standards for infectious waste control and the identification of contaminated materials.

- Discuss the guidelines for infection control in the practice of dentistry.

- Determine the various immersion chemicals used in dentistry, their advantages, and their disadvantages.

- Determine the chemicals used for hard-surface disinfection, their advantages, and their disadvantages.

- Discuss the difference between disinfection and sterilization.

- Describe the steps involved in preparing the packaging of dental instruments for sterilization.

- Compare the steam autoclave with the chemical vapor sterilizer.

Introduction

There are many procedures that DHCWs (dental health care workers) need to adhere to in compliance with infection control measures. Complying with the use of barriers in the dental treatment room, decontamination of surfaces, and use of personal protective equipment (PPE) to prevent cross-contamination are of prime concern. The DHCW needs to be knowledgeable about hazardous chemicals present in many dental materials, methods of use and disposal for each chemical, implementation of disinfection and sterilization techniques,

and overall compliance with Occupational Safety and Health Administration standards.

Government Regulating Agencies

The dental community needs to realize it must comply with certain government standards imposed on them for the safety of dental patients and DHCWs. Some agencies have developed standards and policies that affect the manner in which daily routines are conducted. There are four primary agencies with which each health care worker should be familiar.

- The Occupational Safety and Health Administration (OSHA), a federal agency that provides information and enforcement for the health and safety of employees in the work area

- The Centers for Disease Control and Prevention (CDC), an agency based in Atlanta, Georgia, that studies infectious diseases and provides reports and recommendations regarding them

- The Environmental Protection Agency (EPA), a federal regulatory agency that studies and controls environmental issues and public safety

- The Food and Drug Administration (FDA), a federal agency that controls the use and manufacture of drugs and chemicals

Hazard Communication in the Dental Office

There are two broad categories of materials that DHCWs should be aware of: biohazardous and hazardous (flammable, corrosive, and toxic).

Biohazardous

Biohazardous materials are potentially infectious and include any material that has come in direct contact with blood or body fluids in sufficient amount to cause disease. Some of these are considered to be the **sharps** that have the characteristic of puncturing or cutting tissue, such as needles, orthodontic wires, broken anesthetic cartridges, microscope slides, scalpel blades, and small endodontic instruments (Table 8-1).

Hazardous

Hazardous materials may pose a problem to the DHCW's health and/or may harm the environment when discarded and can be put in the following categories:

- **Flammable.** In dentistry most materials in this category are alcohol based, including chemical sterilizing solution and isopropyl alcohol. Other examples of solutions include acrylic monomers, acetone, and the copal varnish solvents that contain ether. In addition to the liquid flammable materials, oxygen and nitrous oxide gases are known to support combustion but not initiate it.

- **Corrosive.** Materials in this category are those either above or below 7.0 pH, such as alkalies or strong acids, and are reactive when the two combine. Hydrochloric acid and pickling solution are examples of this category. Injuries caused by these materials include **contact dermatitis** (skin irritation or allergy) and eye, nose, throat, and respiratory irritations.

- **Toxic.** This category of materials are known to cause systemic problems if ingested or inhaled and can also cause contact dermatitis. Examples are cold sterilization glutaraldehyde solutions, photo chemicals, and mercury vapor. The effects of these materials could cause immediate harm or may become chronic.

Table 8-1	Guidelines for Infection Control
General Guidelines	**Biohazardous Waste Disposal**

General Guidelines

1. Sterilize everything that can be sterilized.
2. Use disposables wherever possible to eliminate microbial life from the area and prevent additional handling during cleanup. It takes far less time to discard disposables than to completely disinfect the operatory.
3. Use barriers wherever possible to prevent contamination of surfaces. It is easier to dispose of them rather than disinfect or sterilize surfaces.

Barriers

Personal Protective Equipment
- Disposable treatment gloves
- Disposable face masks
- Protective eyewear with side shields
- Professional uniform, covered by a protective garment

Patient Barriers
- Protective eyewear
- Dental dam
- Patient drape/napkin
- High-volume evacuation

Disposable Surface Barriers (plastic barriers)
- Full-chair covers
- Dental light handle covers
- Air/water syringe covers
- Tray and cabinet covers
- Tubing covers/sleeves
- Self-stick barrier film

Biohazardous Waste Disposal

- Blood or blood-soaked items that, when compressed, release blood or known infectious materials capable of causing disease
- Tissue and extracted teeth
- Contaminated needles, surgical blades, wires, sharp items, disposable syringes, and glass cartridges must be discarded in a puncture-proof biohazard sharps container.

Items that are potentially infectious enough to cause disease are discarded in clearly marked biohazard leak-proof bags.

Nonregulated or General Waste Disposal

Included in this category are:
- Disposable gowns
- Protective masks
- Disposable eyewear
- Patient bib if not saturated with body fluids
- Paper towels
- All plastic covers
- Applicable barriers
- Gauze square sponges, cotton rolls, pellets, dental floss and any disposable items that have touched blood and/or saliva, not soaked

Contaminated items that do not possess enough biohazardous material to cause disease are not considered to be infectious.

These items should be discarded in a refuse bag labeled as contaminated waste. Once it leaves the office, it is considered regular waste.

Hazardous Chemicals/Materials. Several hazardous chemicals and materials are found in the dental environment. Some of these will be discussed in greater detail.

Mercury (Hg) is perhaps the best known of the chemical hazards in dentistry. Because mercury is odorless and vaporizes at 10°F, its vapors can easily be inhaled and not be detected. The American Dental Association's (ADA's) Council on Dental Materials and Devices offers guidelines for achieving good mercury hygiene in the dental office.

Because the most serious hazard associated with mercury in dental practice is accidental spills from bulk containers of mercury, employers should consider changing to premeasured amalgam capsules. Rubber treatment gloves should be worn when handling mercury or amalgam, because it can be absorbed through the pores of the skin.

Formaldehyde, another best-known chemical hazard in dentistry, is one of the substances in solutions used in chemical vapor sterilizers. Routes of entry for the vapors of this chemical are inhalation, ingestion (swallowing), and skin contact. It is classified by OSHA as a human carcinogen and should be handled with care. The area where formaldehyde is used *should be well ventilated*. Rubber treatment gloves should be worn if skin contact is likely to occur when pouring solution into a sterilizer. Should the solution come into contact with the skin, the skin should be washed with soap and water immediately.

The manufacturer's instructions for chemical vaporizer sterilizer use must be closely followed to reduce the possibility of vapors escaping into the dental environment. Ideally, these sterilizers should be placed under hoods that are vented to the outside.

Dentistry uses many respiratory irritants. Methyl methacrylate, alcohol-based preparations, and photographic chemicals used to develop radiographs are some of the most common.

Alginate (irreversible colloid) contains diatomaceous earth (a finely ground silicate filler) that can be inhaled, producing a health hazard. Wearing a dental mask when dispensing or mixing alginate should protect the DHCW.

Gypsum (plaster or stone) may cause **silicosis** (a condition in the lungs due to inhaled silica) when enough material is inhaled. A protective mask should be worn whenever working with gypsum products.

OSHA Standards for Biological Hazards

The Occupational Safety and Health Administration has spelled out requirements for infection control in the dental office. Among these are written procedures for the proper handling of chemicals.

A loose-leaf procedures manual will provide the basis for policy and training of dental personnel. Such a manual can be easily revised to meet the dental office needs.

The Procedures Manual. A procedures manual can be in either printed or computerized form. Both are available, thus eliminating the necessity of writing one.

A manual contains the procedures needed to meet OSHA rules that cover labeling, chemical handling, containers, storage, and ordering chemicals. The manual can also include documented Material Safety Data Sheets required by OSHA. These help in the event of an OSHA inspection to prove that OSHA-required procedures and practices are in place.

Standard procedures for sterilization, surface disinfection, and ordering supplies should be included in the manual.

The prime concern of OSHA is that of safe chemical handling and how staff is protected from bloodborne diseases. Both OSHA and the EPA require safe disposal techniques for infectious wastes.

The Material Safety Data Sheet. Basically, OSHA requires a **Material Data Safety Sheet (MSDS)** for any chemical that is supplied in a bottle, can, or bag.

Items requiring an MSDS can be listed in alphabetical order. The list should include the product name, manufacturer's name and telephone number, and the work area where the product is used. The list can be easily updated if new hazardous materials are introduced or can result in the disposal of materials that are no longer useful.

If a manufacturer fails to provide an MSDS for a hazardous product, it is the responsibility of the employer to request it. The vendor is required by law to provide the latest MSDS for that substance.

As the MSDSs are collected, a checkmark is made in the appropriate box to indicate the MSDS is on file. An MSDS for each substance listed is required by OSHA.

When the MSDS arrives, the name of the material and any first-aid instructions should be highlighted with a colored felt-tipped pen. The pages are then inserted in the appropriate section of the procedures manual. Should an emergency occur, that particular MSDS should be easily found.

It is well to remember that MSDSs need to be kept only for materials that are biologically hazardous, not for regular household cleansers and detergents.

OSHA Regulations for Infectious Waste Materials

The Occupational Safety and Health Administration has requirements for infectious waste, also called **regulated waste** or biohazard waste materials. These regulations are designed to protect employees from accidentally or mistakenly coming in contact with hepatitis B virus (HBV) or human immunodeficiency virus (HIV). (Refer to Chapter 6.)

Biohazard Labeling

Requirements set down by OSHA cover labeling when removing hazardous materials from original containers and placing them in a more convenient dispenser. For instance, a surface disinfectant bottle must be labeled with the MSDS number, the contents of the bottle, and the major health hazards the disinfectant may present.

In addition to the requirements of the Department of Health Services, OSHA has regulations for infectious materials. The OSHA standards for infectious waste control emphasize identification of contaminated materials:

- Biohazard warning tags or labels are used as a means to prevent accidental injury or illness to employees who are exposed to hazardous or potentially hazardous conditions, equipment, or operations that are out of the ordinary, unexpected, or not readily apparent. Tags or labels are not necessary when signs or other means of protection are used.

- All warning tags or labels contain a signal word or a major message. The signal word shall be *BIOHAZARD* or the biological hazard symbol, and the major message shall indicate the specific hazardous condition or the instruction to be communicated to the employee. Bags or other receptacles contaminated with potentially infectious material, including contaminated disposable items, are tagged or otherwise identified (Figure 8-1). If warning tags or labels are not used, other equally effective means of identification shall be used for example, red bagging (Figure 8-2).

Training Requirements

In compliance with OSHA regulations, training employees in all aspects of occupational exposure is mandatory. New employees in particular must verify they are knowledgeable in occupational exposure procedures that require proficiency prior to becoming involved in their management. It is required that employers provide training for their staff at no cost to the employee. Training should take place annually, more often as needed, or when new materials are introduced (see Chapter 9).

Disinfection

Disinfection is the process of using chemicals, ultraviolet light, or ionizing radiation as a means to kill bacteria with the exception of spores and resistant microorganisms.

Surface Disinfection

Liquid chemicals used for hard-surface disinfection should be suitable for wiping all surfaces in the treatment room contaminated with **bioburden** (blood, saliva, and debris) (Table 8-2).

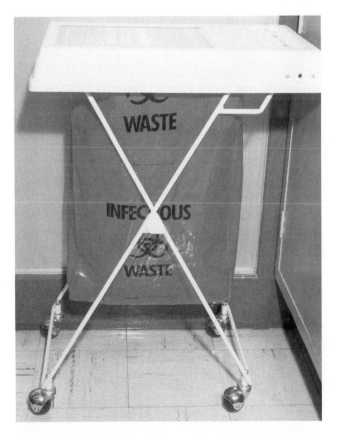

Figure 8-2 Biohazard waterproof bag used for disposal of infectious waste.

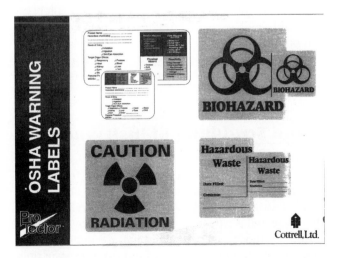

Figure 8-1 OSHA warning labels (Courtesy of Cottrell Ltd.).

Table 8-2	Disinfection Agents

Surface Disinfecting Chemicals

(Not to be rinsed off)

- Iodophors EPA registered: relatively inexpensive; good residual action; recommended
- Sodium hypocholite (bleach) 1–10%: odorous, irritating
- Complex (synthetic) phenol compounds

Immersion Chemicals

(For instrument holding)

- Glutaraldehyde liquid: 2.5% and 3.4%
- Complex phenol compounds: nontoxic, nonirritating
- Sodium hypochlorite 1% solution: corrosive with bleaching capability

Not Recommended for Immersion or Surface Disinfectng

- Alcohol
- Quaternary ammonium compounds

Disinfectants

Disinfectants are chemical agents capable of destroying most bacteria except for spores and resistant microorganisms:

- *Iodophor hard-surface disinfectants* are tuberculocidal and EPA registered, with an EPA number on the label, and consist of certain other chemicals in combination with iodine and a surface-active agent that is continuously released after the surface appears to be dry. This remaining action provides continued protection throughout patient treatment. They dilute according to manufacturer's instructions. Color change, from amber to light yellow, signals loss of potency. This material should be kept away from any light source as it deteriorates faster in the presence of light.

- *Sodium hypochlorite 1–10% solution* is inexpensive but useful, highly irritating to eyes and skin, and damaging to clothing. It has an objectionable odor and is not to be used in areas where space is limited and ventilation restricted. It is highly unstable and must be mixed on a daily basis.

- *Complex (synthetic) phenolic compounds* may be purchased in concentrate or diluted forms. They claim to be tuberculocidal and are EPA registered.

- *Not recommended as disinfectants:* alcohol and quaternary ammonium compounds.

  For accepted brand names, refer to *Accepted Dental Therapeutics*, a publication of the ADA.

Procedure. Surface disinfection requires the application of an EPA-approved surface disinfectant to equipment or working surfaces of the dental treatment room. Chemicals used for surface disinfection constitute only a portion of the process. Friction created during vigorous wiping results in reduction of numbers of microorganisms.

Effective surface disinfection is accomplished by using 4 x 4-in. square gauze sponges, open-cell plastic foam sponges, or disposable paper towels. (The 2 x 2-in. square gauze sponges are not large enough to accommodate the wiping process.) Gauze sponges and disposable paper towels or wipes should be discarded with hazardous waste. Plastic sponges used on contaminated objects must be thoroughly rinsed with cold water, squeezed dry, sprayed with surface disinfectant, and set aside to dry.

Spray-Wipe-Spray Technique

- Clean the surface with a spray bottle of aqueous iodophor solution to remove gross debris.
- Vigorously wipe with a 4 x 4-in. gauze sponge, plastic sponge, or disposable paper towel or wipe.
- Spray the surface or saturate a fresh sponge or paper towel with the disinfecting solution and apply to the surface. Allow to dry from 2 to 10 minutes.

Immersion Chemicals for Chemical Disinfection

- Alkaline glutaraldehyde 2–5% and 3.4% solution
- Synthetic phenol compounds
- Sodium hypochlorite 1% solution

Transporting Contaminated Instuments

When the dental procedure is completed, the DHCW, wearing PPE that includes puncture-resistant utility gloves, removes soiled contaminated instruments from the operatory in a leak-proof container with a solid bottom and solid sides and transports them for manual scrubbing or ultrasonic cleaning and sterilization. This should be done as soon as possible before instruments begin to dry out and in a manner that prevents exposure to others and the environment.

Hand Scrubbing of Instruments

It is of utmost importance to adhere to the use of ultrasonic cleaners rather than hand scrubbing, due to the danger of **aerosolization** (infecting the atmosphere with airborne pathogens) and possible injury. However, there are times when hand scrubbing may be used. Proper methods of hand scrubbing are outlined here. The DHCW should use PPE and puncture-resistant utility gloves and proceed as follows (Figure 8-3):

Procedure 2 Hand Scrubbing Instruments

1 Hand scrubbing of instruments should take place in a basin of soapy water.

2 Instruments should be scrubbed with a long-handled brush while scrubbing only one or two instruments at a time just above the waterline. This will ensure visibility of sharp instruments and prevent injuries.

3 Instruments should be rinsed under cold running tap water, avoiding splashing that could spread pathogens. Cold water easily removes the soap residue.

4 Instruments are dried with disposable paper towels and prepared for sterilization.

Ultrasonic Cleaning

To minimize the amount of handling instruments and aerosolization, an ultrasonic cleaner is used. This cleaning process involves the use of sound waves, causing **implosion** or the formation of minute bubbles that collapse into themselves in the special solution. The mechanical action, also known as **cavitation** of the specialized solution, produces the necessary process that removes debris from the instrument surface. The ultrasonic cleaner is capable of reaching areas that hand scrubbing cannot.

Soiled loose instruments that are not in cassettes are transferred from the holding solution and placed into the insert basket of the ultrasonic cleaner, rinsed thoroughly, and drained. The basket is then gradually lowered into the ultrasonic solution to prevent splash. The level of the solution must be enough to completely submerge the instruments. With the cover closed, the cleaner unit is run for 4–6 minutes for loose instruments and 16 minutes for cassettes. See Figure 8-4.

Following ultrasonic cleaning, the basket, with instruments still in it, is thoroughly rinsed under cold running tap water, taking care not to splash onto surrounding areas. Instruments from the ultrasonic basket are rolled out onto a disposable paper towel and pat dried with a second paper towel. If any debris still remains on the instruments, further manual scrubbing may be necessary.

Frequent changing of the cleaner solution is an absolute necessity, at least once per day. The inside of the container and the cover are rinsed and wiped clean with a disinfecting agent when the solution is changed.

Processing Instrument Cassettes

Instrument cassettes come in various sizes and have taken the place of procedure trays. Instruments are kept intact within the cassettes and are handled as a unit. Cassettes do take up a larger space in the ultrasonic cleaners and sterilizers, therefore, these larger units need to already be in place.

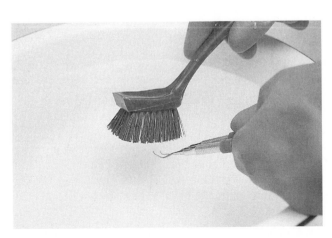

Figure 8-3 Hand scrubbing instruments wearing heavy-duty puncture-proof utility gloves and using a long-handle brush.

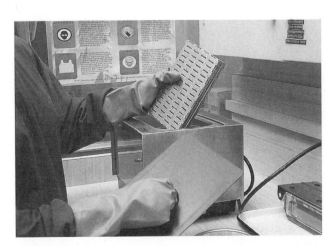

Figure 8-4 Ultrasonic cleaner unit.

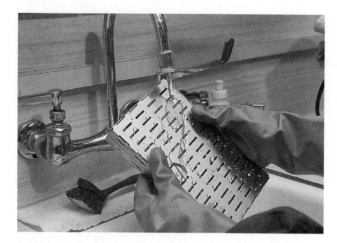

Figure 8-5 Rinsing the instrument cassette taking care to minimize splashing of contaminated solution.

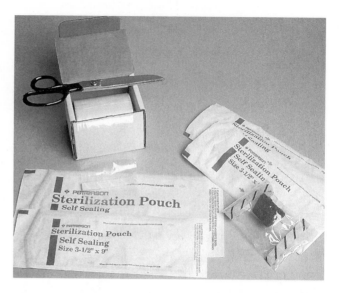

Figure 8-6 Sterilizing bag or pouch and sensitive tape.

The cassette is placed in the ultrasonic cleaner taking care that the solution completely covers it. An enzymatic cleaner solution is preferred, as it dissolves bioburden (visible organic material) and other debris. The ultrasonic cleaner lid is in place to prevent splatter and aerosolization of pathogens. Cassettes are rinsed carefully under running water. They should be held at an angle allowing the water to run into the sink and eliminate splashing of contaminated solution onto the walls, floor, or counter top (Figure 8-5). Cassettes are opened at this time to check for cleanliness. If debris is still present on one or two instruments, they may need to be hand scrubbed.

Ultrasonic Cleaner Reminders

- Only approved cleaning solution should be used.
- The solution should be replaced on a daily basis.
- The solution should be at the proper level, covering the instrument.
- The tank should not be overloaded with instruments.
- The machine should be kept closed.

Sterilization

Sterilization is the process of destroying all microorganisms and their pathogenic products. It is accomplished by moist heat (steam) under pressure or by dry heat.

Methods of sterilization include:

- Steam under pressure (autoclave)
- Chemical vapor under pressure (Chemiclave)
- Dry heat (oven)

- Ethylene oxide (uses a germicidal gas)
- Hot bead (uses small beads or salt)

Packaging Instruments/Objects and Labeling

Instruments should be wrapped and packed loosely enough to allow steam penetration of all surfaces during autoclaving. It is recommended that all instruments be prepackaged before sterilizing. Inexpensive one-use sterilization bags (Figure 8-6) and perforated plastic wraps are available. Paper bags are used for small items, and plastic wraps that can be folded around larger items are used. Bags and wraps must be carefully sealed, with the contents indicated on the packet and the date of sterilization clearly marked. A soft-lead, dull pencil should be used rather than a pen. Care must be taken in labeling a paper packet; a sharp pencil may perforate the paper. Ink used in pens may be dissolved by the vapor or "bleed" and the residue deposited on the instruments and walls of the autoclave chamber.

It is advisable not to mix differing metals in a packet, since a strong galvanic action tends to increase corrosion (i.e., high-carbon steel and chromium-plated handles on instruments).

Hinged instruments (forceps, scissors) or those with movable parts need to be opened during sterilization. Autoclavable contra-angles and handpieces should be sterilized in a chemical vapor sterilizer. Refer to Chapter 31.

1. Prepare the disposable sterilizing bag or pouch.
2. Indicate the contents and date of sterilization (Figure 8-7).

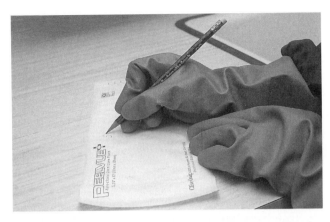

Figure 8-7 Preparing a sterilization bag using a lead pencil indicating date and bag contents.

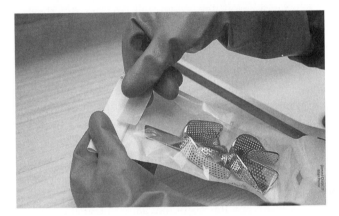

Figure 8-8 Double folding ends of sterilizing bag.

3. Insert sharp surfaces of small instruments into paper coin envelopes (with gummed flap removed), then into the paper wrapper.

4. Seal packet with sensitive tape. Double fold the ends of the bag; then with the tape, seal over the fold and around the reverse side of bag (Figure 8-8). Plastic wraps are sealed over the outside fold and around the entire packet.

Cassette Packaging

Since cassettes come in various sizes, they require something that will cover the entire cassette and allow the steam or vapor to penetrate. To provide sterility to cassettes after sterilization, autoclave wrap is used beforehand. The wrap is supplied in several sizes, from 12 x 12 in. to 24 x 24 in..

To wrap the cassette, it is best to place it in the center of the autoclave wrap and fold the sides over the top, ensuring that the edges of the wrap overlap each other, similar to wrapping a gift. Once wrapped, heat-sensitive tape is applied to seal and hold the edges together. It should be labeled using the same guidelines for labeling as for sterilization bags (Figure 8-9A–C).

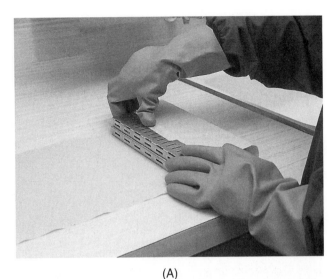

(A)

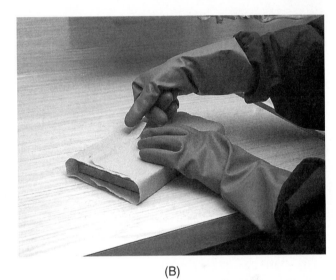

(B)

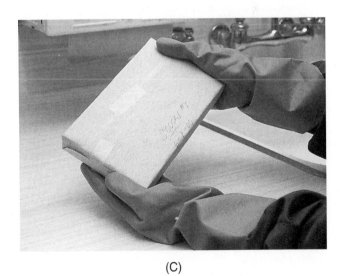

(C)

Figure 8-9 Steps in wrapping an instrument cassette for sterilization: (A) wrapping the cassette; (B) applying sensitive tape; (C) labeling the cassette.

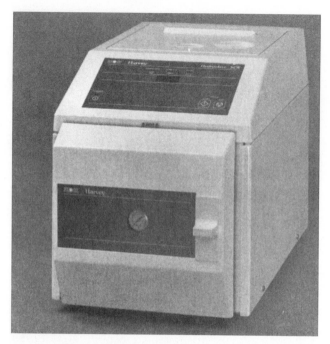

Figure 8-10 Steam autoclave uses steam under pressure (Courtesy of MDT Corporation, Torrance, CA).

Steam Autoclave Sterilization

A pupil (name unknown) of Louis Pasteur, a French chemist, invented the steam autoclave in 1873. Pasteur is known for his discoveries in immunology and microbiology. The autoclave remains the oldest and most widely accepted dental sterilization method (see Figure 8-10). The highest temperatures that can be obtained (250–270°F, 121–132°C) and 15 pounds per square inch (psi) pressure for 30–40 minutes are commonly accepted.

Shorter periods of time for *flash* emergencies, when a fast instrument turnaround is necessary, may be used. This shortened sterilization time is not intended for routine practice but is limited to emergencies only. Instruments are unwrapped for quick sterilization, about 5 minutes (Table 8-3).

When operating the autoclave, be certain that:

1. An adequate distilled water supply is present.
2. All air is allowed to escape and is replaced by steam.
3. The pressure of the steam reaches at least 15 psi and remains there.
4. The thermometer reads at least 250°F (121°C) without fluctuating downward. It is important to remember that this is the optimum combination of temperature and pressure for sterilization. At 15 psi and 250°F (121°C), *saturated steam* is generated. If too little water is used, the steam will become superheated rather than saturated, and its action is the same as hot air. Saturated steam is on the boundary between the liquid and the vapor phase. As this steam strikes colder objects, it condenses to water. This condensation causes a shrinking of volume and local reduction of pressure that draws in more surrounding steam. As objects are heated, the temperatures are equalized, and condensed water returns to the vapor phase.

Steam displaces all air. The increase in temperature from 212 to 250°F (100 to 121°C) gives the added destructive power that will kill spores. Air pockets must be eliminated by the pistonlike action of steam itself. In other words, steam must enter the chamber at one end and drive out air at the lower side of the opposite end. Factors adversely influencing the efficiency of autoclave sterilization are:

● *Superheated steam.* This condition occurs in office autoclaves if there is insufficient water in the sterilizer to retain some water in the liquid state at the temperature the autoclave is used. Superheating may be

Table 8-3	Sterilization Factors		
Sterilizer	*Temperature*	*Pressure*	*Time Required*
Steam autoclave	250°F (121°C)	15 psi	30–40 min
Flash steam	270°F (132°C)	30 psi	5 min
Chemical vapor	260°F (127°C)	20 psi	20 min
Dry heat (oven)	320°F (160°C)		2 hr
	340°F (170°C)		1 hr
	250°F (121°C)	N/A	4 hr
Ethylene oxide	Room temperature	N/A	10 hr
Newer automatic	120°F (49°C) N/A	N/A	1–3 hr
Hot bead	425°F–475°F (218°C–246°C)	N/A	15–30 sec

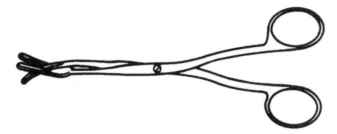

Figure 8-11 Transfer forceps used in handling sterile instruments.

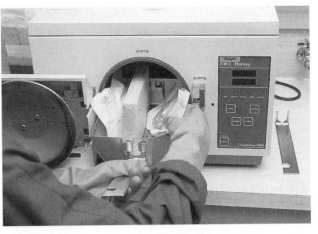

Figure 8-12 Chemical vapor sterilizer uses chemicals under pressure.

caused by carrying a higher pressure in the outer jacket than in the chamber or by placing moist items in the autoclave.

● *Trapped air.* Air becomes trapped in the chamber by an improper air-ejecting device or by faulty packing and improper loading of objects in the autoclave. Air reduces the penetrating power of steam into the depth of packets and prevents contact between steam and microorganisms.

Steam autoclaves create the need to dry the "load" after completion of the cycle. The following steps may be followed:

1. Allow the pressure gauge to return to zero.

2. Open the door slightly to release any steam remaining in the chamber.

3. Remove the packets from the autoclave tray with sterile transfer forceps (Figure 8-11).

4. Place the packets on a clean, dry, sterile towel without touching the packets. The heat of the instruments drives off excess moisture.

5. When dry, store the packets in an appropriate clean, dry drawer or cabinet until ready to use.

6. The exact technique calls for resterilization of instruments that will penetrate soft tissue just before using.

The transfer forceps is often the weakest link in the sterilization process. Therefore, several pairs of large transfer forceps should be sterilized with each load of instruments. A sterile forceps should be used not only for sterilized instruments but also for such items as plastic saliva ejectors when they are removed from a bulk package. This practice will minimize the contamination of the other items remaining in the package. Transfer forceps should not be stored in a glutaraldehyde solution; only dry, sterile forceps are acceptable.

Sterilizers must be listed by Underwriters Laboratories. The manufacturer provides a manual with illustrations to explain proper operation and loading. All instructions are written in easily understandable language.

Chemical Vapor Sterilization

The system used for chemical vapor sterilization depends on heat, water, and chemicals working in **synergy** (substances acting to achieve an effect of which each is individually incapable) (Figure 8-12). The solution in the system is comprised of specific amounts of alcohol, organic solvents, chemical disinfectants, and water. The water is kept below the level (approximately 15%) at which rust, corrosion, and dulling of metals occur. Pressure is used to evacuate air pockets and to raise the internal temperature to the point at which the liquid solution turns to chemical vapor.

Since the solution used in the sterilizer produces a chemical odor, the manufacturer of the chemical vapor sterilizer offers a filtration unit that removes most of the chemical odor after the cycle is completed. The area should be well ventilated and, if possible, placed under a hood that is vented to the outside.

The fact that chemical vapor sterilization does not harm metals is of utmost importance, as this method offers more protection to carbon steel instruments, burs, knives, and other sharp-edged instruments than does a steam autoclave. It can be said that the chemical vapor sterilizer offers a practical method for sterilization, thus eliminating any cross-contamination of instruments and other items that may have been only disinfected.

After sterilization is complete, and when the pressure gauge has returned to zero, the door is opened slightly to evaporate all remaining vapor. Objects should be dry and ready for removal after 3–4 minutes.

Unloading and storing of sterile packets do not vary from that of the steam autoclave.

Dry Heat (Oven) Sterilization

Dry-heat sterilization is a low-cost device. The units are of simple construction, with few moving parts, and maintenance is minimal. In offices where patient load is such that instrument turnaround time is not of primary concern, dry heat may be used in some instances. However, an alternative method of sterilization should be used for high-heat sensitive items, such as instruments.

Dry-heat sterilizers require 2 hours at 350°F (160°C) for a complete cycle. Temperatures above 300°F begin to damage metals and other materials; cutting edges on instruments are destroyed with repeated cycling in dry heat.

Added to the limits of time and temperature, heat distribution tends to be irregular. Dry-heat sterilizers must be loaded loosely and carefully to achieve maximum penetration around instruments. Instruments must be clean, dry, and placed on a metal oven tray or wrapped in a sealed foil bag. Inexpensive paper wraps will scorch and char. Definite procedures for loading and unloading must be observed (Figure 8-13).

Ethylene Oxide Sterilization

To sterilize items that cannot tolerate elevated heat, ethylene oxide may be used. It uses a germicidal gas that has a remarkable penetrating power, allowing it to destroy all microorganisms, including spores and hepatitis viruses. The gas is available in cartridge form, which is wrapped in plastic, broken open, and placed in an enclosed plastic bag with items that need to be sterilized. The plastic bag with its contents is then placed in an enclosed locked chamber where it is allowed to stand overnight for 10 hours at room temperature. Plastic, cloth, or rubber items that are sterilized in this manner need to be aerated for 24 hours to dissipate the toxic gas; metal instruments may be used immediately.

There are newer automatic ethylene oxide sterilizers that use heat in combination with the germicidal gas to speed up the sterilizing process, about 1–3 hours for one cycle. The temperature used is 120°F (49°C) below what other sterilizers use, making it possible to sterilize items that are unable to tolerate elevated temperatures (Figure 8-14).

Hot-Bead Sterilization

The device used for hot-bead sterilization consists of an electrically heated cup containing glass beads or table salt granules. The cup must be preheated for 20 minutes before use.

Burs, reamers, broaches, absorbent points, and other instruments used in the practice of endodontics are sterilized by submersion into such a medium. Burs and root canal instruments require 15–20 seconds. Surfaces of absorbent points require from 5 to 10 seconds and will change from white to a slight yellowish color when they are sterile. The hot-bead sterilizer is not intended for other than limited use (Figure 8-15).

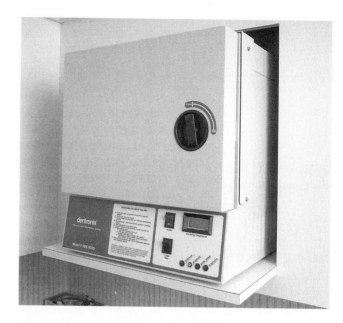

Figure 8-13 Dry-heat (oven) sterilizer uses high heat.

Storage of Sterile Packets

Taped-seal sterile bags, wraps, and trays should be stored unopened, preferably in a closed drawer or cabinet, until ready to use. Tightly sealed paper packets, if well protected, will remain sterile for as long as three months at most, and for about two months, even though storage is in a drawer or cabinet that is frequently opened and closed. In either case, the seal must remain unbroken. Sealed foil bags will remain sterile longer than paper packets because of the resistance of the packaging material.

Monitoring

From time to time, equipment can malfunction and human errors occur. It is advisable to monitor sterilization methods at least once a week. A record of monitoring should be kept for legal purposes.

There are three methods of monitoring: process indicators, biological monitoring, and control indicators.

1. *Process indicators* confirm that the indicator has been exposed to a certain temperature of heat and steam or chemical vapor, as occurs with the stripe on the paper sterilizer bag and sensitive tape. The color change does not guarantee that the items are sterile but only that the load was processed.

2. *Biological monitoring,* the more reliable method, consists of a strip of paper on which resistant spores have been impregnated. The strip is encased in a sealed bag that is placed in the sterilizer just prior to beginning the sterilizing cycle. A strip is placed in

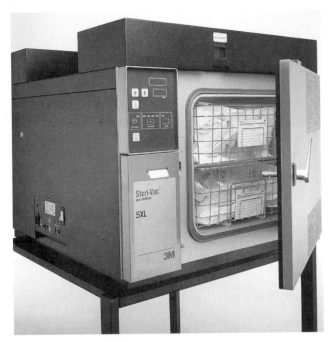

Figure 8-14 Ethylene oxide sterilizer uses a germicidal gas for items that do not tolerate heat. (Photo courtesy of 3M Health Care, St. Paul, MN).

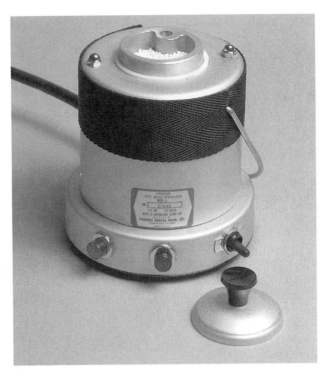

Figure 8-15 Hot-bead sterilizer used for quick sterilization of very small instruments.

the center of the load. On completion of the sterilizing cycle, the strip of spores is cultured to determine if the spores are still vital (alive). Although this simple procedure can be done in the dental office, several companies and institutions (dental schools) will provide the strips, culture them, and keep legal records for a reasonable fee. Ideally, biological monitoring should be performed on a weekly basis in a large-practice office or institution. Once a month is probably sufficient for a private office.

3. *Control indicators* determine if the time, temperature, and pressure were appropriate during the cycle. These vary from the process indicator and biological monitor.

Failure of a biological monitoring test could be due to improper cleaning of instruments, improper or excessive packaging material, overloading the sterilizer, incorrect operation of unit, timing errors, improper temperature, and improper method of sterilization.

The High-Risk Patient

High-risk patients may be classified into two groups: (1) the *suspected high-risk patients*, who may have had or are presently carriers of a disease, and (2) the *known high-risk patients*, who are either carriers or in an active stage of a disease. Infection control procedures must be followed in the treatment of either category as well as with all other patients.

Emergency Patients

Patients not on record should be screened most carefully, as many high-risk groups, including drug users, neglect any preventive care of their teeth and seek help only on an emergency basis.

New emergency patients must be considered high risk; therefore, special precautions must be taken, and only procedures to relieve pain should be performed on the initial visit. Radiographs necessary for diagnosis may be completed. Further treatment should be postponed until the dentist's medical questionnaire is completed and a medical clearance from the patient's physician is obtained.

SUGGESTED ACTIVITIES

● Practice the spray-wipe-spray technique for disinfection.

● Practice placing barriers, including wrap materials, on the operatory equipment.

● Select a mouth mirror, explorer, and cotton pliers (forceps); assume the instruments are contaminated. Follow the steps of procedure for disinfection. Include placing them in a holding solution, then into the ultrasonic cleaner.

- Using all precautions, test the efficiency performance of the ultrasonic cleaner.
- Package the instruments for sterilization. Label the package.
- Package a loaded cassette. Label the package.
- Study the manufacturer's instructions for using a high-heat sterilizer.
- Under the supervision of the instructor, complete a sterilization cycle. Check the color of the heat-sensitive tape.
- Select proper storage for the sterilized instruments.

REVIEW

1. Indicate which two well-known chemical hazards are used in the practice of dentistry: (1) sodium hypochlorite, (2) glutaraldehyde, (3) formaldehyde, or (4) mercury.
   a. 1, 2
   b. 2, 3
   c. 3, 4
   d. 1, 4

2. Indicate two prime concerns of OSHA for dental personnel: (1) safety from chemical handling, (2) protection from bloodborne diseases, (3) working extra hours without compensation, or (4) not being covered by medical insurance.
   a. 1, 2
   b. 2, 3
   c. 3, 4
   d. 1, 4

3. Alkaline glutaraldehyde 2.5 and 3.4% is considered to be:
   a. A surface disinfectant
   b. A sterilizing solution used in a chemiclave
   c. A holding solution for instruments
   d. An immersion chemical for disinfection or sterilization

4. What is bioburden?
   a. Handling of instruments prior to sterilization
   b. Visible organic materials such as blood, saliva, and debris
   c. The removal of debris
   d. The act of becoming infected

5. Aerosolization of pathogens may take place when: (1) instruments are hand scrubbed using a brush several inches above the water line, (2) instruments are cleaned using the ultrasonic cleaner, (3) instruments are rinsed under cold tap water where splashing takes place prior to sterilization, and/or (4) instruments are dried with disposable towels following ultrasonic cleaning.
   a. 1, 2
   b. 2, 3
   c. 3, 4
   d. 1, 3

6. Describe the purpose for MSDS forms.
   a. Provided by the manufacturer and describe the use of the product
   b. Provided by the manufacturer and describe how to handle the product
   c. Provided by the manufacturer and describe hazardous materials in a product
   d. Packing forms from the manufacturer that state the number of items shipped

7. Why is high heat the preferred method of sterilization?
   a. It destroys all forms of microorganisms and its efficiency can be monitored.
   b. It takes less time than surface disinfection.
   c. It prevents any possibility of rusting of instruments.
   d. It is an excellent sterilizer for all plastic materials.

8. Ethylene oxide sterilizers are useful for:
   a. Quick sterilization
   b. Items that cannot withstand elevated temperatures
   c. surgical instruments
   d. endodontic instruments

Occupational Safety and Health Administration (OSHA) Regulations

CHAPTER 9

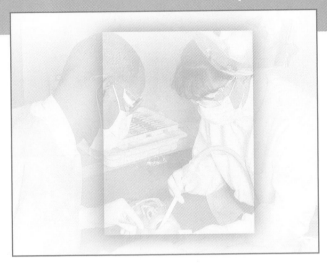

OBJECTIVES

After studying this chapter, the student will be able to:

- Cite the health agencies involved in establishing the infection control standards for dentistry.
- Discuss the principal requirements of the regulations determined by OSHA.
- Describe the elements that are identified in the exposure control plan.
- Discuss why eating, drinking, applying lip balm, and so on are forbidden in the dental treatment room and laboratory.
- List all the personal protective equipment (PPE) that employees are required to wear when splashes, spray, splatter, or droplets of blood or saliva are generated.
- Describe what consists of "regulated waste."
- Describe what types of records should be kept during occupational exposure training programs.
- Cite the agency that approves the disposal of infectious waste materials.
- Determine the necessary documentation for a dental office to be in compliance with OSHA regulations.
- Discuss the primary reasons for a complaint-generated OSHA inspection.
- Discuss the means by which an OSHA inspection may be avoided.

Introduction

The OSHA General Duty Clause requires an employer to furnish employees with "employment and a place of employment, which are free from recognized hazards that are causing or likely to cause death or serious physical harm."

Dentists were notified by OSHA that "health care employers must provide their staff members with the materials and information they need to comply with the infection-control guidelines recommended by the Centers for Disease Control & Prevention (CDC) and the American Dental Association (ADA)." (Anderson, 1995)

Further, an OSHA spokesperson is credited with saying, "Health care professionals are obliged under the law to provide staff members with a safe, sanitary workplace." OSHA interprets its responsibility as ensuring that dental practices are in compliance with CDC and ADA guidelines.

OSHA has issued the "Bloodborne Pathogen Standard," "Hazard Communication Standard," and "Medical Waste Management" aimed at protecting employees in dental offices from the risks of bloodborne disease, including hepatitis B, hepatitis C, and the virus that causes acquired immunodeficiency syndrome (AIDS) or human immunodeficiency virus (HIV). **Bloodborne pathogens** pertain to disease-causing microorganisms that are present in human blood.

OSHA described the action of the requirements as "necessary and appropriate" to prevent transmission of disease in the workplace. A timetable for the new standards was published in 1991 in the *Federal Register*, an official record of government business. Individual states were required to adopt comparable plans within six months of publication of the regulation.

The ADA has been very active working with OSHA in bringing the regulations affecting dentistry into perspective. The ADA advised employers to follow the existing regulations, which took effect in 1992.

OSHA, a U.S. Department of Labor agency, issued the rules with the backing of the Bush administration budget and health agencies and under considerable pressure from Congress to enforce CDC guidelines.

The guidelines in this chapter reflect aspects of infection control for the purpose of protecting dental health care workers (DHCWs).

The Bloodborne Pathogens Standard

OSHA developed the bloodborne pathogen standards for the protection of health care workers, in particular, employees of a health care facility. This standard applies to all occupational exposures to blood or **other potentially infectious materials (OPIM).**

Exposure Control Plan

One of the first requirements to take effect, and the one OSHA inspectors will be checking on, is that every employer develop a written exposure control plan (ECP), identifying workers with occupational exposure and other potentially infectious materials (OPIM) and specifying means to protect and train them. What needs to be included in such a plan is outlined below:

Exposure Control Plan

- Occupational exposure that is specific to each person's job classification should be stated, whether an employee has limited or excessive occupational exposure and is made without regard to the use of personal protective equipment (PPE).

- Implementation and methods of compliance and control are outlined for each circumstance surrounding exposure incidents.

- Compliance with hepatitis B vaccination to include postexposure evaluation incidents with follow-up procedures.

- Hazard communication to employees and record keeping of such training.

- Updating the exposure control plan on a yearly basis that is acceptable to all employees or whenever new incidences of occupational exposure take place or when new or modified procedures are used that compromise the DHCW's safety.

Compliance with Bloodborne Pathogen Standards

To effectively comply with the bloodborne pathogens standards, DHCWs must observe the following:

Universal Precautions. Universal Precautions means that all patients are treated as if they had a contagious infectious disease. Using universal precautions

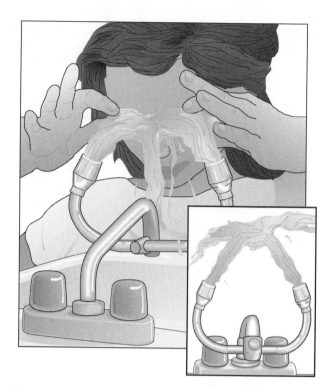

Figure 9-1 Eyewash station uses cold water to flush eyes.

with *all* patients means preventing contact with blood or OPIM such as all body fluids.

Engineering and Work Practice Controls. Engineering controls means controls that isolate or remove the bloodborne pathogen hazard from the workplace.

Using PPE will eliminate or minimize occupational exposure and should be removed prior to leaving the premises.

Thorough hand washing using running water and antiseptic soap must be routine in the care of patients as well as following the removal of PPE. Hand-washing facilities should be readily accessible to employees.

An eyewash station, located on the premises, capable of thoroughly flushing both eyes continuously with running cold water is required (Figure 9-1).

The standard prohibits recapping of needles. Only a one-handed or mechanical device may be used to recap. Contaminated needles must never be bent, recapped, or cut. Sharps must be placed in properly labeled, puncture-resistant containers with leak-proof sides and bottom (Figure 9-2).

Eating, drinking, smoking, applying lip balm, handling contact lenses, and storing food and drink in areas of possible exposure to blood, saliva, tissue, or OPIM

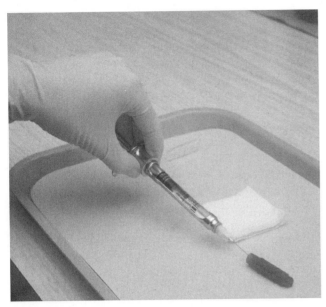

Figure 9-2 Recapping syringe needle using a one-handed technique.

are forbidden. The dental treatment room, laboratory, sterilization area, and darkroom are included.

Procedures involving blood or OPIM shall be performed in such a way that will minimize contamination during splashing, spattering, spraying, and droplet generation of contaminated substances.

Transferring material into a new container for storage, transport, or shipping must be closed, labeled, and color coded accordingly. If the outside of the primary container becomes contaminated, it must be placed within a second container, labeled, and color coded accordingly.

Equipment that will be shipped for repair must be examined and decontaminated of possible infectious materials prior to leaving the premises, unless feasibility of decontamination is not possible; thereupon a label stating possible contamination shall be attached to ensure appropriate precautions.

Personal Protective Equipment. To protect from possible occupational exposure, the employer shall provide employees with necessary and appropriate PPE that will not permit blood or OPIM to cross over and reach the employee's personal clothing, skin, mouth, or other mucous membranes under normal conditions of use.

Employers shall ensure that employees are protected with PPE, unless an employee, exercising professional judgment, declines to wear PPE in a rare circumstance that otherwise would prevent health care delivery or may have posed an increased hazard to the safety of the employee. This situation shall be investigated and documented to determine if changes should be instituted to prevent recurrences in the future.

Employers shall ensure that appropriate sizes of PPE are made available to all employees, to include glove liners and gloves for latex-sensitive employees.

When penetrated by blood or OPIM, the protective garment shall be removed immediately or as soon as feasibly possible.

All PPE shall be removed prior to leaving the work area. The PPE that is removed shall be placed in the appropriate container for storage, washing, decontamination, or disposal.

Gloves shall be worn when it is expected that employees will have contact with blood, OPIM, mucous membranes, and nonintact skin and when handling infectious items or surfaces. Single-use disposable gloves shall not be washed or decontaminated for reuse.

Utility gloves may be reused and decontaminated if the integrity of the glove is not compromised (cracks, torn, punctured); otherwise they must be discarded.

Employees are required to wear masks and protective eyewear or a face shield when splashes, spray, splatter, or droplets of blood, body tissue, or saliva may be generated and eye, nose, or mouth contamination can be reasonably anticipated. Protective eyewear must have solid side shields.

Protective garments such as gowns, laboratory coats, aprons, or clinic jackets shall be worn whenever occupational exposure is anticipated. The degree of occupational exposure will determine the type of garment used.

Housekeeping Management

General Requirements. The work site must be maintained clean and sanitary. A written schedule for maintaining a safe, clean, and decontaminated facility should be determined by the employer based on the type of surface to be cleaned, the type of soil present, and the procedures being performed.

Decontamination. All equipment and working surfaces that come in contact with blood or OPIM shall be cleaned and **decontaminated** (removal or destruction of bloodborne pathogens by the use of physical or chemical means) with an appropriate disinfectant.

● Protective barrier coverings that have been overly contaminated or at the end of a work shift shall be removed and replaced as soon as feasible.

● Receptacles that are reused and have been contaminated with blood or OPIM shall be inspected and decontaminated.

● Contaminated broken glassware shall not make contact with hands but shall be picked up by mechanical means.

● Contaminated reusable sharps shall not be stored or processed such that an employee would be required to reach by hand into containers that housed them.

Regulated Waste. Regulated waste pertains to sharps and items that have been contaminated with body fluids, such as blood or saliva, that may leak during handling, storage, transporting, or shipping.

Sharps. All contaminated materials that cut or puncture the skin such as needles, blades, wires, or broken glass are included in this category. They are regarded as regulated waste.

Contaminated sharps must be discarded immediately in containers that are:

● Closable

● Puncture resistant

● Leak proof on sides and bottom

● Labeled clearly with a biohazard sign

Sharps containers should be easily accessible, maintained upright, not overfilled, and replaced routinely (Figure 9-3).

A **sharps injury** is any injury caused by a sharp object.

A **sharps injury log** is a written or electronic record involving any sharps injury. The exposure incident shall be recorded on a log within 14 working days of the date the incident is reported to the employer. It should contain the following information:

● Date and time of exposure incident

● Type and brand of sharp involved in the exposure incident

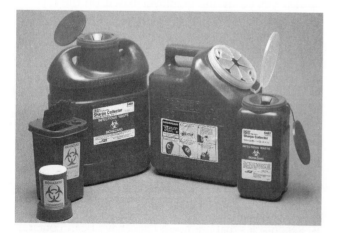

Figure 9-3 Assortment of puncture-resistant sharps containers.

● A description of the exposure incident such as:
1. Job classification of the exposed employee
2. Department or work area where the exposure occurred
3. The procedure performed by the employee when the exposure occurred
4. How the incident occurred
5. The body part involved in the exposure incident
6. If the sharp had engineered sharps injury protection
7. If the sharp had no engineered sharps injury protection and the employee's opinion on how it could have been prevented
8. The employee's opinion about whether other engineering, administrative or work practice control could have prevented the injury

● The sharps injury log shall be maintained for 5 years from the date the exposure incident occurred.

Other Regulated Waste (Medical Waste). Waste-handling requirements oblige employers to handle certain waste as infectious:

● Blood and body fluids

● Items saturated with enough blood or OPIM that can be squeezed out producing drops of liquid substance

● Items caked with dried blood, body fluid, or saliva if they are capable of releasing these materials during handling

● Pathological waste

These waste products shall be placed in containers that are:

● Closable

● Leak proof during handling, storage, transporting, and shipping

● Closed prior to handling, storage, transporting, and shipping

● Labeled clearly with a biohazard sign and color coded

For disposal of dental waste materials, the local Environmental Protection Agency (EPA) should be contacted, who will direct the dentist in how to obtain an EPA-approved system.

Nonregulated Waste. Waste that is not infectious or hazardous is placed in this category. These waste products are discarded in a separate unmarked lined container that may include paper towels, autoclave chamber paper liners, paper products generated from using dental materials, patient napkins if not soaked or contaminated with blood or body fluids, and disposable protective gowns if not soaked or contaminated with blood or body fluids.

Laundry. Contaminated laundry shall be:

- Handled as little as possible, wearing protective gloves
- Placed in closable, labeled, or recognizable color-coded bags
- If soaked or wet, be placed in bags or containers that prevent leakage of fluid to the exterior

Hepatitis B Vaccination. All employees in a health care facility must be protected by hepatitis B vaccination. It is the employer's responsibility to provide the vaccine within 10 working days of initial employment and also to provide a postexposure evaluation to employees who have been exposed to hepatitis B under the following stipulations:

- At no cost to the employee
- At a reasonable place and time
- Performed by a physician or under his or her supervision or the supervision of another licensed health care professional
- An accredited laboratory, at no cost to the employee, does all laboratory tests.

Hepatitis B vaccine shall be made available to employees after reviewing the exposure control plan, indicating that they have been informed and trained in occupational exposure to pathogens.

The employee may consent or decline the vaccination. If the employee declines the vaccination, it shall be documented and signed by that person verifying its refusal.

Postexposure Evaluation and Follow-up. When the employee is exposed to hepatitis B virus (HBV), hepatitis C virus (HCV), HIV, or OPIM while performing duties in the work place, it is termed **occupational exposure**. It must be reported to the employer immediately. It is then the responsibility of the employer to make a confidential medical evaluation and follow-up to include the following:

- The route of exposure and how it occurred
- Identification of the **source individual**, the person whose blood or OPIM may have infected the employee, unless prohibited by state or local law

- The blood of the source individual must be tested as soon as possible with consent unless that individual is already known to be infective. Results of the test are documented and furnished to exposed employee.
- The exposed employee's blood is tested with consent as soon as possible.
- Postexposure prophylaxis (titer) when indicated, as hepatitis B immune globulin, hepatitis vaccine, and tetanus booster, is administered.
- Counseling
- Evaluation of reported illnesses is made available to the employee.

Medical Record Keeping. The standard also imposes certain record-keeping, labeling, training, and waste-handling requirements that oblige employers to ensure that all employees with occupational exposure participate in a training program, at no cost to the employee, during working hours. The training program shall be on a continued basis, at least once annually. Detailed records of training must be maintained for three years.

The employer shall maintain an accurate record for each employee with occupational exposure. It must include:

- Employee's name and social security number
- A copy of the hepatitis B vaccination report to include all dates of vaccination
- A copy of all examination results, medical testing, and follow-up procedures
- Employer's copy of the health care professional's written opinion of employee's duties related to the exposure incident
- Confidentiality of employee's medical records—not disclosed or reported to anyone without employee's written consent
- Employer shall maintain records for at least the span of employee's employment plus 30 years.

Training Records. The standard also imposes certain record-keeping, labeling, training, and waste-handling requirements that oblige employers to ensure that all employees with occupational exposure participate in a training program, at no cost to the employee, during working hours. The training program shall be on a continued basis, at least once annually. Detailed records of training must be maintained for three years. Training sessions should include the following:

- Dates of training session
- Contents of training session

- Names and qualifications of individuals conducting the training session

- Names and titles of persons attending the training sessions

Communication of Hazards to Employees

- Warning biohazard labels that are predominantly visible in fluorescent orange or orange-red with lettering and symbols in contrasting color must be used on containers that hold regulated waste. Red bags or red containers may be substituted for warning labels.

OSHA Inspection

OSHA has indicated that it would respond to complaints immediately, now that health care professionals know the guidelines. The strong OSHA position on the matter takes the guidelines out of the voluntary realm and makes compliance mandatory. The responsibility for instructing employees and ensuring that infection control procedures are followed rests with the employer. Dentists who fail to educate their office employees risk the possibility of an OSHA inspection and a sizable monetary fine.

An OSHA inspection of a dental office most generally occurs as the result of an employee complaint.

What is expected during a complaint-generated inspection?

- The OSHA representative would request infection control records from the employer. Documentation of needle sticks and injury or illness records, if available, would also be requested.

- Following review of the records, the OSHA representative would interview employees, then inspect the dental office. Areas of concern would be those of direct patient care, such as the dental operatory and x-ray area. When the inspection visit to the dental office is complaint generated, the area of complaint is also inspected.

- In addition to inspection of records, employee interviews, and site inspections, the compliance officer would also evaluate the hazard communication program in the office. Areas of concern would include the presence of Material Safety Data Sheets (MSDS) for all chemicals used in the office, a written program of identification of hazardous materials, and verification of employee training in the use of materials and of provisions for continual training of employees.

To minimize the chance of an OSHA inspection:

- CDC and ADA infection control guidelines should be followed.

- Current infection control practices should be documented.

- All employees should be informed, be trained, and follow all precautionary measures of infection control.

- Open communication should be established among all dental personnel. This will encourage employees to discuss and address complaints and problems with the employer, thus eliminating the necessity for OSHA to become involved.

All dental personnel are aware of OSHA. However, there are currently no established guidelines on how to deal with this office.

SUGGESTED ACTIVITIES

- Compare regulated waste with nonregulated waste and determine the disposal of each.

- Make a list of all items in a dental office that qualify as sharps.

REVIEW

1. What three health agencies establish infection control standards for dentistry?
   a. OSHA, EPA, CDC
   b. CDC, ADA, ANSI
   c. ADA, CDC, OSHA
   d. ECP, ADA, OSHA

2. Describe the exposure control plan that OSHA requires of every dental office.
   a. Identifies workers with occupational exposure and specifies how each will be protected and trained
   b. Concerned with universal precautions whereby all patients are treated as if they had a contagious infectious disease
   c. A plan instituted to protect patients from contamination of instruments and materials
   d. Identifies diseases that cause infection

3. What four PPE must be included when performing operative procedures?
   a. Goggles, undergloves, exam gloves, face shield
   b. Goggles, face mask, exam gloves, protective garment
   c. Exam gloves, face shield, goggles, protective garment
   d. Protective garment, face shield, exam gloves, overgloves

4. Who is the "source individual" when occupational exposure takes place?
   a. The dental assistant who was cut by an instrument used on an infected patient
   b. The dentist who accidentally cut the dental assistant while performing a dental procedure
   c. The patient with an infectious disease

5. Indicate which of the following items are considered to be infectious waste materials: (1) the patient's bib, (2) items caked with blood, (3) sharps, and/or (4) pathological wastes.
   a. 1, 2, 3
   b. 2, 3, 4
   c. 1, 3, 4
   d. 1, 2, 4

6. What agency must approve disposal of infectious waste materials?
   a. OSHA
   b. CDC
   c. ADA
   d. EPA

Medical and Dental Emergencies

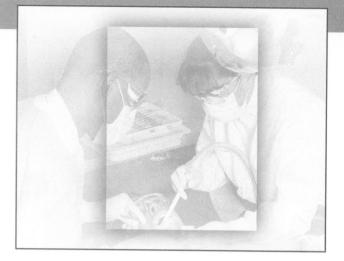

OBJECTIVES

After studying this chapter, the student will be able to:

● List the purposes of a health history.

● Take and record vital signs.

● Recognize medical emergencies, their symptoms, and treatment.

● Use good judgment and prompt action in responding to medical emergencies.

● Describe the legal aspect of medical emergencies in the dental office.

● Instruct a patient with a dental emergency involving an avulsed tooth.

● Determine how to schedule dental emergencies.

Introduction

With more and more individuals seeking dental treatment, the chance of a medical emergency arising in the dental office also increases. Advances in medical technology present situations unknown just a few decades ago. Patients who have organ transplants or implants or who may be undergoing extensive drug therapy bring the dental team a wide variety of challenges. The dental assistant should be prepared to recognize emergency situations that may arise and assist in caring promptly and responsibly for the patient.

Health History

Knowing the dental and medical history of a patient provides valuable information for the dentist (Figure 10-1). Most often, the new patient is asked to complete the history form in the reception area. Once in the treatment room, the dental assistant may review the health history with the patient and explain the importance of an accurate patient history. The purpose of the health history is fourfold:

1. To determine if there are any chronic health conditions or illnesses that may interfere with dental treatment

2. To determine if any medications that the patient is currently taking will have a potential drug interaction with the local anesthetic

3. To have a list of the patient's allergies

4. To be familiar with the patient in case of a medical emergency.

Vital Signs

Prior to the start of treatment, the patient's vital signs should be taken and recorded for the dentist to evaluate. These include blood pressure, pulse (heart rate), respiration, and temperature.

Blood Pressure

Blood pressure is the pressure created by the force of the blood on the artery walls. The **systolic pressure** arises from the contraction of the ventricle that pushes oxygen-rich blood through the arteries. The **diastolic pressure** occurs when the heart is relaxing and the ventricles begin to fill with more blood. Blood pressure is measured in millimeters of mercury (mm Hg). When recording blood pressure, systolic pressure is written over diastolic pressure, much like a fraction as 130/70 mm Hg. Normal blood pressure for an adult ranges from a systolic pressure of 100 to 140 mm Hg and a diastolic pressure from 60 to 90 mm Hg.

Medical History Form

Name _____ Last _____ First _____ Middle _____ Date _____

Address _____ Number, Street _____ Home Phone ( )

City _____ State _____ Business Phone ( )

Occupation _____ Zip Code _____

Date of Birth ___ mo. / ___ day / ___ yr. Sex M F Height ___ Weight ___ Social Security No. _____

Name of Spouse _____ Single Married

Closest Relative _____ Phone ( )

If you are completing this form for another person, what is your relationship to that person? _____

Referred by _____

For the following questions, circle yes or no, whichever applies. Your answers are for our records only and will be considered confidential. Please note that during your initial visit you will be asked some questions about your responses to this questionnaire and there may be additional questions concerning your health.

1. Are you in good health? ... Yes No
2. Has there been any change in your general health within the past year? ... Yes No
3. My last physical examination was on _____
4. Are you now under the care of a physician? ... Yes No
   If so, what is the condition being treated? _____
5. The name and address of my physician(s) is _____

6. Have you had any serious illness, operation, or been hospitalized in the past 5 years? ... Yes No
   If so, what was the illness or problem? _____
7. Are you taking any medicine(s) including non-prescription medicine? ... Yes No
   If so, what medicine(s) are you taking? _____
8. Do you have or have you had any of the following diseases or problems? ... Yes No
   a. Damaged heart valves or artificial heart valves, including heart murmur or rheumatic heart disease
   b. Cardiovascular disease (heart trouble, heart attack, angina, coronary insufficiency, coronary occlusion, high blood pressure, arteriosclerosis, stroke)
      1. Do you have chest pain upon exertion? ... Yes No
      2. Are you ever short of breath after mild exercise or when lying down? ... Yes No
      3. Do your ankles swell? ... Yes No
      4. Do you have inborn heart defects? ... Yes No
      5. Do you have a cardiac pacemaker? ... Yes No
   c. Allergy ... Yes No
   d. Sinus trouble ... Yes No
   e. Asthma or hay fever ... Yes No
   f. Fainting spells or seizures ... Yes No
   g. Persistent diarrhea or recent weight loss ... Yes No
   h. Diabetes ... Yes No
   i. Hepatitis, jaundice or liver disease ... Yes No
   j. AIDS or HIV infection ... Yes No
   k. Thyroid problems ... Yes No
   l. Respiratory problems, emphysema, bronchitis, etc. ... Yes No
   m. Arthritis or painful swollen joints ... Yes No
   n. Stomach ulcer or hyperacidity ... Yes No
   o. Kidney trouble ... Yes No
   p. Tuberculosis ... Yes No
   q. Persistent cough or cough that produces blood ... Yes No
   r. Persistent swollen glands in neck ... Yes No
   s. Low blood pressure ... Yes No
   t. Sexually transmitted disease ... Yes No
   u. Epilepsy or other neurological disease ... Yes No
   v. Problems with mental health ... Yes No
   w. Cancer ... Yes No
   x. Problems of the immune system ... Yes No

Medical History Form

Name _____ Last _____ First _____ Middle _____ Date _____

Address _____ Number, Street _____ Home Phone ( )

City _____ State _____ Business Phone ( )

Occupation _____ Zip Code _____

Date of Birth ___ mo. / ___ day / ___ yr. Sex M F Height ___ Weight ___ Social Security No. _____

Name of Spouse _____ Single Married

Closest Relative _____ Phone ( )

If you are completing this form for another person, what is your relationship to that person? _____

Referred by _____

For the following questions, circle yes or no, whichever applies. Your answers are for our records only and will be considered confidential. Please note that during your initial visit you will be asked some questions about your responses to this questionnaire and there may be additional questions concerning your health.

1. Are you in good health? ... Yes No
2. Has there been any change in your general health within the past year? ... Yes No
3. My last physical examination was on _____
4. Are you now under the care of a physician? ... Yes No
   If so, what is the condition being treated? _____
5. The name and address of my physician(s) is _____

6. Have you had any serious illness, operation, or been hospitalized in the past 5 years? ... Yes No
   If so, what was the illness or problem? _____
7. Are you taking any medicine(s) including non-prescription medicine? ... Yes No
   If so, what medicine(s) are you taking? _____
8. Do you have or have you had any of the following diseases or problems? ... Yes No
   a. Damaged heart valves or artificial heart valves, including heart murmur or rheumatic heart disease
   b. Cardiovascular disease (heart trouble, heart attack, angina, coronary insufficiency, coronary occlusion, high blood pressure, arteriosclerosis, stroke)
      1. Do you have chest pain upon exertion? ... Yes No
      2. Are you ever short of breath after mild exercise or when lying down? ... Yes No
      3. Do your ankles swell? ... Yes No
      4. Do you have inborn heart defects? ... Yes No
      5. Do you have a cardiac pacemaker? ... Yes No
   c. Allergy ... Yes No
   d. Sinus trouble ... Yes No
   e. Asthma or hay fever ... Yes No
   f. Fainting spells or seizures ... Yes No
   g. Persistent diarrhea or recent weight loss ... Yes No
   h. Diabetes ... Yes No
   i. Hepatitis, jaundice or liver disease ... Yes No
   j. AIDS or HIV infection ... Yes No
   k. Thyroid problems ... Yes No
   l. Respiratory problems, emphysema, bronchitis, etc. ... Yes No
   m. Arthritis or painful swollen joints ... Yes No
   n. Stomach ulcer or hyperacidity ... Yes No
   o. Kidney trouble ... Yes No
   p. Tuberculosis ... Yes No
   q. Persistent cough or cough that produces blood ... Yes No
   r. Persistent swollen glands in neck ... Yes No
   s. Low blood pressure ... Yes No
   t. Sexually transmitted disease ... Yes No
   u. Epilepsy or other neurological disease ... Yes No
   v. Problems with mental health ... Yes No
   w. Cancer ... Yes No
   x. Problems of the immune system ... Yes No

Figure 10-1 Medical history questionnaire, long form (Courtesy of the American Dental Association, Chicago, IL).

Procedure 3 Taking Blood Pressure

Materials Needed

Stethoscope (instrument used to hear sounds within the body)
Aneroid (uses atmospheric pressure) or mercury-type **manometer** (Figure 10-2 and 10-3)
Patient's chart
Pen
Gauze
Disinfectant

Instructions

1 The patient should be comfortably seated in an upright position in the dental chair and allowed to relax for a minimum of 5 minutes. Because many patients may be apprehensive and thus have higher blood pressure than normal, this gives them time to calm down. During this time, the assistant can explain the purpose for taking vital signs.

2 The patient's arm is placed at a level of the heart, slightly flexed, palm upward, and supported on the arm of the chair. If the patient has a tight-cuffed sleeve, it should be loosened and rolled above the elbow.

3 The center of the inflatable portion of the deflated cuff should be placed over the brachial artery approximately 1 in. above the **antecubital fossa** (small depression on the inner arm). The rubber

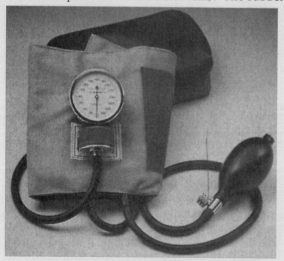

Figure 10-2 Aneroid-type manometer (Courtesy of Omron Healthcare, Inc.).

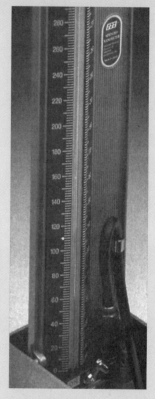

Figure 10-3 Mercury-type manometer (Courtesy of Omron Healthcare, Inc.).

tubing will follow along the inside of the arm (Figure 10-4).

4 The cuff is wrapped around the arm and fastened snugly. Two fingertips should fit under the lower edge of the deflated cuff. It is important that the cuff is neither too tight nor too loose.

Taking the Palpatory Systolic Pressure

1 With the operator's left fingertips, the patient's **radial artery** (artery located at the inner wrist) is located to find the pulse.

2 The rubber bulb is located and the valve is closed.

3 Using the right hand while the left hand feels the pulse, the operator pumps the rubber bulb to inflate the cuff until the pulse can no longer be felt.

continued

continued from previous page
Procedure 3 Taking Blood Pressure

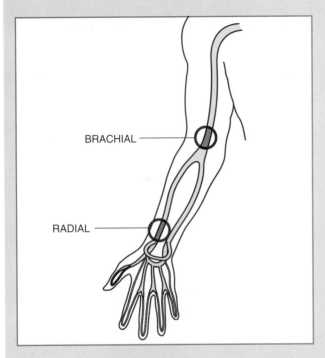

Figure 10-4 Brachial and radial artery sites on arm.

4 The valve on the rubber bulb is opened slowly, allowing the mercury to drop at 2 mm/sec (2 mm equals 1 notch on the gauge of the manometer). A mental note is made of the reading when the radial pulse is felt again. This is the *palpatory systolic pressure*. Now the valve can be opened completely.

Taking the Blood Pressure

1 The stethoscope is placed in the operator's ears with the earpieces facing anteriorly (Figure 10-5).

2 The **brachial artery** (artery located at the inside of the upper arm) is **palpated** (feeling for arterial pulse) in the antecubital fossa. When it is felt, the diaphragm of the stethoscope is positioned over it and below the blood pressure cuff.

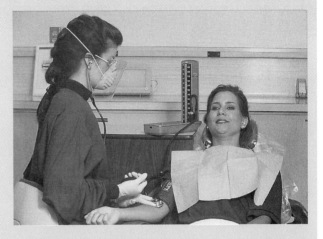

Figure 10-5 Taking the blood pressure on a patient at the chair.

3 The valve of the bulb is closed and cuff is inflated to 30 mm Hg above the palpatory systolic pressure.

4 The pressure of the cuff is released slowly and gradually at 2 mm Hg/sec. Operator should listen for the first heartbeat sound. This is the systolic pressure. A mental note is made of this reading.

5 The cuff continues to be deflated until the sounds become muffled and the heartbeat sound is no longer heard. This is the diastolic pressure.

6 The cuff is completely deflated rapidly.

7 The blood pressure is recorded in the patient's chart, indicating on which arm it was taken, right or left arm. A reading on the left arm is generally higher.

8 The blood pressure cuff is removed gently. The earpieces and diaphragm of the stethoscope are cleaned and disinfected with a suitable disinfectant. *Important:* If the blood pressure needs to be retaken, the operator should wait for a period of at least 15 seconds before reinflating the cuff, as blood may be trapped in the arm and cause an inaccurate reading.

Pulse

The pulse, or *heart rate*, is the rhythmic expansion of the artery when the blood is pushed through with each heartbeat. Generally, the pulse is taken at the radial artery on the thumb side of the wrist. In an emergency, however, it is best to use the carotid artery in the neck.

The assistant should check for three conditions of the pulse:

● Heart rate (number of beats per minute)

● Heart rhythm (whether regular or irregular)

● Quality of the beats (strong, thready, or weak)

Procedure 4
Taking the Pulse

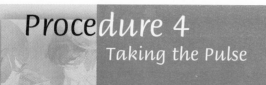

Materials Needed

Watch with a second hand
Patient's chart
Pen

Instructions

1 The radial artery is located at the wrist toward the thumb side (Figure 10-4).

2 The operator's index and middle fingers are placed over the artery. Thumb is not used as it has its own pulsating artery and may cause an inaccurate reading.

3 When the radial pulse is located, the beats are counted for 1 minute. Regularity and quality of the pulse are noted.

4 The pulse rate per minute is recorded in the patient's chart. Normal readings would be between 60 and 80 bpm (beats per minute).

Respiration

Respiration, or *respiratory rate*, indicates how fast the patient is breathing in and out. Patients should not be aware that their respiration is being monitored, because they may alter the normal pattern of breathing. The respiratory rate is often observed immediately after the pulse rate is taken while the operator's hand is still over the patient's radial artery. The assistant watches the chest rise and fall for 1 minute and records the result as breaths per minute. Normal respiratory rate in an adult is between 14 and 18 breaths per minute and in young children between 20 and 25 breaths per minute.

Temperature

The body temperature is usually not taken prior to dental treatment; however, the dental assistant should be prepared to take a patient's oral temperature if the need arises.

Emergency Equipment and Preparation

Every dental office should have some form of emergency kit and oxygen-delivery system on hand (Figure 10-6A, B). The emergency kit should be stocked at all times. It is useless to have a kit in an emergency with-

Procedure 5   Taking Oral Temperature

Materials Needed

Oral thermometer
Plastic sheath for thermometer
Watch with a second hand
Patient's chart
Pen
Suitable disinfectant
Gauze sponge

Instructions

1 Thermometer is disinfected by wiping it from the stem end to the mercury-filled bulb in one motion.

2 Thermometer is rinsed under cool water and dried.

3 Thermometer is held firmly, shaking it until the reading is below 96°F.

4 Plastic sheath is placed on the thermometer.

5 The patient is asked if he or she has had anything to eat or drink or smoked within the past 15 minutes as this may alter the reading. If so, wait 15 minutes to allow the reading to be closer to normal.

6 The patient is instructed to lift his or her tongue while the bulb of the thermometer is inserted sublingually and the patient is asked to close the lips around it. A patient who needs to cough or sneeze should be instructed to remove the thermometer.

7 The thermometer is removed after 3 minutes, the plastic sheath is removed, and a reading is taken.

8 The temperature is recorded in the patient's chart. Normal temperature is 98.6°F, or 37°C.

9 The thermometer is disinfected.

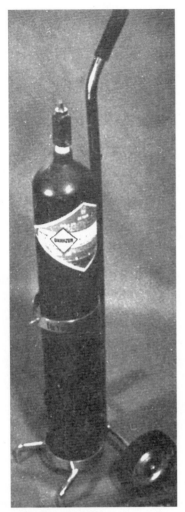

Figure 10-6A Oxygen cylinder.

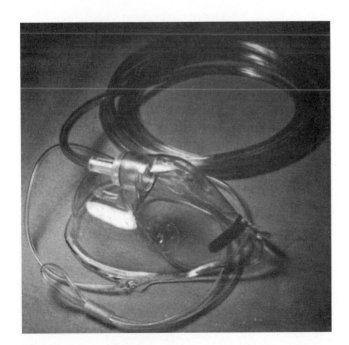

Figure 10-6B Oxygen mask.

out the necessary drugs. Important information for each drug, such as indications for use, standard dosages, adverse reactions, and the expiration date, can be kept handy on a notecard. The oxygen tank should be housed in a portable unit with a demand valve attached to it. This will enable oxygen to flow into a person's lungs even though he or she is unable to breathe.

Having the necessary equipment in an emergency and knowing how to react are the keys to avoiding a crisis. The rule of thumb in any emergency is not to panic! Emergency numbers should be posted near all telephones. Every member of the dental team should be currently certified in basic life support procedures, and each office member should know their role in an emergency. Above all, the patient should *never* be left alone.

Medical Emergencies

Syncope

Perhaps the most frequent medical emergency in the dental office is *syncope*, or *fainting*. Syncope is defined as a momentary loss of consciousness due to a decrease in blood flow to the brain. Patients who are anxious, upset, or in pain are susceptible to fainting. Symptoms include a feeling of warmth, pale skin, perspiration, and clamminess.

Procedure 6
Managing a Syncope

- The dental chair should be put in a **supine** position (patient lying down, face up) to increase blood flow to the brain. Previously, the **Trendelenburg position** (head lower than chest and knees) was recommended.

- Tight clothing should be loosened.

- Aromatic spirits of ammonia, a stimulant, may be passed underneath the patient's nostrils. (*Note:* The ampule should not be held directly under nostrils, as the odor is very strong.)

Following these steps, the patient should respond within a few minutes.

Shock

Shock is a condition that occurs when there is a considerable reduction of blood to the brain, dilation of capillaries in the peripheral areas such as the extremities and the skin, and decreased volume of blood returning to the heart, and therefore decreased blood output from the heart. It may be caused for several reasons: hemorrhage, trauma, drug reaction, poisoning, infection, dehydration, or myocardial infarction (heart attack). The patient's pupils become dilated; breathing becomes shallow and increased; the pulse is rapid, weak, or nonexistent; and the skin is moist, cool, and pale with bluish discoloration on the lips, ear lobes, and fingertips. Frequently, the patient experiences nausea.

Procedure 7
Managing Shock

- Place the patient in a supine position to return blood flow to brain.

- Place a blanket on the patient to prevent heat loss from the body. Do not use external heat.

- Administer oxygen.

- Monitor vital signs.

- Keep airway open

- Call an **EMS (Emergency Medical Service)**: emergency care made available to persons who are experiencing life-threatening conditions.

Orthostatic Hypotension

Orthostatic or postural hypotension (decrease in blood pressure when returned to a seating position after reclining) is often seen in patients who have been in a supine position for a lengthy period of time. When the chair is returned to the upright position, the patient's blood pressure drops suddenly, and he or she becomes lightheaded.

Procedure 8
Managing Orthostatic Hypotension

- Return the chair quickly to the supine position.
- To prevent cases of orthostatic hypotension, raise the chair slowly, pausing for a short period of time between elevations.

Angina Pectoris

Angina pectoris, a suffocating pain in the chest (angina = "pain," pectoris = "chest"), is characterized by acute constriction or narrowing of the coronary arteries that surround the heart, causing decreased blood flow to the heart muscle. It is often associated with physical or emotional stress. The patient may experience **substernal** (under the sternum bone) pain that may radiate to the arms, shoulder, neck, mandible, and teeth or any combination. The patient may also appear **cyanotic** (bluish complexion) and experience shortness of breath. This condition may lead to a heart attack. If the patient experiences an angina attack during dental treatment, the following measures should be taken:

Procedure 9
Managing Angina Pectoris

- Return patient to an upright position. This will alleviate pressure on the chest.

- Administer the patient's own nitroglycerine, placing it under the tongue for 2–3 minutes. If patient does not have a supply of nitroglycerine, amyl nitrate may be used. These are **vasodilators** (cause dilation in blood vessels) and should dilate the coronary blood vessels. Do not use if hypotension is present.

- Administer 100% oxygen to oxygenate tissues.

- If the patient does not experience relief from nitroglycerine, a myocardial infarction (heart attack) may be taking place.

- Call the EMS.

Myocardial Infarction

A heart attack, or **myocardial infarction**, is the death of a part of the heart muscle due to partial or complete cessation of blood flow. This occurs because clogged coronary blood vessels are unable to provide sufficient blood to the heart muscle. Symptoms of a heart attack include intense substernal pain that may radiate to the shoulder, neck, mandible; cold perspiration; shortness of breath; **arrhythmia** (irregular heart rate); cyanotic lips; and anxiety.

Procedure 10
Managing Myocardial Infarction

- Call the EMS.
- Return patient to an upright position to lessen strain on the heart.
- Loosen tight clothing.
- Administer 100% oxygen to oxygenate tissues.
- Administer 1 regular or 4 chewable baby aspirin (325 mg.) and have patient chew but not swallow them until later. This will allow diffusion of aspirin effects through the oral mucosa and blood vessels to break down freshly formed blood clots within 20 minutes.
- Monitor vital signs. If breathing and heartbeat stops, return patient to supine position and perform CPR (cardiopulmonary resuscitation).

Cardiac Arrest

Cardiac arrest, or clinical death, occurs when the heart stops beating. The patient will lose consciousness; become cold and clammy; not breathe; not have a heartbeat or pulse in the large arteries; exhibit dilated pupils; and become cyanotic.

Procedure 11
Managing Cardiac Arrest

- Call the EMS immediately.
- Place patient in a supine position.
- Administer CPR until medical assistance arrives.

Stroke (CVA)

A stroke, or **cerebrovascular accident** (cerebro = "brain," vascular = "blood vessel"), is caused by an abrupt change in blood flow to the brain tissues. In older patients it is caused by a change in the blood vessels brought on by age or hypertension. The affected blood vessels may cause hemorrhaging in the cerebral tissues or vessels may be blocked by a blood clot. If the stroke is slight, the symptoms may include dizziness, headache, or confusion. If the stroke is massive, the symptoms may be unconsciousness, paralysis of one side of the body, impaired speech if conscious, unequal size of pupils of the eyes, and clammy skin.

Procedure 12
Managing Stroke

- If the stroke is slight, the patient should be seated comfortably and reassured.
- Oxygen may be administered.
- If the stroke is massive, the patient should be seated or supine with head and shoulders elevated. Avoid giving patient any stimulants such as an *ammonia ampule*.
- Call the EMS.

Hyperventilation

Hyperventilation (hyper = "excessive," ventilation = "respiration") can be characterized by rapid breathing brought on by a stressful situation. The patient becomes nervous and takes rapid and deep breaths, causing excessive elimination of carbon dioxide from the blood. This alters the body pH (alkalosis).

Procedure 13
Managing Hyperventilation

- Raise the chair to an upright position to ease breathing.
- Instruct the patient to take slow breaths, usually 4–7 breaths per minute.
- If patient is unable to take slow breaths, then a paper bag or headrest cover is placed over the mouth and nose. Tell patient to breathe in and out of the bag. The exhaled air contains additional carbon dioxide to aid in recovery.

Airway Obstruction

Aspiration (inhalation) of objects is the leading cause of airway obstruction in a dental office. These objects may include burs, endodontic files, large pieces of tooth, pieces of amalgam, crowns, or cotton rolls. An obstruction may cause partial or complete blockage. The patient may grab at his or her throat while gasping for air or may cough to try and dislodge the foreign object. If the patient cannot cough or speak and is wheezing, then abdominal thrusts, known as the Heimlich maneuver, are recommended. If the patient can breathe and speak, there is no need for abdominal thrusts (Figure 10-7).

Prevention is the best way to avoid airway obstruction. When performing restorative procedures, a dental dam should be used. The dental dam clamp should be attached to several inches of dental floss so that it can be easily retrieved in case it breaks or slips off from the tooth. A throat pack should be used during surgery or whenever a dental dam is contraindicated. To pack the throat, an opened 2 x 2-in. gauze square is laid toward the back of the throat.

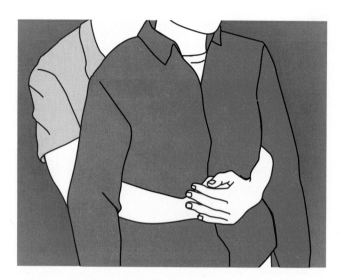

Figure 10-7 Heimlich maneuver.

Procedure 14
Managing Airway Obstruction

- When the patient signals that he or she is unable to breathe or speak due to an obstruction, have him or her stand up to administer abdominal thrusts.
- The dental assistant should summon help.
- Standing behind the patient, placing one fist with thumb side at the top of the stomach or base of the sternum or xiphoid process and the other hand over the fist, give 6–10 quick upward thrusts. Repeat thrusts until object is dislodged.

Unconscious Patient

- If patient becomes unconscious, place him or her in a supine position with head tilted backward to open the airway. The dental assistant should ventilate first or give breaths of air. If unable to ventilate, straddle over the patient's body. Place the heel of one hand over the stomach area above the navel and place the other hand over the first one and give 6–10 upward thrusts. Check the mouth to see if anything has appeared. If so, do a finger sweep using the index finger to remove the object.
- Continue to ventilate and give upward thrusts until the object is in view. Do a finger sweep and remove it.

Pregnant or Obese Victim

- The procedure remains the same, except that the rescuer's hand placement is over the patient's chest instead of the stomach area.

Convulsive Seizure

A central nervous system disorder called **epilepsy** may lead to a convulsive seizure. Epilepsy is an interrupted flow of messages to the brain, causing unexpected behavior. Epileptic seizures may be either **petit mal** or **grand mal**. In petit mal seizures, the patient may become disoriented and stop talking for a few seconds. Seizures of this type are mild and need no treatment. Grand mal seizures are more intense. The patient may experience an **aura**, or warning, of an impending seizure. Involuntary muscle contractions occur along with unconsciousness and possible **incontinence** (loss of bladder control) lasting 3 minutes or more. Although a seizure cannot be stopped or treated, the dental assistant should protect the patient from injury. The patient usually sleeps after muscles are relaxed.

Procedure 15
Managing Seizures

1 Move objects away from the patient to prevent injury.
2 Remove any objects from the mouth, e.g., cotton rolls, saliva ejector, etc.
3 Do not insert objects or fingers in the patient's mouth.
4 A family member or friend should transport patient home and the dental appointment should be rescheduled.

Allergic Reactions

An allergic reaction occurs when the body has developed sensitivity to an **allergen** (a foreign substance). With each exposure to the allergen, the response is more intense. Symptoms include **edema** (swelling), **urticaria** (rash), **wheals** (large welts), and **erythema** (redness of the skin). A more immediate reaction includes swollen and watery eyes, runny nose, and respiratory distress. In an acute reaction, the throat becomes swollen to the point where the patient is unable to breathe. This is known as **anaphylaxis** and it is life threatening.

Procedure 16
Managing Allergic Reactions

1 Epinephrine is the drug of choice, and it should be administered immediately. Other drugs are the antihistamines and should be prescribed as a follow-up measure.

2 The patient's airway must be maintained open to assist the patient's breathing.

3 If the patient is conscious, oxygen should be administered.

4 Call an EMS immediately in a life-threatening situation.

Diabetic Hyperglycemia: Diabetic Coma

Hyperglycemia (hyper = "increase," glycemia = "blood sugar") is a condition that occurs when there is excessive sugar in the blood and urine, causing an increase in the body's demand for insulin. If left untreated, the patient may progress to a **diabetic coma**. Symptoms of diabetic coma are dry mouth and excessive thirst; red lips; flushed and dry skin; rapid and weak pulse; "acetone" (sweet) breath odor; drowsiness; and weakness. If the patient is left untreated, unconsciousness ensues. If the patient is conscious, the dental assistant needs to determine (1) when the patient last ate and (2) if the patient took insulin. Whether the patient is conscious or not, his or her physician should be notified immediately.

Procedure 17
Managing Diabetic Hyperglycemia

Conscious Patient

1 Notify the patient's physician immediately.
2 Have patient take his or her insulin if accessible.
3 Administer glucose (orange juice is best) orally. (Glucose should not harm the patient.)

Unconscious Patient

1 Call the EMS immediately.
2 Place the patient in a supine position.
3 Provide basic life support as needed and monitor vital signs.
4 Administer oxygen.
5 Transfer the patient to a hospital.

Diabetic Hypoglycemia: Insulin Shock

Hypoglycemia (hypo = "decrease," glycemia = "blood sugar"), or **insulin shock**, is caused by low blood sugar. The patient may have taken an overdose of insulin, did not eat, or ate later than usual. A patient who is hypoglycemic appears nervous and hungry. There is an increase in perspiration, causing the skin to be moist. The pupils are dilated, and the patient is pale and weak.

Procedure 18
Managing Diabetic Hypoglycemia

Conscious Patient

1 Candy, sugar cube, or orange juice may be given to the patient while conscious.
2 Notify the patient's physician immediately.

Unconscious Patient

1 Call the EMS immediately.
2 Place the patient in a supine position.
3 Maintain airway open, provide basic life support, and monitor vital signs.
4 Administer oxygen.
5 Intravenous glucose will need to be administered.

Legal Ramifications of Medical Emergencies

It has been shown that 7–8 % of dentists are sued annually. If a lawsuit is served against the dentist, the patient (plaintiff) must prove the following:

1. That the dentist was at fault

2. That the dentist's fault caused injuries to the patient

3. That damages (financial compensation) must be paid to the patient. An *expert witness* is called in on behalf of the plaintiff to describe the appropriate standard of care and to determine whether the dentist followed that course of treatment. If the jury decides that the standard of care was less than what was to be expected, then it claims that the dentist was *negligent* (failed to use ordinary care).

Res Ipsa Loquitur

Res ipsa loquitur means "the thing speaks for itself." Applied to the dentist, this means that the dentist must have performed an injustice to the patient for the result to occur or the patient would not have been harmed.

Good Samaritan Law

The Good Samaritan Law states that health care workers cannot be held liable for death or injury if they acted in good faith when treating someone other than their patient. For example, a patient's elderly neighbor is in the waiting room to drive the patient home and suffers a heart attack. The office staff tries unsuccessfully to resuscitate the individual using standard CPR. In such a case liability on the part of the dental team will be difficult to prove.

Respondeat Superior

Respondeat Superior means "let the master answer." In this case, the dentist is responsible for any actions that are performed by his or her staff during their employment.

Prevention

There are several ways to avoid a malpractice suit in the dental office:

1. The dentist should have a complete medical/dental history on every patient and update it at each visit.

2. The dentist should ensure the patient (or patient's legal guardian, if underage) is aware of the diagnosis, treatment, and subsequent results if the patient does not follow proper home care procedures or

follow the doctor's orders.

3. Everything should be documented completely in the patient's chart. Any unusual situations and treatment should be included. *Nothing* should be left to memory.

4. The office staff should be trained for their roles in an office emergency and practice them periodically.

5. Office staff should attend continuing education seminars to stay abreast of current trends in dentistry.

Dental Emergencies

Dental emergencies may be brought on for several reasons: trauma, bleeding, pain, tissue swelling, and esthetics. The dentist is the only person in the dental office who can offer treatment suggestions. The dental assistant may act on the dentist's advice, especially when conversing with the patient by telephone.

Trauma

Trauma may be due to an accident in which the individual suffered blows to the jaws and dentition. Many times, these cases, depending on severity, are referred to an oral and maxillofacial surgeon for reconstructive repair.

According to the article "Sports-Related Dental Injuries and Sports Dentistry" in the May/June 1998 issue of the *Journal of the American Dental Assistants Association*, it is estimated that more than 5 million teeth are knocked out each year. It is also reported there that 13–29% of all dental injuries are sports related.

When a patient calls to inform the dentist of an accidental traumatic injury, the dental assistant should ask for information on the severity of the accident and if any teeth were lost or **avulsed** (forcibly knocked out of its socket) and give the caller instructions to follow. It is possible that the patient would be sent to a hospital, referred to a local oral surgeon, or instructed to come in to the general practitioner's office. If a tooth was avulsed, every effort to find it should be made. When found, it should be rinsed gently, not scrubbed, and kept moist in a wet paper towel until brought in for replantation in the socket. The sooner this takes place, the better the success rate for replantation.

If the injuries included a broken or dislocated jaw, the caller should be instructed to stabilize it with a sling, securing the lower jaw to the maxillary jaw and tying it at the top of the head.

Bleeding

Bleeding may occur after an extraction, surgical procedure, or accident. Patients who are bleeding substantially should be seen immediately. If bleeding is due to an extraction, the dental assistant should inquire if the bleeding is profuse or slight. The patient should be made to understand that some bleeding may occur that would tinge the saliva and that it would be considered to be "normal." If, however, there is substantial bleeding, the patient should be instructed to fold a gauze square twice and apply pressure to the site by biting on it. A wet tea bag applied to the site has been used for its tannic acid activity, reducing blood flow.

Pain

Pain is usually the chief complaint for an individual who is not a regular patient seeking professional care. A tooth with advanced caries that involves the pulp may bring this on. It is important to know how severe the pain is and whether the patient knows which tooth is causing the pain. The patient should be asked if pain medication has been taken, what type, and how much. This information should be helpful when arranging the emergency appointment, possibly requiring another person to drive the patient if enough medication was taken that may alter the patient's consciousness.

When the patient comes in, it is very likely that the dentist will open the tooth in question after concluding through the use of radiographs and other tests that the pulp is involved. This being the case, a root canal or pulpotomy may be performed and the tooth temporized. The patient should be instructed to return at another time for reevaluation or completion of the procedure.

Tissue Swelling

Tissue swelling may take place overnight whereby the individual exhibits puffiness in a localized area, possibly due to an abscessed tooth or an infected impacted third molar. This is a possible indication of infection, and the patient should be seen as soon as possible. The dentist may wish to prescribe an antibiotic prior to performing any operative dentistry.

Esthetics

Esthetics may involve a broken tooth located in the anterior area of the mouth. It may be sharp to the touch and may or may not be painful. In this case, however, whether the patient is experiencing pain or not, an effort to schedule an emergency appointment is appreciated due to the fact that the patient will not wish to be seen in public.

SUGGESTED ACTIVITIES

- Following the guidelines of this chapter, take and record the vital signs of a fellow student. Include blood pressure, pulse, respiration, and oral temperature.
- After deflating the cuff, wait at least 15 seconds, reinflate the cuff, and proceed to retake the blood pressure. Record it.
- Compare the first blood pressure reading with that of the second. Was there a difference?
- Compare the blood pressure reading using the right and left arms. Was there a difference?
- Continue to perfect your technique for taking blood pressure until the procedure becomes routine and exact.

REVIEW

1. The pulse is taken using the _____ artery, whereas, blood pressure is taken using the _____ artery.
   a. Ulnar, radial
   b. Brachial, radial
   c. Brachial, carotid
   d. Radial, brachial

2. A normal heart rate for an adult is in the range:
   a. 80–100
   b. 16–20
   c. 60–80
   d. 12–18

3. A normal respiration rate for an adult at rest is in the range:
   a. 14–18
   b. 60–70
   c. 18–20
   d. 80–90

4. What condition occurs when there is a hemorrhage in the brain?
   a. Stroke
   b. Shock
   c. Syncope
   d. Epilepsy

5. What takes place systemically when hyperventilation occurs?
   a. Lack of nitrogen
   b. Lack of carbon dioxide
   c. Excess carbon dioxide
   d. Excess nitrogen

6. Name three signs/symptoms of a heart attack: (1) cyanotic lips, (2) shortness of breath, (3) flushed appearance, or (4) intense substernal pain.
   a. 1, 2, 3
   b. 2, 3, 4
   c. 1, 2, 4
   d. 1, 3, 4

7. Name two ways that may prevent airway obstruction during a dental procedure: (1) using a saliva ejector, (2) using a high-volume evacuator (HVE), (3) using throat packs, or (4) using a dental dam.
   a. 1, 2
   b. 2, 3
   c. 3, 4
   d. 1, 4

8. Match each term with its meaning:
   a. Erythema
   b. Edema
   c. Trendelenburg position
   d. Supine
   e. Urticaria
   f. Wheals
   g. Cyanotic

   1. swelling
   2. Rash with welts
   3. Large welts
   4. Redness of skin
   5. Lying down, head lower than chest and knees
   6. Lack of oxygen causing bluish skin
   7. Lying down on back facing up

Preventive Dentistry

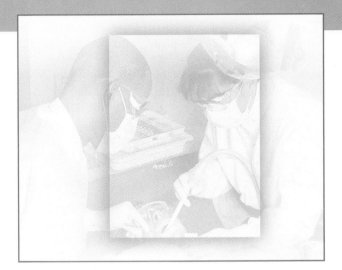

OBJECTIVES

After studying this chapter, the student will be able to:

● Describe dental plaque and its relationship to tooth decay and periodontal disease.

● Explain the role of diet and caries susceptibility tests in preventive dentistry.

● Discuss the use of fluoride and of pit and fissure sealants.

● Differentiate between methods of toothbrushing.

● List and describe auxiliary aids in preventive dentistry.

● Describe at which stages of tooth development fluoride intake occurs.

● List the three types of topical fluoride and describe each one.

● Outline a plan for patient education in preventive dentistry.

● Describe the measures taken when a person experiences fluoride overdose.

Introduction

Unlike early beliefs that tooth loss was part of the aging process, it is now an accepted fact that the teeth were designed to last a lifetime. Prevention of any problems is a key in order to fulfill that goal. To avoid destruction of the teeth and supporting structures, the patient must understand how to maintain optimum oral health. For this reason, the dental assistant must have a thorough knowledge of the fundamentals of preventive dentistry—the *etiology* (cause) of dental decay and periodontal disease and the measures that preserve the oral cavity.

Dental Plaque

Dental **plaque** is a soft, sticky accumulation of bacteria and products of saliva. It is responsible for the development of tooth decay and periodontal disease. Plaque formation occurs in four stages. Initially, a thin, bacteria-free, translucent film called acquired pellicle forms on the teeth. Second, microorganisms that inhabit the oral cavity adhere to the **acquired pellicle**. The bacteria then begin to multiply and grow in layers forming **colonies** (clusters of bacteria). By the end of three weeks, the plaque has become a completely developed mass of microorganisms (see Chapter 6).

Plaque and Tooth Decay

Figure 11-1 shows a simplified diagram of the development of tooth decay.

One of the first microorganisms to attach to the acquired pellicle is ***Streptococcus mutans***. These bacteria grow and multiply by consuming carbohydrates, especially sugars, from the foods that are eaten. Acids are then produced as a waste product. The acid begins **decalcification** (removal of calcium elements from the enamel) of the tooth. As the plaque thickens, the acid is trapped against the tooth and cannot be neutralized by saliva. Decalcification of the tooth continues and another microorganism called ***Lactobacillus*** begins to form inside the carious area (see Chapter 6).

> BACTERIA + SUGAR = ACID
> ACID + TOOTH = DECAY

Figure 11-1   The process of tooth decay (frame).

Plaque and Periodontal Disease

As plaque develops, the highest concentration occurs at the cervical third of the tooth along the gingival margin. Bacteria invade the **gingival sulcus** and attack the gingiva. These bacteria cannot be easily removed. Left undisturbed, **calculus** (mineralized layers of plaque) forms and acts as a further irritant to the tissue (see Chapter 6).

Dietary Control

The effect of diet in preventive dentistry is twofold. As the tooth grows and develops, it needs several vitamins and minerals that promote resistance to tooth decay. Of particular importance are vitamins A, C, and D and the minerals fluoride and calcium. In addition, certain foods promote caries development and gingival destruction. Sticky foods, which are predominantly carbohydrates, adhere to the tooth and provide sugar for the bacteria. Soft diets that lack fibrous foods helpful in stimulating the gingiva encourage the production of plaque and the deterioration of the periodontal structures. For this reason, it is important that the patient understand the significance of diet and nutrition in order to maintain a healthy oral cavity.

Caries Susceptibility

There is no single cause of dental caries, but it can be identified by the decalcification of the inorganic salts of the tooth. Bacterial infection caused by acid-producing organisms results in fermentation of refined carbohydrates retained in the mouth as food debris in undisturbed areas around the teeth. The organic acids formed by the organisms attack the enamel and give bacteria the opportunity to work unmolested, with no danger of the acids produced being washed away by the saliva.

The tendency to develop a carious condition may be caused by faulty diet. To inhibit the development of dental caries, proper home care procedures should be reinforced, such as toothbrushing and flossing, with emphasis on an adequate diet.

Fluoride

Fluorides have been instrumental in reducing tooth decay and promoting general oral health at all ages. It has also had a significant therapeutic effect in controlling periodontal infections. There are two ways that fluoride may be administered: systemically and topically.

Systemic Fluoride

One of the best preventive methods for tooth decay, fluoride has significantly reduced the amount of caries in school-age children. When ingested *systemically*, fluoride works by causing the crystal structure of the enamel to become more resistant to acids produced by bacteria and by preventing the acid-producing bacteria from developing. Fluoride intake occurs during three stages of tooth development: the **mineralization** stage, after mineralization and before eruption, and after eruption. It is normally ingested in drinking water in 1 ppm (1 part fluoride for every million parts of water), and fluoride supplements can also be given from birth to age 14. These can be in liquid or tablet form. Excessive fluoride, however, is detrimental to the teeth. Both **fluorosis** (brown staining) and **mottling** (pitted enamel surfaces) have been seen in such instances. **Hypocalcification** (a condition of diminished calcium during tooth development) may also take place, especially when excess fluoride of over 2 ppm is present in drinking water.

Topical Fluoride

There are three types of *topical* fluoride used in dental offices: sodium fluoride, stannous fluoride, and acidulated phosphate fluoride.

Sodium Fluoride. A 2% aqueous solution is used during a series of four applications each time it is administered. The patient benefits greatly when treatments are administered to newly erupted teeth at ages 3, 7, 10, and 13. It is relatively stable if kept in a polyethylene bottle and the taste is not objectionable. It does not stain teeth or cause gingival inflammation.

Stannous Fluoride. An 8% aqueous solution is used approximately 1 or 2 times annually or more frequently if needed. This preparation is highly unstable; therefore a new solution has to be prepared each time. It has an unpleasant taste and may stain **demineralized** (excessive loss of mineral or inorganic salts from body tissues) areas on teeth as well as tooth color restorations. Furthermore, it may cause sloughing of gingival tissue if inflammation was present during application.

Acidulated Phosphate-Fluoride (APF). A 1.23% sodium fluoride with 0.1 M orthophosphoric acid that may be used in an aqueous solution, gel, or thixotropic forms. **Thixotropic** is a type of gel that becomes fluid when it is placed under stress such as when the material is forced interdentally or agitated in the bottle; later it returns to the gel state. It is recommended to use it 2 times a year. The length of application has been 4 minutes; however, newer preparations use 1 minute. Flexible trays are used when applying this type of topical fluoride (Fig 11-2A).

Fluoride gels and solutions for topical application are preparations of stannous fluoride and acidulated

Procedure 19 Applying Topical Fluoride°

Materials Needed

Basic tray setup

Cotton rolls

High volume evacuator (HVE) tip

Toothbrush and dental floss

Preformed commercial trays, either two single trays placed separately or two trays connected as one (Figure 11-2A)

Liners for trays (if necessary)

Fluoride gel

Saliva ejector tip

Infection control barriers

Instructions

1 Explain the procedure to the patient.

2 Brush, floss, and rinse the teeth. (Research shows that it is no longer necessary to "coronal polish" the teeth prior to administering a fluoride treatment.)

3 Position the patient in an upright position.

4 Dispense the fluoride solution into the tray.

5 Isolate teeth with cotton rolls.

6 When doing both arches simultaneously, dry the maxillary arch first.

7 Remove cotton rolls and Insert tray(s) into the mouth (Fig 11-2B). Using thumb and index finger, squeeze fluoride gel interproximally.

8 Instruct the patient to close down so that all surfaces are adequately covered. Insert saliva ejector and time the procedure.

9 Use the saliva ejector inside the mouth to remove the excess fluoride.

10 Remove tray(s) after adequate timing (from 1 to 4 minutes). Do not rinse the mouth. Use the HVE or saliva ejector to suction out any excess fluoride.

11 Instruct the patient not to swallow fluoride and not to rinse, eat, or drink for 30 minutes to allow the fluoride to be absorbed into the teeth.

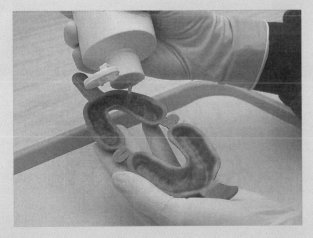

Figure 11-2A Fluoride tray.

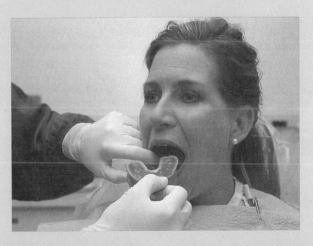

Figure 11-2B Inserting fluoride tray into patient's mouth.

phosphate. Because stannous fluoride solution is unstable, a combination of acidulated phosphate and stannous fluoride is commercially prepared and is available in gel form.

Depending on the carious condition of the patient's mouth, the doctor may prescribe a stannous fluoride application or a topical fluoride gel application. Stannous fluoride treatments are completed in a single application and may be repeated every six months.

Fluoride Overdose

Fluoride has been found to be beneficial when used in small quantities. Problems arise when an excess amount of fluoride is ingested. Potential toxicity does exist when a concentrated fluoride preparation is accidentally swallowed. Dental team members should know how to respond to such an emergency.

Symptoms of Fluoride Overdose.
Onset of symptoms may occur within 30 minutes and may continue for 24 hours. Patient may exhibit the following symptoms:

- Abdominal pain
- Nausea, vomiting, diarrhea
- Excessive salivation and thirst
- Convulsions
- Paresthesia (numbness)
- Cardiovascular and respiratory depression (If not treated, the patient may die in a few hours due to cardiac and respiratory failure.)

Emergency Management

- Vomiting should be induced by stimulating the back of the throat using a finger or taking an emetic (substance to induce vomiting) such as *syrup of Ipecac* orally.
- Emergency Medical Service (EMS) should be called and the patient transported to hospital.
- Administer milk when patient is not vomiting.
- Airway should be kept open and vital signs checked. Cardiopulmonary resuscitation (CPR) should be performed if necessary.
- At the emergency room:
  a. Gastric lavage (stomach should be pumped).
  b. Patient should be given calcium gluconate for muscle tremors.
  c. Endotracheal intubation should be used.
  d. Heart should be monitored.
  e. Patient's blood should be monitored and the patient given calcium, magnesium, potassium.
  f. Intravenous feeding should be given to replace blood volume and calcium.

Fluoride Mouthrinses

Individuals who are considered to be at high risk of acquiring caries should employ fluoride mouth rinses. There are several fluoride mouth rinse preparations on the market. Some may be purchased over the counter, such as the "low-potency rinses," whereas others must be purchased with a prescription, such as the "high-potency rinses." The American Dental Association, Council on Dental Therapeutics, should approve these preparations. Fluoride mouth rinses are used at home or

schools that have a program for its use. Statistics have shown the effectiveness in reduction of cavities by as much as 42.5% in school-age children.

Indications for Use

- For reduction of tooth decay in adolescents, persons with root exposure, teeth with demineralized areas, and all school-age children
- Patients who wear appliances that trap plaque, such as orthodontic appliances, partials, and space maintainers
- Patients who suffer from xerostomia (dry mouth) due to radiation exposure or drugs that inhibit saliva production

Precautions

- Children under 6 years of age should not use rinses due to their inability to expectorate and may tend to swallow instead.
- Some preparations that contain alcohol should not be recommended to a recovering alcoholic.

Fluoride Dentifrices

Fluoride dentifrices are available as pastes or gels. They usually contain sodium fluoride or sodium monofluorophosphate. Patients who are prone to decay or who suffer from sensitivity should be advised to brush their teeth 2 or more times daily using a fluoride dentifrice.

Pit and Fissure Sealants

Pit and fissure sealants are indicated when there are deep pits and fissures in the occlusal surfaces of the teeth that may be difficult to clean. The sealant bonds to the surface and protects the tooth from an accumulation of bacteria that produce acids. Chapter 42 discusses pit and fissure sealants in more detail.

Toothbrushes and Toothbrushing

The single most important instrument in plaque control is the toothbrush. Because of the variety of toothbrushes, it is necessary to be familiar with each patient's needs. Sizes, shapes, and type of bristles are just a few characteristics of toothbrushes. Generally accepted toothbrushes vary from pedodontic (small) to adult sizes. Bristles may be in two or three rows and range from soft to medium-hard. In addition, the toothbrush should be sturdy, easily cleaned, economically priced, and easy to use. Because of the microorganisms existing in the oral cavity, toothbrushes should be discarded after two to three months of use. In the event of a heavy cold or viral infection, a more frequent replacement will help to prevent recurrent disease.

To make the best selection, several factors should be considered. These include (1) the patient's current oral hygiene conditions; (2) the recommended brushing technique; (3) personal and professional preferences; (4) the patient's manipulative ability; and (5) the desire to follow suggested methods.

Battery-powered or electrical toothbrushes can be used for all patients, but they are especially helpful for those who are unable to use a manual toothbrush. **Geriatric** (elderly) patients and the physically and mentally compromised have been successful in cleaning the teeth with such a brush. The same principles apply in using a powered toothbrush as a manual toothbrush for each brushing technique.

Toothbrushing

There are several methods of toothbrushing that can be used for plaque control. In order to decide which technique to recommend to the patient, one must take into account two considerations: (1) the specific technique should remove plaque and (2) there should be no detrimental effects to the gingivae.

Bass or Sulcular Method. The *Bass*, or *sulcular*, method is recognized as one of the most efficient techniques, because it advocates cleaning along the gingival margin and interproximal areas where periodontal disease is likely to begin. It is also recommended for patients who have had periodontal surgery.

A soft bristle brush is used to avoid damage to the gingiva by overzealous or incorrect brushing.

Roll or Rolling Stroke Method. The *roll* or *rolling stroke* method is recommended when concentration on cleaning the gingival sulcus is not of primary concern. Young children and adults with healthy gingiva use this technique.

Procedure 20   Toothbrushing: Bass, or Sulcular, Method

Materials Needed

Toothbrush
Toothpaste (optional)
Infection control barriers
Personal protective equipment (PPE)

Instructions

1 Place the brush on the last two or three teeth in the arch.

2 Position the brush at a 45° angle to the **long axis** (vertical length) of the tooth (Figure 11-3A).

3 Gently guide the bristles into the gingival sulcus (gingival space between tooth cervix and gingiva).

4 Move the brush in short strokes back and forth at least 10 times without moving the tips of the bristles away from the sulcus.

5 Move the brush anteriorly over the next two or three teeth. Be sure to overlap on the previous area.

6 Repeat steps 2–5 continuing along the entire facial surface.

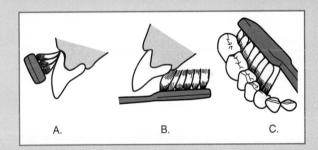

Figure 11-3 Bass method of brushing.
(A) Bristles are placed in the gingival sulcus at 45° to the long axis of the tooth. (B) Position of brush for the maxillary anterior teeth, lingual surface. (C) Position of brush for the mandibular posterior teeth, lingual surface.

7 Move the brush to the lingual surface (Figure 11-3B). Follow steps 1–5.

8 When cleaning the maxillary and mandibular anterior lingual areas, hold the brush vertically and push the bristles into the sulcus.

9 Finish each arch by brushing the occlusal surfaces (Figure 11-3C).

Procedure 21 Toothbrushing: Roll or Rolling Stroke Method

Materials Needed

Toothbrush
Toothpaste (optional)
Infection control barriers
Personal protective equipment (PPE)

Instructions

1 Hold the brush with the bristles pointing apically (Figure 11-4A).
2 Position the side of the brush (bristles) on the gingiva and the brush handle even with the occlusal plane of the teeth.
3 Flex the bristles by pressing against the side of the teeth and gingiva (Figure 11-4B).
4 Roll the brush over the teeth by turning the wrist (Figure 11-4C).
5 Repeat this 5 times.
6 Move to the next area. Be sure to overlap the previous area.
7 Continue along the facial surfaces.

8 Move to the lingual surfaces and repeat steps 1-5.
9 To clean the maxillary and mandibular anterior lingual surfaces, hold the brush lengthwise.
10 Press the bristles against the teeth and gingiva.
11 Roll down for maxillary teeth and up for mandibular teeth. Do this 5 times in each area.
12 Clean the occlusal surfaces. (*Note:* Brushing too high on the gingivae during initial placement can lacerate the gingival mucosa.)

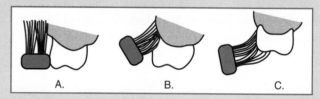

Figure 11-4 Rolling stroke brushing method.
(A) Brush handle is even with occlusal plane, and bristles are pointing apically. (B) Brush pushed against both tooth and gingiva to flex bristles. (C) Brush rolled over the teeth.

Modified Stillman Method. The *modified Stillman* technique is used to stimulate and massage the gingiva in addition to cleaning the cervical third of the tooth.

Charters Method. The *Charters method* stresses cleaning and massaging of the gingiva, especially in patients who have had periodontal surgery. It is not used when the interdental papilla is normal.

Procedure 22 Toothbrushing: Modified Stillman Method

Materials Needed

Toothbrush
Toothpaste (optional)
Infection control barriers
Personal protective equipment (PPE)

Instructions

1 Hold the brush with the bristles pointed apically Figure (11-5A).

2 Place the brush against the tooth, pushing lightly against both tooth and gingiva. This will cause the tissue to *blanch* (turn pale in color).
3 Angle the bristles of the brush at 45° to the long axis (Figure 11-5B).
4 Vibrate the brush to the count of 10; then roll it along the crown of the tooth (Figure 11-5C).
5 Do this 5 times before moving to the next area.
6 In the anterior lingual region, hold the brush lengthwise (Figure 11-5D).

continued

continued from previous page
Procedure 22 Toothbrushing: Modified Stillman Method

7 Press and vibrate the brush, roll, then repeat.

8 Clean the occlusal surfaces as in the sulcular method (Figure 11-5E). (*Note:* without careful brush placement, tissue lacerations can result. Choose a soft-bristle brush rather than one with hard bristles.)

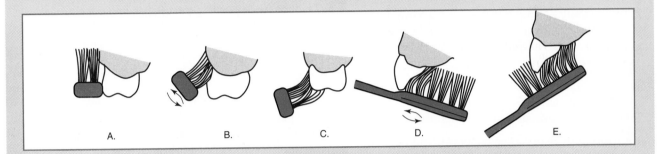

A.   B.   C.   D.   E.

Figure 11-5 Modified Stillman brushing method. (A) Handle positioned even with occlusal surface and bristles pointed apically. (B) Bristles angled at 45° to the long axis and the brush vibrated. (C) Brush rolled over the crown. (D) Mandibular anterior lingual toothbrush placement. Brush pressed and vibrated. (E) Brush rolled over the crown.

Procedure 23   Toothbrushing: Charters Method

Materials Needed

Toothbrush
Toothpaste (optional)
Infection control barriers
Personal protective equipment (PPE)

Instructions

1 Place the brush against the tooth with the bristles pointing toward the occlusal surface.

2 Place the brush at the neck of the tooth, and angle the brush at 45° to the occlusal surface (Figure 11-6).

3 Press the bristles lightly against the margin of the gingiva.

4 Vibrate the brush slowly while counting to 10.

5 Because the Charters method is difficult to perform on the lingual surfaces, the modified Stillman toothbrushing method is often employed for these areas.

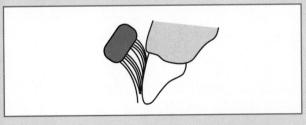

Figure 11-6 Charters brushing method. Toothbrush angled at 45° to the long axis with the tips of the bristles directed toward the incisal or occlusal surface.

General Information Regarding Toothbrushing

Regardless of the type of toothbrushing method used, certain general considerations apply.

1. *Cleaning occlusal surfaces.* The bristles should be firmly pressed into the pits and fissures. The back-and-forth method should be used to scrub these areas (Figure 11-7).

2. *Overlapping.* As the brush is moved to an unclean area, it should overlap partially onto the previously cleaned area. This reduces the possibility of missing any teeth during brushing.

3. *Counting strokes.* Patients can count the number of strokes (such as 5 or 10) or use a timer to encourage concentration on a thorough cleaning.

4. *Cleaning sequence.* The patient should begin by focusing on areas where problems in cleaning may exist. In this way, if time is limited, the critical areas are cleaned well. Generally, the patient should begin on the facial surface and proceed from one side to the other then continue to the lingual surface. The occlusal surface is cleaned prior to moving on to the opposing arch.

5. *Timing routine of brushing.* As in all instances, the frequency of brushing and the time of day depend on the individual patient's needs. It is recommended that most patients brush at least twice daily with a thorough cleaning prior to bedtime.

Dentifrice

A **dentifrice** is used in conjunction with a toothbrush to clean the teeth. Most commonly known as *toothpaste*, it can be either a paste or powder. Ingredients may include *fluoride* (to inhibit tooth decay), *flavorings* (to provide an agreeable taste), *abrasives* (to clean and polish), *coloring agents* (to enhance appearance), and *detergents* (to produce a foaming action). Other chemi-

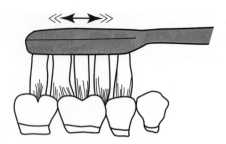

Figure 11-7 Occlusal brushing. Back-and-forth motion while pushing the bristles into the occlusal surface.

cals may lessen sensitivity to the cementum of the tooth, reduce mouth odors, or chemically aid in plaque removal. Professional recommendations are geared to the patient's gingival condition, caries susceptibility, and need for desensitization of the cementum. It is the method of toothbrushing and flossing, however, not necessarily the type of dentifrice used, that should be of primary concern in home care.

Dental Floss

Toothbrushing can only clean three tooth surfaces well—facial, occlusal, and lingual. In order to reach the interproximal surfaces—mesial and distal—dental floss, dental tape, or super floss is used.

Dental floss is round and can be either waxed or unwaxed. Waxed floss is used for tight contacts, since it will not fray as unwaxed floss does. Unwaxed floss is recommended for easy-to-clean tooth surfaces, smooth restorations, and areas without calculus. Dental tape is flat and has sharp edges. It can be used for the same purpose as waxed floss. Super floss is made to resemble yarn. It is very effective where large interdental spaces occur.

Flossing can be performed either before or after brushing. When flossing is done first, the fluoride in the toothpaste will cover the interproximal areas where plaque was removed. Flossing should be performed at least once a day and preferably before retiring to bed.

Procedure 24 Flossing

Materials Needed

Dental floss
Infection control barriers
Personal protective equipment (PPE)

Instructions

1 Use a piece of floss approximately 15–18 inches in length. Wrap most of the floss around the middle finger on one hand and just a small amount on the middle finger of the other hand. When moving

continued

continued from previous page
Procedure 24 Flossing

from tooth to tooth, floss can be unwrapped from one finger and onto the other (Figure 11-8A).

2 Begin in the maxillary right quadrant on the most distal surface. With no more than 2 inches of floss between the fingers, guide the floss with both thumbs or thumb and index finger (Figure 11-8B).

3 Pull the floss around the distal surface of the tooth. Starting at the sulcus, move the floss up and down several times.

4 Before moving to the next area, use a clean piece of floss. Unwrap the floss from one finger and onto the other.

5 Hold floss in a diagonal position over the teeth at the insertion point. Seesaw the floss between the contact areas. Do not force or snap the floss as the interdental papilla may be injured in the process (Figure 11-8C).

6 Pull the floss around the mesial surface of the tooth. Starting at the sulcus, move the floss up and down several times. Cross the interdental papilla, and wrap the floss around the distal surface of the neighboring tooth. Slide the floss up and down several times (Figure 11-8D).

7 Remove the floss using a seesaw motion. If the contact is too tight or the floss begins to shred, hold it against the proximal surface and pull the floss through, unwrapping it from the opposite finger.

8 Move to the mandibular arch. Guide the floss with both forefingers (Figure 11-8E). Continue with steps 3–7.

9 Move from tooth to tooth until all teeth have been flossed.

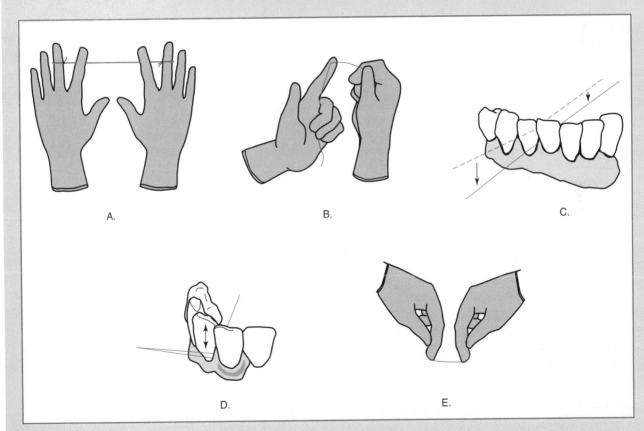

A.   B.   C.

D.   E.

Figure 11-8 Use of dental floss. (A) Floss wrapped around the middle two fingers. (B) The floss can be guided in one of two ways for the maxillary arch: with thumb and forefinger or with both thumbs. (C) Floss seesawed interproximally. (D) It is necessary to floss into the sulcus. (E) When flossing in the mandibular arch, floss is guided with both index fingers.

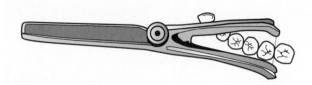

Figure 11-9 Floss holder.

Precautions

Flossing incorrectly could result in floss cuts and trauma to the interdental papilla. Problems may be avoided when proper instruction and precautions are brought to the patient's awareness. Examples of causes are as follows:

- Allowing too much floss length between fingers when inserting interproximally
- Snapping the floss between the contacts without using a finger rest
- Seesawing the floss once it is in the interproximal area

Interproximal Aids

If a patient experiences difficulty flossing, a *floss holder* may be used (Figure 11-9). Patients who lack the manual dexterity to floss will benefit most from using a holder. In the event that the patient has a fixed bridge, a *floss threader* is a convenient way to guide the floss under the *pontic* (an artificial tooth that replaces a missing tooth) to clean the space and the cervical portion of the crown. It resembles a needle with a large eye (Figures 11-10 and 11-11).

A *perio-aid* is a device that has two angled ends and round toothpick tips inserted into either end (Figure 11-12). It is recommended for removing plaque in *furcation*-involved (division in multirooted tooth where supporting bone has been lost) teeth or at the gingival margin.

A 2-inch triangular wooden tip known as a *Stim-U-Dent* is suggested for use when there is lack of interdental papilla. The Stim-U-Dent is inserted interproximally with the base of the triangle positioned on the gingiva. By moving it back and forth, the proximal tooth surfaces are cleaned simultaneously (Figures 11-13A,B).

When areas of the mouth are inaccessible or where there are open contacts or bridgework, it is advisable to use an *interproximal brush*. Consisting of a handle that is straight or curved and a minibrush that may be tapered or straight, the interproximal brush is inserted and moved back and forth (Figure 11-14).

To revive unhealthy gingivae, a *rubber-tipped stimulator* is available. By massaging the diseased area, blood flow is increased. A rubber-tipped stimulator

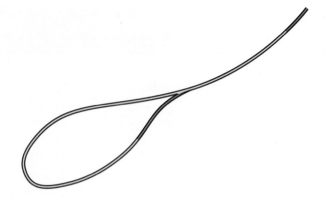

Figure 11-10 Floss threader.

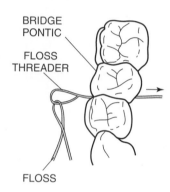

BRIDGE
PONTIC

FLOSS
THREADER

FLOSS

Figure 11-11 Use of floss threader with a fixed bridge.

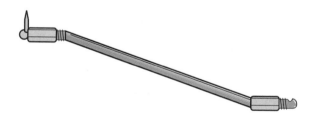

Figure 11-12 Perio-aid.

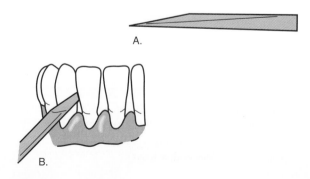

A.

B.

Figure 11-13 Stim-U-Dent.

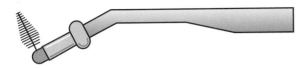

Figure 11-14   Interproximal brush.

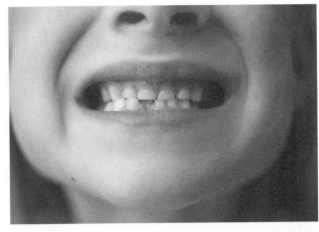

(A)

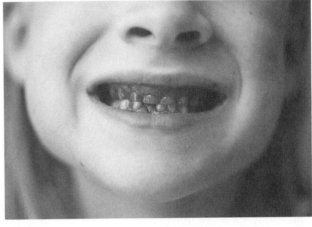

(B)

Figure 11-16   (A) Teeth as they appear before disclosing. (B) Appearance of teeth after disclosing.

should *never* be used on healthy gingiva to avoid damaging the existing interdental papilla and disturbing the periodontal ligament attachment (Figure 11-15).

Other Oral Hygiene Aids

Because dental plaque is usually colorless, a **disclosing solution** or **disclosing tablet** is used to identify the deposits (Figures 11-16A, B). The disclosing agent can be either a liquid mixture or a tablet that contains a dye or coloring chemical. Solutions are used most often in dental offices, because they are too messy to use at home. The solution is swabbed directly onto the teeth. The advantage of using disclosing solutions is that they stain plaque deposits more readily. Tablets are recommended for home use. They are chewed and mixed with the saliva by swishing them around in the mouth. The main disadvantage of using these agents is that they stain not only the teeth but the lips, tongue, and gingiva. For this reason, patients are encouraged to disclose, floss, and brush before bedtime. The stain should disappear by morning.

   Oral irrigation is a process whereby water is forced continuously or periodically through an irrigation tip (Figure 11-17) into the interproximal areas to eliminate debris. Most systems used at home are either power-driven pumps or attached to a water faucet. The unit is turned on, and the water flow is adjusted. The irrigation tip is directed at the interproximal space and not into the gingival sulcus (Figure 11-18). If a high pressure is used, damage to the gingival tissues may occur, or bacteria may be forced into the gingival sulcus. Other chemical agents such as mouthwashes, *chlorhexidine alexidine* (an anti-infective agent used topically) can be used in lieu of water to reduce the number of bacteria in the oral cavity. Oral irrigation is advantageous for patients undergoing orthodontic treatment or those who have fixed bridges to clean hard-to-reach areas. It should be stressed in all situations, however, that oral physiotherapy is not a replacement for daily toothbrushing and flossing.

Oral Rinses or Mouthwashes

Oral rinses or mouthwashes can be categorized as either breath fresheners (cosmetic) or as an aid in reducing bacteria (therapeutic). They can be prepared at home or purchased in a store. Mixtures prepared at home usually

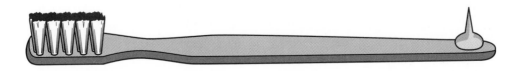

Figure 11-15   Rubber-tipped stimulator.

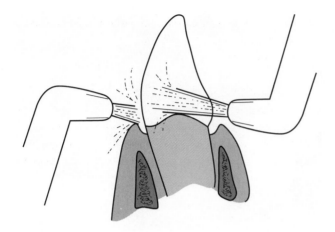

Figure 11-17 Oral irrigation tips.

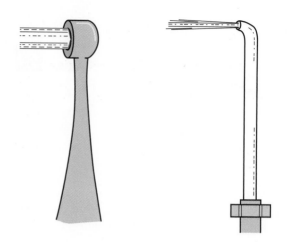

Figure 11-18 Water irrigation. Note horizontal spray to avoid forcing bacteria into the sulcus.

consist of plain water, saline (salt) solutions, or bicarbonate of soda (baking soda). Commercial rinses contain water, sweetener, alcohol, flavoring, and coloring. Mouthwash is often used as a rinse before dental procedures to reduce microorganisms. Patients use mouthwash at home for a "quick cleaning" when they do not have the time to brush and floss, for care following surgery, for reduction in decay-producing bacteria, or just to eliminate breath odors. Therapeutic mouthwashes that contain chlorhexidine alexidine or sanguinarine aid in controlling plaque and mouth odors. Unfortunately, chlorhexidine alexidine may alter the taste of some foods or stain the teeth. Patients using these rinses should have regular prophylaxis appointments.

Patient Education as a Part of Preventive Dentistry

No matter how much time and money are invested in restoring an unhealthy mouth, if the patient does not understand the need for adequate home care, then all is lost. During the initial patient education counseling session, the role of plaque and diet should be discussed. The patient should then be given a plan of personal oral hygiene based on his or her needs. Once the patient understands the first two steps, he or she should be encouraged to return for recall appointments in order to monitor home care.

The patient education plan is divided into three sections: motivation, education, and reinforcement.

In order to develop a patient education program, the patient must show the desire to learn. This includes being made aware of the problem and subsequently being willing to change behavior.

After the patient is motivated to learn, he or she needs to be educated. Always encourage the patient, correcting mistakes in a positive manner. Involve as many of the senses as possible. This is more stimulating to the patient than just hearing a lecture. Pamphlets with pictures or videotapes can be excellent tools when they address the patient's individual needs. Actively engaging the patient in participation is by far the best method for learning. The patient learns faster and retains the information longer.

Once learning is complete, the patient must practice these skills. Reinforcement is essential in making these activities a habit.

SUGGESTED ACTIVITIES

- Compare the types of fluoride in dentistry and the pros and cons for the use of each.
- Compare the several methods of toothbrushing. Use a typodont to demonstrate each method, taking into account the consideration that the technique should remove plaque, with no detrimental effects to the gingivae.
- Select a piece of floss and using a typodont demonstrate the procedure for flossing the mandibular arch.
- Select a piece of floss, and using a fellow student, demonstrate the procedure for flossing both the maxillary and mandibular arches.
- Assume that some of the contacts are too tight to allow the floss to slide up and down interproximally as intended. What would your approach be to complete the flossing?

REVIEW

1. Name the vitamins and minerals that promote resistance to tooth decay:
   a. Vitamins B, K and minerals iron, potassium
   b. Vitamins A, C, D and minerals calcium and fluoride
   c. Vitamins C, K, E and minerals fluoride and phosphorus
   d. Vitamins A, D and minerals calcium and iron

2. Indicate what two problems are caused by excessive fluoride intake: (1) mottled enamel, (2)calculus build-up, (3) fluorosis, or (4) gingivitis.
   a. 1, 2
   b. 2, 3
   c. 1, 3
   d. 3, 4

3. Pit and fissure sealants are used on:
   a. Smooth surface cavities
   b. Teeth that have beginning cavities on occlusal pits and fissures
   c. Teeth with deep pits and fissures on occlusal surfaces

4. A device used to guide floss under the pontic of a bridge is a:
   a. Floss threader
   b. Floss holder
   c. Flosser

5. What is the recommended fluoride content in drinking water?
   a. 5 ppm (parts per million)
   b. 3 ppm
   c. 10 ppm
   d. 1 ppm

6. After a fluoride treatment, the patient is instructed not to rinse, eat, or drink for:
   a. 15 minutes
   b. 30 minutes
   c. 5 minutes
   d. 1 minute

7. Indicate some symptoms associated with systemic fluoride overdose that may exhibit: (1) abdominal pain; (2) nausea, vomiting, diarrhea; (3) excessive salivation; and/or (4) headache.
   a. 1, 2, 3
   b. 2, 3, 4
   c. 1, 3, 4
   d. 1, 2, 4

8. Match the toothbrushing method to the correct description
   a. Bass
   b. Rolling stroke
   c. Modified Stillmans
   d. Charters

   1. Stimulates and massages gingiva as well as cleans the cervical third of the tooth
   2. Cleans the gingival margin, recommended for postsurgical patients
   3. Used on children and adults with healthy gingiva
   4. Cleans the gingival area; not recommended when the interdental papilla is intact. Bristles are pointed occlusally.

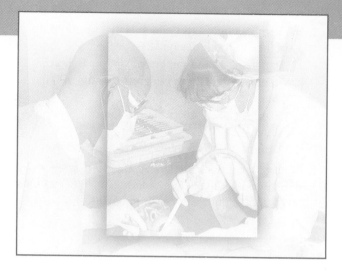

OBJECTIVES

After studying this chapter, the student will be able to:

● Describe the digestive changes that occur in the mouth, stomach, small intestine, and large intestine.

● Name the six key nutrients required by the body for total health.

● Discuss the meaning of Recommended Dietary Allowances (RDAs) and how they are established.

● Explain the importance of protein in the diet.

● Explain the difference between essential and nonessential amino acids.

● Determine what carbohydrates are, their source, and why they are essential to body functions.

● Explain the importance of fats in the diet.

● State three conditions or health problems associated with too much fat in the diet.

● Describe the functions of vitamins in human nutrition.

● Name the three minerals that have a direct relationship in the formation of teeth.

● Give the two minerals most prominent in bone and tooth structures and the functions of each.

● Give the five main functions of water in maintaining proper body water balance.

Introduction

Nutrition is a complex and often debated subject. Theories without scientific basis continue to prevail. Much information tends to confuse the public rather than present proven principles.

Dentistry retains a respected tradition for providing patients with sound nutritional advice. Consider the fact that dentists routinely see many more healthy persons than do physicians. As a result, dental personnel have more time to discuss reliable nutritional information.

To better understand what happens to the food we eat, a review of the human digestive system is in order.

The Digestive System

Digestion involves both mechanical and chemical processes. *Mechanical processes* include the chewing of food, the churning actions of the stomach, and the muscular contractions of the intestinal tract. This regulated pattern of contractions is known as **peristalsis**. Peristalsis breaks up food into smaller and smaller particles, mixes them with digestive juices, and continually moves the food mass through the intestinal tract.

Chemical processes involve substances affecting the organs of the body, the **enzymes**. An enzyme is usually a protein that initiates and accelerates a chemical reaction. Enzymes are responsible for chemical changes that break down foods into simpler forms that can be absorbed. As **catalysts**, enzymes bring about these changes without having their own composition changed in the process. Enzymes have a specific action. A particular enzyme will act only on one kind of foodstuff and will react with no other. For instance, an enzyme that digests starch will not digest fat.

Digestive Process

The **alimentary canal**, known as the digestive tube from the mouth to the anus, consists of the mouth, pharynx, esophagus, stomach, small and large intestines, rectum, and anus.

Mouth. In the mouth begins the mechanical and some chemical breakdown of foods (Figure 12-1):

● Teeth grind food.

● Saliva adds moisture to food, acts as a lubricant, and forms a small, round ball of food (bolus).

● The tongue helps food bolus along the way and to cross the trachea (windpipe).

● The epiglottis, a trap door that closes the trachea, forces the food into the esophagus.

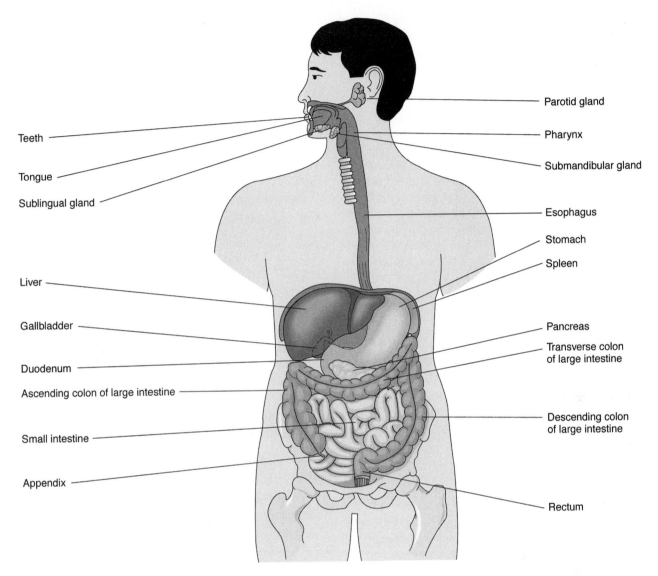

Figure 12-1 The digestive system.

Digestion of some carbohydrates begins because of the chemical action of the enzyme *salivary amylase,* formerly called ptyalin.

Pharynx (Throat). The pharynx is connected to the esophagus and moves finely chopped food as puree to the stomach.

Esophagus. The esophagus is a tube leading to the stomach:
- Nerve endings along the esophagus cause waves of constriction (unusual narrowing), or peristalsis, as food moves to the stomach.
- The **cardiac sphincter**, a band of muscle between the esophagus and stomach, allows food to enter the stomach and prevents **reflux** of food back into the esophagus.

- The brain alerts the stomach to start the release of gastric juices, hydrochloric acid (HCl) and pepsin, a protein-specific enzyme.

Stomach. Food in the stomach is churned and mixed with gastric juices (HCl and pepsin) until it reaches a liquid consistency. The food will spend approximately one-half hour in the stomach. Partial digestion of some nutrients occurs:
- Carbohydrates—minor action
- Fats—minor action
- Protein—action of HCl forms *polypeptides* (two or more amino acids combined with water)

In the stomach HCl stimulates intestinal hormones from the liver and pancreas; the liver releases bile that has been stored in the gallbladder; the pancreas releases pancreatic juice. Both juices are alkaline and will neutralize the HCl remaining in the food mass. Before food enters the small intestine, the **pyloric sphincter**, a band of muscle, regulates food entering the small intestine and prevents reflux or backflow.

Small Intestine. In the first 10 inches of small intestine, where nutrients are absorbed into the body system, food, having been churned and bathed in digestive juices, is now sent on a 4–8-hour journey through the small intestine. Peristalsis waves twist and wrench the intestine and swish food solution back and forth. Millions of nearly microscopic fingers, called villi, in the intestine stir the solution and transfer the usable nutrients into the blood and lymph systems. The small intestine is composed of the *duodenum*, the first part, the *jejunum*, the middle portion, and the *ileum*, the last portion.

Chemical Reactions in Digestion/Absorption of Nutrients

- All carbohydrates convert to monosaccharides (simple sugar that cannot be broken down to a simpler substance).
- All fats are emulsified by bile (combined with glycerin). Emulsified fats are further converted to monoglycerides (glycerol) and fatty acids.
- All proteins convert to amino acids. Cellulose, fiber, and some fats resist digestion and move on!

Large Intestine. The large intestine consists of the ileocecal valve, which permits the chyme (semifluid mass of partly digested food) to enter the colon and prevents backflow into the ileum. The cecum, a blind pouch located at the lower right area of the abdomen, and the vermiform appendix, a fingerlike projection, extend into the abdomen and the colon. The colon (large intestine) is further divided into the *ascending colon, transverse colon, descending colon*, and *sigmoid colon*.

- In the large intestine (colon), remains of food solution will spend approximately 10–12 hours. Large quantities of water and some nutrients wait here to be absorbed into the system.
- Food solution remaining in the colon is fed by colonies of bacteria to decay remains; intestinal contents take on a solid consistency.
- Fecal matter is excreted as body waste.

Rectum. The rectum is located below the sigmoid colon and its primary function is to control the internal and external anal sphincters for the purpose of defecation (bowel movement).

Anus. The anus is the outside opening located below the rectum. Body waste or defecation is excreted through this opening.

Therefore, orange juice, buttered toast, egg, and milk for breakfast will leave the body as heat, carbon dioxide (CO_2), water (H_2O), and nitrogenous waste!

Liver and Its Function

The liver is the first station through which blood passes after leaving the small intestine, where it has picked up absorbed compounds (nutrients).

Carbohydrates

- Carbohydrates come from the intestine and reach the liver in the form of monosaccharides.
- The liver transforms monosaccharides to glycogen (for storage).
- From glycogen the liver produces **glucose** (blood sugar); glucose is sent in a steady amount to all cells of the body via blood circulation.
- The liver keeps blood glucose (sugar) level constant; the liver may convert more glycogen into blood glucose as needed—should there be too much glucose, it will convert back to glycogen.
- The liver is responsible for keeping glycogen and glucose in chemical equilibrium.
- Excess glycogen is stored as *fat*.

Fatty Acids and Glycerin (Glycerol)

- Fatty acids and glycerin reach the liver from the intestine.
- The liver recombines fatty acids and glycerin into fats.
- Liver fats may be sent via the blood system to all cells of the body.
- Fats may be stored under the skin, along membranes of the abdomen, and around the heart, kidneys, and other organs.
- Liver and fat deposits communicate via the blood system; if too much fat is in the liver, remaining fat is deposited elsewhere; if there is too little fat in the liver, fats from other areas of the body can replenish the reduced fat in the liver.

Protein. Any amino acids not passed to the body cells via blood are chemically removed as carbon dioxide (CO_2) during respiration (breathing); nitrogen that is left is removed in the urine.

Metabolism. Metabolism is the sum total of the physical and chemical processes and reactions taking place among the ions, atoms, and molecules of the body. For instance, metabolism involves the way nutrients are absorbed into the blood following digestion. Refer to Chapter 14.

Chemical Reactions. The chemical reactions in metabolism require the activity of *enzymes*. Many of these enzymes require other substances, or **coenzymes**. Where an enzyme substance is usually made of protein, a coenzyme is an organic substance that is *not protein*. It is one that can unite with a given protein to form an active enzyme system. One of the important functions of vitamins, certain minerals, and hormones is to act as coenzymes.

Basic Metabolic Rate (BMR). The *basic metabolic rate* is the minimal rate at which the body must produce energy to continue its essential life processes. It is the measure of how quickly an individual converts food into energy.

The BMR is calculated from the person's rate of metabolism while at complete rest and in a fasting state. The rate expressed is in a percentage that indicates how far it varies from the norm, or from the average range for a person of the same age, sex, and size.

Basic Metabolic Need. Basic metabolic need is the amount of energy required to carry on the involuntary work of the body and to maintain the body temperature:

● One-third of energy is maintained in functional activities of various organs—heart, kidneys, and lungs.

● Two-thirds of energy is needed for oxidation in the resting tissues, especially the maintenance of muscle tone.

Key Nutrients

Nutrients are substances that supply the body with essential nourishment. The key nutrients are described in Table 12-1.

Key nutrients are necessary for:

● Growth, maintenance, and repair of tissues

● Energy requirements

● Regulating body processes

● Maintaining a constant internal environment

Good nutrition depends on an ample supply of all the essential nutrients found in the food of a well balanced diet. *Diet* is the total of all food taken into the body and includes both liquid and solid forms. Each nutrient has a key role to play, but it is important to remember that all the nutrients work together in an intricate metabolic balance. An extra supply of one nutrient cannot make up for the shortage of another. In fact, a deficiency of one nutrient may interfere with maximum use of others.

Recommended Dietary Allowances

Recommendations for the average daily amounts of nutrients that population groups (by age and sex) should consume over a period of time are termed *Recommended Dietary Allowances* (RDAs) and are established by the Food and Nutrition Board of the National Academy of Sciences—National Research Council.

Table 12-1 Key Nutrients

Nutrients	Dietary Benefits and Sources
Proteins	Furnish energy The only nutrients capable of building body tissues Sources are plants and animals
Carbohydrates	Energy nutrients Source is primarily plants
Fats	The highest calorie nutrient Provide energy and other nutritional needs Source is plants and animals
Vitamins	Necessary in minute amounts for growth, development, and optimum health Source is organic (living) substances
Minerals	Necessary in minute amounts for growth, development, and optimum health Inorganic substances whose source is neither organic life nor any product of organic life
Water	An important nutrient which is the principal constituent of the body

Calories

One calorie (spelled with a small *c*) is the amount of heat required to raise the temperature of 1 gram of water by 1°C. A Calorie (spelled with a capital *C*) is 1000 times larger than the calorie and is used in metabolic studies. In common usage, a *calorie* pertains to the amount of energy contained in food required for activity and growth in daily life. The term *energy* is used interchangeably with calorie. Body requirements mainly depend on body size, basal metabolic rate, activity, age, sex, and environmental temperature. Calories come from carbohydrates, protein, fat, and alcohol:

- 1 gram of protein = 4 calories
- 1 gram of carbohydrate = 4 calories
- 1 gram of fat = 9 calories
- 1 gram of alcohol = 7 calories (and no nutritional value)

Basal metabolic need is based on 1 Calorie per hour per kilogram of body weight (1 kilogram = 2.2 pounds).

Food Groups

Food can be classified into *food groups* that provide essential nutrients in about the same quantities. Systems for dividing food into groups may vary. For the purposes of this chapter, four essential food groups plus a nonessential group (sometimes referred to as five groups), will be discussed.

All the food from each of the four food groups work together to supply the necessary energy and nutrients for growth, maintenance, and health. It is recommended that a wide variety of foods from each group be selected. Adjustment in size and number of servings should be based on individual RDA needs. A description of the four groups is presented in Tables 12-2 to 12-5.

The Nonessential Group

Because these foods are not included in any other official group, they are classified as the *nonessential group*. Refined sugars, in all forms, are carbohydrates that provide no nutrients; these are empty calories. Carbohydrate needs can be best met from foods that provide other nutritional benefits.

Fats are needed in the diet. However, this nutritional need should not be met by selecting foods that provide mostly fat calories (such as butter and lard). Many of the available foods have fat in them; these fill the need for dietary fats. Consequently, foods that contain primarily fat calories are included in the nonessential group (Figure 12-2).

Table 12-2 Milk Group

Major nutrient contributions	Calcium, phosphorus, protein, riboflavin, vitamins A and D
Recommended daily servings	Children under 9: 2–3 cups
	Children 9–12: 3+ cups
	Teenagers: 4+ cups
	Adults: 2+ cups
	Pregnant women: 3+ cups
	Nursing mothers: 4+ cups
Serving size	1 cup = 8 oz fluid milk
	(whole, skim, buttermilk, nonfat, lowfat) or designated milk equivalent
	Equivalents (based on equal content of calcium)
	11/2 oz cheddar/swiss cheese
	11/2 cups cottage cheese
	1/4 cup dry skimmed milk powder
	11/2 cups ice cream
	1/2 cup evaporated milk
Food found in this group	Fluid milk (skim, whole, nonfat, buttermilk, lowfat), condensed, evaporated, powdered milk
	Cheeses
	Ice cream
	Yogurt
	Dishes made with milk products

Table 12-3 Meat Group

Major nutrient contributions	Protein, iron, thiamin, riboflavin, vitamin B_{12} (animal products only)
Recommended daily servings	2 or more servings
Serving size	2–3 oz lean, boneless cooked meat, poultry or fish 2 eggs 1 cup cooked dry beans or peas 4 tablespoons peanut butter 1/2–1 cup nuts, sesame, or sunflower seeds
Food found in this group	Beef, lamb, veal, pork (except bacon), organ meats (liver or sweetbreads), poultry (chicken, turkey, goose, duck), fish, shellfish, lunch meats (bologna, liverwurst) ***Meat alternatives*** 　Eggs 　Dried beans, peas, lentils 　Nuts, peanuts and peanut butter 　Soybeans, soybean flour

Table 12-4 Vegetable and Fruit Group

Major nutrient contributions	Carbohydrates, vitamins A and C
Recommended daily servings	Vegetables: 3–5 servings Fruit: 2–4 servings
Serving size	1/2 cup vegetable or fruit 1 medium apple, banana, orange, potato, 1/2 medium grapefruit or melon 1 small salad
Foods found in this group	All fruits and vegetables (cooked or raw)

Table 12-5 Bread and Cereals Group

Major nutrient contributions	Carbohydrates, thiamin, niacin, iron, riboflavin
Recommended Daily Servings	6–11 servings
Serving size	1 slice bread, 1 roll, 1 biscuit 1 cup ready-to-eat cereal, flake or puff varieties 1/2–3/4 cup cooked cereal 1/2–3/4 cup cooked pasta (macaroni, spaghetti, noodles) 5 saltines 2 square graham crackers
Foods found in this group	All breads and products made with flour Breakfast cereals Rice, pasta Grits, Bulgar (granulated wheat) Oats, barley, buckwheat, rye

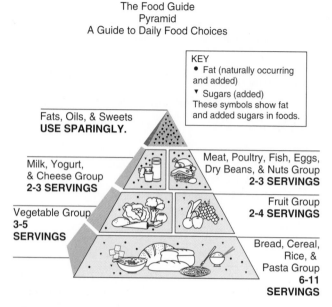

The Food Guide
Pyramid
A Guide to Daily Food Choices

KEY
• Fat (naturally occurring and added)
▼ Sugars (added)
These symbols show fat and added sugars in foods.

Fats, Oils, & Sweets
USE SPARINGLY.

Milk, Yogurt, & Cheese Group
2-3 SERVINGS

Meat, Poultry, Fish, Eggs, Dry Beans, & Nuts Group
2-3 SERVINGS

Vegetable Group
3-5 SERVINGS

Fruit Group
2-4 SERVINGS

Bread, Cereal, Rice, & Pasta Group
6-11 SERVINGS

Figure 12-2 The food pyramid: a guide to daily food choices. (Source: U.S. Department of Agriculture, Washington, D.C.).

Protein

A group of organic compounds containing carbon, hydrogen, oxygen, and nitrogen form proteins. *Protein* substances in the body are essential to its structure and function. None of the cells of the body can survive without an adequate supply of protein.

The end products of protein digestion are *amino acids*. Amino acids constitute about 20% of the cell mass and are the chief constituent of protein. Amino acids occur naturally in plant and animal tissues. More than 20 different amino acids are commonly found in proteins. Some of them can be produced in the body, but the human organism cannot manufacture others. These essential amino acids must be provided by protein foods in the diet.

Food proteins are of great nutritional importance, because they are necessary for the building and repair of all kinds of body tissues, especially of muscles and organs, heart, liver, and kidneys.

Functions of Proteins

The main function of protein is *tissue synthesis*, or tissue regeneration. **Synthesis** is a reaction, or series of reactions, in which a complex compound is created from elements and simple compounds.

Structural Protein (Synthesized by Body)

● Structures such as cell walls, various membranes, connective tissue, and muscles are mainly protein.

● Hormones, so important in the regulation of metabolism, are proteins.

● Enzymes that act as catalysts in the chemical reactions of metabolism are proteins.

● One molecule of protein is composed of 22 different amino acids. To make body protein, the cell must have 22 of the amino acids simultaneously.

● Protein is the only nutrient that can *make new cells* and *repair tissues.*

Dietary Protein (supplied to the body from food)

● Builds new body tissues for growth during pregnancy, infancy, childhood, and for repair after injury or illness

● Maintains body structure

● Produces compounds essential for normal body functions, such as enzymes, hormones, and hemoglobin

● Regulates body water balance

● Supplies an alternate energy source of protein (4 calories per gram)

Types of Amino Acids

Essential. Eight must be supplied by the diet.

● Used for growth and repair of tissues

● Cannot be stored for reserve; must be available simultaneously for tissue synthesis and maintenance

Source of Essential (High-Quality or Complete) Amino Acids

● Animal—lean meat, fish, poultry, dried beans, eggs and cheese. Egg is designated as the perfect protein against which other proteins are measured as a good source in human nutrition.

Nonessential. *Twelve to 14 are synthesized by the body.*

● Can supply some essential amino acids, BUT are not used for tissue synthesis; are oxidized and nitrogen content excreted.

Source of Nonessential (Low-Quality or Incomplete) Amino Acids

● Natural—grains (bread and cereal products), vegetables (peas, beans), small amounts of fruits

Nonessential amino acids are lacking in one or more essential amino acids and cannot perform the function of synthesis.

Protein Quality. The quality of dietary protein depends on whether:

● It supplies all eight essential amino acids.

● The amount supplied will provide each amino acid in the amount needed for protein synthesis.

Amino Acid Balance. Dietary protein needs to supply each amino acid in the amount needed for protein synthesis in the body. When amino acids are supplied in amounts smaller than those needed, the total amount of protein that can be synthesized or used by other amino acids will be limited.

Although a daily supply of protein is essential to good nutrition, excess protein tends to put a strain on the liver and kidneys, as they process the excess. Protein intake greater than the RDA increases the urinary excretion of calcium and reduces the amount of calcium available for use by the body.

Carbohydrates

Carbohydrates are a chemical compound of carbon, hydrogen, and oxygen. Carbohydrates are present, at least in small amounts, in most foods. Chief sources are sugars and starches.

Functions of Carbohydrates

Carbohydrates provide the major source of energy for the body:

● They convert carbohydrates into glucose, for use by tissues, cells, nerves, blood sugar, and muscular energy.

● They aid in oxidation of fats by combining with oxygen and removing hydrogen.

● They help to maintain body temperature.

● They store excess glycogen in the liver.

Types of Carbohydrates

Carbohydrates are chemically classified as:

● Monosaccharides (simple sugar)

● Disaccharides (each molecule yields 2 molecules of monosaccharide—double sugar)

● Polysaccharides (may yield 10 or more molecules of monosaccharides—complex sugar)

Carbohydrate Conversion

● Sugar—yields simple carbohydrates (monosaccharides and disaccharides)

● Starches—yield complex sugar (polysaccharides) in digestible form for humans

● Dietary fiber—cellulose (polysaccharides) no enzyme can break it down; is not digestible

Digestive Process of Carbohydrates

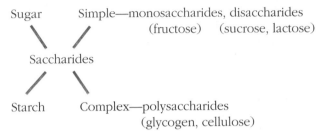

Sugar

Simple—monosaccharides, disaccharides
(fructose)   (sucrose, lactose)

Saccharides

Starch

Complex—polysaccharides
(glycogen, cellulose)

Carbohydrate Sources

● *Sugar* sources include refined table sugar (sucrose), syrups, honey, molasses, bread, cookies, and cakes. Naturally occurring sugars are found in fruits, vegetables, and milk. Milk and dairy products contain carbohydrates in the form of milk sugar (lactose). Sugar is the only food that is nearly 100% carbohydrate.

● Starch sources include grains, grain products, and starchy vegetables (such as potatoes and root vegetables).

Body Requirements

The body needs about 100 grams of carbohydrate, estimating 4 calories per gram, or 400 calories of carbohydrate, each day for energy and to ensure body maintenance and growth. Of all the major nutrients, carbohydrate is consumed in the greatest amount in the human diet.

Metabolism of Carbohydrates

Energy is needed for specific processes of metabolism: glucose for tissue cells, mainly the nervous system, depends solely on sugar for energy and must be in continuous supply.

● Brain cells are continually active whether a person is awake or asleep and need a continuous supply of glucose (sugar) in the fluid surrounding the cells.

● The brain and other nerves cannot make use of another energy source and are vulnerable to temporary deficiency in blood sugar.

● As mental processes originate in the brain, attitudes toward life are affected by the amount of glucose present in brain cells.

● The brain controls muscle reflexes.

Physical Conditions and Sugar Balance

- *Hypoglycemia*—abnormally low level of blood sugar

- *Hyperglycemia*—abnormally high blood glucose level

- *Diabetes mellitus*—a disorder of carbohydrate metabolism in which the ability to oxidize and utilize carbohydrates is lost as a result of disturbances in the normal *insulin* mechanism (protein hormone, secreted by pancreas)

- *Diabetic coma*—insulin insufficiency (administer insulin to patient)

- *Insulin shock*—insulin insufficiency (provide patient with orange juice or sugar)

Fats

Fats (lipids) are a group of oily organic substances insoluble in water but soluble in alcohol. The two basic units of fats in the human mechanism are fatty acids and **glycerol** (a sugar alcohol). Fats are a normal component of every living cell wall and membrane within the cell.

Functions of Fats

Fats are a source of body fuel and provide efficient energy in a relatively small amount of food. Humans cannot synthesize fat; therefore, it must be supplied by the diet.

Dietary fat is the most concentrated source of energy, 9 calories per gram. Normal tissue function is dependent on an adequate supply of fatty acids. Fat carries the fat-soluble vitamins A, D, E, and K.

Fats also help to maintain body temperature. They act as a cushion mechanism to protect vital organs and to pad various areas such as the buttocks, palm of the hands, and soles of the feet.

Types of Fats

The greatest portion of body and dietary fats are composed of complex molecules, called *triglycerides*. These fatty acids are of two types: *saturated* and *unsaturated*. Saturation is based on the number of hydrogen atoms a certain fatty acid contains.

Saturated Fatty Acids. **Saturated fatty acids** contain a greater number of hydrogen atoms and are often naturally solid at room temperature.

- Saturated fats are not an essential part of the diet.

- Saturated triglycerides tend to increase the amount of serum cholesterol in the blood.

Source of Saturated Fatty Acids

- Animal—fatty meats, whole milk (cream), egg yolk, animal organs (liver, kidney), butter, yellow (hard) cheese

- Plant—palm oil, coconut oil

Unsaturated Fatty Acids. Unsaturated fatty acids contain fewer hydrogen atoms and are often liquid at room temperature.

- Unsaturated fats provide essential fatty acids required by the body.

- Unsaturated triglycerides tend to lower the serum cholesterol when used to replace part of the saturated fat in the diet.

Source of Unsaturated Fatty Acids

- Vegetable—oils of safflower, sunflower, corn, soybean, cottonseed, peanut

Unsaturated fats are further divided into *monounsaturated* and *polyunsaturated fats*, depending on the hydrogen atoms present.

- **Monounsaturated fats** are those of olive oil and peanut oil. They neither raise nor lower serum cholesterol.

- **Polyunsaturated fats** include the common vegetable oils. Safflower and sunflower are the least saturated (10%). Corn and soybean are a bit more saturated (14%). Peanut oil is the most saturated (20%).

Hydrogenated oils are higher in saturated fat because of the process of adding hydrogen atoms to the oil. *Hydrogenation* is a process whereby polyunsaturated oils are changed into solid fats, for example, the chemical change from vegetable oil (liquid) to margarine (solid).

Cholesterol. **Cholesterol** (sterols) is an essential body element that is present in nerve tissue, body fluids, blood, and bile. Cholesterol is important in body chemistry. The body's own production of cholesterol is necessary in the functioning of certain systems, for example, the nervous system.

- The greatest portion of cholesterol is converted into bile salts by the liver.

- It serves as the main building block of male and female sex hormones in the body.

- It is involved with vitamin D in calcium metabolism.

- There is a likely relationship between tension and cholesterol in blood.

- Reduced saturated fats in the diet may help to control blood cholesterol.

Vitamins

The term *vitamin* comes from the Latin word *vita* which means *life*, and is used to name a group of chemically unrelated compounds that are necessary for proper metabolism. Vitamins consist of various relatively complex substances occurring in plant and animal tissues and are smaller than the energy nutrients.

Vitamins cannot be made in sufficient quantities by the body and must be consumed through the diet. Very small amounts (milligrams) of vitamins fill the need for this essential nutrient.

Functions of Vitamins

Vitamins are organic substances necessary for proper growth, development, and good health.

- They assist enzymes in the digestion, absorption, and metabolism of proteins, carbohydrates, fats, and minerals; they are termed *coenzymes*.
- They help enzymes convert fuel food into energy needed for life-sustaining body functions.
- They participate in the formation of blood cells, genetic material, hormones, and chemicals of the nervous system.

Types of Vitamins

Vitamins are identified according to their solubility. There are 13 vitamins, divided into two types: *fat-soluble* and *water-soluble* vitamins (Table 12-6).

Fat-Soluble Vitamins. *Fat-soluble vitamins* can be dissolved in fat rather than water.

- They include vitamins A, D, E, and K.
- They are not destroyed by cooking and are stored in body fat and fatty tissue.
- It is not essential that they be consumed daily.
- Excessive amounts may build up to toxic (poisonous) levels.

Water-Soluble Vitamins. *Water-soluble vitamins* will dissolve in water.

- They include vitamin C and eight B vitamins.
- They cannot be stored in the body and must be consumed in the daily diet.
- They are naturally present in foods, are fragile, and may be washed away or destroyed during food preparation.

Minerals

Minerals are inorganic (do not occur in the plant or animal worlds) substances. Various minerals are distributed throughout the body tissues.

Minerals must be supplied in the diet and generally can be obtained by a varied or mixed diet of animal and vegetable products that meet the energy and protein needs of the body. Minerals work together to maintain the health and well being of the individual.

Functions of Minerals

When minerals are taken into the body as nutrients, they are absorbed through the gastrointestinal tract and excreted via the kidneys, bile, and other intestinal secretions as waste products.

- Minerals are a component of teeth and bones and give rigidity to their structure.
- They form compounds essential for normal metabolism.
- They activate cellular enzyme systems and hormones found in the body.
- They maintain the pH (acid-base balance) of body fluids and osmotic cell balance. *Note: Osmosis* is the process whereby molecules in two different solutions are separated by a semipermeable (allows passage) membrane. Molecules are capable of passing through the membrane inside the cell (intracellular) and outside the cell (extracellular).
- Minerals regulate the transmission of nerve impulses and the contraction of muscles.

Types of Minerals

Minerals may be classified into two groups: *macrominerals* and *microminerals*, or *trace minerals* (Table 12-7). Minerals that occur in large amounts in nature are needed in greater quantities by the body. Some authorities advocate the need for 100 milligrams (mg) or more of the macrominerals daily for optimum health. Microminerals (trace minerals) are those needed in only small amounts or a few milligrams per day.

Characteristics of Minerals. Minerals retain their chemical identity throughout the entire digestive process:

- Minerals will work together as long as a balance is maintained.
- One mineral, as a rule, cannot be administered without affecting the absorption and metabolism of other minerals.
- Increasing excess amounts of minerals beyond the RDA may in some cases be harmful.
- Serious risks are associated with megadose (excessively large amounts) of minerals.

Table 12-6	Vitamins		
Vitamins	**Sources**	**Important Functions**	**Deficiency Symptoms**
Fat Soluble			
Vitamin A	Fish liver oils. Liver. Vegetables (green and yellow). Fruits (yellow). Butter, margarine. Whole milk, cream. Cheese. Egg yolk.	Needed for growth. Health of the eyes, night vision. Structure and functioning of the cells of the skin and mucous membranes. Clear, smooth skin.	Retarded growth. Night blindness. Increased susceptibility to infections. Changes in skin and mucous membranes.
Vitamin D	Vitamin D–enriched milk. Sunshine. Fish liver oil.	Absorption of calcium from digestive tract. Responsible for the body's assimilation of calcium and phosphorous.	Soft bones. Poor tooth development. Rickets. Osteoporosis and osteomalacia (softening of bones).
Vitamin E	Wheat germ oil. Vegetable oil. Vegetable greens. Egg yolk, milk, fat, butter. Meat.	An antioxidant that helps to protect other nutrients from destruction by oxidation. Unites with oxygen to build the resistance of blood cells to ruptures.	Severe deficiency would result in the degeneration of body's skeletal muscles, paralysis of legs, and reproductive failure.
Vitamin K	Vegetable greens. Cabbage. Cauliflower. Soybean oil.	Normal clotting of blood. Normal liver function.	Delay in blood clotting (hemorrhages).
Water Soluble			
Vitamin B_1 (thiamine)	Yeast. Pork, organ meats. Wheat germ. Meat. Dried beans and peas. Whole-grain or enriched products.	Important in glucose metabolism. Normal function of nervous system. Promotion of normal appetite and digestion. Functioning of the heart, nerves, and muscles.	Retarded growth. Loss of appetite. Nerve disorder. Less resistance to fatigue. Impairment of digestion. Disease (beriberi).
Vitamin B_2 (riboflavin)	Liver. Meat. Milk. Vegetable greens. Yeast. Fish, poultry, eggs. Enriched or whole-grain bread and cereals.	Needed for growth. Health of skin and mouth. Well-being and vigor. Functioning of the eyes. Important in energy and protein metabolism.	Retarded growth. Lesions at corners of mouth (cheilosis). Dimness of vision. Cataractlike symptoms. Intolerance to light. Premature aging. Dermatitis.
Niacin (nicotinic acid)	Meat, fish, poultry. Milk. Whole-grain or enriched Products. Peanut butter.	Component of two enzymes. Helps cells to use other nutrients. Health of skin. Functioning of digestive and nervous systems.	Smoothness of tongue, (glossitis). Skin eruptions. Digestive disturbances. Mental disorders. Disease (pellagra).
Vitamin B_{12}	Organ meat. Eggs. Saltwater fish.	Blood-regeneration cells in bone marrow and gastrointestinal tract.	Pernicious anemia.
Folic acid (folacin)	Yeast. Spinach.	Antianemic factor. Component of certain enzymes active in formation of red blood cells. Found in liver.	Megaloblastic anemia.
Vitamin B_6	Liver. Pork. Muscle meat. Whole-grain cereals. Vegetables.	Functioning coenzyme in metabolism of all energy-yielding nutrients. Requirement dependent on protein intake.	Rare.
Pantothenic acid	Yeast. Liver. Kidney. Eggs. Nuts. Whole-grain products.	Metabolism of protein.	Rare.
Biotin	Egg yolk. Organ meat, muscle. Milk. Whole grains. Many vegetables. Some fruits.	Function for several enzyme systems. Involved in metabolism of protein, carbohydrates, and fats. Synthesized by intestinal bacteria.	Unlikely.
Vitamin C (ascorbic acid)	Citrus fruits, Melons. Berries. Other fruits. Tomatoes. Vegetables (especially raw).	Important role in formation and maintenance of collagen. Helps resist infection. Aids in healing. Cell activity. Maintaining strength of the blood vessels. Health of gingival tissue (gums).	Sore gingivae (gums). Hemorrhage around bones. Tendency to bruise easily. Disease (scurvy).

Table 12-7 Minerals

Minerals	Sources	Important Functions	Deficiency Symptoms
Macrominerals			
Calcium (Ca)	Milk, cheese, sardines, and other whole canned fish. Vegetable greens. Some fruits.	Normal development and maintenance of bones and teeth. Clotting of the blood. Normal heart action. Iron assimilation. Nerve and muscle action.	Retarded growth. Poor tooth formation. Rickets. Slow clotting of blood. Osteoporosis. Osteomalacia.
Phosphorus (P)	Meat, poultry, fish. Milk. Cheese. Dried beans and peas. Whole-grain products.	Formation of normal bones and teeth. Maintenance of normal blood reaction. Maintenance of healthy nerve tissue. Normal muscle activity.	Retarded growth. Poor tooth formation. Rickets. Osteoporosis. Osteomalacia.
Magnesium (Mg)	Whole-grain cereals. Nuts. Small amounts in milk, meat, fish, eggs, and green vegetables.	Found in large amounts in bones. Major extracellular electrolyte. Controls body fluid concentration and volume.	Heavy perspiration or excessive water ingestion. Severe vomiting and diarrhea.
Potassium (K)	Fruit. Vegetables. Meat Milk.	Major intracellular electrolyte. Controls normal pH of body.	Loss from large doses of certain drugs. Dehydration. Muscular weakness, paralysis, rapid heart beat. Low blood pressure, diarrhea, and intestinal distention.
Chlorine (Cl)	Salt, salty foods. Seafood and other animal foods.	Major extracellular electrolyte. Formation of hydrochloric acid found in digestive tract. Control of blood pH. Activator for enzymes necessary for carbohydrate metabolism.	Occurs with dehydration.
Sulfur (S)	Eggs. Protein-rich foods.	Present in every cell in body. Present in hair, skin, and nails. Associated with protein, is a constituent of two amino acids. Active in energy metabolism.	Unlikely.
Microminerals			
Iron (Fe)	Liver, organ meat. Oysters. Vegetable greens. Dried beans and peas. Egg yolk. Whole-grain or enriched products.	Formation of hemoglobin in the red blood cells. Carrying oxygen to body tissues.	Anemia, characterized by weakness, dizziness, loss of weight, gastric disturbances, pallor.
Copper (Cu)	Liver. Dried beans and peas. Meat. Nuts. Cereals.	Essential, occurs in all body tissues. Concentrated in brain, liver, heart, and kidneys. Necessary for normal absorption and utilization of iron.	Rare—severe malnutrition.
Iodine (I)	Seafoods. Iodized salt.	Formation of thyroxine, a hormone that controls metabolic rate.	Anemia. Enlargement of thyroid gland (goiter).
Fluorine (F)	Fluoridated water (1 ppm— one million parts of water). Plants and animals.	Formation of teeth. Resistance to dental caries.	Heightened tooth decay. *Excess amounts will result in mottled enamel.*
Zinc (Zn)	Meat. Liver. Eggs. Seafood.	Found in most body tissues, particularly liver, voluntary muscles and bones. Needed for several body enzymes.	Retards sexual development. Severely stunts growth.
Chromium (Cr)	Animal protein. Whole-grain products. Brewers yeasts.	Needed for normal glucose metabolism and a cofactor for insulin.	Disturbances of glucose metabolism associated with old age and/or pregnancy.

continued

Table 12-7	Minerals (continued)		
Minerals	**Sources**	**Important Functions**	**Deficiency Symptoms**
Manganese (Mn)	Nuts. Whole grains. Fruits. Vegetables.	Large concentration in bones. Present in pituitary gland, liver, pancreas, gastrointestinal tissues. Essential for normal bone structure, reproduction, normal function of central nervous system and enzyme action.	Unknown.
Cobalt (Co)	Liver. Kidney. Oysters, clams. Lean meat. Salt water fish. Milk.	Integral component of vitamin B_{12}. Needed for the function of all cells, particularly those of the bone marrow, nervous system, and gastrointestinal tract.	Rare.

Water

Water is the most abundant nutrient in the body. In fact, 65–70% body weight is water. Water is found in the plasma and lymph and surrounds each cell. Bone is one-third water; muscle is two-thirds water; and whole blood is four-fifths water.

Water is a critical and often forgotten nutrient, second only to oxygen as being essential for life. Humans can live longer without food than without water.

Functions of Water

In the circulatory system, water acts as a solvent (capable of dissolving other substances) for nutrients and hormones:

- It serves to transport waste products away from various parts of the body.
- It maintains blood volume.
- It serves as a catalyst in metabolic reactions.
- It acts as a lubricant.
- It regulates body temperature (perspiration helps to release excessive body heat and assists in the even distribution of heat in the body).

Water Sources for the Body

- Drinking water and beverages consumed
- Metabolic end-products of carbohydrates, protein, and fats
- Water formed through oxidation of foods

Water Balance

The distribution of water inside and outside the cells depends on adequate protein and balanced mineral intake. Sodium (salt) and potassium are minerals largely responsible for water balance.

- Body maintains water balance through respiration, evaporation at the skin surface, and urinary excretion.

Conditions Arising from Water Imbalance

- Excessive water loss, which leads to severe alteration in body function.
- Reduction of 10% in volume of body fluids, which results in dehydration. This is fatal if left untreated.
- Heat exhaustion as a result of water depletion occurs when replacement of water is inadequate, coupled with prolonged sweating.
- Liquid intake of coffee, tea, and alcohol are diuretics and cause water to be excreted by the kidneys.

Symptoms of Water Imbalance

- Thirst, fatigue, infrequent urination, and fever occur.
- Severe cases lead to delirium, coma, and possible death.

Excessive Intake of Water

- This may occur during exposure to heat.
- Adequate replacement of salt is lost through perspiration—it is essential to avoid salt depletion heat exhaustion.

Symptoms of Salt Depletion

- Fatigue, nausea, vomiting, exhaustion, weakness
- During periods of heavy labor or exercise, intake of adequate water and salt is recommended. One and one-half to two quarts of water should be consumed on the daily diet. The sodium content in prepared foods is generally adequate for sodium replacement.

Dietary Analysis

Dietary analysis is the primary tool used to determine the nutritional adequacy of a person's diet.

Limitations of Dietary Analysis

It is important to recognize the limitations of dietary analysis. There may be:

- Difficulty in getting an accurate recording of food intake
- Variability in food stuffs and nutrient contents
- Individual variations in the absorption of nutrients

The Diet Diary

A diet diary is used to gather information necessary to diet analysis. A person records everything consumed by himself or herself throughout the day. The entry should list all foods, both solid and liquid, as well as snacks. The entry should be specific as to what food was eaten, how it was prepared, the size of portion, and when it was eaten (Figure 12-3).

Water, black coffee, tea without sugar, and diet soft drinks (nonessential foods) should be included, but not extended into any food group. Coffee with cream and sugar is still considered a nonessential.

DIET DIARY

Name _____ Date _____ Day _____

Instructions

Details are important! Be certain to list everything you ate, how much you ate of each item, how it was prepared, and when you ate it.

Start each day with a new page. Use as many pages as necessary per day.

TIME	FOOD (Note quantity and how it was prepared.)

Figure 12-3 Diet diary.

The Diet Analysis

Use a prepared dietary analysis form (Figure 12-4), and do the following:

- List each food, and determine the food group in which it belongs.

- Compare the amount eaten with the amount allowed for a serving of that food. For example, one apple is considered one serving. If only half an apple is consumed, it would be listed as a half serving. If two apples were eaten, the amount would be listed as two servings.

- Total the number of foods eaten in each group during the day. Compare this with the number that should have been eaten. This will help evaluate how well the person did in meeting the needs of all food groups.

- Review the nonessential foods eaten.

- Look for excesses, frequency of intake, and amount of cariogenic foods consumed.

DIET ANALYSIS FORM

Name _____ Date _____ Day _____

FOOD EATEN	FOOD GROUP					CARIOGENICITY
	MILK	MEAT	F&V	B&C	OTHER	HIGH/LOW
TOTAL SERVINGS						

FREQUENCY OF EATING (times per day) _____
CARIOGENIC FOODS SCORE _____
BASIC NUTRITION SCORE

Figure 12-4 Diet analysis form. (F&V, fruits and vegetables; B&C, breads and cereals).

SUGGESTED ACTIVITIES

● Apply your knowledge of the four food groups. Determine the food group in which each food recorded on your diet diary belongs.

● Prepare a written plan for a well-balanced diet for one day.

● Determine the nutritional needs for one day (making an entry each time a food is consumed). Use a prepared diet diary form for the entries.

● Record all information on a prepared dietary analysis form. Evaluate the nutritional adequacy of the one-day diet.

REVIEW

1. In what area of the digestive system are nutrients absorbed into the body system?
   a. Stomach
   b. Duodenum
   c. Esophagus
   d. Large intestine

2. The first internal organ through which blood passes after leaving the small intestine is the:
   a. Pancreas
   b. Gallbladder
   c. Liver
   d. Stomach

3. Which key nutrient is responsible for building body tissues?
   a. Protein
   b. Carbohydrates
   c. Vitamins
   d. Minerals

4. Fats, oils, and sweets pertain to which food group?
   a. Meat
   b. Milk
   c. Nonessential
   d. Breads and cereals

5. What is the source of essential amino acids?
   a. Meats, eggs, cheese
   b. Grains, cereals, breads
   c. Carbohydrates
   d. Fruits and vegetables

6. Which vitamins are fat soluble?
   a. B_1, C
   b. B_{12}, folic acid
   c. B_6, biotin
   d. A, D

CHAPTER 13

Coronal Polishing

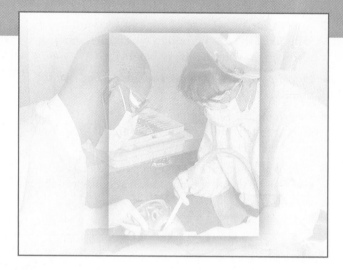

OBJECTIVES

After studying this chapter, the student will be able to:

● Give rationale for performing coronal polishing.
● Explain what selective polishing means.
● Indicate what specific areas of tooth structure should be avoided when coronal polishing.
● Describe which abrasive agents are used intraorally.
● Describe which abrasive agents are used in the laboratory.
● Explain how dental stains are classified.
● Give some examples of extrinsic stain.
● Describe how stains become intrinsic.
● Indicate how the patient is positioned for performance on the maxillary arch.
● Indicate how the patient is positioned for performance on the mandibular arch.
● Give the fundamental techniques for operator positioning.
● Explain the procedure for polishing teeth.
● Describe what the airbrasive machine is and why it is used.

Introduction

In some states it is within legal limits to have patients' teeth polished by a dental assistant who is licensed to perform this procedure. It may be the registered dental assistant (RDA) or the expanded functions dental assistant (EFDA) that would render this service.

Coronal polishing is meant only to remove plaque and extrinsic stains from the natural teeth; it does not involve removal of calculus nor does it take the place of a prophylaxis. To perform coronal polishing, the dental hygienist or dentist should have removed calculus from the teeth, and the gingiva should be in a healthy state, not bleeding.

Principles of Coronal Polishing

Teeth are polished for the purpose of removing plaque and extrinsic stain from the **clinical crown** (the crown portion of the tooth that is visible in the mouth) of the teeth (Figure 13-1). However, the operator must always

be alert to certain other clinical manifestations that might alter the manner of polishing. Other considerations that would affect the patient's health and well-being would be the presence of artificial joints or heart valvular damage requiring antibiotic premedication.

Rationale for Performing Coronal Polishing

● Prior to the placement of dental dam
● Prior to acid etching teeth for placement of orthodontic brackets or pit and fissure sealants
● Prior to fluoride treatment
● Prior to cementation of orthodontic bands
● After removal of orthodontic bands provided there is no calculus present

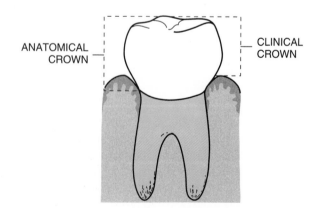

ANATOMICAL CROWN

CLINICAL CROWN

Figure 13-1 Clinical crown is the visible part of the anatomic crown.

Selective Polishing

Prior to polishing the teeth, an assessment to determine the areas of concern should be conducted. The operator should be aware that when polishing tooth structures for 30 seconds with pumice paste, as much as 4 **millimicrometers** (1 millionth of a millimeter) might be removed.

Therefore, certain types of dentition to be *avoided* are:

- Exposed cementum, softer and more **porous** (has more open spaces within the structure) than enamel
- Newly erupted teeth, incompletely mineralized
- Demineralized areas that exhibit white spots on teeth
- Teeth classified with amelogenesis imperfecta (thin enamel)

Abrasive Agents

The term **abrasive** pertains to hard particles with sharp or rounded edges that produce scratches when applied to a surface. The amount of frictional heat generated when using abrasives is directly proportional to the following, all of which generate more frictional heat:

- *Particle size.* The larger the particles, the more abrasive.
- *Quantity* of particles. The more particles, the more abrasive.
- *Dry powders.* Abrasive particles used to polish natural teeth are suspended in paste that act as lubricant and reduce the amount of frictional heat created by the act of polishing.
- *Rapidity* or circular motion plus abrasives. Slow speed must be used when polishing teeth. Refer to Chapter 32.
- *Excessive pressure* used with application. Light pressure is indicated for polishing teeth.

Abrasive agents are available in several grades and are used in accordance to their purpose. For example, some abrasive agents are used exclusively in the laboratory for polishing precious metals or acrylic materials. Other abrasives are used intraorally for polishing and removing stain on enamel surfaces and for polishing metallic restorations.

Abrasive Agents Used in Dentistry

- *Pumice.* Of volcanic origin, composed of complex silicates of aluminum, potassium, and sodium. Supplied in the following particle sizes:
  a. Pumice flour or superfine pumice—least abrasive used on enamel
  b. Fine pumice—moderately abrasive
  c. Coarse pumice—not used intraorally
- *Silex (silicon dioxide)*
  a. XXX Silex—fairly abrasive
  b. Super-fine Silex—used for enamel stain removal
- *Calcium carbonate (chalk).* May be used to polish intraoral metallic restorations.
- *Tin oxide.* Used on intraoral metallic restorations.
- *Corundum (emery).* Used in the laboratory:
  a. Aluminum oxide—used to polish porcelain restorations
  b. Levigated alumina, a fine powder—used to polish precious metals
- *Rouge.* Iron oxide, in the form of a fine red powder—used to polish precious metals in the laboratory.
- *Diamond Particles.* A paste made of diamond particles to be used on porcelain surfaces.

Abrasive Preparations

Abrasive preparations for the purpose of polishing natural teeth are commercially made and are available in different forms such as pastes, powders, or tablets. To meet individual needs, some are more abrasive than others. The more commonly used preparations are pastes, known as *prophy* paste, premeasured in sufficient quantities to polish one person's full complement of teeth. Pastes contain an abrasive of sufficient hardness to qualify as coarse, medium, or fine; other ingredients are water, a moistening agent such as glycerin, artificial sweetener, flavoring, and a binder to prevent separation of ingredients and spatter, usually agar-agar or sodium silicate powder. Fluoride is also added to abrasive pastes; however, this should not be considered an alternative to a fluoride treatment.

Dental Stains

Dental stains are classified according to source and location. Stains that develop according to location are either *extrinsic* or *intrinsic.* Stains that develop from a source are known as *exogenous* and *endogenous.*

- Extrinsic stains occur on the *external* surfaces of teeth and may be removed by mechanical means such as brushing, scaling, or polishing.
- Intrinsic stains occur on the *internal* surfaces of teeth and may not be removed by mechanical means.
- Exogenous stains develop or originate from sources *outside* of the teeth. They are extrinsic for the most part, but may become intrinsic by becoming incorporated within the tooth structure.

● Endogenous stains develop or originate from sources *within* the teeth. They are *always* intrinsic due to their incorporation within the dentin.

Extrinsic Stains

● *Yellow stain.* The appearance is a dull yellow exhibiting the presence of bacteria, occurring at any age. Located throughout the mouth, it is associated with the presence of bacteria due to uncleanliness.

● *Green stain.* May vary from a light or yellowish green to very dark green, usually occurring on the cervical third of maxillary anterior teeth. Seen primarily in children but could occur at any age. Enamel under the stain may be demineralized due to bacterial plaque exhibiting a rough appearance.

● *Black line stain.* Seen as a thin brown or black line located at the cervical third, pits, and fissures of all teeth except on facial surface of maxillary anterior teeth affecting primary or permanent teeth. More common in females and children, but could affect all ages. Generally, teeth are clean with lower incidence of decay.

● *Tobacco stain.* Varies from a light to dark brown or black. Found primarily on cervical third and lingual portions of teeth. Smokeless tobacco leaves heavy stains that may penetrate enamel and become an intrinsic stain.

● *Orange and red stains.* Appears as orange or red stain on the cervical third of teeth. Occurs more frequently on facial and lingual surfaces of anterior teeth. Thought to be caused by chromogenic bacteria.

● *Other extrinsic stains.*

1. Stannous fluoride imparts a light brown to yellow stain.

2. Chlorhexidine and alexidine mouthrinses used against plaque result in a brownish stain.

3. Foods/drinks such as coffee, tea, and soy sauce contribute to brownish stains.

4. Betel leaf, common in eastern countries, discolors teeth a dark brown to black color.

Endogenous Intrinsic Stains

When intrinsic stains occur, they are usually due to a breakdown of the pulp causing the dentinal tubules to be affected, transmitting the stain to the enamel, or the stain was acquired during tooth development. These types of stains are not removable by mechanical means. Bleaching is one alternative to stain removal; however, it may not always be satisfactory. Another alternative that has been effective is the bonding of composites or other materials onto the teeth.

● *Pulpless teeth stain.* The decomposition and bleeding of the pulp may cause the penetration of such substances through the dentinal tubules to the enamel, causing a wide range of dark colors to occur that make up the stain.

● *Tetracycline stain.* Appears as a light green to dark yellow or gray-brown band on all affected teeth. Teeth are affected according to the period of time and the length of time **tetracycline** (an antibiotic) was administered. If discoloration appears on primary teeth on a child, it would be assumed that the mother took the antibiotic in her third trimester of pregnancy. If discoloration appears on permanent teeth, it would be assumed that the affected person took the antibiotic during early childhood, at a time when formation of permanent teeth was occurring. It has been documented that the tetracycline antibiotic has an affinity for bones and teeth and is therefore absorbed by them.

● *Defective tooth development.* Several conditions fall in this category due to genetic or abnormal formation:

1. *Amelogenesis imperfecta.* This condition occurs when the *enamel* is not properly formed. The appearance of teeth is yellowish-brown or gray-brown due to the visibility of the dentinal color and the absence of the enamel.

2. *Dentinogenesis imperfecta.* A hereditary condition marked by imperfect formation and calcification of *dentin*, giving the teeth a gray to bluish-brown opalescence of the enamel due to the absence of dentin.

3. *Enamel hypoplasia.* Takes place when there was a short period of disturbance in the formation of enamel, causing the teeth to appear with white spots that usually discolor brown with food pigments.

4. *Dental Fluorosis.* Exists when excessive fluoride, more than 1 part per million (ppm), was systemically ingested during a period of time when *mineralization* of the teeth was occurring. Affected teeth erupt with white spots that later become brown due to food pigments. If the teeth were severely affected, they may exhibit cracking or pitting, also called **mottled enamel**.

Exogenous Intrinsic Stains

The teeth affected by stains that originate outside the teeth but that become a permanent stain within the teeth are termed intrinsic exogenous stains. Restorative silver amalgam materials, smokeless tobacco stain, endodontic therapy restorative materials, and certain drugs such as stannous fluoride or silver nitrate placed within the teeth are the primary culprits.

Polishing the Teeth

To polish teeth adequately, the operator should be familiar with all instruments, materials, procedure, and technique required for effective coronal polishing. Patient positioning and operator positioning are of great importance for easy access and comfort. Using the third finger of the hand that holds the instrument, the operator should establish convenient locations for **fulcrum** (a point of rest and support that provides stability) positions while holding the handpiece or instrument in the patient's mouth. A **finger rest** (a pivot point that allows the hand to turn and move the instrument) is also applied while fulcruming (Figures 13-2A to D). These elements are essential in providing:

● *Stability* by controlling the action of the instrument

● *Control* by providing a focal point to allow the hand to move as a unit

● *Injury prevention* by providing controlled movement that would disallow uncontrolled movements

● *Patient comfort* by giving the patient a sense of confidence and security in the operator's performance.

Positioning of the Patient

The patient must be positioned for easy access, plus patient and operator comfort. The operator will make final adjustments for the elevation of the chair and patient positioning for performance on the *maxillary* vs. *mandibular* areas.

● For maxillary arch, place the patient in a supine position so that the maxilla is perpendicular to the floor when the mouth is open.

● For mandibular arch, place the patient in a supine position with head slightly raised so that the mandible is parallel with the floor when the mouth is open.

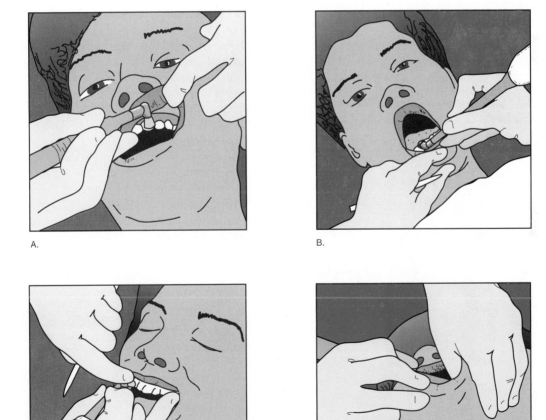

A.

B.

C.

D.

Figure 13-2 Fulcrum, using third finger. (A) Fulcruming on the same arch close to polishing area. (B) Using the index finger of opposite hand as a fulcruming point. (C) Fulcrum across the arch. (D) Extraoral fulcrum on bony surface.

Positioning of the Operator

The operator needs to be positioned in a comfortable, **ergonomic** (concerned with the design and structure of machines and facilities that contribute to the well-being of an individual's body), and workable place to deliver optimal care to the patient without self-injury or possible long-term debilitation; see Chapter 35. Some fundamental techniques are:

- The operator's chair should be adjusted at a height that allows the feet to be placed flat on the floor with the thighs parallel to the floor and the body weight centered on the seat of the chair.

- The backrest should support the operator's back, placing it in a straight, upright position supporting the head in alignment with the back.

- The position of the operator in relation to the patient, using the hands of the clock as a guide, are (Figure 13-3):

  1. For *right-handed* operators, the area of function primarily would be from the 8:00 to the 12:00 o'clock position with some deviations for special situations.

  2. For *left-handed operators*, the area of function primarily would be from the 12:00 to the 4:00 o'clock position with some deviations for special situations.

Coronal Polish Armamentarium

The Handpieces. When performing coronal polishing, the straight low-speed handpiece together with a right-angle (prophy angle) or a contra-angle handpiece is used (Figure 13-4). Right angles may be autoclavable or disposable. When the autoclavable type is selected, it will need to be heat sterilized and lubricated appropriately prior to reuse. Disposable-type right-angle handpieces already have rubber cup or brush attachments, minimizing cross-contamination.

Rubber Polishing Cups. Rubber polishing cups and brushes designed for the autoclavable handpieces are used only once and discarded after each patient to prevent cross-contamination. There are several types of rubber polishing cups: snap-on for the button-type right angle; threaded for the screw-on-type right angle; and latch type for the contra-angle handpiece. The shape and size of polishing cups may vary. Some cups are larger in diameter and fit over most of the crown portion of permanent teeth, while other cups are smaller in diameter and fit primary teeth and surfaces of teeth that have orthodontic brackets. Rubber polishing cups are designed to be flexible enough to flare while polishing in close proximity to the gingiva. They should be able to adapt to the contour of the tooth and carry enough polishing material to polish three teeth. If not used properly, they could abrade gingival tissues.

Prior to applying disclosing solution, the patient's lips should be protected with a nonpetroleum lotion to avoid discoloration of the lips. Use of petroleum-based jelly may destroy the operator's latex gloves.

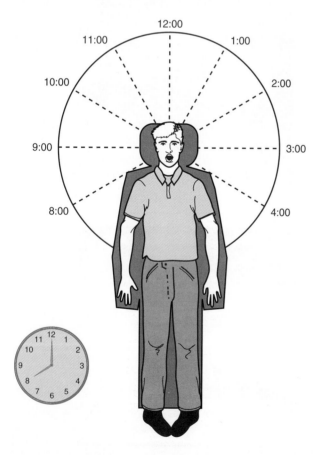

Figure 13-3 Using clock face; position of operator: For right handed operators from 8:00 to 12:00 position. For left handed operators from 12:00 to 4:00 position.

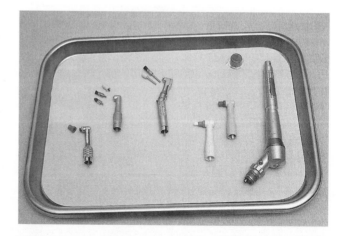

Figure 13-4 Handpieces. Autoclavable straight, right-angle, contra-angle, and disposable angles with rubber cups and brushes.

Disclosing Solution. Erythrosin red dye is most commonly selected, which is useful in disclosing the patient's teeth to detect where bacterial plaque is located. It may be applied to the teeth using a cotton-tipped applicator or by having the patient swish a few drops in very little water to coat the teeth. The excess is then suctioned by the saliva ejector or evacuator (Figure 13-5).

Prophy Paste (Abrasive). There are several from which to choose. The operator should evaluate the condition of the patient's teeth to determine if there is sufficient stain to select a *coarse* as opposed to a *medium* or *fine* preparation.

Bristle Brushes. Bristle brushes are used to polish and remove stain from pits and fissures as found on occlusal surfaces of posterior teeth. They are made of synthetic material and must be wet when used.

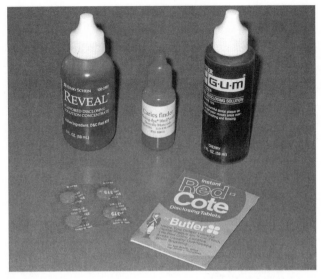

Figure 13-5 Disclosing solution used to stain the teeth.

Procedure 25 Polishing Using Rubber Cups

Materials Needed

Disclosing solution
Applicator tips
Nonpetroleum lotion
Straight handpiece
Prophy or right-angle handpiece
Assorted rubber cups and bristle brushes
Polishing agent (prophy paste)
Dental floss or tape
Air and water syringe
Saliva ejector/HVE
Infection central barriers
Personal protective equipment (PPE)

Instructions

1 Medical history and oral inspection are completed.

2 Procedure is explained to the patient.

3 Patient and operator are positioned according to stated criteria.

4 Disclosing solution is applied to the teeth for plaque detection. (Patient's lips should be protected with nonpetroleum lotion). (See Chapter 11).

5 Polishing should begin at the most posterior tooth of the quadrant and move forward toward anterior teeth.

6 The polishing cup is filled with polishing agent and distributed over approximately three teeth at a time.

7 The handpiece should be used at the slowest setting to avoid heat production and aerosolization of particles.

8 Fulcrum (finger rest) should be established intraorally on solid tissue such as teeth, not mobile teeth or soft tissue (see Figure 13-2A). If established extraorally, it should be on a bony surface such as the chin (see Figure 13-2D).

9 The handpiece should rest in the "V" of the hand between the thumb and index finger for operator comfort (Figure 13-6).

10 Pressure applied to the cup should be light, just enough to flare the edges of the rubber cup. The inner edge of the cup is used for polishing, not the center (Figure 13-7).

11 The stroke should be an intermittent wiping motion moving from the gingiva toward the occlusal or incisal surface with overlapping

continued

continued from previous page
Procedure 25 Polishing Using Rubber Cups

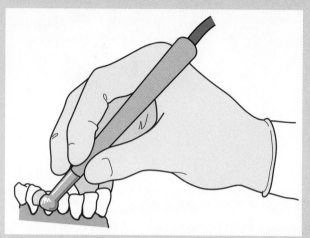

Figure 13-6 Handpiece resting in "V" of hand for operator comfort.

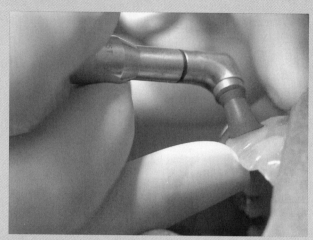

Figure 13-7 Rubber cup flared when applied to tooth.

strokes. Never leave the cup in only one area of the tooth for any length of time, as heat will be generated that may contribute to pulpal death.

12 A sequence of polishing should be maintained to avoid missing any teeth. The operator may use sextants or quadrants as guides.

13 When two polishing agents are used, two polishing cups are also used.

14 Polishing cups are discarded after each use.

15 Flossing is performed after polishing is completed. While prophy paste is still in place, dental floss or tape is used to polish the interproximal areas.

16 Teeth and gingival areas are flushed with water several times to remove polishing agent.

Procedure 26
Using Bristle Brushes

1 Soak the brush in hot water to soften bristles.

2 Carry the polishing agent on the brush and distribute over occlusal surfaces of posterior teeth.

3 When applying the brush on the tooth surface, take caution to avoid aerosolization of particles; therefore use the slowest speed to rotate the brush.

4 Finger rest, pressure applied, and the use of intermittent strokes follow the procedure for polishing cups.

5 Discard brushes after each use.

Airpolishing

This is known as an airbrasive, airabrasive, or air-powder abrasive machine that uses sodium bicarbonate particles together with warm water and air delivered with a force to the tooth surface using 65–100 pounds per square inch (psi) and water pressure of 20–60 psi. This procedure is used in removal of stain and heavy plaque (Figure 13-8). Several factors may be of interest:

● There is greater risk of cross-contamination due to increased aerosolization of particles. Therefore, it is wise to have the patient rinse with a mouth rinse to reduce bacterial count of the oral cavity.

● The patient should remove contact lenses and wear protective eyewear, hair cover, and complete coverall drape for safety precaution. Lips should be lubricated to avoid drying effect of the sodium bicarbonate.

● The operator should wear the usual protective clothing, gloves, mask, face shield, protective eyewear, plus hair cover for optimum protection.

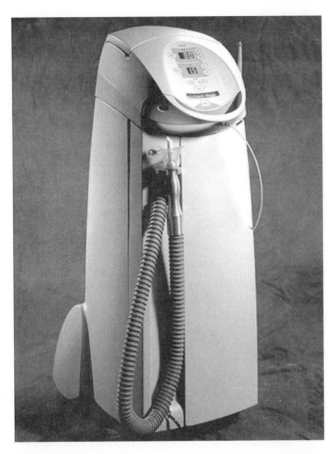

Figure 13-8 Air abrasive unit. May be used in removal of stain and heavy plaque (Courtesy of Midwest Dental Products Corporation, a Division of DENTSPLY International).

- High-volume oral evacuation should be employed due to the high level of aerosol production.
- Contraindications for use are:
  1. Patients with restricted sodium diet
  2. Patients that are afflicted by respiratory diseases that would limit their breathing and swallowing
  3. Patients that are known to have communicable infectious conditions that would infect the aerosol produced
  4. On exposed cementum or dentin
  5. On nonmetallic restorations such as composite resins where pitting or removal may occur

SUGGESTED ACTIVITIES

- Assemble the slow-speed straight handpiece. Affix the selected right-angle handpiece and rubber polishing cup.
- Select a polishing agent.

- Using a mounted typodont, position the mandibular for polishing.
- Observing the criteria, establish a fulcrum intraorally, making certain the straight handpiece rests in the "V" of the hand, between thumb and forefinger, and apply the polishing agent to the designated teeth. Follow the stated procedure; include flossing the mandibular arch.
- Reposition the mounted typodont for maxillary polishing.
- Follow the criteria for fulcruming, coronal polishing, and flossing.
- Using a fellow student as a patient, practice the following steps for coronal polishing. Position the patient in the chair, adjusting the backrest. Observe the criteria for position of the operator in relation to the patient. Apply fulcrums for maxillary and mandibular teeth. (*Note:* To actually polish the teeth, the patient must comply with all criteria of calculus removal and medical health status.)
- Complete all the stated criteria of the procedure in accordance with the guidelines.

REVIEW

1. Indicate three reasons for performing coronal polish: (1) prior to dental radiography, (2) prior to dental dam placement, (3) prior to acid etching for orthodontic band placement, and/or (4) after removal of orthodontic bands.
   a. 1, 2, 3
   b. 2, 3, 4
   c. 1, 3, 4
   d. 1, 2, 4

2. Dental stains located on the external surfaces of teeth that may be removed by mechanical means are termed:
   a. Endogenous
   b. Exogenous
   c. Intrinsic
   d. Extrinsic

3. What are dental stains originating from sources within the tooth called? Give an example.
   a. Endogenous; tetracycline
   b. Exogenous; pulpless teeth
   c. Intrinsic; yellow
   d. Extrinsic; tobacco

4. Selective polishing means that the following teeth should be avoided except:
   a. Newly erupted teeth
   b. Demineralized areas that exhibit white spots
   c. Endodontically treated teeth
   d. Exposed cementum

5. A point of rest and support that provides stability while holding the handpiece in the patient's mouth is termed:
   a. Focal point
   b. Thumb rest
   c. Modified pen grasp
   d. Fulcrum

6. For what reason is disclosing solution used?
   a. To ease the polishing procedure
   b. To stain oral tissues
   c. For plaque detection
   d. For calculus detection

7. To polish interproximal areas of teeth, one should:
   a. Floss interproximally while the abrasive material is in place.
   b. Use the bristle brush interproximally.
   c. Use a stimudent.
   d. Use a toothbrush.

Human Cell Structure and Function

CHAPTER 14

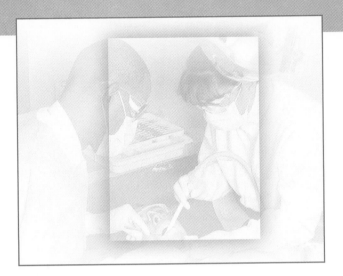

OBJECTIVES

After studying this chapter, the student will be able to:

- Discuss the role of genes in the development of body cells.
- Describe the sequence of cell division (mitosis).
- Describe the basic structure of human body cells.
- Discuss the role of proteins in cell development and maintenance.
- Describe the four basic tissues of the body.
- State the single most important substance of the body and its function.
- Discuss the development and life span of the red blood cells (erythrocytes).
- Discuss the development and life span of the white blood cells (leukocytes).
- Describe the human circulatory system.
- Compare the human lymphatic system with the circulatory system.
- Discuss antigen-antibody reactions as they pertain to immunity.
- Discuss blood clotting.
- State the difference between active immunity and passive immunity.

Introduction

The understanding of cell structure and function does not consist of learning a vast number of scientific names but in comprehending the process that is taking place in the body. This chapter is meant to be functional rather than anatomical. It is intended for those who have had no previous contact with **anatomy** (study of structures and parts of the body) and **physiology** (study of the functions of the body systems) and provides only a review for those who have. Microscopic descriptions have received little emphasis, as they are apt to be meaningless to one who has not himself or herself studied changes under the microscope.

Any study of human body systems must have a logical place to start. Having established that fact, the logical place to start is at the beginning, with the cell, the basis of life. The **cell** is a unit of structure, of development, and of function, both normal and abnormal.

Cells

Each human adult body, "that miracle of mechanical perfection," is composed of minute units of life, or cells, too numerous to measure. Together these cells give the body its appearance, shape, and form. Each human cell, except for mature red blood cells that lose their nucleus soon after their cell division is completed, has a potential capability of forming a complete human being.

The cells are controlled by **genes** (units of heredity), and every cell in an individual has the same set of genes. There are many thousands of genes within each cell, just how many is uncertain.

The genes are biologic blueprints that form and shape the body on a production line making identical cellular models, millions of them every day. In the internal world of the body, there are no new cellular models; each new cell is a replica of an old one.

Cell Division and Differentiation

All the cells of the body originate from a solitary cell created by the union of a sperm from the father and an **ovum** (fertilized egg) from the mother. This cell divides to create more cells that, in turn, divide and subdivide. The process of cell division is called **mitosis**.

The first cells formed by the fertilized ovum are identical. Then a complicated, almost endless, process called differentiation occurs. **Differentiation** is a series of changes whereby the cells acquire completely different individual characteristics. Thus, cells of different shape, size, and texture are created, each with a specific task. All the cells of the body become specialized in form and function, with the exception of the sex cells that are set aside at a very early stage of development for the purpose of reproduction of the race.

Cell Structure

Although cells may be highly specialized in their function, they all have the same basic structure. That is to say, they have an outer covering called the *cell membrane*, a main substance called the **cytoplasm**, and a **nucleus** (Figure 14-1).

The cell membrane is a very fine layer of tissue that regulates entry of raw materials into and discharge of waste material from the cells. Tissue comes from the French word *tissu*, which means fine gauze or weave. The cell membrane possesses membrane gateways or minute perforations through which substances such as oxygen pass into the cell and waste products such as carbon dioxide pass out. Cell membranes are capable of selection in the passage of substances into and out of the cell. This mechanism is termed diffusion.

Beneath the cell membrane is the cytoplasm (*cyt-* = "cell," *plasm-* = "basic material of the cell"), or cellular fluid. Cytoplasm is a watery gelatin like substance that gives the cell its bulk and provides the medium in which chemical changes occur.

The nucleus is the control center of the cell and influences growth, repair, and reproduction of the cell. The nucleus is where the blueprints of life are stored in a "library" composed of 46 chromosomes arranged in 23 pairs of different shapes and sizes. A **chromosome**, a large collection of genes, may be thought of as one volume in this library, and the genes as the pages that provide building instructions.

The cytoplasm and the substance of the nucleus are collectively termed **protoplasm**. Protoplasm is composed of water (75%) and protein (25%), along with various minerals. Proteins are any group of organic compounds (combined natural elements) containing carbon, hydrogen, oxygen, nitrogen, and usually sulfur and phosphorus. Proteins exist in the cell in the form of **molecules**, the smallest units of a compound.

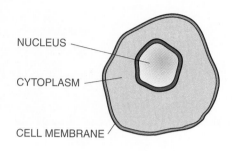

Figure 14-1 Structure of a cell.

Proteins, named from the Greek word meaning "first importance," are the chemical basis of life on earth. They account for about 12% of body weight and shape the characteristics of individual cells. Proteins also control the multitude of chemical changes taking place simultaneously within cells. None of the body cells can survive without an adequate supply of proteins.

Products such as hormones and enzymes are formed from proteins. **Hormones** are chemical messengers produced by cells of the body and transported by the bloodstream. Hormones regulate growth, the biologic clock, and basic drives and emotions. *Enzymes* are catalysts that stimulate biochemical reactions (chemistry of vital processes), without taking any direct part in them. Every cell contains several thousand kinds of enzyme molecules, all of which are essential for building up the cell, maintaining it, and helping it carry out its specific duties.

Proteins are formed by linking together hundreds of amino acid molecules. Twenty-three different sorts of *amino acids* (building blocks) are found inside the body, and all but 10 can be manufactured by cells. During digestion, the proteins consumed are broken down into simpler compounds (amino acids) with the release of energy and improved cell function. The *catabolic phase* (*cata-* = "down"; *bol-* = "food"), or chemical change that food undergoes, is also referred to as catabolism. The *anabolic phase* (*ana-* = "upward") converts the simpler compounds obtained from the nutrients into organized substances of living matter. This chemical change is also referred to as anabolism.

These two phases combine as the process of body metabolism. *Metabolism* (*meta-* = "changed, involving change") is the total of the complex physical and chemical processes involved in the maintenance of life.

Types of Cells and Tissues

The various types of cells that make up the tissues of the body possess the general features common to all cells; but each kind has, in addition, certain characteristics and specialized functions (Figure 14-2).

A. EPITHELIUM

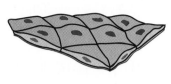

SQUAMOUS

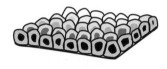

CUBOIDAL

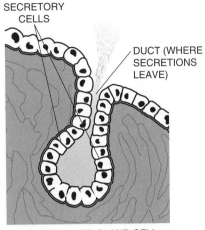

SECRETORY CELLS

DUCT (WHERE SECRETIONS LEAVE)

EXOCRINE (DUCT) GLAND CELL (SWEAT AND MAMMARY GLANDS)

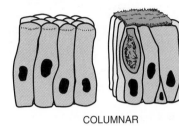

COLUMNAR

B. MUSCLE

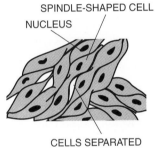

SPINDLE-SHAPED CELL

NUCLEUS

CELLS SEPARATED FROM EACH OTHER

SMOOTH

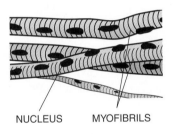

NUCLEUS   MYOFIBRILS

SKELETAL

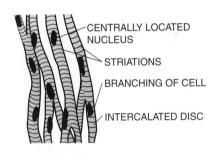

CENTRALLY LOCATED NUCLEUS

STRIATIONS

BRANCHING OF CELL

INTERCALATED DISC

CARDIAC

C. CONNECTIVE

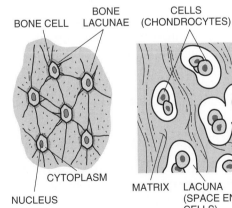

BONE CELL

BONE LACUNAE

CELLS (CHONDROCYTES)

FIBROBLAST CELL

CYTOPLASM

COLLAGEN FIBERS

CYTOPLASM

NUCLEUS

MATRIX

LACUNA (SPACE ENCLOSING CELLS)

CLOSELY PACKED COLLAGEN FIBERS

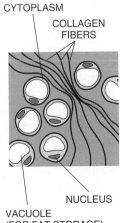

VACUOLE (FOR FAT STORAGE)

NUCLEUS

BONE   CARTILAGE   DENSE FIBROUS   FAT

(continued)

Figure 14-2 Common types of cells and tissues in the human body: (A) epithelium, (B) muscle, (C) connective, and (D) nerve.

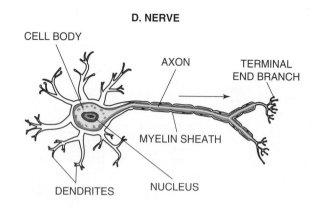

D. NERVE

CELL BODY

AXON

TERMINAL
END BRANCH

MYELIN SHEATH

DENDRITES   NUCLEUS

Figure 14-2 (continued).

Epithelium (Covering Tissue)

Epithelium is made up of cells that may be thin and flat, or tall, in the shape of columns, or varied shapes between the two (Figure 14-2A). Epithelium may be a single layer in thickness or it may be composed of several layers of cells. It covers the exposed surfaces of the body—the skin, the eyes, the lips; it also lines the cavities, the ducts (passageways) of glands, tracts, vessels and makes up linings in the interior of the body. It lines the digestive tract, the blood vessels, the abdominal and chest cavities, as well as the secretory cells of glands. Epithelial tissues serve to protect, absorb and secrete (to generate and separate out a substance from cells of body fluids). For secretion, there are groups of cells that have grown down from the surface epithelium to form glands. A **gland** is composed of a specialized group of cells that draws specific substances from the blood and alters them for later release. Epithelial tissue is characteristic in that one of its surfaces is usually "free", exposed either to the exterior of the body or to the cavity of a hollow structure.

Muscle (Contracting Tissue)

There are three varieties of muscle tissue: the *striated* or skeletal muscles, which move the skeletal parts; the *smooth* muscles of the internal organs and blood vessels; and the *cardiac* or muscle of the heart (Figure 14-2B).

Striated or skeletal muscle (voluntary) is composed of bundles of long, thin, cylindrical fibers arranged parallel to one another. Each fiber is an arrangement of several cells that are fused into a single unit; each fiber has many nuclei. Skeletal muscle is attached to bones, and the contractions of this muscle cause the parts of the skeleton to move.

Smooth muscle (involuntary) is so named because of the absence of stripes. The cells of smooth muscle are positioned with their cells lying parallel to one another, so that a contraction of each cell results in a shortening (and thickening) of the groups of cells in a particular tissue. Examples are muscles in the digestive

system that help in moving the food through the alimentary canal.

The **cardiac** (heart) muscle somewhat resembles the striated muscle but lacks the elasticity of the skeletal muscle.

Connective and Supporting Tissue

Under this heading are grouped a variety of cells of common embryonic origin. These tissues are characterized by the large amount of extracellular or nonliving materials they contain. The *connective tissue* proper is made up of cells somewhat resembling smooth muscle cells. These cells have the peculiar property of manufacturing long fibrous strands that make up the bulk of the tissue. These fibers are interlaced with one another, giving the tissue a tough, fabriclike consistency. The tissue also possesses a degree of elasticity that varies with the numbers of elastic fibers included in it. Connective tissue, as the name implies, connects the cells of the body to one another and binds together the tissues of all the organs. It is found almost everywhere in the body. It binds the nerve and muscle fibers of nerve trunks or muscles into compact bundles and holds together the cells of the internal organs (Figure 14-2C).

Bone and Cartilage. *Bone* and *cartilage* (gristle) are living tissues composed of living cells that are capable of manufacturing the extracellular rigid parts of the tissues. In the case of bone, this consists of calcium and phosphorus compounds. It is these cellular products that give bone and cartilage their properties of rigidity and strength, on which depend their more obvious functions.

Fat Tissue. Fat tissue is composed of specialized cells that have the ability to take up fat and store it—a single droplet within each cell. The bulk of the cell is simply inert fat, which has no ability to move or act, and is compressed into a thin covering wall surrounding the fat droplet. A number of fat cells are bound together in a more or less structural mass by connective tissue. Fat tissue is found especially under the skin, and much of it is located in and about a number of internal organs.

Nerve (Conducting Tissue)

The characteristic structural feature of nerve cells is the extension of long, thin processes from the main body of the cell. Bundles of these extensions make up the nerves of the body and serve as pathways in the brain and spinal cord. Nervous tissue is highly specialized with long hair-like processes and will instantly transmit sensation, depending on the degree of irritability or stimulation causing the response. It may be well to remember that a nervous system that is not irritable (does not respond to stimulation) is completely valueless (Figure 14-2D).

Water and Salt

The single most important substance in the body is water. An individual can endure hunger for days but will not survive without water. The water of the body dissolves salts to form electrolytes. An **electrolyte** is a substance that undergoes chemical change to form ions in solution. An ion has a charge of positive or negative electricity through gaining or losing an electron in the chemical process. Because of the formed ions, an electrolyte is capable of conducting electricity within the body.

Electrolytes in the body play an essential role in the workings of the cell and in maintaining balance in the fluids, or acid-base balance. An *acid-base balance* is a state of chemical balance in which the tissues of the body contain the proper proportions of various salts and water. A normal acid-base balance is a state of equilibrium (balance) between acidity and alkalinity of the body fluids. This acid-base balance is referred to as the hydrogen ion (H+) concentration or pH. An optimal pH between 7.35 and 7.45 on a scale of 0–10 must be maintained; otherwise, the body will not function properly.

The chief electrolyte ions are formed from sodium, potassium, and calcium salts. *Sodium* is a key regulator in water balance and is also necessary to normal function of muscles and nerves. *Potassium* is one of the main components of cell protoplasm. *Calcium* is essential for normal muscle physiology and blood clotting.

Sodium and chloride salts are found in large amounts in the fluid outside the cell (*extracellular fluid*). Potassium, magnesium, and phosphate salts are found in large amounts in the fluid inside the cell (*intracellular fluid*).

Blood

Blood is the body's internal transport system from major organs to every living cell. Blood is composed of cells and fluid. **Plasma** is the fluid, a faintly straw-colored substance, which consists of at least 90% water, with the balance in cells. Plasma accounts for 55% of blood volume and the cells for 45%.

Blood Cells

Erythocytes. Erythrocytes are produced in the red bone marrow and comprise the vast majority of oxygen-carrying cells (Figure 14-3). Because of the **hemoglobin** (red color of the blood protein) these cells contain, they are called erythrocytes (*eryth-* = "red"; *cyt-* = "cell"), or *red blood cells*. Hemoglobin is the principal protein in the erythrocyte. Hemoglobin picks up oxygen from the lungs and releases it to every living cell in the body. The blood's most important function is to carry oxygen.

Erythrocytes are biconcave disks, meaning that they have a rounded, hollowed-out surface on either side. They are the most numerous of any of the blood cells. During the early stages of formation, before they pass into the circulating blood, the red cells possess a nucleus, but the nucleus is lost before the cell becomes a functioning unit. In view of this, it may be more accurate to refer to these structures not as cell but as **corpuscles**, or "little bodies" (Figure 14-4).

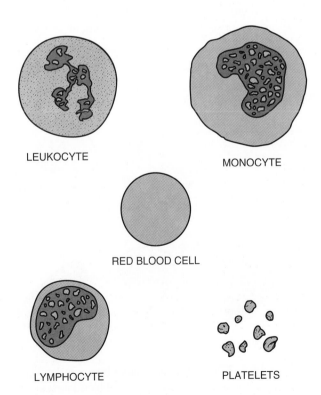

LEUKOCYTE

MONOCYTE

RED BLOOD CELL

LYMPHOCYTE

PLATELETS

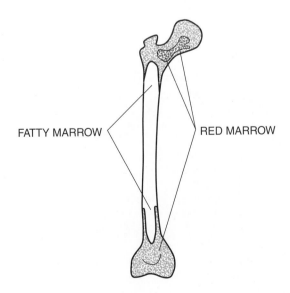

FATTY MARROW

RED MARROW

Figure 14-3 Cross section of the femur bone to show the large space in the shaft filled with fatty marrow and the ends of the bone filled with red bone marrow.

Figure 14-4 Blood cells in humans vary in size and shape.

Red cells possess remarkable elasticity and tend to bend and twist as they are forced through the smaller blood vessels. However, as soon as a larger channel is reached, they resume their original shape. The cell may reach a fork in the blood vessel and be bent by the stream on either side, then slide on and go back to its original shape (Figure 14-5).

The lack of a nucleus in the circulating red cells makes cell division impossible. Actually, the production of new red cells occurs outside the blood stream in the red bone marrow. Red cells are produced at the rate of 200 billion per day. Red cell production depends on a sufficient supply of iron and two main B vitamins, B_{12} and folic acid, in the body. (Refer to Chapter 12.) Deficiencies in these two vitamins occur as a result of poor diet or from failure of the small intestine to absorb them.

Red blood cells remain in circulation for about 110–120 days. If so, an individual red blood cell can make more than 40,000 journeys around the body in a month. Based on the average life of a red blood cell, it can be calculated that two million cells are destroyed—and formed—every second of our lives.

Leukocytes. Leukocytes (*leuko-* = "colorless") are semitransparent and contain no hemoglobin; they are referred to as *white cells* (see Figure 14-4). They are always **nucleated** (have a nucleus) even in the mature form and when circulating in the blood.

Leukocytes are formed in the red bone marrow, in the same regions from which red cells arise. It is thought by some scientists that in the development of the two

different cells, one becomes a red cell while the other results in a white cell. Whether or not this is the case, it is clear that red corpuscles and leukocytes differentiate in the same tissue, the red bone marrow. Although the circulating white cells contain nuclei, white cell division does not occur in the blood stream; they grow and multiply outside the blood stream.

White blood cells are larger than erythrocytes and lack the uniform structure of the red corpuscles. Seventy percent of all leukocytes have numerous small granules in their cytoplasm and are classified as *granular leukocytes.* Their estimated life span varies from 9 to 13 days. Unlike red cells that are simply carried along in the blood, white cells have freedom of movement. Rapidly activated by infected or injured tissue, leukocytes squeeze their way through the blood vessel walls and engulf foreign particles, such as bacteria.

Because the number of white cells increases three- to fourfold during infection, leukocytes are of major importance in a laboratory diagnosis of disease. White cells provide the body with a line of defense that is second only to the skin. There are several types of white cells, each programmed to perform a specific task.

Lymphocytes. Lymphocytes are termed *agranular white cells* (*a-* = "without") because they lack granules in their cytoplasm. Lymphocytes possess a single nucleus, a thin rim of clear cytoplasm, and a cell membrane (Figure 14-4). Lymphocytes are produced in the red bone marrow and develop in the lymphatic tissue, found in many regions of the body, for example, the tonsils and adenoids (Figure 14-6).

Lymphocytes are slightly larger than red cells and are concerned with immunity (protection against a particular disease) and combating infection. Lymphocytes

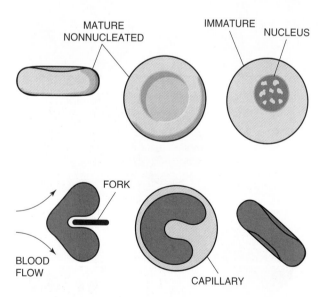

Figure 14-5 Red blood cells. Note how a red cell may be bent when it strikes a fork in a blood vessel or become twisted as it is forced through a narrow capillary, then resumes its original shape.

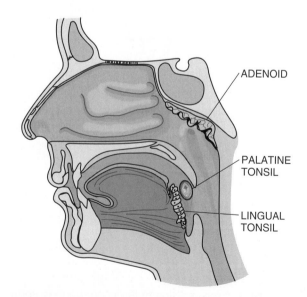

Figure 14-6 Tonsils and adenoids are composed of lymphatic tissue.

are said to be *thymus dependent.* The thymus is a gland-like mass of tissue lying on the midline of the upper chest region, beneath the sternum and over the heart. The thymus manufactures its own characteristic material (thymosin) that it releases directly into the blood and lymph system.

Platelets.   Platelets, also called **thrombocytes** (*thrombo-* = "clot"), are small platelike structures, the smallest formed elements of the blood. They are produced in the red bone marrow, have no nucleus, and possess a very thin membrane (Figure 14-4). Platelets tend to stick fast to damaged surfaces and help with the clotting of blood.

Blood Vessels

There are three major types of blood vessels in the body: arteries, capillaries, and veins.

Arteries.   Arteries are the vessels through which the blood passes away from the heart to various parts of the body. The wall of an artery is well jacketed, with three coats (layers) to withstand the high pressure of the blood flowing through them. The outer coat is white fibrous connective tissue, covering a middle layer of smooth muscle and elastic tissue. Beneath the middle coat lies an elastic membrane that is lined with a smooth

endothelium (inner covering). Together, these walls maintain pressure through the arterial system. The muscular and elastic tissues in artery walls ensure that the surges of blood from the heart are converted into a more steady flow (Figure 14-7).

Capillaries.   Capillaries are the smallest blood vessels in the body. These tiny vessels are the last link in the chain of delivery from the lungs to the cells. The blood stays in the capillaries, while oxygen and other essential substances are exchanged for carbon dioxide and other waste products. This exchange and just how it occurs is one of the miracles of biochemistry (the science of living organisms and of vital processes). It is known that the exchange is made through the capillary walls that are only one cell thick. Capillaries join with tiny veins known as **venules** that unite to form larger and larger veins.

Veins.   Veins are vessels through which blood passes from various organs to the heart, carrying away blood that has given up most of its oxygen. Veins, like arteries, have three coats: an outer, middle, and an inner. These coats are not so thick and collapse when the vessel is cut (Figure 14-8).

Blood is able to flow uphill through veins because of the valves inside them—two-flap valves—that operate rather like river lock gates. These prevent the blood from flowing backward (Figure 14-9). Cell waste is discharged into the veins for excretion through the kidneys or through the lungs. The veins take blood back to the heart and the heart pumps it to the lungs, where it receives fresh oxygen.

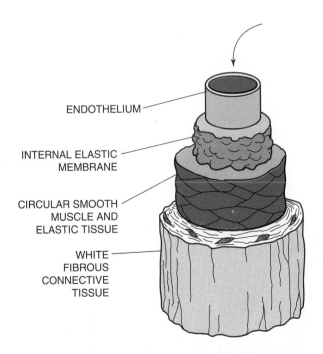

ENDOTHELIUM

INTERNAL ELASTIC MEMBRANE

CIRCULAR SMOOTH MUSCLE AND ELASTIC TISSUE

WHITE FIBROUS CONNECTIVE TISSUE

Figure 14-7 Structure of arteries. Well-jacketed arteries are able to withstand the high pressure of the blood flowing through them and to maintain pressure throughout the arterial system. [Source: Miller, B.F. & Keane, C. (1992). *Encyclopedia and dictionary of medicine, nursing, and allied health* (2nd ed.). Philadelphia: Saunders.]

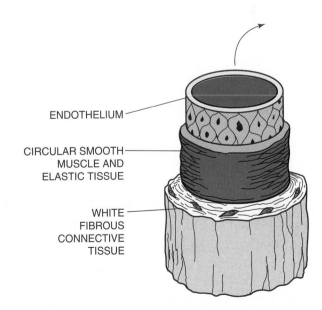

ENDOTHELIUM

CIRCULAR SMOOTH MUSCLE AND ELASTIC TISSUE

WHITE FIBROUS CONNECTIVE TISSUE

Figure 14-8 Structure of veins. Veins carry oxygen-depleted blood back to the heart and lungs and do not have to withstand the same pressure as the arteries.

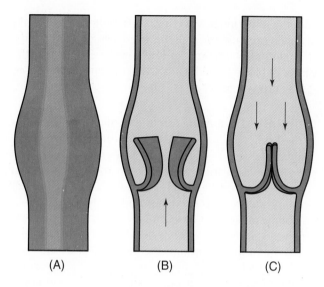

(A)   **(B)**   **(C)**

Figure 14-9 Veins have two-flap valves inside them to prevent backward flow of venous blood. (A) External view of the vein showing wider area where valve is located. (B) Internal view of open valve that allows blood to flow through. (C) Internal view of closed valve preventing backward flow of blood.

The Circulatory System

The fact misunderstood by physicians and philosophers until 350 years ago was that the body has a double circulatory system. William Harvey concluded that the blood moves in a continuous onward motion and direction from the heart to the arteries to the veins and back to the heart. But at some point, blood must pick up oxygen from the lungs. This means that blood returning from the body must be pumped to the lungs from the heart, and that is why the heart has four chambers, not two.

From the earliest of times our ancestors have realized the importance of the heart to life itself. It seems appropriate in any review of blood circulation that a brief consideration of the workings of the heart be made.

The heart is a hollow, muscular organ whose function is to cause the blood to circulate through the body. The heart lies within the thorax (chest region), enclosed in a sac of fibrous tissue called **pericardium** (*peri-* = "around"; *cardi-* = "heart").

Heart Structure

The heart is composed of muscles or **myocardium** and valves. It is completely divided by a septum (partition) into two parts, the so-called left heart and right heart. Each part is divided into two chambers. The valves, made up of extraordinarily thin membranes, or **endocardium**, also line the heart cavity. Although very thin, the valves in a healthy heart prevent even a single drop of blood from leaking through when closed.

On the right side of the heart the *tricuspid valve* divides the chamber into an **atrium** and a **ventricle**, (Figure 14-10). The tricuspid valve has three segments

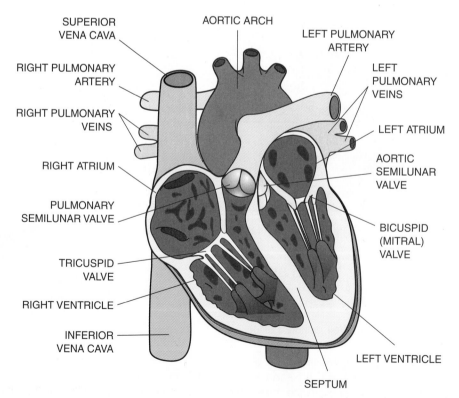

Figure 14-10 Interior of the heart.

or triangular parts (*tri-* = "three"; *cuspid* = "segment"). The atrium receives the venous blood from the body; the venous blood passes through the tricuspid valve into the ventricle. The tricuspid valve prevents any backflow of venous blood. The ventricle sends the impure blood to the lungs by way of the *pulmonary artery* (*pulmon* = "lung"). The mouth of the pulmonary artery is guarded by the *pulmonary valve.*

The left chamber of the heart is divided by the *mitral valve*, which separates the left atrium from the left auricle and regulates the flow of blood from one chamber to the other. The atrium receives the purified blood from the lungs, and the ventricles send the blood into the great artery, the *aorta.*

The aorta is the main trunk of the arterial blood system, carrying blood from the left side of the heart to the arteries of all limbs and organs, except the lungs.

Blood Circulation

Leading from the left heart, the aorta branches upward, backward, and then downward; this is referred to as the *aortic arch.* Along its course to the lower abdominal cavity, the aorta gives off *arteries* that branch into smaller and smaller vessels extending to all parts of the body (Figure 14-11). The smallest of the arteries are **arterioles**. **Capillaries** branch into the very smallest vessels of the arterial system. Capillaries unite with minute

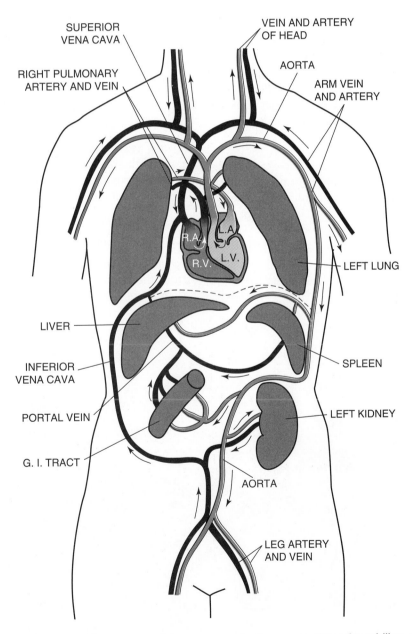

Figure 14-11   Circulatory system. The aorta and vena cava actually course along the midline of the body. Vessels containing oxygen-poor blood are in black. Arrows indicate direction of flow.

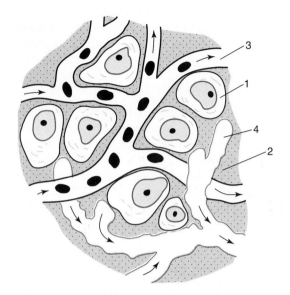

Figure 14-12 Tissue fluid bathing body cells: (1) tissue cell; (2) tissue fluid; (3) blood vessel; (4) lymphatic flow. [Source: Boyd. (1962). *An introduction to the study of disease* (5th ed.). Philadelphia: Lea & Febiger. After Rabin. *Pathology for nurses.* Courtesy of Saunders.]

veins, called venules, which, in turn, form larger and larger veins. The veins of the lower portion of the body empty into the *inferior vena cava.* The veins of the head and neck flow into the *superior vena cava.* These two venous channels empty into the right heart to complete the *systemic circulation.*

From the right heart arises the *pulmonary artery,* which soon divides into two, one for each lung. Each

pulmonary artery divides into smaller and smaller arteries that enter the lung via the *pulmonary capillaries.* These capillaries penetrate all parts of the lung(s), then collect into larger and larger veins, finally forming the *pulmonary veins,* which empty into the left heart. This makes up the *pulmonary circulation.*

The Lymphatic and Immune System

The *lymphatic system* makes up the secondary transport system of the human body. This functional unit is composed of lymph vessels, lymph fluid, lymph nodes, and spleen. The main function of the lymphatics is to drain the tissue fluids of the body.

As explained, blood carries oxygen and nutrients to the cells and waste products away from them. However, not all the plasma is reabsorbed into circulation. Some is left behind in the tissue fluid and is removed by the lymphatics.

Lymph Vessels

Lymph vessels, like blood vessels are distributed to all parts of the body. The lymphatic system does not have a continuous closed circulation but appears to have a closed end at the point of origin (Figure 14-12).

Lymph Capillaries

Lymph capillaries are thin-walled tubes that carry lymph from the tissue spaces to the larger lymphatic vessels (Figure 14-13).   Lymph vessels can be compared to

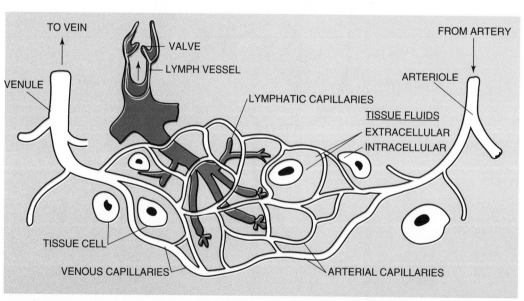

Figure 14-13   A capillary bed of arterial, venous, and lymphatic flow. [Source: Miller, B.F. & Keane, C. (1992). *Encyclopedia and dictionary of medicine, nursing, and allied health* (2nd ed.). Philadelphia: Saunders.]

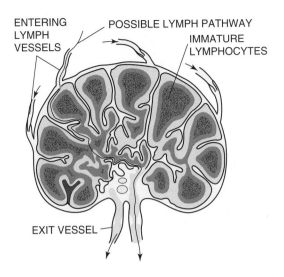

ENTERING LYMPH VESSELS

POSSIBLE LYMPH PATHWAY

IMMATURE LYMPHOCYTES

EXIT VESSEL

Figure 14-14 Cross section of a lymph node. Lymph flows slowly through a series of channels within the node. Certain of the white cells (lymphocytes) are formed in the node and added to the lymph as it flows through the node.

veins, in that they conduct the flow toward the thoracic region. As do veins, lymphatic vessels have valves to prevent the backflow of fluid. Small lymph vessels join others lying next to them to form larger channels.

Lymph Fluid

Lymph fluid is a clear, colorless liquid consisting of about 95% water and the remainder plasma. Lymph flows in the spaces between the cells and body tissues. When the plasma seeps through the capillary walls and circulates among body tissues, it is known as tissue fluid. When tissue fluid is drained from the tissues and collected by the lymphatic system, it is called *lymph*.

Since the tissue fluid is constantly being added to, there must be some means of escape. Excess tissue fluid, containing the waste products from the body's living cells, passes through the thin walls of the lymphatics and is carried away as lymph.

Lymph Nodes

Lymph then passes through a series of filters known as lymphatic glands or *lymph nodes* (Figure 14-14). Major lymph nodes are found along the medium-size lymph vessels at the knee, elbow, armpit, groin, neck, chest, and abdomen.

Lymph nodes act as filters to trap bacteria and other debris and vary greatly in size (Figure 14-15). Normal lymph nodes can be felt in the groin. Swollen lymph nodes may be felt in the armpit of an individual with an infected hand or in the neck of a person with

infected tonsils. It is in the lymph nodes that bacteria and other injurious agents that may have gained access to the tissue fluid are strained out and usually destroyed, (Figure 14-16). Larger and larger channels join in the left shoulder region in the thorax, near the heart. The lymphatics form one or two main ducts that open into the large veins of the upper body.

The Spleen

The *spleen* is located in the upper left quadrant of the abdomen, just below the diaphragm and behind the stomach. The spleen produces lymphocytes and monocytes that are important cells in the immune system.

The spleen also filters microorganisms and foreign debris from the blood. Other functions of the spleen include storing red cells, maintaining appropriate balance between blood cells and blood plasma, and destroying and removing worn-out red blood cells.

Immune Responses

The mechanisms of immunity are concerned with the body's ability to recognize and dispose of substances that it interprets as foreign or harmful to its well-being. When such a substance enters the body, complex mechanical and chemical activities are set in motion to protect and defend the body's cells and tissues.

The foreign substance, usually a protein, is called an **antigen**. An antigen may consist of soluble substances, such as toxins (poisons), foreign proteins, or particles of bacteria and tissue cells. The most common response to the antigen is the production of an **antibody**. The antigen-antibody reaction is an essential component of the overall immune response.

Antigen-Antibody Reaction

Antigen-antibody reaction occurs as the substance interpreted as a foreign invader gains entrance into the body. Any antigen, be it bacteria or foreign matter, induces the production of antibody that will affect only the specific antigen for which it was created.

Antibodies. Antibodies, also called *immune* bodies, are soluble proteins produced by the white cells. Most all antibodies are proteins. A fraction of the protein consists of gamma globulin. *Gamma globulin* is a specific protein developed in the lymphoid tissues in response to harmful agents. Gamma globulins are essential to the establishment of immunity, because nearly all antibodies contain gamma globulin molecules.

The antigen-specific property of the antibody is the basis of the antigen-antibody reaction that is essential to an immune response.

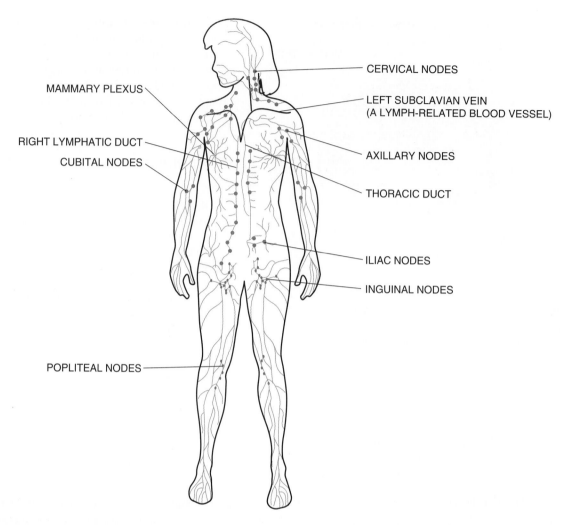

CERVICAL NODES

LEFT SUBCLAVIAN VEIN
(A LYMPH-RELATED BLOOD VESSEL)

AXILLARY NODES

THORACIC DUCT

ILIAC NODES

INGUINAL NODES

MAMMARY PLEXUS

RIGHT LYMPHATIC DUCT

CUBITAL NODES

POPLITEAL NODES

Figure 14-15 Major lymph nodes are found in the torso, head, neck, and armpits. Lymph nodes that drain infected areas of the body are liable to become inflamed and tender to the touch.

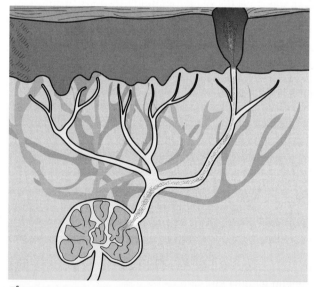

Figure 14-16 Prevention of the spread of bacteria. Bacteria enter the lymph vessels (white channels) and many are filtered out and destroyed in the lymph nodes.

Cells of the Immune System

Highly specialized cells are involved in the body's immune system. Along with *lymphocytes*, there are *phagocytes, macrophages, monocytes,* and *thrombocytes.*

Lymphocytes. Lymphocytes are cells with a nucleus but no granules in their cytoplasm. Lymphocytes adapt to the functions of the immune system.

T-lymphocytes, also called *T-cells,* originate in the red bone marrow as "stem cells" and are converted by the thymus (Figure 14-17). They are stimulated by thymosin, secreted by the thymus, before becoming circulating lymphocytes. Because of this stimulation, T-cells have a dual role; they control immune mechanisms and kill alien cells and organisms. *Helper T-cells* are a type of T-cell that stimulates antibody production in the B-cells.

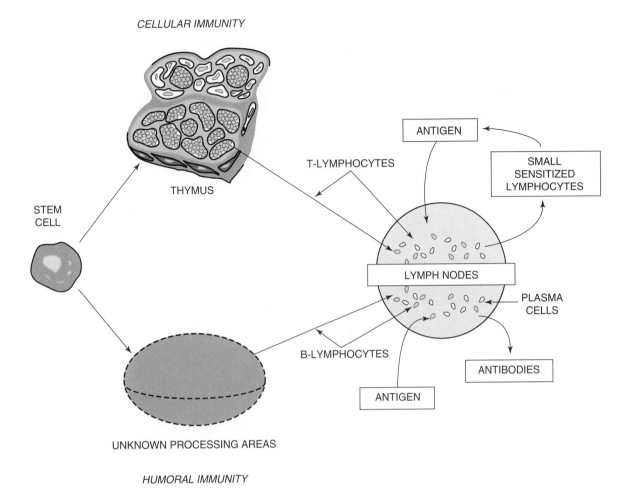

CELLULAR IMMUNITY

THYMUS

STEM CELL

T-LYMPHOCYTES

ANTIGEN

SMALL SENSITIZED LYMPHOCYTES

LYMPH NODES

PLASMA CELLS

B-LYMPHOCYTES

ANTIGEN

ANTIBODIES

UNKNOWN PROCESSING AREAS

HUMORAL IMMUNITY

Figure 14-17 Formation of antibodies and sensitized lymphocytes by a lymph node in response to antigens. [Source: Miller, B.F. & Keane, C. (1992). *Encyclopedia and dictionary of medicine, nursing, and allied health* (2nd ed.). Philadelphia: Saunders.]

Phagocytes. Phagocytes (*phago-* = "eating") are white cells, commonly referred to as "cell eaters," and the mechanism involved is called *phagocytosis.* The word element, *-osis,* means disease. These cells are found everywhere throughout the tissues. Like leukocytes, they normally collect in great numbers in infected areas. It is a scientific fact that phagocytes circulate through the system and eat diseased and dead cells (Figure 14-18).

Macrophages. Macrophages (*macro-* = "large") are large, highly phagocytic cells in the walls of blood vessels and in loose connective tissue. They are usually immobile, or *fixed,* but, when stimulated by inflammation, they become actively mobile, or *free.* When erythrocytes (red cells) are no longer useful, they are destroyed by macrophages in the spleen and liver. Macrophages are said to provide the janitorial services of the immune system.

Monocytes. Monocytes are phagocytic leukocytes that are formed in the red bone marrow and are carried

to other parts of the body, where they mature into macrophages.

Thrombocytes. Thrombocytes (blood platelets) are principally concerned with the clotting of blood and contraction of the blood clot. The clotting process is complex. The reactions involved in converting the fluid (blood) into a solid (clot) are always set off when blood vessels are ruptured.

When an injury occurs, the blood platelets collect on surfaces of the ruptured vessel and quickly disintegrate, and clotting begins. Apparently, platelets and tissue cells alike yield clot-inducing materials when they are injured. Both cells and platelets release similar substances.

Blood Clotting

Fibrinogen, a protein always present in blood plasma, is necessary for blood clotting. Another agent important to clotting is called thrombin. Thrombin (a catalyst) is

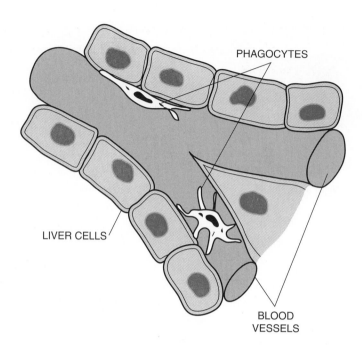

Figure 14-18 Phagocytic cells in the walls of blood vessels of the liver. These cells engulf and destroy worn-out red blood cells.

released by injured tissues or platelet disintegration and reacts with fibrinogen, converting it into *fibrin* (an insoluble protein). Entangled, interlacing threads of fibrin form a meshwork for the basis of the blood clot. Between the meshes, the formed elements (red and white blood cells) become entrapped in a solidifying mass. As it solidifies, the clot also shrinks, squeezing from the small spaces within the mass a straw-colored liquid known as *serum*. The great number of red cells give the clot its color but do not otherwise contribute either to the formation or the final internal structure of the clot. Red cells are simply caught in the fibrin meshwork.

Clotting is a plasma phenomenon rather than a blood mechanism.

Types of Immune Response

Cellular Immunity.
Cellular immunity, dependent on T-lymphocytes, is primarily concerned with a delayed type of immune response. These responses may be due to slowly developing bacterial diseases, viral infections, and tumor cells, such as cancer.

Some of the sensitized T-cells combine with an antigen, causing the antigen to become inactive. Other sensitized T-cells, with the help of lymphokines, destroy the antigen. Another protein called interferon is produced by the T-cells following a viral infection. Some of

the T-cells are transformed into "killer cells." Killer cells produce a chemical toxin that damages the cell membrane of the antigen, causing it to rupture and lose its contents.

Lymphocytes that have been converted into T-cells but are not used in the immune response may revert back to lymphocytes. If later they are needed to react with an antigen, they can become sensitized again.

Humoral Immunity.
Humoral immunity is a broad category of immune response that takes place in the body fluids (humors). *Humor* refers to any fluid or semifluid of the body. Humoral immunity is concerned with antibody and complement activity. *Complement* is a group of enzymatic proteins that are present but inactive in blood serum.

Active and Passive Immunity.
Individuals whose own tissues have produced the antibodies are said to possess *active immunity*. This immunity may be acquired by a person who had the disease and recovered from it. Immunity can also be induced by the introduction of weakened or dead antigens into the body. The latter is called *vaccination*. The vaccinated individual is said to possess *artificial active immunity*, because the antibodies of the blood and tissues have been self-produced with the help of an artificial antigen. *Artificial passive immunity* is acquired when antibodies are *borrowed* from another host, conferring temporary immunity.

SUGGESTED ACTIVITIES

● Compare the origin of erythrocytes, leukocytes, and lymphocytes and their functions.
● Compare the structural characteristics of the three major types of blood vessels.
● Compare active and passive immunity.

REVIEW

1. Match the term to its definition:

____ a. Chromosome   1. An element in the basic structure of a cell
____ b. Genes   2. Cell division
____ c. Nucleated   3. The smallest units of a compound
____ d. Mitosis   4. A large collection of genes
____ e. Diffusion   5. Also referred to as the basis of life
____ f. Differentiation 6. Cell changes whereby they acquire different characteristics
____ g. Cell   7. Units of heredity
____ h. Molecules   8. The mechanism whereby substances go into and out of a cell
____ i. Nucleus   9. Cells that have a nucleus

2. Indicate the three functions of hormones: (1) regulate growth, (2) help cells to carry out their duties, (3) maintain the acid-base balance of body fluids, and/or (4) regulate the biologic clock.
   a. 1, 2, 3
   b. 2, 3, 4
   c. 1, 2, 4
   d. 1, 3, 4

3. Which type of cell has the characteristic of being exposed to the exterior of the body or to the cavity of a hollow structure?
   a. Muscle
   b. Epithelium
   c. Connective
   d. Fat

4. Where are erythrocytes produced?
   a. Red bone marrow
   b. Liver
   c. Spleen
   d. Pancreas

5. Leukocytes are responsible for:
   a. Providing the body with defense against infection
   b. Regulating hormone levels
   c. Building tissue cells
   d. Regulating optimal pH

6. What does the term phagocytosis mean?
   a. A diseased phagocyte
   b. A forming phagocyte
   c. A phagocyte responsible for clotting blood
   d. A phagocyte that eats diseased and dead cells

7. The blood vessels that are able to withstand great pressure are:
   a. Capillaries
   b. Arteries
   c. Veins
   d. Venules

8. Antibodies are produced by the body in response to:
   a. Erythrocytes
   b. Leukocytes
   c. An antigen
   d. Gamma globulin

Bones of the Head

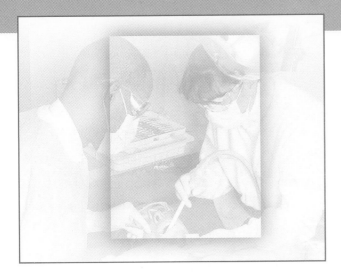

OBJECTIVES

After studying this chapter, the student will be able to:

- Name the two parts of the skull.
- Describe the shape and function(s) of the skull.
- Identify the eight bones that form the cranium.
- Identify the movable bone of the skull.
- Identify the bones that form the skeleton of the face.
- Locate the vomer bone.
- Name the smallest and most fragile bones of the face.
- Locate the four processes of the maxilla.
- Describe the function of the alveolar process.
- Locate and name the four bony parts of the roof of the oral cavity.
- Identify the median and transverse palatine sutures.
- Locate and describe the anterior palatine foramen.
- Describe the anatomy of the mandible.
- Locate the name of three processes of the mandible.
- Locate, then describe the mental protuberance.
- Identify and locate the two sets of foramina found on the mandible.

Introduction

The skull is divided into two parts: the cranium and the skeleton of the face. Since we are concerned with the teeth and the tissues that cushion the teeth in the skull,

it is necessary to become familiar with the entire skull in detail.

The skull is the bony framework of the head that rests on the spinal column. It is oval in shape and wider in the back (posterior) than in the front (anterior). The **cranium** provides protection for the brain and support for the structures attached to it. The 22 bones that make up the skull are irregular in shape and, with one exception (the lower jawbone, or mandible), are immovably joined. Where two bones are joined with a seam, the line formed is termed a **suture**. Sutures are identified by the region where the bones are joined, such as coronal suture (the line formed by the frontal and two parietal bones in the crown; **corona** = "of the head").

The skull consists of three parts:

- The cranium, which is composed of 8 bones that contain and protect the brain
- The face, which is composed of 13 bones
- The mandible, which is composed of 1 bone

Cranium

Eight bones form the cranium (Figure 15-1):

- Frontal
- Parietal (two)
- Temporal (two)
- Sphenoid
- Ethmoid
- Occipital

The *frontal* bone forms the forehead, a portion of the roof of the eye sockets, or orbits, and part of the nasal cavity. The orbits are the irregular, cone-shaped cavities in which the eyes are located. The arch formed by the frontal bone over the eyes is thick, sharp, and prominent. It protects the eyes and is called the supraorbital margin (**supra** = "over"; *orbital* = "the eyes"; *margin* "the ridge"). The frontal **sinuses** (large hollow spaces) are located just above the supraorbital margins.

The two *parietal* bones (right and left) form the greater part of the sides and roof of the skull (**parietal-**

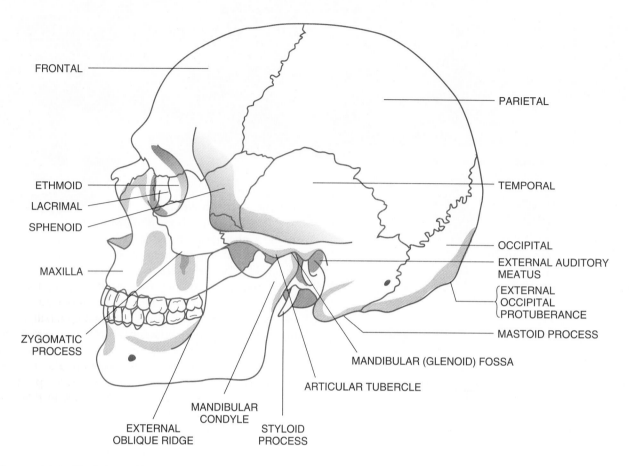

FRONTAL

PARIETAL

ETHMOID

LACRIMAL

SPHENOID

TEMPORAL

OCCIPITAL

EXTERNAL AUDITORY MEATUS

MAXILLA

EXTERNAL OCCIPITAL PROTUBERANCE

MASTOID PROCESS

ZYGOMATIC PROCESS

MANDIBULAR (GLENOID) FOSSA

ARTICULAR TUBERCLE

MANDIBULAR CONDYLE

EXTERNAL OBLIQUE RIDGE

STYLOID PROCESS

Figure 15-1 Skull, lateral aspect.

"forming the walls of a cavity"—in this case, the walls of the skull cavity). Each parietal bone is irregularly four sided in shape with its external surface convex and its internal surface concave.

The *temporal* bones (right and left) form the sides and base of the skull. Each temporal bone is bounded in front by the sphenoid bone, above by the parietal, and in back by the occipital. Each temporal bone has a pit or depression, called the mandibular or glenoid fossa (**glenoid** = "shallow or slightly cupped"), into which the lower jawbone, or mandible, fits, thus allowing movement of the mandible (Figure 15-1). The sharp projection on the undersurface of the temporal bone is the styloid process (**styloid** = "slender and pointed"; *process* = "prominence or outgrowth"), see Figure 15-1. The rounded projection at the back of the temporal bone is the mastoid process, a bony projection behind the external ear. The temporal bone also contains the external auditory canal, or external auditory meatus, and the middle and inner ear.

The *sphenoid* bone (**sphenoid** = "wedge shaped") is situated at the anterior (front) portion of the base of the skull. It is shaped somewhat like a bat with its wings outspread and its body joined to the occipital bone in

the back and to the ethmoid bone in the front. Air spaces in the body are the sphenoid sinuses, which connect with the nasopharynx, as do the other sinuses of the skull. At the center of the sphenoid, a cradlelike structure, the **sella turcica**, which cradles the pituitary gland, is found. The wings of the sphenoid bone extend downward and are identified as the pterygoid process (**pterygoid** = "wing shaped"; *process* = "projection"). Two pterygoid plates are located at its inferior aspect, the lateral and medial. From the medial plate, the **hamulus**, a spiny projection, is found (Figure 15-2).

The *ethmoid* bone is a thin bone at the anterior base of the cranium. It is located between the orbits, and helps form the roof, sides, and septum of the nose. The bone is very light and spongy, or honeycombed. The air spaces in the side (lateral) portions of the bone are the ethmoid sinuses (Figure 15-3).

The *occipital* bone is located at the back and base of the skull (**occiput** = "back part of the head"). It is characterized by a large opening called the foramen magnum (**foramen** = "opening or hole"; *magnum* = "large"). Through the foramen magnum pass the spinal cord, spinal nerves, and vertebral arteries. If you feel the back of your scalp, you can note a projection or protuberance.

This is midway between the top of the occipital bone and the foramen magnum. It is called the external occipital **protuberance** (rounded projection).

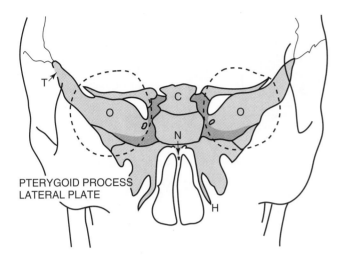

Figure 15-2 Sphenoid bone, showing pterygoid process and surfaces of bone: T = temporal; O = orbital; C = cranial; N = nasal; H = hamulus.

Bones of the Face

There are 14 bones that form the skeleton of the face:

- Nasal bone (two)
- Vomer
- Inferior nasal conchae (two)
- Lacrimal bone (two)
- Maxillae (two)
- Zygomatic bone (two)
- Palatine bone (two)
- Mandible

The facial bones are identifiable in Figure 15-4.

The *nasal* bone consists of two small, oblong bones placed side by side to form the bridge of the nose. They are situated at the middle and upper part of the face and lie close to the upper part of the maxillae.

The *vomer* is a single bone within the nasal cavity. It is found at the lower and back part of the nasal cavity and forms a part of the nasal septum (the partition between the two nasal chambers). The interior portion is usually bent to one side or another, making the nasal chambers of unequal size.

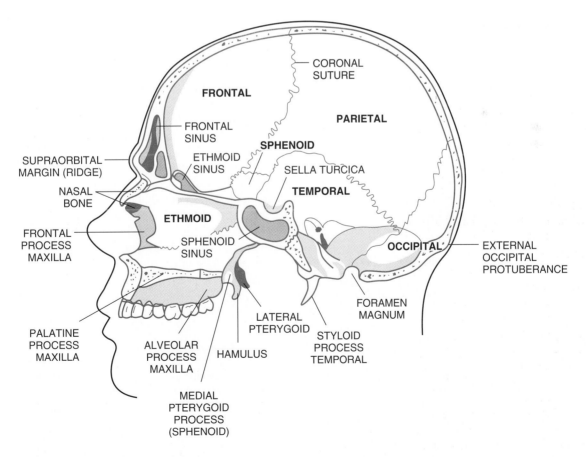

Figure 15-3 Cranium (cross section).

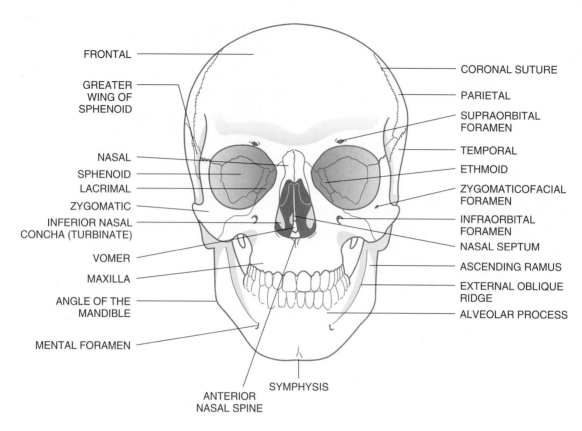

FRONTAL

GREATER
WING OF
SPHENOID

NASAL
SPHENOID
LACRIMAL
ZYGOMATIC
INFERIOR NASAL
CONCHA (TURBINATE)

VOMER

MAXILLA

ANGLE OF THE
MANDIBLE

MENTAL FORAMEN

CORONAL SUTURE

PARIETAL

SUPRAORBITAL
FORAMEN

TEMPORAL

ETHMOID

ZYGOMATICOFACIAL
FORAMEN

INFRAORBITAL
FORAMEN

NASAL SEPTUM

ASCENDING RAMUS

EXTERNAL OBLIQUE
RIDGE

ALVEOLAR PROCESS

ANTERIOR
NASAL SPINE

SYMPHYSIS

Figure 15-4 Skull, anterior aspect.

Situated on the outer wall of each nostril are the inferior nasal conchae, also known as turbinate. Each consists of a thin layer of cancellous bone (**cancellous** = "spongy, having a latticelike structure"). This bone appears to be curled on itself to resemble a scroll, or spiral coiled form.

The *lacrimal* bones (**lacrimal** = pertaining to tears) are found at the front part of the inner wall of each orbit. They are the smallest and most fragile bones of the face. They resemble a fingernail in form, thickness, and size. A part of the tear duct passes through a canal in the lacrimal bone.

The *maxilla* (maxillary arch) is formed by the union of the two maxillae. It helps to establish the boundaries of the roof of the mouth, the floor and outer walls of the nose, and the floor of each orbit. The maxilla is the largest bone of the upper face and is often referred to as the upper jaw. Each maxilla has a body (the main mass of the bone) and four processes. The body resembles a pyramid, and within its thin walls is a large cavity, the **maxillary sinus** (antrum of Highmore). On the lower part of the posterior surface of the body is the maxillary **tuberosity** (a rounded prominence or projection).

The four processes of the maxilla are named as follows: zygomatic, palatine, frontal, and alveolar. The zygomatic process joins the zygomatic bone to form the zygomatic arch, thus making up the cheek bone. The palatine process joins the opposing palatine process at the palatine suture to form the front part of the floor of the nasal cavity and the roof of the mouth. The frontal process extends upward and backward along the side of the nose. The alveolar process extends downward from the body of the maxilla. The sockets for the maxillary teeth are found in the alveolar process of the maxilla.

The *palatine* bones are L shaped and are in the back part of the nasal cavity. They help form the roof of the mouth, the floor and outer walls of the nasal cavities, and the floor of each orbit. The vertical portion of the palatine bones extends to the orbit, and the horizontal part helps form the floor of the nasal cavity and the roof of the mouth.

The Hard Palate

The oral cavity is only partially surrounded by bones. The lateral and interior walls are formed by the inner surface of the alveolar processes and join at the midline. The inner (lingual) surfaces of the teeth complete these walls.

The roof of the oral cavity (Figure 15-5) is formed by the hard palate, which consists of four bony parts.

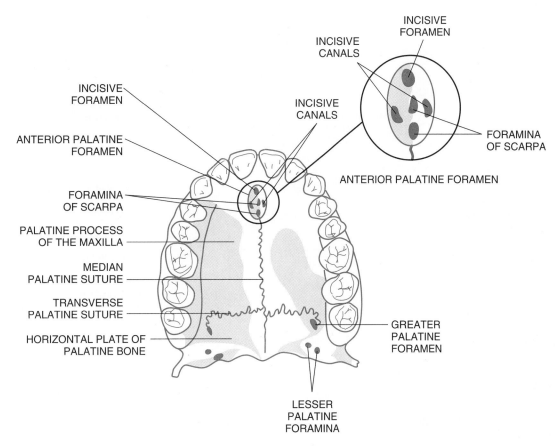

INCISIVE
FORAMEN

INCISIVE
CANALS

INCISIVE
CANALS

INCISIVE
FORAMEN

FORAMINA
OF SCARPA

ANTERIOR PALATINE FORAMEN

INCISIVE
FORAMEN

ANTERIOR PALATINE
FORAMEN

FORAMINA
OF SCARPA

PALATINE PROCESS
OF THE MAXILLA

MEDIAN
PALATINE SUTURE

TRANSVERSE
PALATINE SUTURE

HORIZONTAL PLATE OF
PALATINE BONE

GREATER
PALATINE
FORAMEN

LESSER
PALATINE
FORAMINA

Figure 15-5 Palatine bone with sutures and foramina.

These include the palatine processes of the maxillae and the horizontal plates of the palatine bones. Between the bones of the right and left halves of the palate is found the median palatine suture; between the maxillae and the palatine bones, the transverse palatine suture (**transverse** = "a process that projects across the palate"). The bony processes are joined together by means of this cross-shaped suture.

At the midline, immediately behind the incisors, is the opening of the incisal or anterior palatine foramen. It appears to be funnel shaped and serves as a common opening for the two incisive canals, two foramina of Scarpa, and the incisive foramen. The incisive foramen is the most anterior of the group. Posterior to the incisive foramen are two foramina, situated at the median line, called the foramina of Scarpa. Located laterally to the anterior palatine suture are the incisive canals.

Close to the posterior border of the hard palate and near the transverse palatine suture are other openings in the bone. Each palatine bone has three foramina. Just lingual to the third molar area is the greater palatine foramen. Behind this are found two smaller or lesser palatine foramina.

The Mandible

The *mandible* is the only bone of the skull that is movable; it is the longest and strongest bone of the face. The mandible is sometimes referred to as the lower jaw. It consists of a body, a curved horizontal bone, and two perpendicular portions, the ascending **rami** (ramus, singular) branch. The rami unite with the ends of the body, forming the angle of the mandible. The upper border of each ramus presents two distinct processes: the coronoid process on the anterior and the condyloid process on the posterior. The posterior process is sometimes referred to as the mandibular condyle (a condyle is a round projection at the end of a bone that fits into a depression on another bone). The condyloid process consists of a neck and a condyle. The condyle of the mandible normally rests in the mandibular (glenoid) fossa of the temporal bone. Between the coronoid and the condyloid processes is the sigmoid notch (or mandibular notch). It is a saddlelike depression in the bone (Figure 15-6).

The body is curved somewhat like a horseshoe with its external surface concave (possessing a curved, depressed surface). There is a thick ridge at the median

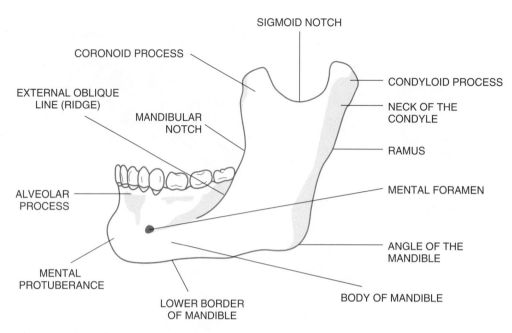

Figure 15-6 Mandible, lateral aspect.

line. This ridge, or **symphysis**, is the line of fusion where the two distinct bones of the mandible blend together into one. The symphysis divides below and fuses with the lower border of the mandible to enclose a triangular projection called the mental protuberance (**mental** = "pertaining to the chin"). From either side of the mental protuberance a ridge extends backward and upward and is continuous with the anterior border of the ramus. This ridge is called the external oblique line or ridge (**oblique** = "on a slant, neither perpendicular nor horizontal"), see Figure 15-7.

The superior border of the body contains the **alveoli** (sockets for the teeth) and is called the alveolar process. Each alveolar process is composed of two compact bony plates known as **cortical plates**: the external [buccal or labial (buccal = "the cheek"; labial = "the lips")] and internal (**lingual**), or the surface nearest the tongue. Joining these surfaces are partitions, or **septa**, that make up the sides of the alveoli.

Foramina of the Skull

On the face of the skull are several important foramina. Above the eye orbits are the supraorbital foramina (*supra* = "above"); under the orbits of the eye on the maxilla are the infraorbital foramina (**infra** = "inferior or below"). On the zygomatics are the zygomaticofacial foramina (Figure 15-4). The incisive or anterior palatine foramen found just behind the maxillary central incisors includes the incisive foramen, incisive canals, and

foramina of Scarpa. On the posterior part of the palate are the lesser palatine foramina and the greater palatine foramina. On the lateral surface of the mandible are the mental foramina (Figure 15-6). On the lingual surface of the mandible (next to the tongue) are the mandibular foramina (Figure 15-7), and at the midline at the center of the mandible, the lingual foramen.

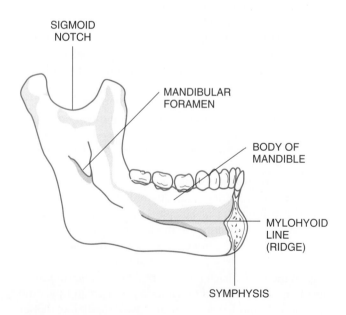

Figure 15-7 Mandible, medial aspect.

SUGGESTED ACTIVITIES

● Using a skull, identify the eight bones that form the cranium.

● Locate, then identify, the bones that form the skeleton of the face.

● Locate, then identify, the four processes of the maxilla.

● Locate the two sets of mandibular foramina. Name them.

REVIEW

1. Identify the lettered parts of the illustration. Select from the following list:
   1. Occipital
   2. Temporal
   3. Styloid process
   4. Sphenoid
   5. Ethmoid
   6. External auditory meatus
   7. Frontal
   8. Mandibular condyle
   9. Parietal
   10. Mandibular (glenoid) fossa
   11. Mastoid process

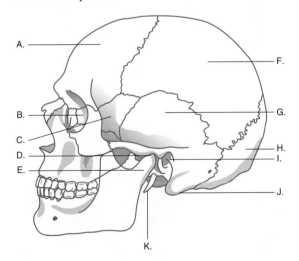

   a. _____
   b. _____
   c. _____
   d. _____
   e. _____
   f. _____
   g. _____
   h. _____
   i. _____
   j. _____
   k. _____

2. A marked prominence or projection of the bone is termed:
   a. Fossa
   b. Process
   c. Suture
   d. Conchae

3. The hamulus is a projection that extends downward from the:
   a. Temporal bone
   b. Maxillary process
   c. Palatine process
   d. Pterygoid process

4. A foramen is defined as:
   a. An opening or hole
   b. A rounded projection
   c. A shallow depression
   d. A slender pointed process

5. The four processes of the maxilla are:
   a. Styloid, frontal, pterygoid, palatine
   b. Alveolar, frontal, zygomatic, pterygoid
   c. Zygomatic, palatine, frontal, alveolar
   d. Frontal, alveolar, pterygoid, palatine

6. On which bone is the external auditory meatus located?
   a. Parietal
   b. Temporal
   c. Maxillary
   d. Sphenoid

7. On which bone are the mental foramina located?
   a. Mandibular
   b. Frontal
   c. Zygomatic
   d. Sphenoid

8. Name the term pertaining to the chin.
   a. Protuberance
   b. Glenoid
   c. Mastoid
   d. Mental

9. Name the term that means wall or partition, which separates two chambers.
   a. Suture
   b. Septa
   c. Foramen
   d. Symphysis

10. Name the two processes located at the superior portion of the mandibular bone.
    a. Sigmoid, ramus
    b. Mental, symphysis
    c. Condyle, coronoid
    d. Mylohyoid, mandibular

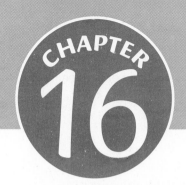
CHAPTER 16

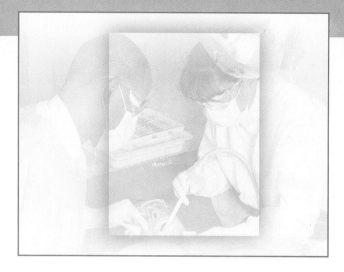

OBJECTIVES

After studying this chapter, the student will be able to:

- Locate and name the air cells of the anterior group of paranasal sinuses.
- Locate and name the air cells of the posterior group of paranasal sinuses.
- Identify the largest of the paranasal sinuses.
- Discuss the various sizes and shapes of the sinuses.
- List the functions of the paranasal sinuses.

Introduction

Air cavities in the bones above and on each side of the nasal cavities are termed paranasal sinuses. They vary in shape and size in individuals and are normally lined with a mucous membrane that is continuous with that of the nasal cavities (Figure 16-1).

Groups of Sinuses

The air cells of the nose are the frontal, ethmoidal, sphenoidal, and maxillary. They are named after the bones in which they are located and consist of two groups:

1. Anterior group, or those opening into the middle meatus (opening or passage) of the nose:
   - Maxillary sinus (antrum of Highmore)
   - Frontal sinus
   - Anterior and middle ethmoid cells
2. Posterior group
   - Sphenoidal sinus (opens into the sphenoethmoidal recess)
   - Posterior ethmoid cells (open into the superior meatus)

Anterior Group

Maxillary Sinus. This is a pyramid-shaped cavity in the body of the maxilla and is the largest accessory sinus of the nose. The base is formed by the lateral wall of the nasal cavity, and its apex extends into the zygomatic process. The size of the sinus varies from side to side in the individual but is situated usually below the floor of the nose. In some cases, the floor is perforated with the apical portion of some of the maxillary teeth. The roof of

the maxillary sinus is often ridged with elevations of the infraorbital canal (Figure 16-2).

Frontal Sinus. The frontal sinus is situated behind the superciliary arch (above the eyebrow). Such a cavity is rarely symmetrical because of the placement of the septum. It drains through the frontonasal duct into the main cavity of the middle meatus and opens from either the right or left, according to its lateral position.

Anterior and Middle Ethmoid Cells. Ethmoid cells consist of a number of thin-walled cavities and are

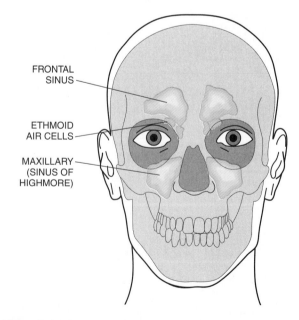

Figure 16-1 Paranasal sinuses, front cross-sectional view.

FRONTAL SINUS

ETHMOID AIR CELLS

MAXILLARY (SINUS OF HIGHMORE)

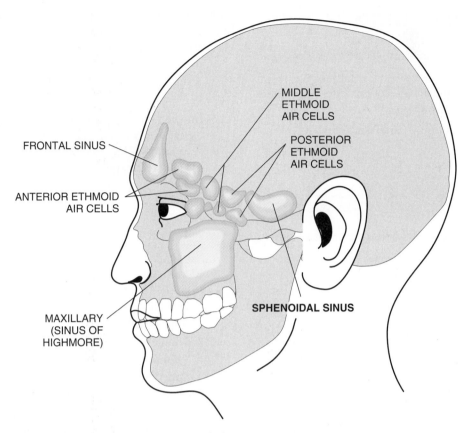

FRONTAL SINUS

ANTERIOR ETHMOID
AIR CELLS

MIDDLE
ETHMOID
AIR CELLS

POSTERIOR
ETHMOID
AIR CELLS

MAXILLARY
(SINUS OF
HIGHMORE)

SPHENOIDAL SINUS

Figure 16-2 Paranasal sinuses, side cross-sectional view.

situated between the upper parts of the nasal sinuses and orbits. They are separated from these cavities by thin bony plates.

Posterior Group

Sphenoidal Sinuses. Contained within the body of the sphenoid, the sphenoidal sinuses vary in shape and size and, as in the case of other sinuses, are rarely symmetrical. If they are exceptionally large, they may extend into the great wing of the sphenoid or the roots of the pterygoid process; they may also enter the base of the occipital bone. An opening is found in the superior part of the anterior wall of sphenoidal sinuses.

Posterior Ethmoid Cells. The posterior ethmoid cells open into the superior meatus under the superior nasal concha. They may, in some cases, connect with the sphenoidal sinus.

Functions

1. Reduce the weight of the skull.

2. Give resonance to the voice.

3. Act as reserve chambers for warm air during the physiologic process of respiration. During inspiration, the warmed air from the sinuses is drawn into the lungs.

Sinusitis

Proper ventilation and drainage of the sinuses are important because of their close proximity to the roots of the maxillary bicuspids and molars. Any physiologic dysfunction may result in serious sinus infection, which is often directly related to the maxillary teeth (dentogenic), sinuses, or both: maxillary sinus inflammation or maxillary **sinusitis** (a bacterial infection or inflammation of the mucous membranes that line the sinuses). Symptoms of sinusitis include:

● Pressure buildup due to **exudate** accumulation

● Nasal discharge

● Pain in the area of the sinus

● Tenderness of some of the maxillary teeth.

Usual recommendations for this type of infection are decongestants and analgesics until the sinuses are well drained. Antibiotics are also recommended to eradicate bacterial infection.

SUGGESTED ACTIVITIES

● Using a hinged-cranium skull, locate the paranasal sinuses.

● Locate and name the air cells of the anterior group, then the posterior group.

● Identify the largest of the paranasal sinuses.

REVIEW

1. Identify the lettered parts of the illustration. Select from the following list:
   1. Ethmoid air cells
   2. Maxillary (sinus of Highmore)
   3. Frontal sinus

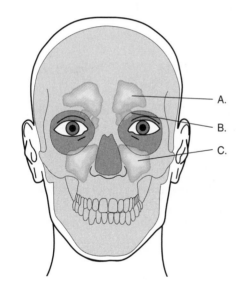

   a. _____
   b. _____
   c. _____

2. Which is the largest paranasal sinus of the skull?
   a. Anterior and middle ethmoid cells
   b. Frontal
   c. Sphenoidal
   d. Maxillary

3. Name the membrane that lines the paranasal sinuses.
   a. Paranasal membrane
   b. Mucous
   c. Cilia

4. Symptoms of sinusitis include (1) pressure buildup due to exudate accumulation, (2) pain in the lower jaw, (3) pain in area of the sinus, and/or (4) tenderness of some maxillary teeth.
   a. 1, 2, 3   c. 1, 3, 4
   b. 2, 3, 4   d. 1, 2, 4

5. Indicate the three functions of the paranasal sinuses: (1) act as reserve chambers for warm air during respiration (2) reduce the weight of the skull, (3) give resonance to the voice, or (4) filter out impurities.
   a. 1, 2, 3
   b. 2, 3, 4
   c. 1, 3, 4
   d. 1, 2, 4

6. Identify the lettered parts of the illustration. Select from the following list:
   1. Frontal sinus
   2. Anterior ethmoid air cells
   3. Middle ethmoid air cells
   4. Posterior ethmoid air cells
   5. Sphenoidal sinus
   6. Maxillary sinus (antrum of Highmore)

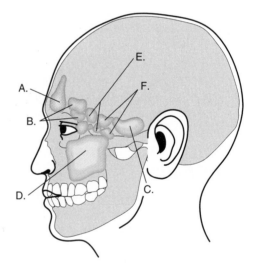

   a. _____
   b. _____
   c. _____
   d. _____
   e. _____
   f. _____

Muscles of Mastication

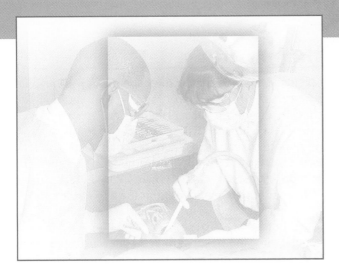

- Locate the external pterygoid muscle and state its function.
- Determine the muscles that control the movements of the mandible and temporomandibular joint.

OBJECTIVES

After studying this chapter, the student will be able to:

- Define muscle contraction and relaxation.
- Locate the masseter muscle and determine its insertion.
- Define the word synergist and identify the muscles involved.

Introduction

Movements of the mandible are controlled principally by four pairs of muscles known as the muscles of **mastication** (*masticate* = "chew or grind with the teeth"). These muscle pairs are the temporals, masseters, internal pterygoids, and external pterygoids. Some knowledge of the function and action of these muscles is necessary to fully understand their importance (Figure 17-1).

Muscles, generally, have two reactions or reverse movements, termed contraction and relaxation. Contraction is the change in muscles by which they become thickened and shortened. During relaxation, muscles become less tense or rigid. Even when there is no visible movement, not all fibers of the muscles are

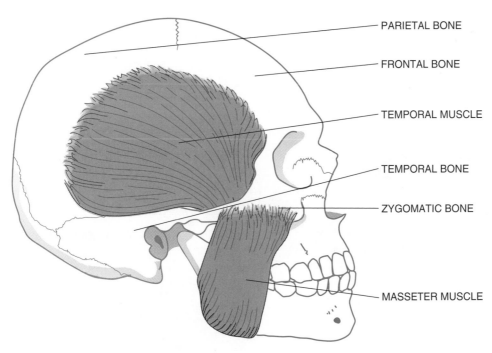

PARIETAL BONE

FRONTAL BONE

TEMPORAL MUSCLE

TEMPORAL BONE

ZYGOMATIC BONE

MASSETER MUSCLE

Figure 17-1 Muscles of mastication.

completely relaxed. Instead, some remain in a slight state of contraction called muscle tone, or **tonus**.

Most muscles extend from one bone to another bone, and each is attached to one of these bones by **tendons** (fibrous cords). The muscles of mastication are found chiefly in the face and are attached at one end to the skin, causing it to move. The point of attachment at the other end of the muscle is more or less stationary and is called the **origin**. The point of attachment that moves is called the **insertion**.

The Temporals

The temporal muscle, the largest muscle of mastication, is a broad, radiating, or fan-shaped muscle. Situated on the lateral surface of the skull, its origin is a wide field that tends to fill the temporal fossa. This field is composed of a narrow strip of the parietal bone, the temporal surface of the greater frontal bone, and the temporal surface of the greater wing of the sphenoid bone. Its fibers converge as they descend and are inserted into the medial surface, the **apex** (or pointed end) and anterior border of the coronoid process, and the anterior border of the ramus nearly to the third molar area.

The temporal muscle is built for movement rather than power and serves mainly to elevate the mandible and close the jaws. Its posterior fibers have a retracting action because of their slanting direction downward and forward. The zygomatic process acts as a pulley. Below

this process, the action of the muscle is very significant (Figure 17-2).

The Masseters

The masseter muscle is the most superficial (**superficial = "on or near the surface"**) muscle of mastication and stretches as a rectangular plate from the zygomatic arch to the outer surface of the mandible. It consists of two portions that can be separated, although not completely, into a superficial and a deep portion. The superficial portion, the larger of the two, arises by a thick, strong bundle of tendinous fibers from the zygomatic process of the maxilla and from the anterior two-thirds of the lower border of the zygomatic arch. The fibers have a general direction downward and backward; their insertion is the angle and lower half of the ramus. The deep portion is smaller and more muscular by nature; its origin is the posterior third of the lower border and the whole of the medial surface of the zygomatic arch. Its fibers pass downward and forward and are inserted in the upper half of the ramus and lateral surface of the coronoid process of the mandible. Refer to Chapter 15.

The masseter is composed of long, parallel fibers and is primarily a muscle of great power and fast contractility. It is capable of exerting much pressure upon the teeth, especially in the molar region. As the superficial fibers protract, or extend, in the closing movement of the jaw, the deep fibers retract.

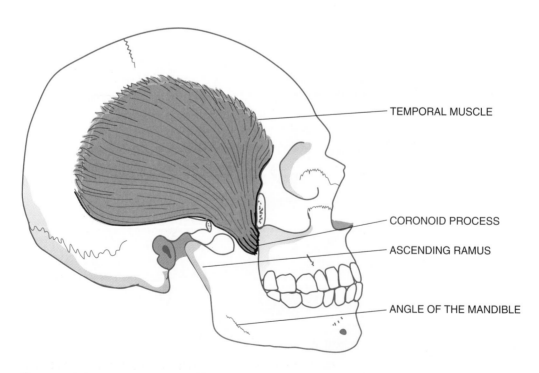

TEMPORAL MUSCLE

CORONOID PROCESS

ASCENDING RAMUS

ANGLE OF THE MANDIBLE

Figure 17-2 Muscles of mastication (view with zygomatic arch removed).

The Internal Pterygoids

The internal pterygoid muscle (also known as the medial pterygoid muscle) is rectangular in shape, is powerful, and acts as a counterpart to the masseter. It is positioned on the medial side of the ramus of the mandible with its origin in the pterygoid fossa. Three points of origin, or heads, are apparent: one on the medial surface of the lateral pterygoid plate of the sphenoid bone, another at the palatine bone, and a third at the maxillary tuberosity.

The internal structure of the internal pterygoid muscle is an intricate combination of both fleshy and tendinous fibers that arise from one tendon and end on another. These fibers are arranged at an angle to the general direction of the muscle. It is this braided arrangement that tends to increase the power of the muscle.

From the pterygoid fossa, the internal pterygoid muscle runs downward, backward, and outward; its insertion is the medial surface of the angle of the mandible and the medial surface of the ramus, as high as the mandibular foramen. Fibers of the internal pterygoid may meet fibers of the masseter behind and below the angle of the mandible. Its superficial part is a **synergist** of (works with) the masseter muscle and assists in closing the jaws.

Because the main pull of the internal pterygoid is directed upward, this muscle is not able to shift the mandible to one side or the other except in synergism with the masseter muscle. They are so placed that they suspend the angle of the mandible in a sling, which functions in the articulation of the maxilla and mandible; this is termed the mandibular sling (Figure 17-3).

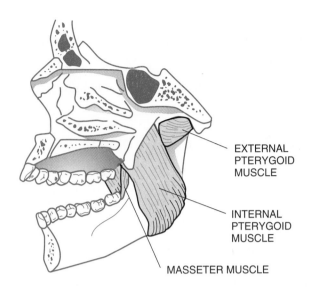

Figure 17-3 Internal pterygoid muscle, medial aspect.

The External Pterygoids

The external pterygoid muscle (lateral pterygoid muscle) is a thick, short muscle that arises with two heads. The larger and inferior head arises from the outer surface of the lateral pterygoid plate; the smaller and superior head arises from the lower part of the lateral surface of the greater wing of sphenoid and from the infratemporal fossa. The fibers of the upper head run horizontally backward and outward. The fibers of the lower head converge upward and outward; the upper fibers run more horizontally, and the lower fibers ascend more steeply (Figure 17-4). The two heads are separated anteriorly by

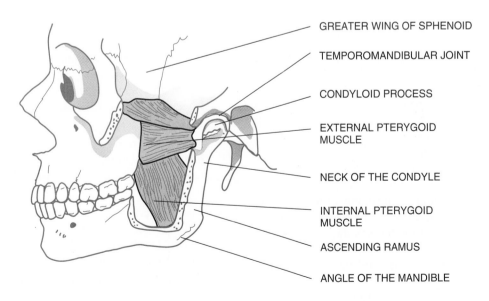

Figure 17-4 External and internal pterygoid muscle, lateral aspect (view with zygomatic arch and coronoid process removed).

a gap that varies in width, but they may fuse in front of the temporomandibular joint and can be separated only artificially.

The external pterygoid muscle's action is to open the jaw and protrude it (*protrude* = "to thrust forward").

The Temporomandibular Joint

The temporomandibular joint (TMJ) is so named because of the two bones that form the joint, the temporal bone and the mandible. It is the connection between the mandibular and maxillary jaws. It is located between the glenoid fossa and the articular tubercle (**tubercle** = "a small, rounded elevation on a bone for attachment of a tendon"). On the condyle lies a disc of tough, fibrous tissue called the **interarticular disc**, often referred to as the **meniscus** (a fibrous cartilage within a joint). The thickness and curvature of the disc are varied and conform to the shape of the bones.

Surrounding the meniscus is a dense, **fibrous capsule** (enclosed sac), the capsular ligament, which completely surfaces the TMJ and is attached to the neck of the condyle and to the nearby surfaces of the temporal bone. The disc divides the space between the glenoid fossa and the condyle into two cavities. These cavities lie above and below the meniscus and are filled with synovial fluid (**synovia** = "a thick, sticky fluid found in joints of bones").

The three osseus (**osseus** = "bony") portions making up the TMJ are (1) the glenoid fossa, an oval depression in the temporal bone lying anterior to the ear canal external acoustic meatus; (2) the articular tubercle, a raised portion of the temporal bone just anterior to the glenoid fossa; and (3) the condyloid process of the mandible. The condyloid process lies in the glenoid fossa with the meniscus separating the bones. The mandible, the only movable bone of the face, is attached to the cranium by the ligaments of the joint.

The majority of the fibers of the capsular ligament are inserted into a depression on the anterior surface of the neck of the condyle. The uppermost fibers of the external pterygoid muscle are attached to the anterior surface of the articular tubercle and the anterior border of the interarticular disc (meniscus). The posterior fibers of the temporal retract the mandible (Figure 17-5).

Although supported by ligaments, the temporal, masseter, and external and internal pterygoid muscles of mastication control the movements of the mandible and of the TMJ. The left and right TMJs function in unison and are capable of both hinge and gliding actions in mouth opening.

The hinge action of the mouth opening uses only the synovial cavity below the meniscus with the head of the condyle rotating around a point on the underside of

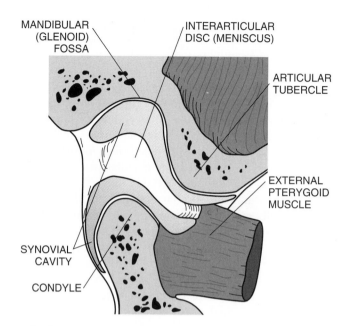

Figure 17-5 Temporomandibular joint.

the meniscus. The body of the mandible drops downward and backward.

The gliding action of the mouth opening involves both the upper and lower synovial cavities of the TMJ. This consists of a gliding of the condyle and meniscus forward and downward along the articular disc during protrusion and lateral movements of the mandible during mastication.

Changes take place within the TMJ when the jaws are closed or open or when it performs lateral or gliding actions. The wider the mouth opens, the further forward the condyle moves (Figure 17-6).

SUGGESTED ACTIVITIES

- Seat a fellow student in an upright position in the dental chair. Adjust the headrest. Assume the position of an operator, seated on a dental stool. Adjust the level of the dental chair, if necessary.

- Place pads of the tips of the index and middle fingers of each hand on the patient's TMJs (right and left). Apply sufficient pressure to feel the movements of the TMJs. Maintain this pressure throughout the exercise.

- Direct the patient to close the lips and bring the teeth into occlusion, exerting pressure on the molar region. Do the right and left TMJs function in occlusion? Which muscles are involved?

- With lips closed, direct the patient to open jaws and move the lower jaw laterally from right to left, then left to right. Do the TMJs function in unison? Which muscles are involved?

A.   B.   C.

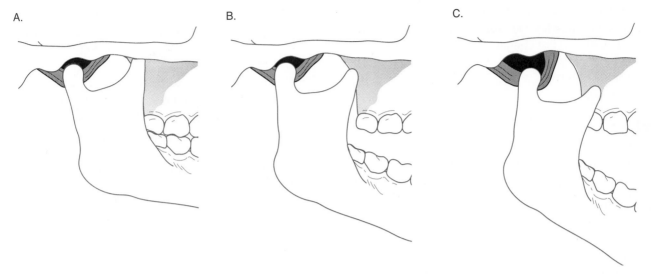

Figure 17-6 Three views of the TMJ: (A) closed jaws, (B) half open, and (C) fully open.

- With lips and jaws open, direct the patient to protrude the lower jaw. Do the TMJs function in unison? Which muscles are involved?

- With lips closed, direct the patient to move the mandible as if chewing food, first on the right side, then on the left. Are the TMJs functioning in unison? Which muscles are involved in mastication?

REVIEW

1. Identify the lettered parts of the illustration. Select from the following list:
   1. Masseter muscle
   2. Temporal muscle
   3. Zygomatic bone
   4. Frontal bone
   5. Parietal bone
   6. Temporal bone

a. _____
b. _____
c. _____
d. _____
e. _____
f. _____

2. Identify the lettered parts of the illustration. Select from the following list:
   1. Internal pterygoid muscle
   2. External pterygoid muscle
   3. Masseter muscle

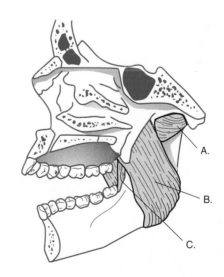

a. _____
b. _____
c. _____

3. Indicate which of the following are actions of the masseter muscles: (1) exerts great pressure upon the teeth, (2) fast contractility, (3) extends the mandibular jaw forward, and/or (4) closes the mandibular jaw.
   a. 1, 2, 3
   b. 2, 3, 4
   c. 1, 2, 4
   d. 1, 3, 4

4. Name the action of the temporal muscle:
   a. Elevates the mandibular jaw
   b. Opens the jaws
   c. Protrudes the mandibular jaw
   d. Moves the mandibular jaw from side to side

5. Indicate which of the following are actions of the external pterygoid muscle: (1) closes the jaw, (2), opens the jaws, (3) protrudes the mandibular jaw, and/or (4) moves mandible from side to side during mastication.
   a. 1, 2, 3
   b. 2, 3, 4
   c. 1, 2, 4
   d. 1, 3, 4

6. Name the action of the internal pterygoid muscle.
   a. Moves mandible from side to side during mastication
   b. Opens the jaws
   c. Protrudes the mandibular jaw
   d. Together with the masseter, suspends the angle of the mandible

7. Name the three bony portions that make up the temporomandibular joint (TMJ): (1) the glenoid fossa (2) the articular tubercle, (3) the condyle, or (4) the coronoid process.
   a. 1, 2, 3
   b. 2, 3, 4
   c. 1, 2, 4
   d. 1, 2, 4

Oral Cavity and Salivary Glands

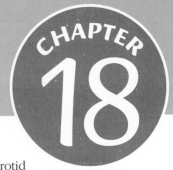

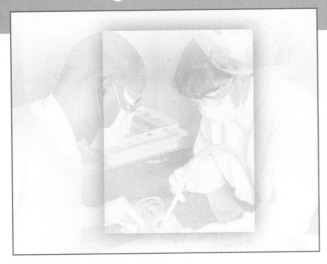

CHAPTER 18

- Locate and describe the parotid gland and parotid duct (Stensen's duct).
- Locate and describe the submandibular gland and submandibular duct (Wharton's duct).
- Discuss the sublingual glands and the ducts found on them.

Introduction

The cavity of the mouth is nearly oval shaped and consists of two parts: an outer and smaller portion, the **vestibule** (an opening, forming an entrance to another cavity), and the inner and larger part, the oral cavity proper. The vestibule is a slitlike opening, bound externally by the lips and cheeks and internally by the gums and teeth.

The mucous membrane that lines the oral cavity is called the oral mucosa. Under the oral mucosa in certain areas, such as the lips, the cheeks, and the palate, are the minor salivary glands. In addition, there are major salivary glands that supply secretions to the oral cavity.

The Oral Cavity Proper

The oral cavity proper is roofed by the hard palate (Figure 18-1). In the posterior is the soft palate, which lacks the bony quality of the hard palate. The greater

OBJECTIVES

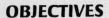

After studying this chapter, the student will be able to:

- Describe the basic parts of the mouth cavity.
- Locate and describe the glossopalatine arch.
- Locate and name the two mucosal attachments (frenum) found in the mouth.
- Distinguish the differences of shape and location of the taste buds on the tongue.
- Determine which taste buds are larger in size.
- Discuss the types of secretions that occur in the salivary glands.
- Describe the functions of saliva.

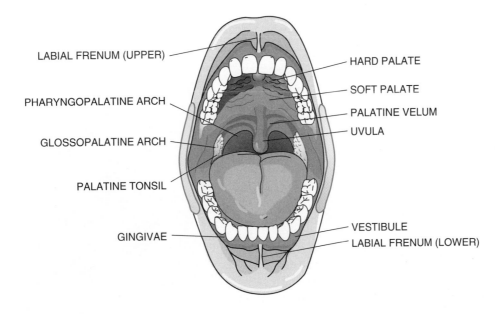

Figure 18-1 The mouth: view A.

LABIAL FRENUM (UPPER)
PHARYNGOPALATINE ARCH
GLOSSOPALATINE ARCH
PALATINE TONSIL
GINGIVAE
HARD PALATE
SOFT PALATE
PALATINE VELUM
UVULA
VESTIBULE
LABIAL FRENUM (LOWER)

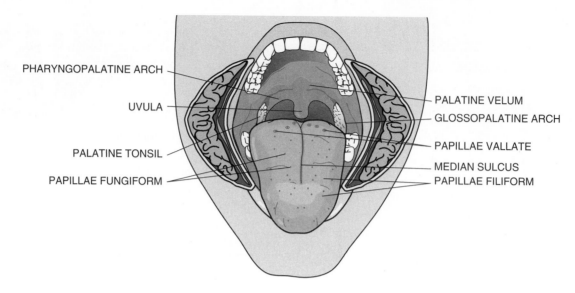

Figure 18-2 The mouth: view B.

part of the floor is formed by the tongue. The entire cavity is covered with mucous membrane, or mucosa. The lips are two fleshy folds surrounding the orifice (**orifice** = "opening") of the mouth. The inner surface of each lip is connected at the medial line by a fold of mucous membrane, the frenulum or labial **frenum**, to the gum tissue (gingivae). The upper attachment, or frenum, is larger and stronger than the lower attachment (Figure 18-2). The cheeks (buccae) form the sides of the face and are continuous in front with the lips.

The soft palate, in a relaxed state and with its lower border free, appears to hang as a curtainlike partition and is referred to as the **palatine velum** (*velum* = "veillike"). It is continuous with the **glossopalatine arch** (*glosso* = "tongue"; *palatine* = "pertaining to palate"). Suspended from the middle of its lower border is a small, conical, fleshy body, the **palatine uvula**. Posterior to the glossopalatine arch is the **pharyngopalatine arch** (**pharyngo** refers to pharynx, the cavity that connects the mouth and nasal passages with the esophagus and stomach). The **palatine tonsils** are two prominent masses located on either side of the oral cavity between the glossopalatine and pharyngopalatine arches. The tonsils consist basically of lymphatic tissue (Figure 18-3).

The tongue (lingua) lies on the floor of the mouth, within the curve of the mandible. The tongue is the principal organ of taste and an important organ of speech. It assists in **mastication** (the act of chewing) and **deglutition** (the act of swallowing) of food. The **dorsum** (the upper surface) of the tongue is marked by a **median sulcus** that divides it into symmetrical halves (corresponding parts in size and form) on either side of the sulcus. Thickly distributed over the anterior two-thirds

of the dorsum are projections, or **papillae** filiform (**filiform** = "cone shaped"). Scattered irregularly and sparingly over the dorsum are large, round projections of a deep red color called papillae fungiform (**fungiform** = "mushroom shaped"). They are narrow at their attachment to the tongue and broad and rounded at their free edges; they are covered with secondary papillae.

At the back of the tongue are the papillae vallate (**vallate** = "cup shape"), large in size and varying in number from 8 to 12. Usually found in two rows, the papillae form a V (inverted form) at the median line.

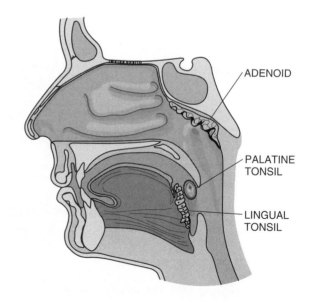

Figure 18-3 The tonsils.

Each papilla is in the form of a truncated cone (a cone-shaped object appearing to have its apex cut off) from 1 to 2 millimeters (mm) wide with the smaller end directed downward and attached to the tongue. The taste buds are scattered over the mucous membrane of the mouth and tongue at irregular intervals. They are found especially in the sides of the papillae vallate.

For a substance to have a taste, it must be soluble; that is, the substance must be dissolved in the saliva and must come in contact with the taste buds. The four primary tastes are sweet, sour, salty, and bitter. Although a specific taste bud transmits only one of the primary taste sensations, most of them respond to a lesser extent to substances that produce one or two of the other primary tastes. It is probably the combination of response on the part of two or three types of taste buds that characterizes the specific taste sensation associated with a particular substance.

The acid taste is usually transmitted through the taste buds on the anterior half of the tongue toward the midline; sweet and salty are on the lateral borders of the tongue in the anterior portion. The bitter taste is transmitted through receptors in the posterior third of the tongue.

Salivary Glands

Some of the salivary glands are serous glands, i.e., secrete **serum** (serous pertains to serum, a clear liquid). Others are mucous glands (**mucous**, or **mucin**, a slimy, gluelike secretion). Some are mixed glands that secrete both serum and mucus. Secretions of the major and minor salivary glands become mixed or blended to form saliva. In this chapter the importance of the major salivary glands is stressed (Figure 18-4).

Secretion is defined as the biological expulsion of material that has been chemically modified by a cell to serve a purpose elsewhere in the body or in some body process. Saliva protects the lining of the mouth (mucous membrane) against drying and aids in **expectoration** (the act of ejecting or spitting out) of injurious or distasteful substances. Saliva makes speech easier through the continuous moistening of the oral tissues and the teeth. Saliva lubricates food, aiding its passage to the stomach. In humans, as in some other mammals, saliva contains a digestive enzyme called salivary amylase (ptyalin). The suffix *-ase* designates an **enzyme** (*enzyme* = "a secretion of living cells capable of causing or accelerating a chemical reaction"). Amylase refers to enzyme action on **amylon** (from the Greek word for starch).

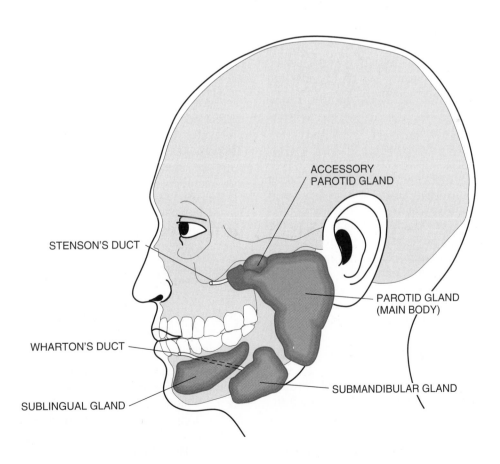

Figure 18-4 Salivary glands.

Salivary amylase is an enzyme that splits cooked starches. It breaks down the complex molecule to simple components. Although this action happens rather quickly, salivary digestion is usually incomplete by the time the food is swallowed, even though the chewing process has been conscientiously prolonged. Most of the enzyme action occurs within the saliva-saturated mass of food during the passage of the food from the mouth to the stomach before the gastric juice of the stomach has been mixed with the food. It is remarkable to note that salivary amylase cannot split starches into simple sugars; and double sugars taken by mouth as such (e.g., ordinary cane sugar) are unaffected by this enzyme. The reason for this is unknown but acceptable when it is realized that double sugars (disaccharides) cannot be absorbed by the body as such. Further enzyme action is necessary for the breakdown of double sugars into absorbable simple sugars; this occurs later in the small intestine.

The salivary glands lie just outside the oral cavity proper and are connected to the cavity by **ducts** (a canal or passage for fluids). Their secretions are controlled under normal conditions by various stimuli, such as touching the oral mucosa and the smell, sight, or thought of food. Many tiny mucous glands lie under the mucosa of the hard and soft palates; see Chapter 15. Some of the largest mucous glands of the palate are found near the base of the uvula (Figure 18-4). The buccal areas also have tiny mucous glands that secrete constantly into the vestibule.

Of the many glands that supply the oral cavity, there are three pairs of major salivary glands: the parotid, submandibular, and sublingual.

Parotid Glands

The parotid (*parotid* = "near the ear") is a serum-secreting gland and lies in front of and below the ear, one on either side of the face; it is the largest salivary gland. It is positioned between the external ear and the angle of the mandible. Above, it is broad and reaches nearly to the zygomatic arch. A small projection of the parotid gland passes over the upper portion of the masseter muscle (refer to Chapter 17). This small part, separated from the main body of the gland by a slight groove, is often referred to as the accessory parotid gland (*accessory* = "a subordinate or added part"). The lower part of the main body is somewhat tapered and reaches below the level of a line joining the tip of the mastoid process and the angle of the mandible. The remainder of the gland is irregularly wedge shaped and extends deeply inward toward the styloid process and the muscles arising from it. The parotid duct (also called Stensen's duct) enters the mouth opposite the buccal surface of the maxillary second molar tooth. The location of the opening of the duct in the oral cavity is marked by a small flap of tissue, the parotid papilla, which varies greatly in size and shape. The secretion of the parotid is almost entirely ptyalin, or amylase.

Submandibular Glands

One submandibular gland is located on each side of the face. The gland is irregular in shape and about the size of a walnut. It is a mixed salivary gland, one that contains both serum- and mucus-secreting cells and that secretes both ptyalin and mucin. The serous cells contribute the major part of the secretion. The submandibular gland lies beneath the lower jaw and discharges its secretion into the oral cavity through the submandibular duct (Wharton's duct) at the anterior base of the tongue and on either side of the lingual frenum. The opening is marked by an elevation, the sublingual **caruncle** (a small fleshy elevation). Occasionally, the duct may become closed due to the formation of **salivary calculus** (a hard mass containing lime salts and found in saliva). This partial or complete closure of the duct produces swelling of the floor of the mouth. On the other hand, stimulation of the gland may induce secretion so forcefully that the liquid is released in tiny streams that spurt completely out of the oral cavity.

Sublingual Glands

The sublingual gland is the smallest of the major salivary glands. It is situated beneath the mucous membrane of the floor of the mouth and is primarily mucus secreting; its secretion does not contain ptyalin. It is situated on either side of the base of the tongue and is shaped somewhat like an almond. The ducts number from eight to twenty. The numerous small ducts (ducts of Rivinus) and the single larger duct (duct of Bartholin) either join the mandibular duct or open directly onto the floor of the mouth. Any infection of the sublingual gland results in swelling of the floor of the mouth and pain during movement of the tongue.

SUGGESTED ACTIVITIES

- Using a fellow student as a patient, locate and identify the mucosa of the oral cavity. Include the palatine vellum, palatine uvula, and palatine tonsils.

- Direct the patient to open the mouth and extend the tongue. Find the median sulcus. Direct the patient to lift the tongue; observe the lingual frenum. Roll the upper lip upward; observe the upper labial frenum. Roll the lower lip downward; observe the lower labial frenum.

● Refer to Figure 18-4; locate and describe the major salivary glands. Determine which are serous and which are mixed. Do each have a duct that empties into the oral cavity? Explain how the salivary glands form saliva.

REVIEW

1. Match the terms with corresponding facts:

___a. Mucosa
___b. Uvula
___c. Papilla filliform
___d. Papilla vallate
___e. Hard palate
___f. Lower frenum
___g. Posterior third
___h. Median line of inner lip surface

1. Continuous with pallatine vellum
2. Covers entire mouth cavity
3. Larger of the taste buds
4. Anterior portion of roof of mouth
5. Middle anterior of the tongue
6. Location of frenum attachment
7. Transmits bitter taste of tongue sensation
8. Smaller and weaker frenum

2. Indicate some functions of the salivary glands not related to chemical digestion: (1) contains enzymes to aid in digestion, (2) lubricates the food and aids in swallowing, (3) protects the lining of the mouth by producing saliva, and/or (4) makes speech easier by keeping mucosa and teeth moistened.
a. 1, 2, 3
b. 2, 3, 4
c. 1, 2, 4
d. 1, 3, 4

3. Another term for the opening of the parotid duct is:
a. Ducts of Rivinus
b. Wharton's duct
c. Sublingual duct
d. Stensen's duct

4. Which of the salivary glands is the largest, and which is the smallest?
a. Parotid, sublingual
b. Parotid, submandibular
c. Submandibular, sublingual
d. Sublingual, parotid

5. Identify the lettered parts of the illustration. Select from the following list:
1. Glossopalatine arch
2. Median sulcus
3. Palatine tonsil
4. Palatine velum
5. Papillae filiform
6. Papillae fungiform
7. Papillae vallate
8. Pharyngopalatine arch
9. Uvula

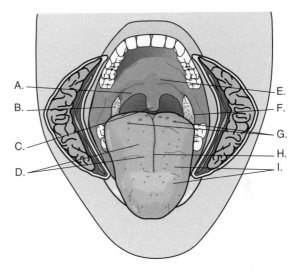

a. _____
b. _____
c. _____
d. _____
e. _____
f. _____
g. _____
h. _____
i. _____

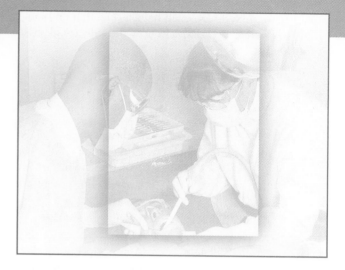

OBJECTIVES

After studying this chapter, the student will be able to:

- Name the three divisions of the trigeminal nerve.
- Discuss the areas of the face and head supplied by the ophthalmic division of the trigeminal nerve.
- Locate the maxillary division of the trigeminal nerve and determine its branches and the areas it supplies.
- Locate the mandibular division of the trigeminal nerve and discuss how it differs with the two other nerve divisions.
- Locate and discuss the four ganglions found with the cranial nervous system of the trigeminal nerve.

Introduction

The nerves that supply the region of the oral cavity and face are called **cranial nerves**. There are three kinds of nerves: **sensory** (those concerned with sensation), **motor** (those that stimulate movement of muscles), and **mixed** (those possessing both sensory and motor nerve fibers).

This chapter is concerned with the trigeminal nerve (*tri* = "three"; *geminal* = "paired, or in twos"), the largest of the 12 cranial nerves. All cranial nerves come in pairs—a right and a left; the trigeminal nerve is paired and has three main branches, or divisions. The trigeminal nerve is called the fifth cranial nerve, the number corresponding to its position on the brain in relation to the other cranial nerves.

Trigeminal Nerve

The fifth cranial, or trigeminal, nerve emerges from the midbrain and passes forward for a short distance. It then spreads fanlike to form a ganglion (**ganglion** = "a mass of nerve cells found outside the brain or spinal canal"). This mass is called the gasserian, or semilunar, ganglion (*semi* = "half"; *lunar* = "moon"; i.e., it is half-moon or crescent shaped). The small motor portion of the trigeminal nerve passes along a course below the semilunar ganglion and joins the mandibular branch, continuing on, beside the otic ganglion (**otic** = "ear)". The sensory

portion that forms the gasserian ganglion receives fibers from three main divisions: the ophthalmic (**ophthalmic** = "eye"), maxillary, and mandibular nerves.

Ophthalmic Division

The *ophthalmic division* (first division) of the trigeminal nerve is the smallest branch from the gasserian ganglion. It passes forward and leaves the cranium through an opening in the posterior wall of the orbit, called the superior orbital fissure (**fissure**, or natural groove, found in the orbit). Before this division leaves the cranium, it divides into three branches: the frontal, lacrimal (**lacrimal** = "tears"), and nasal (**nasociliary**) nerves (Figure 19-1).

This division of the trigeminal nerve supplies (1) the lacrimal gland through the lacrimal nerve; (2) the skin of the eyelids, eyebrows, forehead and nose; (3) part of the mucous membrane of the nasal cavity; (4) the **cornea** (the "window" of the eye) and **conjunctiva** (delicate membrane lining the eyelids and covering the eyeball); (5) the **ciliary body** (muscle attached to the lens of the eye that helps to focus the eye); and (6) the **iris** (pigmented membrane surrounding the pupil), which gives the eye its color and controls the amount of light entering the eye.

Maxillary Division

The *maxillary division* (second division) of the trigeminal, a sensory nerve, leaves the cranial vault by way of the foramen rotundum (**rotundum**, or round; i.e., a large round, natural opening in the bone of the greater wing of sphenoid through which the superior maxillary nerve passes). It then enters the pterygopalatine fossa

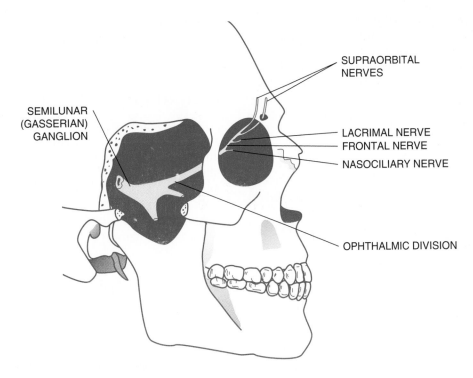

Figure 19-1 Trigeminal nerve, ophthalmic division.

and divides into three main branches: the infraorbital, zygomatic, and sphenopalatine nerves.

Infraorbital Nerve. The infraorbital branch is the largest branch of the maxillary nerve. It passes through the infraorbital canal, emerges from the bone through

the infraorbital foramen, and branches into three superior alveolar nerves: the anterior superior alveolar, middle superior alveolar, and posterior superior alveolar. The terminal fibers of these branches supply the tissues below the orbit, the lateral tissues of the nose, and the upper lip (Figure 19-2).

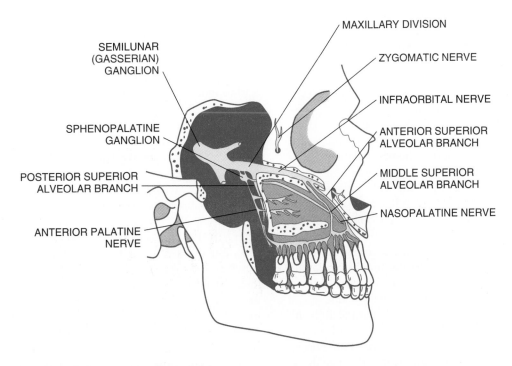

Figure 19-2 Trigeminal nerve, maxillary division.

The *anterior superior alveolar* branch travels forward and downward through the bone beneath the infraorbital foramen and sends its fibers into the pulp chambers of the maxillary central incisor, lateral incisor, and cuspid teeth, the periodontal membrane, and the gingivae of this area. Some fibers pass forward to innervate the mucous membrane of the oral cavity just below the nose and the upper lip.

The *middle superior alveolar* branch moves in a forward direction through the bone and slightly behind the anterior superior branch. Its fibers supply the maxillary first and second bicuspid teeth and the mesiobuccal root of the maxillary first molar. Other small fibers of this branch innervate the periodontal membrane and facial gingivae surrounding these teeth.

The *posterior superior alveolar* branch is composed of two or three branches, coursing down the posterior surface of the maxilla to enter one or several posterior superior dental foramina. This nerve supplies all the roots of the maxillary second and third molar teeth and two roots of the maxillary first molar tooth. (As previously stated, in the majority of cases, the mesiobuccal root of the maxillary first molar is supplied by the middle superior alveolar nerve.) Other small fibers innervate the facial gingiva and periodontal membrane surrounding these teeth.

Zygomatic Nerve. The zygomatic nerve is situated in the lower fissure of the orbit, along with part of the infraorbital branch. The zygomatic sends branches along the orbital surface and pierces the zygomatic bone; it emerges to form the zygomaticofacial branch (so called because of its location). A second small branch, the zygomatic temporal, emerges from a small foramen on the temporal surface to innervate tissues of that region.

Sphenopalatine Nerves. The sphenopalatine nerves branch from the maxillary nerve in a downward direction. A body of nerve tissue found suspended by two short nerves from the maxillary nerve is the sphenopalatine ganglion (Meckel's ganglion). This ganglion lies just below the maxillary nerve in the sphenopalatine fossa. Two nerves of interest here are the *nasopalatine nerve* and the *anterior palatine nerve*. The nasopalatine courses from Meckel's ganglion along the septum of the nose, through the palatine canal, and terminates in the foramina of Scarpa located on the median line and palatally to the maxillary central teeth. This nerve innervates the maxillary anterior mucosal tissues and the palatal mucoperiosteum (the fibrous sheath covering the hard palate) and is directly related to the anterior palatine nerves. The anterior palatine nerve arises from Meckel's ganglion, descends through the posterior palatine canal (in the palatine bone), and emerges on the palate from the posterior palatine foramen. It passes forward on the palate and intermingles with the nasopalatine nerve, opposite the cuspid tooth. It innervates the maxillary

molar and bicuspid mucosal tissues and the palatal mucoperiosteum in that area (Table 19-1).

Mandibular Division

The *mandibular division* (third division) of the trigeminal, a mixed nerve, is the largest branch given off from the gasserian ganglion. It exits from the cranium through the foramen ovale (**ovale** = "egg shaped") and is made up of two roots, a large sensory root, and a small motor root (the motor part of the trigeminal). It differs from the other two divisions of the trigeminal, because it is both sensory and motor. The *mandibular nerve* supplies the teeth and gums of the mandible, the skin of the temporal region, the lower lip, the muscles of mastication, and the anterior two-thirds of the tongue.

The anterior portion, a branch of the mandibular nerve, is basically motor in character. It innervates the temporal, masseter, internal pterygoid, and external pterygoid muscles, as well as the anterior surface of the temporomandibular joint; refer to Chapter 18 and Figure 19-3.

The *buccal nerve*, a continuation of the anterior portion, is sensory only. It passes forward and toward the side and divides into many small fibers that supply the mucous membrane of the cheek. Although this nerve passes through the buccinator muscle, it does not supply the motor stimulation for that muscle.

The *lingual nerve* branches just below the buccal nerve and from the posterior portion of the mandibular nerve. It travels forward and downward to the lingual surface of the mandible. As it nears the area, lingual to the mandibular second or third molar roots, it attaches itself to the submandibular ganglion. The attachments are usually two short nerves by which the ganglion appears to be suspended. This small mass of nerve tissues is **autonomic** (self-controlling) in its work with involuntary nerve impulses that innervate the sublingual and tongue glands. The fiber ends of the lingual nerve supply the lateral and superior surface tissues of the tongue and record sensations of touch and taste and promote glandular function.

The *inferior alveolar nerve* is a continuation of the mandibular nerve and is the largest branch of the mandible. It gives off a branch called the *mylohyoid nerve*, just above the point where it enters the mandibular foramen. The fibers of this branch are motor in character. The inferior alveolar nerve passes through the mandibular foramen and follows the mandibular canal; it sends sensory branches to all the molar and biscupid teeth. At a point approximately between the apices of the first and second bicuspids, the inferior alveolar divides into the mental and incisive branches. The *mental branch* passes through the mental foramen and innervates the chin and lower lip, and the *incisive branch* supplies the mandibular anterior teeth, Table 19-1.

Table 19-1 Innervation of Teeth and Tissues

Nerve	Teeth	Tissues
Maxillary Arch		
Anterior superior alveolar	Centrals, laterals, cuspids	Facial gingiva and periodontal membrane of anterior teeth
Middle superior alveolar	First bicuspid Second bicuspid Mesial buccal root of first molar	Facial gingiva and periodontal membrane of bicuspid area
Posterior superior alveolar	First molar distal buccal and lingual roots Second molar Third molar	Facial gingiva and periodontal membrane of molar area
Nasopalatine		Anterior palatal mucosal tissues Palatal mucoperiosteum from cuspid to cuspid
Anterior palatine		Molar and bicuspid palatal mucosal tissues Palatal mucoperiosteum from posterior of molars to the cuspid area
Mandibular Arch		
Inferior alveolar (the lingual nerve is usually involved)	All mandibular teeth	Labial mucosa anterior of mental nerve including lower lip Anterior two-thirds of the tongue (lingual nerve) Floor of the mouth (lingual) Lingual mucosa of all teeth (lingual)
Incisive	Bicuspids, anterior teeth	Chin and lower lip anterior of mental foramen
Mental		Chin and lower lip anterior of mental foramen
Buccal		Buccal mucous membrane of the cheek and gingiva of molars
Lingual		Lingual mucosa of all teeth Anterior two-thirds surface of tongue Floor of the mouth

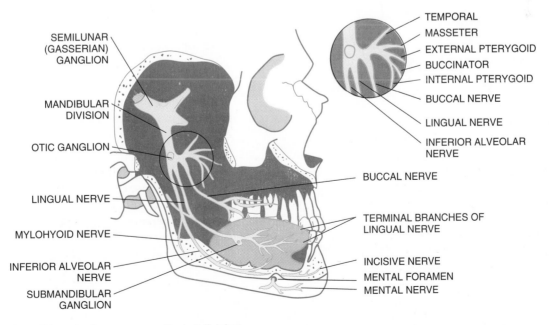

Figure 19-3 Trigeminal nerve, mandibular division.

SUGGESTED ACTIVITIES

● Remembering that all cranial nerves come in pairs, use Figure 19-2 to locate the gasserian ganglion, sphenopalatine ganglion, and infraorbital nerve. Determine which branches of the maxillary division innervate the teeth. Which nerves of the maxillary division innervate the maxillary mucosal tissues and palatal mucoperiosteum?

● Use Figure 19-3 to locate the gasserian ganglion and the mandibular division of the trigeminal. Determine the sensory nerves and those that are mixed. Determine which nerve supplies the teeth and gums of the mandible.

REVIEW

1. Identify the lettered parts of the illustration. Select from the following list:
   1. Ophthalmic division
   2. Semilunar (gasserian) ganglion
   3. Nasociliary nerve
   4. Supraorbital nerves
   5. Lacrimal nerve
   6. Frontal nerve

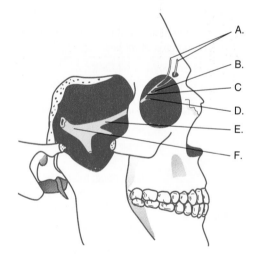

    a. _____
    b. _____
    c. _____
    d. _____
    e. _____
    f. _____

2. Match the cranial nerves with the correct description.
   ___a. Nasopalatine
   ___b. Anterior superior alveolar
   ___c. Mandibular
   ___d. Mental and incisive
   ___e. Maxillary
   ___f. Posterior superior alveolar
   ___g. Infraorbital
   ___h. Inferior alveolar
   ___i. Ophthalmic
   ___j. Middle superior alveolar

   1. Largest branch of the maxillary nerve
   2. Innervates the lingual and distobuccal roots of the maxillary first, second, and third molars
   3. First division of the trigeminal nerve
   4. Innervates the maxillary first and second bicuspids and the mesiobuccal root of the maxillary first molar
   5. Innervates the chin and lower lip
   6. Sensory branch of all mandibular molar and bicuspid teeth
   7. Third division of the trigeminal nerve
   8. Innervates maxillary centrals, laterals, cuspids, and supporting tissues of this area
   9. Second division of the trigeminal nerve
   10. Innervates the maxillary anterior, palatine nerves, and the palatal mucoperiosteum

3. Which maxillary nerves innervate the pulp, periodontal membrane, and gingival tissues of the maxillary central incisor, lateral incisor, and cuspid teeth?
   a. Posterior superior alveolar nerve
   b. Sphenopalatine nerve
   c. Nasopalatine nerve
   d. Anterior superior alveolar nerve

4. Two additional branches of the inferior alveolar nerve are:
   a. Buccal and lingual nerves
   b. Mental and incisive nerves
   c. Mylohyoid and lingual nerves
   d. Incisive and buccal

5. Define the term ganglion.
   a. A mass of nerve cells found outside the brain and spinal canal
   b. A mixed nerve
   c. A motor nerve
   d. A sensory nerve

Blood Supply to the Head and Neck

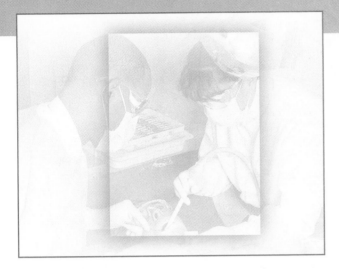

OBJECTIVES

After studying this chapter, the student will be able to:

● Locate the lingual artery, a branch of the internal carotid, and discuss its importance to the oral cavity.

● Locate the internal maxillary artery and determine its importance to the field of dentistry.

● Locate the three branches of the internal maxillary artery and discuss the areas supplied by each.

● Locate the pterygoid plexus and trace the venous flow to the internal jugular vein.

● Determine the importance of the maxillary vein.

Introduction

Many individuals take for granted the fact that blood circulates, and the concept is implied rather than expressly stated, even when the gross anatomy of the circulatory system is discussed. About 300 years ago, however, although much was known about the heart and the blood vessels and their distribution, the nature of blood was unknown. At that time William Harvey demonstrated that the blood moves in a continuous double circulation.

The organs of the blood-vascular (**vaso** = "blood vessel") system are the heart and **blood vessels** (arteries, capillaries, and veins). These organs form a closed passageway of tubes through which the blood circulates. The heart is a muscular pump that propels the blood through the blood vessels. The arteries are elastic tubes that carry the blood away from the heart to the tissues of the body. Capillaries are microscopic, hairlike vessels through which blood passes from arteries to veins. Veins are less muscular than arteries; their walls are thinner, and most have paired valves that prevent the backward flow of blood.

The arteries carry oxygenated blood from the heart to all regions of the body. Because of this high-pressure delivery system, blood flows rapidly. The arteries expand and contract with the pumping beat of the heart. A rupture of the arterial system can be readily detected by the rhythmic spurting of bright red blood. If the blood spurts from a wound as in a severed artery, pressure should be applied against the artery on the side of the wound toward the heart. This helps to control bleeding.

Veins, although similar in form to arteries, serve as the low-pressure system that returns the blood to the heart. Veins are equipped with valves that open in the direction of the flow of blood. This valve arrangement is effective in preventing a reverse flow as the blood is carried to the heart. Venous flow can be detected when blood runs slowly but steadily from a wound. When a vein is severed, pressure should be applied to the vein on the side of the wound away from the heart.

Arteries of the Head

The common carotid arteries (right and left) supply arterial blood to the head. Each divides in the neck (at the upper border of the thyroid cartilage) to form two branches: external and internal arteries. The internal carotid arteries lie deep and supply branches to the brain and the eyes. The external carotid arteries are more **superficial** (situated nearer the surface) and have branches that go to the throat, tongue, face, ears, and the wall of the cranium (Figure 20-1).

The branches of the external carotid artery are named according to the area they supply. The external maxillary (facial) artery arises from the external carotid artery and enters the face at the lower border of the masseter muscle, where it is comparatively superficial. This artery is easily compressed against the lower border of the mandible. At this point, the external maxillary artery passes forward and upward to the angle of the mouth, where it takes a more vertical course to become the angular artery. It travels upward to the middle of the eyelid and terminates.

The lingual artery is the second major branch of the external carotid and is directly related to the oral cavity. From the anterior of the external carotid, the lingual branches in archlike fashion, then travels in a straight course and passes under the mandible. It again divides into four branches. One branch supplies the mucous membrane of the top surface of the tongue, the glos-

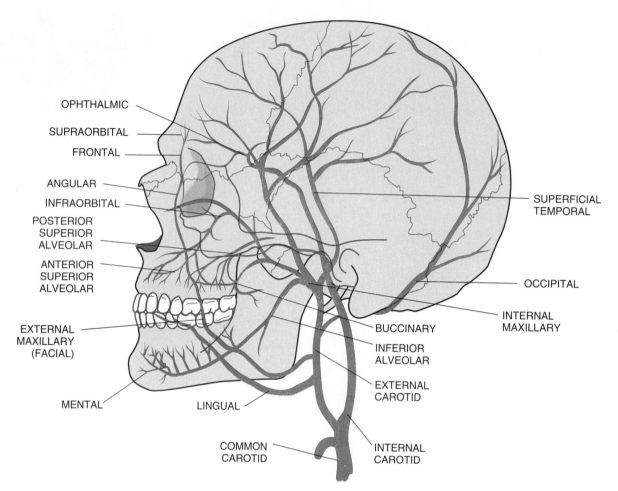

Figure 20-1 Arteries of head and neck.

sopalatine arch, the tonsil, and the soft palate. Others supply muscles, the alveolar process of the mandible, and the mucosa. Yet another, the deep lingual artery, runs along the undersurface of the tongue, ending at the tip.

The superficial temporal artery is the smaller of the two terminal branches of the external carotid artery. It travels behind the neck of the condyle and travels upward in front of the ear. There it branches to supply the frontal and parietal areas of the scalp.

The occipital artery arises from the posterior part of the external carotid, opposite the external maxillary (facial) artery. It runs along the occipital bone and ends in the posterior part of the scalp.

Other arteries of the face are the buccinator and infraorbital arteries from the internal maxillary artery. The ophthalmic artery branches to form the frontal and supraorbital arteries.

The internal maxillary artery (sometimes referred to as the maxillary artery) is the largest of the two terminal branches of the external carotid. Its three branches provide the blood supply for the teeth. The inferior alveolar artery supplies the mandibular teeth; the posterior

superior alveolar artery supplies the maxillary bicuspids and molars; and the anterior superior alveolar artery, a branch of the infraorbital artery, supplies the maxillary central and lateral incisors and cuspids.

Veins of the Head

Blood drains from the head and the interior of the skull into venous channels situated between two layers of the **dura mater** (the outermost membrane) of the brain. These are called **venous sinuses**. In relation to dentistry, the most important of these sinuses are the two cavernous sinuses that are connected with veins of the face (through veins of the orbits). Because of this direct association, infection in and about the nose and cheeks can easily enter the sinuses.

Major veins of the area are the facial vein, the superficial and deep temporal veins, the maxillary vein, the **tributaries** (those that flow into the larger veins), the internal jugular vein, and the external jugular vein (Figure 20-2).

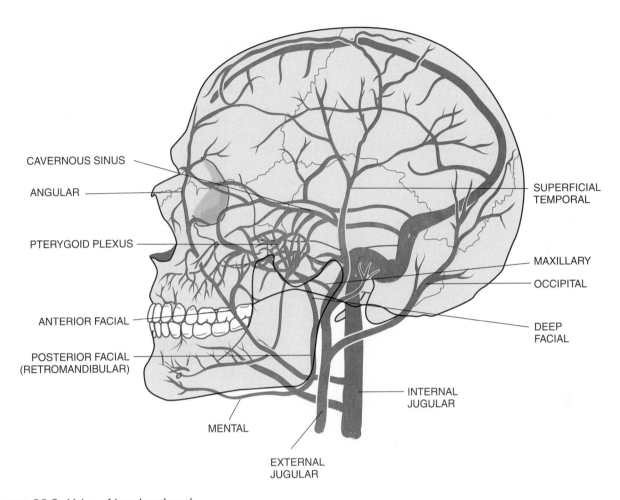

Figure 20-2 Veins of head and neck.

CAVERNOUS SINUS

ANGULAR

PTERYGOID PLEXUS

ANTERIOR FACIAL

POSTERIOR FACIAL
(RETROMANDIBULAR)

MENTAL

EXTERNAL
JUGULAR

SUPERFICIAL
TEMPORAL

MAXILLARY

OCCIPITAL

DEEP
FACIAL

INTERNAL
JUGULAR

The facial vein is divided into sections according to the structures over or through which it courses. At the inner **canthus of the eye** (where the upper and lower eyelids fuse), it arises as the angular vein. It follows a course similar to that of the external maxillary artery. Near its point of origin, it receives blood from the infratrochlear and infraorbital veins. At the root of the nose, and as a continuation of the angular vein, the anterior facial vein runs downward and backward across the face, crossing the border of the mandible at the anterior border of the masseter muscle. Beneath the angle of the mandible, it unites with the posterior facial vein to form the common facial vein. The anterior facial vein unites with the deep facial vein, one of considerable size, from the pterygoid **plexus** (a network of veins). This plexus forms a rather dense network around the external pterygoid muscle. The facial vein carries the blood collected from the facial region to the internal jugular vein. This large blood vessel is found running parallel to the common carotid artery.

The superficial and deep temporal veins join together in the region anterior to the external acoustic meatus and bring blood from the superficial tissue of the skull and the temporal fossa. At a point just below the junction of the temporal vessels, the maxillary vein connects to the main tributary to form a complex union of occipital, posterior facial, and external jugular vessels. The maxillary vein receives blood from the maxillary and mandibular alveolar systems, including all the teeth.

The posterior facial vein is normally a short vessel. The vein is an auxiliary vessel to the external jugular at the junction of the maxillary vein and the common facial vein. It is attached to the common facial vein just behind and below the angle of the mandible. This vessel is otherwise referred to as the retromandibular vein because of its location.

The external jugular vein usually takes a course posterior and superficial to the internal jugular vein. From its junction with the superficial temporal, maxillary, and retromandibular vessels, the external jugular travels downward to join the internal jugular vein under the clavicle (collarbone).

SUGGESTED ACTIVITIES

- Study Chapter 14 for further information regarding the blood vessels and circulatory system.
- Complete the Review of this chapter.

REVIEW

1. Match the listed terms to the corresponding facts.

   ___ a. Artery

   ___ b. Vein

   ___ c. Lingual artery

   ___ d. Common carotid artery

   ___ e. Inferior alveolar artery

   ___ f. Posterior superior artery

   ___ g. Tributaries

   ___ h. Clavicle

   ___ i. Venus sinuses

   ___ j. Canthus of the eye

   1. Supplies the maxillary posterior teeth
   2. Collarbone
   3. Causes blood to spurt from a wound
   4. Supplies arterial blood to the head
   5. Blood runs slowly from a wound
   6. Veins that flow into larger veins
   7. Where upper and lower eyelids fuse
   8. Venous channels located between two layers of the dura mater
   9. Supplies the mandibular teeth
   10. Supplies blood to the tongue

2. Which of the veins receive blood from both the maxillary and mandibular alveolar systems (including all the teeth)?
   a. Occipital
   b. Maxillary
   c. Internal jugular
   d. External jugular

3. What does the term plexus mean?
   a. Network of veins
   b. Cavernous sinus
   c. Tributaries
   d. Below the clavicle

4. Into what two arteries does the common carotid artery divide?
   a. Maxillary, mandibular
   b. Facial, occipital
   c. Internal jugular, external jugular
   d. Internal carotid, external carotid

5. Which vein follows closely the same course as the external maxillary artery?
   a. Angular
   b. Infraorbital
   c. Infratrochlear
   d. Posterior facial

Development of the Face, Nose, Tongue, and Palate

CHAPTER 21

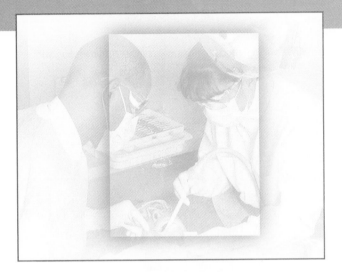

OBJECTIVES

After studying this chapter, the student will be able to:

- Discuss the process of cell division.
- Discuss the specialization process of tissue differentiation.
- List the three distinct cell layers that form in the developing human embryo.
- Distinguish epithelial cells from connective cells with respect to their structure and function.
- Discuss the chronological stages of development of the face and associated structures.
- Determine the time at which the embryonic development of the tongue occurs.
- Determine the time at which the embryonic development of the palate occurs.
- Describe the developmental stages of the tongue.
- Describe the developmental stages of the palate.
- Discuss the reasons for the occurrences of an anomaly.

Introduction

The human body is formed from the division of the fertilized ovum (**ovum** = the female reproductive or germ cell that after fertilization is capable of developing into a new member of the same species). The process of division, **mitosis**, results in the formation of two daughter cells, each of which resembles the original. As division follows division, the daughter cells may exhibit new or altered structures and functions. This process is called **differentiation** (when the original cells take on the duty of forming a particular type of tissue).

Histology is the study of plant and animal tissues and involves the internal structure of organisms and their parts. Their structures are so minute that they must be studied under a microscope. This chapter describes the tissues and internal structure of the teeth and closely related parts of the oral cavity. The development of the face, its associated structures, and the masses of tissue that are directly involved are discussed.

As the external structures of the face develop, other important developments occur internally. The tongue and palate, for example, appear during this time and are also discussed in this chapter.

Differentiation

The first evidence of differentiation in the mass of cells of the developing human embryo (**embryo** = a young organism up to the end of the second month of intrauterine life) is the formation of three distinct cell (germ) layers. An outer layer of cells forms the ectoderm (**ecto** = outer) while a tube develops within the mass and the cells lining it form the endoderm (**endo** = within). This tube forms the basis of the future alimentary canal and the organs that arise from it—lungs, liver, pancreas.

The mesoderm (**meso** = middle) consists of cells lying between the ectoderm and the endoderm of the primary germ layers.

The primitive cells of each germ layer can differentiate along two separate lines to form either epithelium or connective tissue.

Epithelial cells cover surfaces (e.g., skin) or line cavities (e.g., the mouth). In these situations, they are essentially protective in function.

A secondary function that may be performed by covering epithelia, such as the intestinal and respiratory epithelia, is secretion of mucus. A feature common to all epithelial cells is that they are closely **contiguous** (touching along a boundary or at a point) with one another.

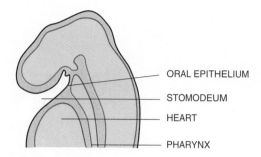

Figure 21-1 Head end of human embryo (three to four weeks).

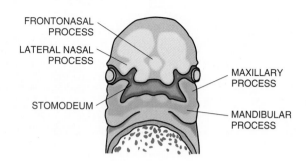

Figure 21-2 Head of human embryo (three to four weeks).

Connective tissue cells are the other cell type present in the body. They are usually widely separated from each other by a zone containing a substance in which fibers are embedded. Collagen fibers (**collagen** = a vital crystalline, protein substance present in all connective tissue) are the most abundant, but in some areas (e.g., the walls of the large arteries), elastic fibers are also present. This type of connective tissue (tendon, bone, cartilage, and fibrous tissue) is primarily supportive in function. Other connective tissue cells have the capability of contraction (muscle fibers) or conduction (nerve cells).

The cells of the body show considerable diversity of structure and function, yet each is remarkably independent. Each receives a supply of oxygen and foodstuffs from the bloodstream with which it will produce its own structural components and secretions. Each cell will also release the energy required for chemical, electrical, or mechanical work (refer to Chapter 14).

Stages of Development

During the chronological development (**chronology** = accepted order of past events) of single systems or parts of systems, it must be remembered that these systems do not arise independently of one another. To simplify the study, we describe the development of isolated structures and their relationships in detail.

Face

An examination of a human embryo reveals, as early as the third or fourth week, the pharynx (upper portion of the digestive tract) and a large cavity known as the stomodeum (**stomodeum** = a depression at the head end of the embryo that becomes the front part of the mouth; Figures 21-1 and 21-2). This completes the first important step in the development of the face. During the same period, two paired structures are evident, the maxillary and mandibular processes; these form the lateral walls of the primitive oral cavity (**primitive** = first in time, original). A lateral view of the embryo shows the relation of these two processes and the line of union between them.

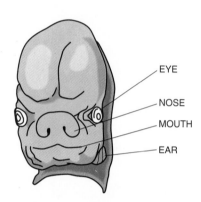

Figure 21-3 Head of human embryo (about eight weeks).

Nose

In the sixth week of development, two additional structures originate; these are known as the nasal processes and are comprised of the frontal and lateral portions. By the end of the seventh week, an inverted U-shaped elevation of tissue surrounds each process and forms the primitive external nares (**nares** = nostrils). As the nasal processes develop, the maxillary processes increase in size and grow toward the midline of the face. At the same time, they tend to push the nasal processes closer together (Figure 21-3). By the 10th week, the maxillary arch is formed and its parts aligned (**aligned**, arranged in a line) from side to side. The two nasal processes migrate medially, meet, and fuse, and the primitive nasal septum is established (**septu** = dividing wall, or partition).

In the meantime, the mandible has continued to develop. As these processes migrate from their lateral position, they fuse at a point in the midline.

Tongue

The tongue develops from mucous membrane composed principally of epithelium and connective tissue.

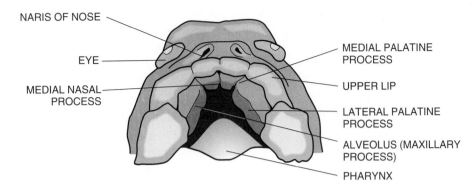

Figure 21-4 Palatal view of human embryo (about 10 weeks).

Mucous membrane coverings of the tongue consist of a swelling along the median floor of the pharynx and can be recognized during the fifth week of embryonic life. Later development of the tongue is involved in a rapid **proliferation**, or multiplication of the cells. By the seventh week, the tongue becomes fairly well separated from the mandible. It becomes elevated from the floor of the mouth because of the infiltration of the muscle as it builds up internally.

Palate

In the sixth week, the beginning of the palate appears. There are several processes, one of which originates from the medial nasal process. The others, which are located laterally, develop from the maxillary tissue. There are two important stages of development. The first is known as the open palate stage. During this stage, the medial migration of the nasal processes and the fusing of the primitive septum occur. The cavity of the palate is H shaped. The upper half of the H represents the future nasal cavity, the lower half, the oral cavity (Figure 21-4).

In the lower (oral) part of the cavity, the position of the tongue is largely responsible for the shape of the opening. Its superior surface projects above the mandibular tissue to such an extent that it lies just below the nasal septum.

The second stage of development is the closed palate stage and consists of two important changes. First, the tongue drops to a lower position in the oral cavity, which permits the fusion of the palatal processes at the medial surface of the palate. This fusion occurs first in the anterior region. The palate fuses posteriorly sometime during the 19th week. Second, during this fusion process, **ossification** (conversion into bone) of the anterior part of the palate begins. This eventually results in the formation of the hard palate. See Chapter 15.

It is important to remember that the processes forming the framework of the primitive nose comprise the central core around which the later development of the soft part of the face is laid down.

At times, anomalies (**anomaly** = any deviation from the normal) occur. Failure of the lateral palatine processes to unite or fuse at the midline is a condition termed cleft palate (**cleft** = an opening or crevice). Variations of this condition are many: clefts in the palatine process usually are evidenced at the midline, and those involving the hard palate may occur on one or both sides of the midline in close proximity to the nares. A condition known as **harelip** (imperfect fusion of the upper lip) is frequently associated with cleft palate and is also a congenital defect.

SUGGESTED ACTIVITY

● Participate in a classroom discussion, stressing embryonic development of the cells and tissues of the face, nose, tongue, and palate.

REVIEW

1. Match the terms with the correct description.

___a. Mitosis	1. Intrauterine human life before the second month
___b. Differentiation	2. Digestive tract
___c. Collagen	3. The study of plant and animal tissues
___d. Histology	4. A vital crystalline protein substance in all connective tissue
___e. Embryo	5. Process of cell division
___f. Stomodeum	6. When original cells take on formation of particular types of tissue

2. An aspect of the function of epithelial tissues is to provide:
   a. Support
   b. Contraction
   c. Protection
   d. Conduction

3. What is another function of epithelium?
   a. Connects to other organs
   b. Secretes mucus
   c. Contracts tissue fibers
   d. Provides oxygen

4. The maxillary arch is formed by:
   a. The 4th week
   b. The 7th week
   c. The 10th week
   d. The 3rd week

5. What does the inverted U-shaped elevation represent on a human embryo?
   a. External nares
   b. Pharynx
   c. Heart
   d. Stomodeum

Early Development of the Teeth and Tooth Buds

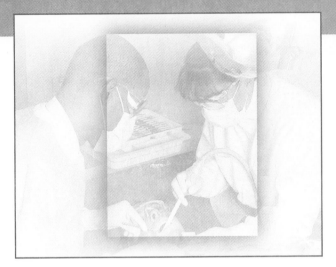

OBJECTIVES

After studying this chapter, the student will be able to:

- Describe the early (embryonic) development of tooth tissues and the beginning formation of tooth buds.
- Discuss the periods of cell development from initiation through morphodifferentiation.
- Define the terminology used in the chapter.
- Describe the stages of development of the tooth buds, including the formation of dentin, enamel, and roots.
- Discuss the order or sequence of organic tissue development.

Introduction

In the study of the structure and development of the teeth, it is appropriate to point out that the teeth are formed by two distinct embryonic tissues: (1) **ectoderm**, or the origin of the enamel organ (crown) portion of the tooth (ectoderm is the outermost of the three primitive germ layers of the embryo), and (2) mesenchyme, from which all the other parts of the tooth and the associated supporting structures develop. **Mesenchyme**, a layer of specialized cells of the **mesoderm** (connective tissue), forms a spongework of cells out of which the dentin, the cementum, and the periodontal ligament originate.

The formation of the teeth begins during the embryonic stage and extends through the **fetal period** (from the second month to full term) and after birth to age 21 (age of complete maturation). At birth there are normally 44 teeth in various stages of development. The deciduous (primary) teeth number 20 and advance in development to the point of eruption. Soon after birth, about the sixth month, they begin to erupt; the majority of teeth erupt by age 2–3 years. The 24 remaining buds are permanent (secondary) teeth, which continue their formation through childhood. It must be emphasized that all eruption schedules are approximations, because no two individuals are alike in their development.

Periods of Development

The development and beginning formation of the tooth buds (at about the sixth week) arise from the oral epithelium tissue, which lines the primitive cavity of the stomodeum. This period of development is termed **initiation**. At first, these dental tissues consist of a continuous ridge of tissue, one for each jaw, and appear as solid **proliferations** (multiplications of cells) of the oral epithelium extending into the underlying mesenchyme. However, these **laminae** (thin layers or plates) are found to be in a position at about right angles to the surface epithelium. They extend around the arch of each jaw and are known as the labiodental laminae (**labiodental** = pertaining to the areas of the lips and teeth).

Differentiation (when the original cells take on the duty of forming each type of tooth tissue) is the second period of development and one that may be further separated into two phases: (1) **histodifferentiation** occurs when the cells of the inner epithelium of the ectoderm prepare to form enamel and become **ameloblasts** (enamel-forming cells) and the peripheral cells become **odontoblasts** (dentin-forming cells) and (2) **morphodifferentiation** occurs when the formative cells are arranged to establish the future shape and size of the organ. Their formation along the future dentinoenamel and dentinocemental junction serves to outline the future crown and root portions of the tooth.

As soon as the labiodental lamina is differentiated, it can be seen as two distinct parts. One part consists of a vertical labial ingrowth, marking off the future lip and vestibule. This structure is termed the **labial lamina** (a thin layer of tissue that forms the lips). The second part continues as an extension toward the tongue. This epithelium gives rise to the enamel organs and is termed the **dental lamina** (thin layer of tooth-producing cells).

Tooth buds form as outgrowths of the dental laminae. Ten of these buds are normally present in each jaw at sites corresponding to the location of the future decid-

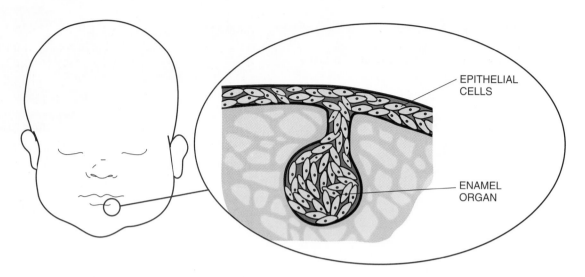

Figure 22-1 Bud stage of tooth development.

uous teeth. As the jaw develops, the dental lamina and the 10 separate tooth buds can be distinguished. At first, these buds appear as solid structures; they then become hollowed out by the further development of the underlying mesenchyme. In this form they serve as molds to fashion the developing crowns of the teeth.

Tooth development begins, as previously mentioned, at about the 5th to 6th week of **intrauterine** (embryonic) life. Within a short time, the development of all the deciduous teeth is initiated. Development of the permanent teeth begins about the 17th week of prenatal life. However, initiation and growth of the various tissues are spread over a period of several years.

Stages of Development

During the first stage of development, or **bud stage** (Figure 22-1), the tooth bud enlarges to become the embryonic **enamel organ**. This organ subsequently develops the enamel of the tooth. A shallow, indented area appears along the lower margin of the enamel

organ; the enamel organ assumes the shape of a cap. This stage of tooth development is called the **cap stage** (Figure 22-2).

The connective tissue within the cap becomes more cellular, because of the proliferation of the cells, and forms what is termed the **dental papilla**. This connective tissue eventually forms the dental pulp and dentin. As the dental papilla becomes further enveloped by the enamel organ, the structure of the enamel organ assumes the shape of a bell. This period of development is called the **bell stage** (Figure 22-3). During this stage, the cells of the enamel organ differentiate and become four separate and distinct layers.

During the bell stage, the cells that have been joined to the oral epithelium begin to disintegrate. At the same time, connective tissue surrounds the enamel organ, and the dental papilla forms a rather dense band of tissue, called the **dental sac**. Development of the cementum, the periodontal ligament (formerly referred to as the "periodontal membrane"), and the lamina dura of the alveolus occurs within the dental sac.

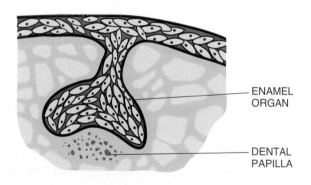

Figure 22-2 Cap stage of tooth development.

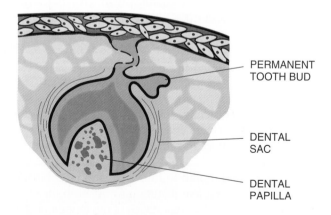

Figure 22-3 Bell stage and dental sac formation.

Formation of the Dentin

The development of the dentin occurs just prior to that of the embryonic enamel. The first step is the formation of a reticular membrane (**reticular** = netlike), the fibers of which appear in a fan-shaped arrangement as they approach the crown area. At the same time, other reticular fibers are developing in the crown area; these pass between the cells arranged on the periphery of the pulp. These specialized cells develop from the outer surface of the dental papilla and are called odontoblasts. They become dentin-forming cells. The process of the formation of dentin is termed **dentinogenesis** (beginning of dentin). Dentin is first differentiated on the tip of the developing crown and gradually envelops the entire pulp cavity (Figure 22-4).

Dentin forms in the shape of small tubes, referred to as **dentinal tubules**. During formation, the dentinal tubules retain a small amount of organic tissues, or collagen (a vital, crystalline, protein substance present in all connective tissue), in their **lumen** (canal of the tubule). These collagenous tissues are called **odontoblastic processes**, or **Tomes' dentinal fibrils**. The area these fibrils occupy during this stage of development is known as **predentin**, an uncalcified layer of material. Once the predentin has been established, the organic framework receives inorganic salts, principally of calcium and phosphorus; this stage is called **apposition** (adding together). The predentin becomes calcified (hard) and is converted to dentin. The growth of dentin is incremental; i.e., the dentin increases layer upon layer. As each additional layer is deposited, the former layer becomes calcified. **Calcification** continues until the entire dentin of the crown has been formed.

In the calcification of dentin, Tomes' dentinal fibrils do not calcify but maintain a metabolic pathway (for the exchange of nutrients and energy, which keep the organ vital) between the pulp and the dentin.

Formation of the Enamel

Immediately after the first layer of dentin is laid down, special epithelial cells (called ameloblasts) begin to form enamel. The process of enamel formation is called **amelogenesis** (beginning of enamel). Many details with regard to enamel formation are uncertain, but it is generally believed that the ameloblasts play approximately the same role as that of the odontoblasts.

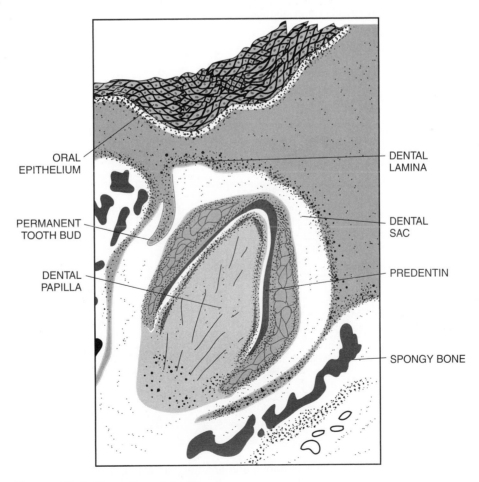

ORAL EPITHELIUM

PERMANENT TOOTH BUD

DENTAL PAPILLA

DENTAL LAMINA

DENTAL SAC

PREDENTIN

SPONGY BONE

Figure 22-4 Formation of dentin.

Enamel formation takes place in two distinct phases: the **formative phase** and the maturation phase. The first, or formative, phase involves the formation of an **enamel matrix** (matrix = a layer of cells that gives form to the crown). The enamel matrix is the detailed development of a wide protoplasmic process (**protoplasm** = the essential constituent of a living cell). These are called Tomes' enamel processes and arise in the region of the future dentinoenamel junction at growth centers corresponding to the location and the number of tips of the cusps. The centers of development are often called **lobes** because they have marked fissures, or divisions. Calcification of Tomes' enamel processes is from the tip of each cusp toward the cervical portion of the tooth (**cervix** = necklike). It is believed that the thickness of enamel is completed in a matrix state before final calcification starts (Figure 22-5).

During the second, or **maturation, phase** in the development of enamel, the matrix undergoes calcification. With calcification, many-sided columns of enamel form; these are called **enamel rods**, or **prisms**. Separating each prism is a calcified substance called **interprismatic substance**.

The ameloblasts retain their structural characteristics until the crown appears, or erupts, in the oral cavity. However, during the later phase of development, the ameloblasts have a horny covering that is firmly attached to the outer enamel surface. The covering, or cuticle, is called **Nasmyth's membrane**. Although some authorities believe this to be a protective covering for the crown, the positive function of the membrane is questionable. When the enamel has completely formed, layers of the enamel organ merge and form the reduced (less vital) enamel epithelium, or Nasmyth's membrane. As the tooth erupts, the part that remains on the crown proper is soon lost.

The remaining reduced enamel epithelium fuses with the epithelial lining of the oral cavity, forming the epithelial attachment.

Root Formation

During morphodifferentiation, the enamel epithelium in the apical portion of the tooth, together with the dental papilla, forms the outline of the root. At this time, the innermost cell layer, or inner enamel epithelium, and the outermost cell layer, or outer enamel epithelium, merge in a loop at the site of the cervix of the tooth. This is called the **cervical loop**. The layers then grow downward for a short distance as a double row of cells termed Hertwig's epithelial root sheath (Figure 22-6). The sheath acts as a limiting membrane for shaping the root of the tooth and is responsible for the formation of root

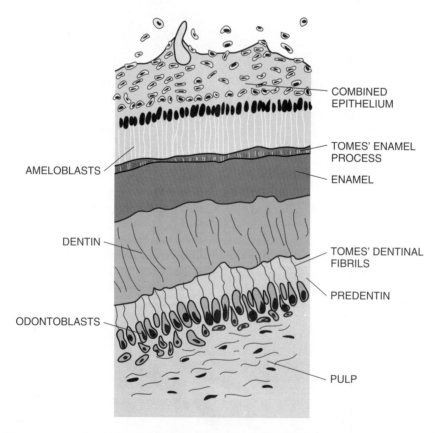

COMBINED EPITHELIUM

TOMES' ENAMEL PROCESS

ENAMEL

AMELOBLASTS

DENTIN

TOMES' DENTINAL FIBRILS

PREDENTIN

ODONTOBLASTS

PULP

***Figure* 22-5** Increments of dentin and enamel (highly magnified).

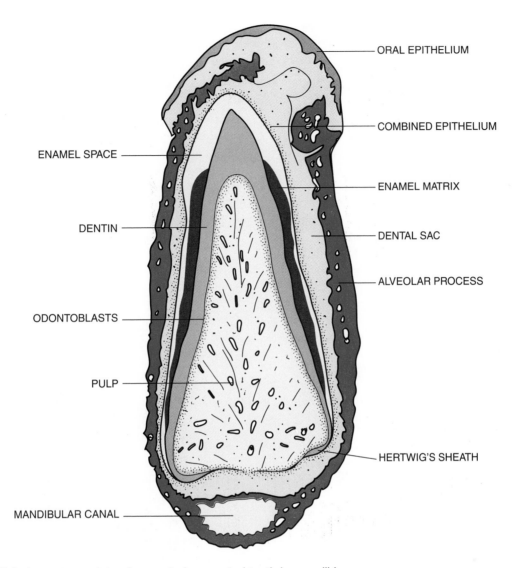

ORAL EPITHELIUM

COMBINED EPITHELIUM

ENAMEL SPACE

ENAMEL MATRIX

DENTIN

DENTAL SAC

ALVEOLAR PROCESS

ODONTOBLASTS

PULP

HERTWIG'S SHEATH

MANDIBULAR CANAL

Figure 22-6 Late stage of development of unerupted tooth in mandible.

dentin. Under the influence of the inner layer of cells, the cells of the dental papilla become odontoblasts, and the formation of the root begins. As the root dentin forms, the tooth moves toward the surface and erupts. Soon after the root dentin begins to form, Hertwig's sheath in that area begins to disintegrate, and the connective tissue of the dental sac grows through the disintegrating sheath and contacts the dentin. As the connective tissues contact the dentin, they become cementoblasts and deposit a layer of cementum on the surface of the dentin.

There is an order to the sequence of events in root formation: (1) the dentin forms, (2) the root lengthens, and (3) cementum is deposited. This sequence is repeated until the root is fully formed.

SUGGESTED ACTIVITIES

● Create a chart to show the periods of development such as initiation and differentiation, and indicate what takes place during each period.

● Create another chart to show the stages of development such as the bud, cap, and bell stages, and indicate what takes place during each stage.

● Create a third chart to show the formation of dentin, enamel, and root, and indicate the primary cells responsible for their development.

● Using all key terms in this chapter, make study cards of each term and use them for basic review.

REVIEW

1. Match each term with the corresponding meaning.

___a. Ectoderm

___b. Mesenchyme

___c. Ameloblasts

___d. Odontoblasts

___e. Initiation

___f. Proliferation

___g. Histo-differentiation

___h. Morpho-differentiation

1. Specialized cells that produce enamel
2. Multiplication of cells
3. Origin of the enamel portion of the tooth
4. When the formative cell arrangement establishes the future shape and size of the organ
5. Specialized cells that produce dentin
6. Origin of parts of the tooth other than enamel
7. Period of development when cells prepare to form enamel and dentin
8. Period of development when the tooth bud begins to form

2. Identify the lettered parts of the illustration. Use the corresponding number from the following list:
   1. Oral epithelium
   2. Dental lamina
   3. Dental sac
   4. Predentin
   5. Spongy bone of mandible
   6. Dental papilla
   7. Permanent tooth bud

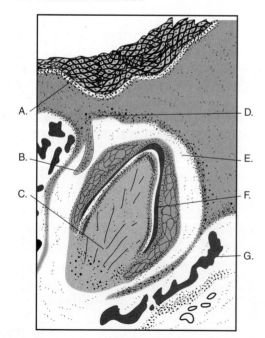

a. _____   e. _____
b. _____   f. _____
c. _____   g. _____
d. _____

3. Identify the lettered parts of the illustration. Use the corresponding number from the following list:
   1. Combined epithelium
   2. Ameloblasts
   3. Tomes' enamel process
   4. Odontoblasts
   5. Pulp
   6. Enamel
   7. Tomes' dentinal fibril
   8. Predentin
   9. Dentin

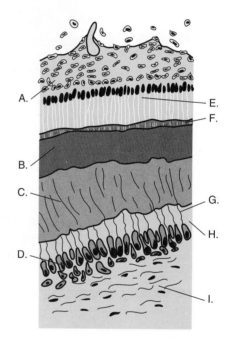

a. _____   f. _____
b. _____   g. _____
c. _____   h. _____
d. _____   i. _____
e. _____

4. Describe the function of the odontoblasts.
   a. Dentin-forming cells
   b. Enamel-forming cells
   c. Cementum-forming cells

5. What type of tissue forms the dental papilla?
   a. Epithelium
   b. Odontoblasts
   c. Ameloblasts
   d. Connective

Composition and Formation of the Teeth

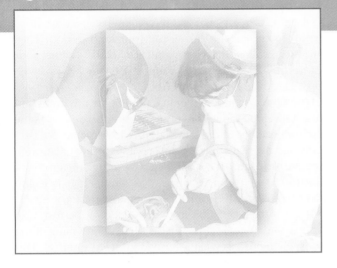

dentin and normally filled with pulp tissue. That portion of the pulp cavity found mainly in the coronal portion is termed the **pulp chamber**. It is always a single cavity. The remaining portion confined within the root is known as the **pulp canal**, or **root canal**. The pulp chamber is comparatively large, and the root canals are small, tapering from the pulp chamber to a minute opening at the apex of the root, which is known as the **apical foramen**.

From a histological point of view, the teeth are made up of four main tissues: enamel, dentin, cementum, and dental pulp. This chapter describes these tissues and the internal structures of the teeth in detail.

OBJECTIVES

After studying this chapter, the student will be able to:

- Recognize the anatomic parts of a typical tooth.
- Discuss the tissue found in the crown of a human tooth.
- Discuss the primary and secondary types of dentin.
- Compare the development, structure, and function of the types of cementum.
- Discuss the structure and functions of the dental pulp.

Introduction

A tooth consists of three parts: the **anatomic crown**, the anatomic root, and the **pulp** cavity. The anatomic crown is that portion that is covered by enamel and is exposed in the oral cavity. The anatomic root is that portion of the root covered by **cementum**; the root is embedded in a bony socket within the maxillae or mandible and surrounded by soft tissue. The narrowed portion, or cervix, and the line denoting the junction of the anatomical crown and the anatomic root are known as the **cementoenamel junction**, or cervical line. The tip of the root is called the **apex**.

Both the crown and the root consist of two layers of hard substance (tissue) surrounding the dental pulp. The crown's outer layer is **enamel**, and its inner layer is **dentin**. The root's outer layer is cementum, and its inner layer is dentin (Figure 23-1).

The **pulp cavity** is a space in the central portion of the crowns and roots of teeth that is surrounded by

Enamel

Enamel is the hardest tissue in the human body and consists of approximately 96% inorganic material and 4% organic material. Calcium and phosphorus are its main inorganic components. Designated carbon compounds are the organic components (Refer to Chapter 22.) Made of this calcified substance, enamel is the hard tissue that covers the entire crown of the tooth and protects the

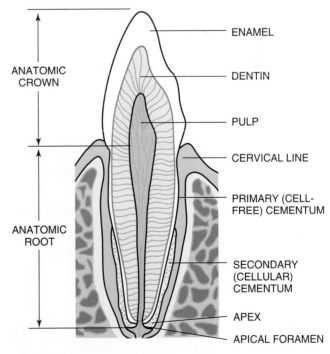

Figure 23-1 Tissues of teeth.

dentin. The morphological structure of enamel is known as the enamel rod or prism (**morphology** = the science of organic form and structure). The enamel rods are continuous structures that originate at the dentinoenamel junction and terminate at the free enamel surface. In a transverse section, human enamel rods are roughly **polygonal** (having many sides) in shape. One or more of the surfaces may be convex or concave. These highly calcified rods are separated by a minute interprismatic space, which is also calcified in mature enamel (Figure 23-2).

The direction of the rods varies in different teeth. In general, they are arranged radially, in a fanlike arrangement, from the tip of the cusp to the dentinoenamel junction. They gradually assume a more acute (sharp) angle in the direction of the dentinal tubules as the cementoenamel junction is approached.

Lines of Retzius

In a longitudinal tooth section (lengthwise cut through the tooth), a number of brown lines may be observed that represent the contour lines of the enamel. These are known as the **lines of Retzius**, or incremental lines. They are areas of diminished calcification caused by brief pauses in the development of the enamel. The lines of Retzius are similar in appearance to the annual developmental rings seen in the trunk of a tree, and they indicate stages of tooth development in much the same way.

Lines of Schreger

The **lines of Schreger**, or enamel lamellae (thin plates of bone), develop as narrow cracks that become filled with organic matter during the formation period. They are the result of the wavy direction of the enamel rods caused by stretching or twisting the enamel as it develops. These lamellae extend from the surface of the tooth toward the dentinoenamel junction. Some are known to reach the junction and even penetrate the dentin. Some authorities believe the lamellae provide an entry for bacteria and make teeth more susceptible to decay. Through **transillumination** (passing a light through the crown of the tooth), these areas appear as alternating light and dark bands and are sometimes mistaken for fractures.

A further variation in the direction of the rods also appears in enamel. This consists of an intertwining of the rods, giving rise to what is termed **gnarled enamel**. This structure apparently increases the strength of the enamel.

Enamel is formed by epithelial cells that lose their functional ability once the tooth has been completed. Mature enamel has no power of further growth or repair and is an **inert substance** (is not active and remains idle).

Dentin

Dentin is the hard, dense, light yellow substance that makes up the bulk of the tooth. It is harder than bone but

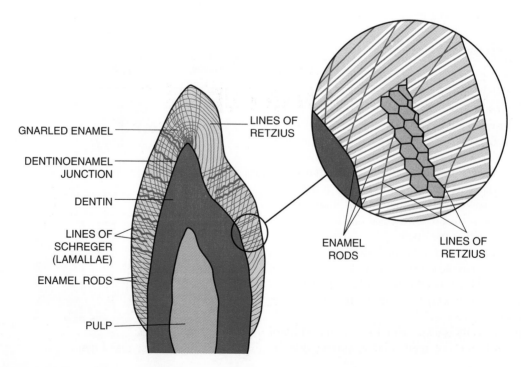

Figure 23-2 Structure of enamel.

softer than enamel. Dentin consists of approximately 70% inorganic matter. The chief inorganic components are calcium and phosphorus.

Structure of Dentin

Morphologically, dentin consists of a calcified matrix and dentinal tubules (Figure 23-3). In the living state, there is no unoccupied space in the dentinal tubule, except for a minute capillary area that allows for the circulation of tissue fluid. Variations in the structure of dentin are numerous.

Generally, the dentinal tubules follow a somewhat S-shaped course, beginning at the surface of the pulp and ending at the dentinoenamel junction. These hollow structures are known as **Tomes' dentinal tubules**. Each tubule contains a fiber called a **Tomes' dentinal fibril**, which is a protoplasmic extension of an **odontoblast** (dentin-forming cell) on the surface of the pulp. Some of the dentinal fibrils pass across the dentinoenamel junction and terminate in the enamel.

The cell bodies of the odontoblasts appear as a layer of columnar cells between the pulp and the dentin. They are considered to be part of the pulp.

Formation and calcification of the dentin begin at the tip of the cusp(s) and proceed inward toward the pulp. Brief pauses between the deposited layers (increments) are marked by fine lines that are at right angles to the dentinal tubules.

Secondary Dentin

All the dentin in a newly formed tooth is called **primary dentin**. Soon after eruption, a layer of dentin adjacent to the pulp cavity forms. This may appear somewhat different in form from the dentin near the periphery and is classified as regular **secondary dentin**. When the dental pulp is irritated as a result of caries (dental decay), cavity preparation, **abrasion** (wearing away), or **erosion** (disintegration of tooth surfaces other than those used in mastication), a layer of secondary dentin begins to form directly under the site of the structural change. This formation, which is a direct result of the irritation or stimulation, is called irregular secondary dentin.

Sensitivity

Dentin is sensitive to various stimuli. It reacts to **tactile** (touch), **thermal** (temperature), and chemical stimulation. Sensitivity is not uniform in all teeth; it varies greatly from person to person. The mechanism transmitting the sensation through the dentin to the pulp is not thoroughly understood in spite of numerous studies that have been made. It is generally agreed upon that dentin does not have nerve fibers and that the sensitivity may be due to changes in the dentinal fibrils.

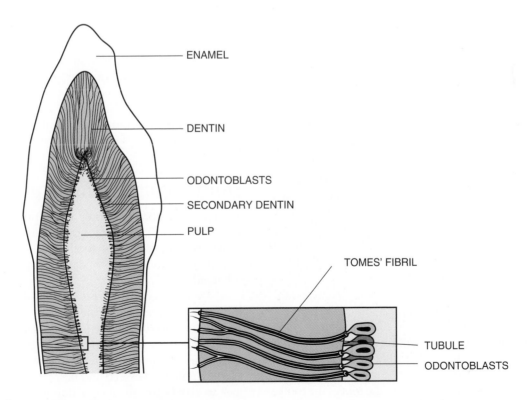

Figure 23-3 Structure of dentin.

Age Changes

It may be noted that layers of dentin form in locations beneath areas of the tooth that have been heavily worn through **attrition** (wearing away by continued friction and chewing). As long as pulp tissue remains sound and unaltered, the apposition of dentin may continue. This causes the pulp chamber to become reduced in size, a condition generally found in the teeth of people in their later years of life.

Cementum

Cementum is the bonelike tissue that covers the roots of the teeth in a thin layer. Its composition is approximately 55% inorganic and 45% organic. The inorganic components are mainly calcium salts. The chief constituent of the organic material is collagen.

Cementum originates in a manner similar to bone. The cells concerned with **cementogenesis** (beginning of cementum) arise from embryonic connective tissue and develop from the dental sac. They differentiate and enlarge to become fairly large round cells that lie adjacent to the root of the tooth. Cementum is deposited in layers. The end product of this deposition is a thin layer of calcified tissue that is deposited on, and firmly attached to, the entire root surface. Embedded in the cementum are the principal (collagenous) fibers of the periodontal ligament. The opposite ends of these fibers are embedded in the alveolar bone and are called Sharpey's fibers. These fibers are responsible for supporting the tooth in the socket.

The cementum joins the enamel near the cervix of the tooth; the cementoenamel junction is somewhat variable. It may extend precisely to the termination of the enamel, it may extend beyond the cervical termination of the enamel, or it may fail to extend to the enamel. In a few teeth, a break is present between the enamel and the cementum, exposing a narrow area of root dentin. Such areas are very sensitive to thermal, chemical, or mechanical stimuli.

Histologically, two types of cementum are recognized: cell-free (primary) and cellular (secondary). Primary cementum does not contain cells and is usually distributed quite uniformly over the surface of the root. Secondary cementum contains cells similar to bone, or **cementocytes**, and is usually confined to the apical third of the root.

Functions of Cementum

The main function of cementum is mechanical. It anchors the tooth to the bony wall of the socket.

In addition to the important function performed by cementum in anchoring the fibers to the root of the tooth, there is another process in which it may take part.

Frequently, the root undergoes resorption; i.e., both cementum and dentin are destroyed. When this happens, new cementum may replace the lost tissue of the root and bring about a functional repair. This situation may arise in cases in which a fracture of the root takes place.

Cementum is formed throughout the life of the tooth. This compensates for the loss of tooth substance due to wear on the **occlusal** (biting and chewing) surfaces of the teeth. This process allows for the attachment of new fibers of the periodontal membrane to the surface of the root. This is discussed in Chapter 24.

Dental Pulp

Blood Supply

The blood supply of the pulp enters through the apical foramen and is accompanied by a lymphatic draining system (Figure 23-4). (Lymph is a clear, colorless fluid that is derived from and closely resembles blood. It is carried by an independent system of vessels, called the lymph system, from the tissues to the heart.) The arteries have narrow lumina with some smooth muscle fibers in their walls. The veins are often more numerous and have exceedingly thin walls and relatively wide lumina. In young teeth, the pulp is filled with blood vessels. In older teeth, some of these blood vessels are replaced with other tissue.

Sensitivity

The nerve supply of the pulp consists of one type of fiber that ends in a dense network below the odontoblast layer. Another type of fiber terminates as fine nerve endings on the surface of the odontoblasts. Depending on their structure and function, these nerve endings transmit sensations of either pain or touch.

Functions of Dental Pulp

The chief function of the pulp is the formation of dentin. However, it also provides nourishment to the dentin, provides sensation to the tooth, and responds to irritation either by forming secondary dentin or by becoming inflamed.

Dental pulp is enclosed within the hard walls of the pulp chamber, which permits no expansion of the pulp tissue. Swelling of the pulp tissue due to inflammation compresses the blood vessels against the walls of the chamber. This results in **thrombosis** (clotting of the blood within the vessels) and may result in strangulation and **necrosis** (death of cells due to disease or injury). These dead cells are referred to as necrotic tissue.

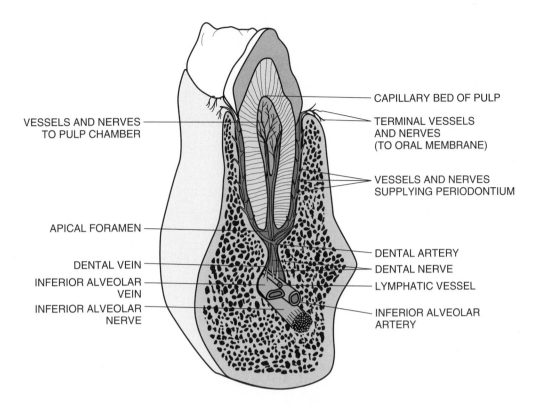

CAPILLARY BED OF PULP

TERMINAL VESSELS
AND NERVES
(TO ORAL MEMBRANE)

VESSELS AND NERVES
SUPPLYING PERIODONTIUM

VESSELS AND NERVES
TO PULP CHAMBER

APICAL FORAMEN

DENTAL VEIN

INFERIOR ALVEOLAR
VEIN

INFERIOR ALVEOLAR
NERVE

DENTAL ARTERY

DENTAL NERVE

LYMPHATIC VESSEL

INFERIOR ALVEOLAR
ARTERY

Figure 23-4 Blood and nerve supply to tooth and surrounding structures.

Age Changes in the Pulp

Other facts concerning the pulp are important to recognize. Pulp tissue is more extensive in young teeth than in the teeth of the mature individual. Furthermore, the thickness of dentin in the coronal (crown) part of the deciduous or young permanent tooth is less than in the tooth of the mature individual.

SUGGESTED ACTIVITIES

● Create a chart to show tooth structures such as enamel, dentin, cementum, and pulp, and indicate the component parts and the purposes for each structure.

● Using all key terms in this chapter, make study cards of each term and use them for basic review.

REVIEW

1. Name the lines that indicate the stages of development in tooth enamel.
   a. Lines of Schreger
   b. Lines of Retzius
   c. Gnarled enamel
   d. Enamel rods

2. Which is the hardest tissue in the human body?
   a. Compact bone
   b. Cancellous bone
   c. Enamel
   d. Dentin

3. Name the cell bodies that appear as a layer of columnar cells between the pulp and the dentin.
   a. Ameloblasts
   b. Osteoclasts
   c. Osteoblasts
   d. Odontoblasts

4. What type of dentin forms as a direct result of irritation or stimulation?
   a. Irregular secondary dentin
   b. Regular secondary dentin
   c. Primary dentin

5. Name some functions of the dental pulp: it (1) forms ameloblasts, (2) provides sensation to the tooth, (3) provides nourishment to dentin, and/or (4) forms dentin.
   a. 1, 2, 3
   b. 2, 3, 4
   c. 1, 2, 4
   d. 1, 3, 4

6. Which two tooth tissues form continuously throughout the life of the tooth?
   a. Enamel and dentin
   b. Dentin and cementum
   c. Cementum and pulp
   d. Pulp and dentin

Tissues Surrounding the Teeth

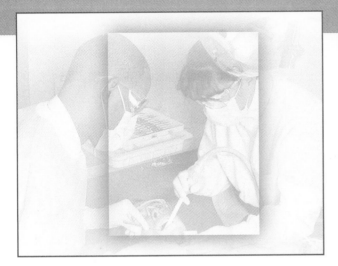

OBJECTIVES

After studying this chapter, the student will be able to:

● Determine the supporting tissues of human teeth.

● Discuss the structure and function of the alveolar process(es).

● Discuss the structure, functions, and importance of the periodontal ligament.

● Identify the types of gingiva and the function of each.

● Discuss the radical changes that may occur in the gingiva(e) and the contributing reasons for the change.

Introduction

In the first chapters of this section, histology has been limited to the development and structure of teeth. However, it must be realized that without the presence and function of a group of structures that immediately surround the cervical part of the crown and root, these teeth would be nonfunctional. Although these structures are closely related and often blend together, it is helpful to consider them separately.

The tissues that surround and support the teeth are the alveolar process, the periodontal ligament (membrane), and the gingivae. Collectively, they are called the **periodontium**.

Alveolar Process

The alveolar process as such develops in connection with the growth of the jaw and the eruption of the teeth.

The alveolar processes are not structures separate from the maxilla and mandible but are parts of them that are especially designed to provide sockets and supports for the teeth. To understand the relationships of the teeth, mandible, and maxilla, it will be helpful to review the structure of these bones. Refer to Chapter 15.

Histologically, the alveolus is made up of compact bone with an inner (lingual) and outer (facial) plate called the **cortical plate**. Between these two plates, the bone is spongy (cancellous). Both the inner and outer cortical plates are continuous with a thin layer of compact bone, the alveolar process proper, or lamina dura. This dense bone lines the root socket and affords attachment for the principal fibers of the periodontal ligament. In some areas of the jaw, the lamina dura and cortical plates are interrupted by perforations (small openings) through which pass blood, lymph vessels, and nerves (Figure 24-1).

The cortical plate provides strength and protection for the supporting bone (maxilla and mandible) and also acts as a site for attachment of skeletal muscles. The cortical plate is covered by **periosteum** (fibrous sheath) and varies slightly in the different regions of the arches. In the labial sections, the cortical plate is attached directly to the **alveolar process proper** (**lamina dura**). Because of this arrangement, the bone overlying the roots of the anterior teeth is of a brittle nature. The cortical plate is more dense in the mandible than in the maxilla and has fewer perforations for passage of vessels and nerves.

Periodontal Ligament

The **periodontal ligament** (membrane) is a term used for a group of connective fibers that suspend the tooth in the socket and support the gingiva. *Note*: Previously, some references have used the term periodontal membrane. However, the term periodontal ligament is widely accepted, because it is more descriptive when reviewing its function. This ligament is made up primarily of **Sharpey's fibers** and principal fibers (Figure 24-2). Sharpey's fibers are bundles of principal fibers anchored in the cementum on one end and in bone on the other. They form bundles of fibers that are arranged so as to withstand the functional stresses of the tooth after it has fully erupted. The fibers are not elastic, but owing to the wavy direction of their course, some slight tooth movement is permitted.

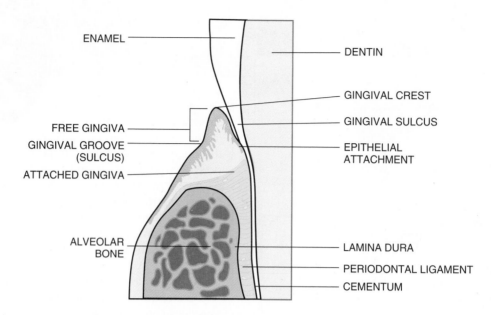

Figure 24-1 Structure of the periodontium.

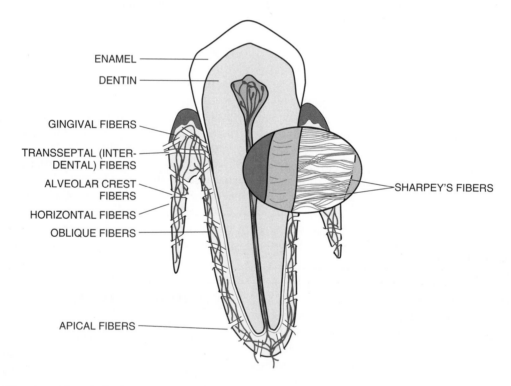

Figure 24-2 Structure of periodontal membrane, principal fibers.

In the erupted tooth, several groups of fibers can be distinguished. The principal fibers are concerned with the support of the gingival tissues and the tooth. They are white collagenous fibers and are arranged as follows: (1) gingival fibers—radiate in the gingiva and are attached to the tooth in the region of the cementoenamel junction; (2) transseptal (interdental) fibers—connect cervical portions and cementum of adjacent teeth; and (3) alveolar group fibers—attached to the alveolar process and to the tooth (Figure 24-3). The alveolar group may be further divided into four subdivisions: (a) cervical crest fibers—extend from the cervical cementum to the crest of alveolar bone; (b) horizontal fibers—extend from the cementum to the alveolar process at right angles to the root of the tooth; (c) oblique fibers—extend obliquely (in a slanting direction) from the cementum to the apical two-thirds of the root to the alveolar process; and (d) apical fiber—radiate from the

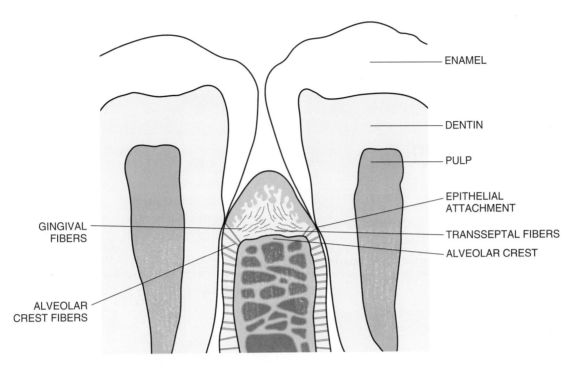

Figure 24-3 Fibers of periodontal ligament.

cementum surrounding the apex of the root to the alveolar process.

The **principal fibers** support the gingival tissue and suspend the tooth in the socket. This type of attachment is termed **gomphosis**.

The blood supply of the periodontal ligament is derived from the vessels in the alveolus. These vessels may enter the ligament by three different routes: (1) some accompany the vessels that supply the pulp and branch just before the pulpal vessels enter the apical foramen; (2) some are extensions of vessels that supply the alveolus; and (3) some are from the deep vessels that supply the gingiva. An adequate lymphatic drainage accompanies the blood vessels. Refer to Chapter 23.

Within the ligaments are **cementoblasts** that form cementum, **osteoblasts** that build bone, and **fibroblasts** that form fibrous tissues. The presence of small nests of slightly modified epithelial cells may be observed in the periodontal ligament. These cells are remnants of the enamel organ and are known as **epithelial nests**.

The functions of the periodontal ligament are formative (cementoblasts and osteoblasts), supportive (principal fibers), sensory, and nutritive (nerves and blood vessels).

Gingiva

The surface of the gingiva consists of various layers of epithelium. The gingiva consists of free gingiva and attached gingiva. The free gingiva (so-called because it is movable) fits snugly around the crown of the tooth just above the cervical part (cervix). The edge, or lip, of the free gingiva is the gingival crest (gingival margin). Between the tooth and the free gingiva is the space called the **gingival sulcus** (*sulcus* = groove) that extends to the point at which the gingiva is attached to the tooth. Below the sulcus, the attachment of the tooth and gingiva is a marked line separating the free gingiva and the attached gingiva; this is called the **free gingival groove**. Triangular folds of gingival tissue between the teeth consist of both free and attached gingiva; these are called **interdental papillae** (*papilla* = cone-shaped projection). The chief function of this tissue is protection; it prevents injury and infection to the deeper tissues.

Changes in the Gingiva

Radical changes can and do occur in both the composition making up the gingiva and the relation of the gingiva to the tooth. These changes may be referred to as **gingival recession**. As the term implies, the gingivae recede rootward, and, as a result, the **gingival crest** recedes from its original position to a more rootward position. Such changes may be the result of advancing age, improper oral hygiene, malocclusion, and physiologic or pathologic disturbances.

Epithelial downgrowth is accompanied by detachment of the periodontal fibers from this portion of the root. Recession may proceed to the degree that the crest of the gingiva may recede to a point below the cementoenamel junction. This type of gingival recession occurs in the absence of any known pathologic disturbance (alterations produced by disease). It results in the exposure of more of the crown in the tooth cavity, and because it is accompanied by a detachment of the gingiva (an extremely wide and deep space in the gingival crevice), it is called a **periodontal pocket**.

SUGGESTED ACTIVITIES

● Create a chart to show the supporting tissues surrounding teeth such as the alveolar process, periodontal ligament, and gingiva, and indicate the component parts of each and their purposes.

● Using all key terms in this chapter, make study cards of each term and use them for basic review.

REVIEW

1. Identify the lettered parts of the illustration. Select the corresponding number from the following list:

   1. Gingival fibers
   2. Dentin
   3. Transseptal (interdental) fibers
   4. Horizontal fibers
   5. Oblique fibers
   6. Enamel
   7. Apical fibers
   8. Alveolar crest fibers
   9. Sharpey's fibers

   a. _____
   b. _____
   c. _____
   d. _____
   e. _____
   f. _____
   g. _____
   h. _____
   i. _____

2. Name the three supporting structures of the teeth: (1) periodontal ligament, (2) gingiva, (3) gingival sulcus, and/or (4) alveolar process.
   a. 1, 2, 3
   b. 2, 3, 4
   c. 1, 2, 4
   d. 1, 3, 4

3. Collectively, the supporting structures of the teeth are called:
   a. Periodontium
   b. Tooth attachment
   c. Supporting bone
   d. Supporting tissues

4. What type of fibers are those that suspend the tooth in the socket and support the gingiva?
   a. Gingival
   b. Alveolar
   c. Vertical
   d. Connective

5. The space between the tooth and free gingiva is called:
   a. Gingival crest
   b. Gingival fibers
   c. Gingival sulcus
   d. Attached gingiva

6. The attachment of the principal fibers to cementum or bone is called:
   a. Gomphosis
   b. Connective fibers
   c. Cervical attachment
   d. Epithelial attachment

Eruption and Resorption of Teeth

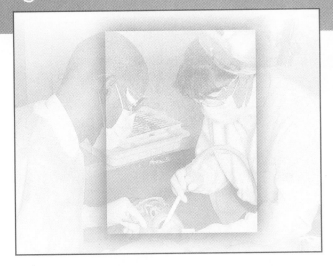

OBJECTIVES

After studying this chapter, the student will be able to:

- Discuss the events that occur prior to the tooth eruption process.
- Determine some of the physiologic symptoms leading to the eruption of deciduous (primary) teeth.
- Explain the sequence and usual times of eruption of deciduous teeth.
- Explain the sequence and usual eruption times of permanent teeth.
- Discuss the progressive changes that occur in the dental pulp of a tooth.
- Review and determine the usual positions of the succedaneous teeth.
- Explain the area of greatest resorption of the deciduous teeth.
- Explain why deciduous roots may be retained and unresorbed as permanent (succedaneous) teeth erupt.
- Discuss the specialized cells involved in the process of root resorption.

Introduction

The eruption of the teeth is a normal physiologic process—a result of growth—during which the crown of the developing tooth and the root are formed. All the factors that allow crowns to escape from their bony surrounding and appear in the oral cavity are not fully understood. Growth results in the enlargement and elongation of the tooth, accompanied by the positioning of the tooth in the oral cavity. Some authorities have speculated that the process is a result of pressure exerted by the roots as they elongate during development. Only recently has it been concluded that the teeth of human beings are in a state of continuous eruption.

Process of Eruption

A review of the events that occur prior to or that accompany eruption may give us a better understanding of this process. In the enamel organ stage of development, the tooth is enclosed in a **fibrous sheath** (the dental sac) that lies within a **crypt** (space within the alveolar bone). Differentiation of the cells results in the formation of the permanent tooth bud. Fibers from the dental sac position themselves in the root of the tooth, and since the crown is virtually complete just preceding eruption, the result is the occlusal movement of the tooth, also referred to as active eruption (*occlusal* = the contacting surfaces of opposing teeth, upper and lower arch).

When the crown emerges through the oral epithelium, a union of the oral and combined epithelia occurs. The portion made up of the oral mucosa is altered somewhat and forms the gingiva. The combined epithelium on the cervical part of the crown is retained and becomes the epithelial attachment. Refer to Chapter 24.

At the time of eruption, the fibers of the periodontal ligaments are not fully formed or attached; this occurs when the teeth are formed sufficiently to **occlude** (biting surfaces of maxillary and mandibular teeth meet).

There are normally 10 deciduous (primary) teeth and 16 permanent teeth in each jaw. During early childhood and before all the deciduous teeth have erupted, the child is said to have incomplete deciduous dentition. Later on, when the child has a full complement of deciduous teeth, the term used is complete deciduous dentition. Loss of the deciduous anterior teeth, and replacement by permanent teeth at about the age of 5 or 6 years, is called **mixed dentition**.

Some deciduous teeth erupt entirely uneventfully, and others erupt with some incident. A study of the symptoms (evident disorder in the functions of the body) of deciduous tooth eruption reveals excessive **salivation** (secretion of saliva), or drooling. This is followed by periods of fretfulness and biting, accompanied by a loss of appetite. In the event that body resistance is lowered, a rise in body temperature, coughing, sneezing, and diarrhea may be evidenced.

Ordinarily, the permanent teeth develop to replace and assume the position of the deciduous teeth after **exfoliation** (involved in the process of shedding the

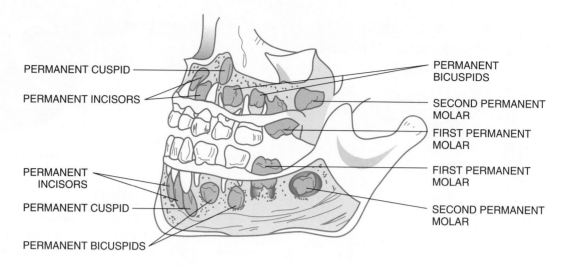

PERMANENT CUSPID

PERMANENT INCISORS

PERMANENT INCISORS

PERMANENT CUSPID

PERMANENT BICUSPIDS

PERMANENT BICUSPIDS

SECOND PERMANENT MOLAR

FIRST PERMANENT MOLAR

FIRST PERMANENT MOLAR

SECOND PERMANENT MOLAR

Figure 25-1 Mixed dentition (approximately age 7).

primary teeth); such teeth are called **succedaneous teeth.** They develop in close proximity to the root(s) of the deciduous teeth (Figure 25-1). As the permanent tooth crown develops, the root of the deciduous tooth undergoes the physiologic process of **resorption** (a loss of substance and reduction of the volume and size of tissues). This results in a loss of attachment, and the tooth is exfoliated. In the areas where the permanent tooth buds do not replace the primary teeth, the permanent tooth buds arise independently.

Eruption of the permanent teeth, although somewhat less dramatic, often presents problems not present in the eruption of deciduous dentition. Tooth buds of the permanent teeth develop in the jaw during the time the deciduous teeth are in their normal positions; they are not situated so that their lengthwise movement alone will bring them into position in the dental arch. They must erupt to pierce the oral epithelium and at the same time assume the relative position of other teeth in the arch. Consequently, these teeth must, and often do, undergo movements in several directions in addition to the occlusal movement.

Eruption of Deciduous (Primary) Teeth

The eruption of deciduous (primary) teeth commences about the seventh month after birth and is completed about the end of the second year. In some individuals there may be considerable variation from the schedule. In most instances, the mandibular teeth erupt before the maxillary teeth; i.e., generally, a mandibular incisor erupts shortly before the incisor of the maxillary arch with which it occludes. The anterior group consists of two central incisors, two lateral incisors, and two cuspids in each arch. Posterior dentition consists of two first molars and two second molars in each arch.

Authorities agree that the explanations of extremes in the eruption sequence cannot be given in every case. However, they have noted that the positions of erupting teeth and the time period involved follow a relatively uniform plan (Table 25-1).

Eruption of Permanent Teeth

The permanent dentition, or teeth that erupt to take the place of the deciduous teeth and those that erupt posterior to the space occupied by the deciduous teeth, should total 32 teeth when fully erupted and complete. These are divided into 2 groups (maxillary and mandibular) consisting of 16 teeth each. The anterior group consists of 2 central incisors, 2 lateral incisors, and 2 cuspids in each arch. The posterior dentition is composed of 2 first bicuspids (premolars), two second bicuspids (premolars), 2 first molars, 2 second molars, and 2 third molars in each arch.

Eruption of the permanent teeth is dependent to some extent on the exfoliation of the deciduous teeth. There is great variation in the sequence of eruption. Table 25-2 is meant as a guide to normal eruption.

Changes in Dental Pulp

After the crown and part of the root are formed, the tooth penetrates the mucous membrane and becomes evident in the mouth. Further formation of the root is thought to be an active factor in pushing the crown toward its final position. Eruption of the tooth is said to be complete when most of the crown is apparent and when it has made contact with a tooth or teeth in the opposing arch.

Actually, eruption continues as more of the crown is exposed; root dentin and cementum continue to form after the tooth is in use. Formation of the root is about

Table 25-1 Deciduous Teeth: Approximate Ages and Most Usual Times of Eruption

Deciduous Teeth	Normal Span (months)	Average Age (months)
Mandibular central incisor	3–9	6
Maxillary central incisor	5–9	7
Mandibular lateral incisor	5–9	7
Maxillary lateral incisor	7–11	9
Mandibular first molar	10–14	12
Maxillary first molar	12–16	14
Mandibular cuspid	13–18	16
Maxillary cuspid	15–20	18
Mandibular second molar	18–22	20
Maxillary second molar	22–26	24

Table 25-2 Permanent Teeth: Approximate Ages and Most Usual Times of Eruption

Permanent Teeth	Normal Span (Years)	Average Age (Years)
Mandibular first molar	5–7	6
Maxillary first molar	5–7	6
Mandibular central incisor	5–7	6
Maxillary central incisor	6–8	7
Mandibular lateral incisor	6–8	7
Maxillary lateral incisor	7–9	8
Mandibular cuspid	8–10	9
Maxillary first bicuspid	9–11	10
Mandibular first bicuspid	9–12	10
Maxillary second bicuspid	9–12	10
Maxillary cuspid	10–12	11
Mandibular second bicuspid	10–12	11
Mandibular second molar	10–13	11
Maxillary second molar	11–13	12
Mandibular third molar	16–25	17
Maxillary third molar	16–25	17

half finished when the tooth emerges. Cementum covers the root. Ultimately, the root is completed.

The pulp tissue continues to function with its blood and nerve supply after the tooth is formed. By this time, the pulp cavity within the tooth has become small in comparison to the tooth size. Its outline is similar to the outline of the crown and the root, with the opening of the pulp cavity constricted at the apex. This opening is called the apical foramen. The pulp continues in its tissue-forming function; it may form secondary dentin as a protection to itself.

The dental pulp is a connective-tissue organ containing a number of structures. Among these structures are veins, arteries, a lymphatic system, and nerves. The primary function of the pulp is to form the dentin structure of the tooth. When the tooth is newly erupted, the dental pulp is large. It becomes progressively smaller as the tooth formation is completed. The pulp is relatively large in deciduous teeth and in newly erupted permanent teeth. For this reason, the teeth of children and young people are more sensitive than the teeth of older persons when exposed to changes in temperature and to dental operative procedures.

As a person ages, the pulp cavity becomes more constricted and smaller in size. Sometimes the pulp chamber within the crown is completely obliterated; in some rare instances, the entire pulp chamber has been found to be filled with secondary deposit. Although deciduous teeth are not usually affected by this process, they may show secondary dentin in the pulp chambers as a result of irritation produced by caries or excessive wear.

Resorption of the Deciduous Roots

The resorption (disintegration) of deciduous roots is a natural phenomenon. The smaller teeth, even though they are well suited for the growing jaw, are replaced with larger teeth that are better able to perform the work of more mature jaws. Because the jaws have become larger, the pressure of mastication has increased, and stronger structures are needed to withstand the stress.

By the time the deciduous teeth have erupted, the permanent teeth are left to occupy a position near the apices of the deciduous anterior teeth and between the roots of the deciduous molars. If the succedaneous tooth is lingual to the root of the deciduous tooth, resorption will be greatest in the area of the root that lies next to the permanent tooth organ; i.e., the lingual surface (refer to Figure 25-1). When the deciduous roots surround the permanent tooth bud, as in molars, the root surfaces of the tooth nearest the permanent (succedaneous) tooth are the first to experience resorption.

In cases where the permanent successor is not in alignment with the deciduous roots, eruption may be along a path that permits a portion of the deciduous root to be retained and unresorbed. This can be revealed by means of a radiographic (x-ray) examination. The deciduous root should be physically extracted to make room for the proper development of the permanent tooth. On the other hand, deciduous roots tend to resorb even when no permanent successor is present. A deciduous tooth may remain in position far beyond its natural shedding time, and resorption occurs because the deciduous tooth is unable to withstand the forces of mastication. In this case, the root is resorbed by traumatic stimulation (*trauma* = damage produced by external force).

The process of shedding (exfoliating) deciduous teeth can be summarized by saying that it is the result of progressive destruction of the roots. Pressure created during growth and eruption of permanent teeth stimulate activity of the osteoclasts, cementoclasts, and dentinoclasts. **Osteoclasts** are specialized cells that destroy the bone between the deciduous tooth and its permanent successor. The **cementoclasts** and **dentinoclasts** then cause general resorption of the roots of the deciduous (primary) teeth until only the crowns remain. As this takes place, the permanent tooth is moving into position. When the deciduous tooth crowns are shed, this space is occupied by the permanent tooth. Permanent molars erupt in the space posterior to the deciduous teeth that have developed during the forward growth of the maxillae and mandible.

SUGGESTED ACTIVITIES

- Create a chart that shows the chronological order of changes that take place during the life of the dental pulp.
- Study a cut-away typodont containing both primary and permanent tooth buds (mixed dentition).
- Using all terms in this chapter, make study cards of each term and use them for basic review.

REVIEW

1. Identify the lettered parts of the illustration. Select the corresponding number from the following list:

Mandibular
1. Permanent incisors
2. Permanent cuspid
3. Permanent biscuspids (premolars)
4. First permanent molar
5. Second permanent molar

Maxillary
6. Permanent incisors
7. Permanent cuspid
8. Permanent bicuspids (premolars)
9. First permanent molar
10. Second permanent molar

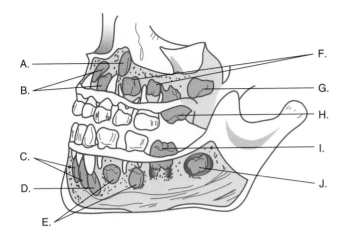

A. _____
B. _____
C. _____
D. _____
E. _____
F. _____
G. _____
H. _____
I. _____
J. _____

2. The process of shedding deciduous teeth is termed:
a. Succedaneous
b. Exfoliation
c. Resorption
d. Mixed dentition

3. Teeth that replace and assume the relative position of the deciduous teeth are called:
a. Primary
b. Exfoliated
c. Succedaneous
d. Nonsuccedaneous

4. Specialized cells that destroy bone are called:
a. Osteoclasts
b. Osteoblasts
c. Cementoclasts
d. Cementoblasts

5. What would be the normal span of months involved in the eruption sequence of deciduous teeth?
a. From 8 to 36 months
b. From 6 to 12 months
c. From 3 to 26 months
d. From 12 to 24 months

6. What would be the normal span of years involved in the eruption sequence of permanent teeth?
a. From 6 to 12 years
b. From 4 to 16 years
c. From 8 to 21 years
d. From 5 to 25 years

External Features of the Teeth

CHAPTER 26

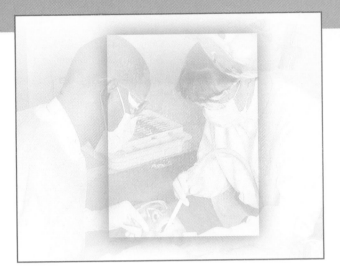

Section 6 determined that man has two series of teeth: (1) deciduous, or sets that are exfoliated (shed), and (2) permanent (succedaneous) teeth that replace deciduous teeth and permanent molars.

To become familiar with terms generally used in describing the external appearance of the teeth is the objective of this chapter. Some of these terms have been used in previous chapters and may be familiar, but they will be repeated to make this chapter complete.

OBJECTIVES

After studying this chapter, the student will be able to:

● Define the term nomenclature.
● Develop terminology for the teeth of human dentition, and be able to define each term.
● Develop a mental image of the crown surfaces of each tooth and their position in the mouth.
● Explain the five surfaces of a tooth and how to divide the crown and root(s) into thirds for study.
● Study each tooth and recognize important landmarks.

Introduction

Section 6 on dental histology described the tissues of the teeth, their surrounding structures, and development. This section deals with the description of the teeth.

Odontology is the study of the descriptive anatomy of teeth, i.e., the external form and relationship of the teeth. Teeth are appendages (added parts) usually found in the mouth and attached to but not forming a part of the skeleton. The main purposes of teeth are to seize and masticate food and to act as "weapons of defense."

Nomenclature of Teeth

A scientific system and terms for the several parts of the teeth, as well as their names and locations in the skull, is called nomenclature. The dental assistant can be of great help to the dentist by becoming well acquainted with all these terms (Figure 26-1).

Maxillary teeth are located in the upper arch of the mouth (bones forming the upper arch are the maxillae), in the maxillary arch, and their roots are embedded in the alveolar processes of the maxillae. They are sometimes referred to as "upper teeth."

The lower arch (formed by the mandible) is called the mandibular arch. Teeth of the lower arch are called mandibular teeth rather than "lower teeth."

The teeth of human dentition are divided into certain groups, according to their function. They are **incisors** (*incise* = to divide or cut) called central and lateral incisors, respectively, and **cuspids** (or **canine**, so named because they are similar in appearance and development with *Canidae*—Latin: family of dogs), used for tearing, piercing, and holding food. These six teeth are collectively called anterior teeth (*anterior* = toward the front).

Bicuspids (or **premolars**, so named because they take an anatomical position in front of the molars) are used to pierce and crush food; **molars** (derived from the word *molaris*—Latin: grindstone) are the grinding teeth. These teeth (a total of 10 in each arch) are called the posterior teeth (*posterior* = toward the rear).

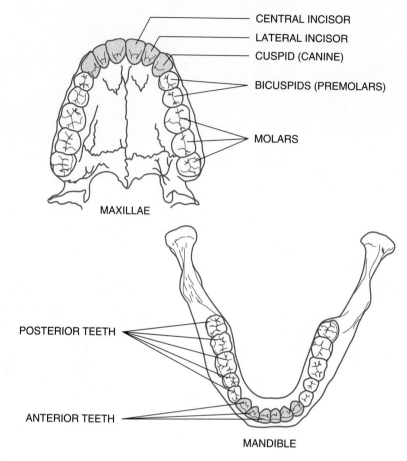

Figure 26-1 Position of teeth in arch.

Crown Surfaces

There is really only one surface on the crown—the **coronal surface** of a tooth (derived from the Latin *corona dentis*, the crown of a tooth). However, because this surface bends over in several directions, areas result that face different directions. These areas receive their names from the direction in which they face. An imaginary line is drawn from the most prominent part of the forehead (the glabella) to a point on the alveolar margin and then between the two central incisors in each arch. This is commonly known as the **median line** (Figure 26-2). Those surfaces that face this line are called **mesial** surfaces; those facing away from it are known as **distal** surfaces.

Collectively, **facial** surfaces are (1) the surfaces of the anterior teeth that face toward the lips (**labial** surfaces) and (2) the surfaces of the posterior teeth that face toward the cheeks (buccal surfaces). The facial surfaces of the anterior teeth are generally seen when a person smiles; depending on the breadth of the smile, some of the posterior facial surfaces may also be evident.

Lingual surfaces are the surfaces of both the anterior and posterior teeth that face toward the tongue (*lin-*

gua = tongue). A term sometimes used to denote those surfaces of the maxillary teeth is **palatal**, since they face the hard palate.

Occlusal surfaces are the horizontal surfaces of the posterior teeth used for masticating food. They

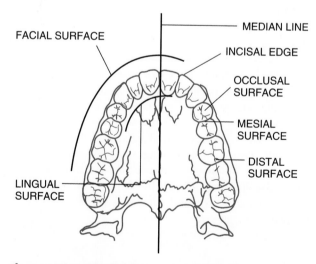

Figure 26-2 Median line and surfaces of teeth.

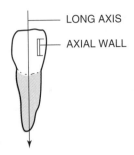

Figure 26-3 Long axis of tooth.

derive their name from occlusion (the relationship between the masticating surfaces of the maxillary and mandibular teeth when they are in contact).

Incisal edges are the cutting edges of the anterior teeth. After these surfaces become flattened from wear, they are called *incisal surfaces.*

The long axis of a tooth is the imaginary line (axial line) around which the structures of the teeth are more or less symmetrically arranged. The amount of deviation from the axial line differs in every individual and in every tooth of the individual. However, any surface of a tooth that is parallel to the long axis of the tooth is called an **axial** surface. The mesial, distal, facial, and lingual surfaces are axial surfaces. The boundary of a cavity lying within the tooth and parallel to the long axis is termed the axial wall (Figure 26-3).

Proximal surfaces are tooth surfaces that lie adjacent to one another in the same arch. Mesial and distal surfaces of adjacent teeth are proximal surfaces. Areas on the proximal surfaces that actually touch each other are called contact areas. The space between proximal surfaces is called **interproximal** space. Part of the interproximal space is occupied by the interdental papilla. The part that is not so occupied is referred to as the **embrasure** (the V-shaped space radiating from the contact areas of the teeth). Embrasures may extend in different directions from the proximal surfaces and are distinguished by their direction: (1) occlusal, (2) facial, (3) lingual, and (4) gingival (Figure 26-4).

Embrasures (1) serve as escapeways for food during mastication, (2) tend to promote "self- cleaning" of the interproximal surfaces by allowing the free passage of food from between the teeth during mastication, and (3) create a well-formed contact that protects the underlying soft tissues in the gingival embrasure by preventing the wedging of fibrous food between the teeth.

Division into Thirds

For descriptive purposes when teeth are discussed, each axial surface of the crown and of the tooth is divided horizontally into thirds, with each third being named in accordance with the area in which it lies (Figure 26-5). When looking at the tooth from the labial or buccal aspect, one sees that the crown and root may be divided into thirds from the incisal or occlusal surface of the crown to the apex of the tooth. Each of the five surfaces (aspects) of a crown may be marked off in thirds when viewing or studying any aspect. There is one middle third and two other thirds that are named according to the area they approach, such as cervical, occlusal, mesial, or lingual. In addition, each axial surface may be divided **longitudinally** (lengthwise) into thirds; i.e., each mesial and distal surface may be divided into a facial (labial or buccal), middle, and a lingual third.

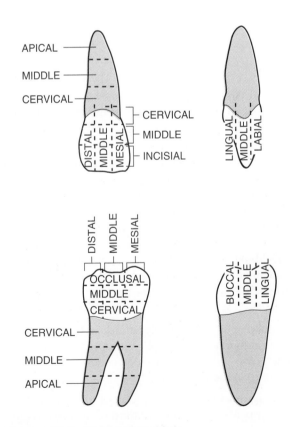

Figure 26-5 Division into thirds.

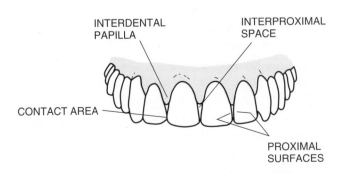

Figure 26-4 Proximal surfaces and contact areas.

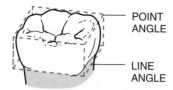

Figure 26-6 Line angle and point angle, shown on molar tooth.

Angles of the Teeth

A **line angle** is formed by the junction of any two surfaces of a tooth crown, and its name is derived by combining the names of the two surfaces. A **point angle** is formed by the junction of any three surfaces of a tooth, and its name is derived by combining the names of the three surfaces (Figure 26-6).

It should be noted here that in combining names to denote line angles, the *al* ending of the first name is dropped and the letter *o* is substituted (as in mesiobuccal or mesiocclusal). In the case of point angles, the letter *o* is substituted in the first two names, as in mesiobuccocclusal. Line angles and point angles are used only as descriptive terms to indicate location.

Other Landmarks of Teeth

To briefly review the subject, each tooth has a crown and a root portion. The **anatomic crown** is that part of the tooth covered with enamel. The **anatomic root** is that part covered with cementum. The **clinical crown** is the part of the tooth that is exposed in the oral cavity. The cervix, or neck, of the tooth is the constricted portion at which the anatomic crown and the root meet. The cervical line (cementoenamel junction) is the slight indentation that encircles the tooth at the cervix and marks the junction of the enamel with the cementum.

A tooth may have a single root, or it may have two or three roots. When a tooth has two roots, the root portion is said to be **bifurcated** (divided into two branches). When it has three roots, the root portion is said to be **trifurcated** (divided into three branches) (Figure 26-7).

To intelligently study each tooth, the dental assistant must be able to recognize the following important landmarks:

- A **cusp** is a rounded elevation, or mound on the working surface of a cuspid, bicuspid, or molar tooth. Each cusp is representative of a center of calcification (a lobe) in the developing tooth.

- A **cingulum** is the lingual lobe of an anterior tooth and appears on the cervical third of the tooth (Figure 26-8).

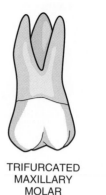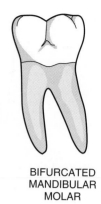

TRIFURCATED MAXILLARY MOLAR

BIFURCATED MANDIBULAR MOLAR

Figure 26-7 Tooth roots.

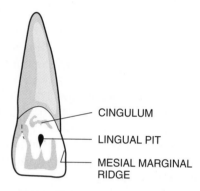

CINGULUM

LINGUAL PIT

MESIAL MARGINAL RIDGE

Figure 26-8 Lingual aspect of maxillary central incisor.

- A **mamelon** is one of the three prominences at the incisal edge of a newly erupted incisor. These prominences will wear away during use, leaving a flattened surface to the incisal portion.

- A **ridge** is any linear elevation on the surface of a tooth that is named according to its location and form, such as a buccal ridge, incisal ridge, and marginal ridge.

- **Marginal ridges** are those rounded borders of the enamel that form the margins of the occlusal surfaces of the bicuspids (premolars) and molars mesially and distally and the mesial and distal margins of the incisors and cuspids lingually (Figure 26-9).

- **Triangular ridges** are the ridges that descend from the tips of the cusps of bicuspids and molars toward the center part of the occlusal surfaces.

- A **transverse ridge** is formed by two triangular ridges that join and cross the occlusal surface of the posterior tooth.

- An **oblique ridge** runs diagonally across the occlusal surface of maxillary molars.

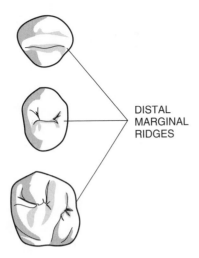

Figure 26-9 Marginal ridges.

- A **sulcus** is a notably long depression or valley in the surface of a tooth between ridges and cusps. It has a developmental groove at the junction of its inclines.

- A **developmental groove** is a shallow groove or line on the surface of a tooth. It represents the junction of two or more developmental lobes. A supplemental groove is also a shallow linear depression on the surface of the tooth, but it does not mark the junction of primary parts. Buccal and lingual grooves are developmental grooves found on the lingual surfaces of posterior teeth.

- A **fissure** is a linear fault occurring along a developmental groove. It is caused by failure of the enamel of the separate lobes to become properly fused, or joined.

- A **fossa** is an irregular depression on the surface of a tooth.

- A **pit** is a small pinpoint depression on the surface of a tooth, usually located at the end of a groove or where two or more grooves join (i.e., the central pit of the mandibular first molar is located where the developmental grooves join in the central fossa).

SUGGESTED ACTIVITIES

- Work with a fellow student to study all the information in this chapter.

- Use a typodont to locate and identify the landmarks of the teeth.

- Use a full arch plaster model and coloring pencils to mark the landmarks outlined in this chapter, i.e., use a green pencil to mark all marginal ridges and a red pencil to mark all fossae.

REVIEW

1. Name the surfaces of an anterior tooth.
   a. Mesial, distal, incisal, buccal, lingual
   b. Mesial, distal, occlusal, lingual, labial
   c. Mesial, distal, lingual, incisal, occlusal
   d. Mesial, distal, incisal, labial, lingual

2. Name the axial surfaces of a tooth.
   a. Mesial, distal, facial, lingual
   b. Mesial, incisal, facial, distal
   c. Mesial occlusal, buccal, distal
   d. Distal, facial, incisal, axial

3. The V-shaped space extending outward from the contact areas of the teeth is termed:
   a. Marginal ridge
   b. Gingival margin
   c. Embrasure
   d. Triangular ridge

4. On which teeth are oblique ridges likely to be most pronounced?
   a. Mandibular first molars
   b. Maxillary first molars
   c. Maxillary third molars
   d. Mandibular third molars

5. What term is used to indicate the root portion of a tooth that has two branches? The root portion that has three branches?
   a. Birooted, trirooted
   b. Double rooted, triple rooted
   c. Bifurcated, trifurcated

6. Indicate the three functions of embrasures: (1) serve as escapeways for food during mastication, (2) tend to promote "self-cleaning" of the interproximal surfaces by allowing the free passage of food from between the teeth during mastication, (3) promote better oral health by allowing the toothbrush to reach interproximally, and/or (4) as well-formed contacts protect the underlying soft tissues in the gingival embrasure by preventing the wedging of fibrous food between the teeth.
   a. 1, 2, 3
   b. 2, 3, 4
   c. 1, 2, 4
   d 1, 3, 4

CHAPTER 27

Descriptions of Individual Teeth

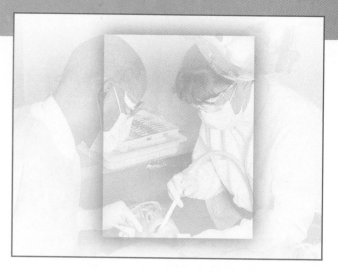

OBJECTIVES

After studying this chapter, the student will be able to:

- Describe individual variations in size, shape, and other characteristics of teeth as well as their basic design and function.
- Compare cusps, roots, and the occlusal aspects of anterior and posterior teeth.
- Define terms and identify anatomical landmarks of individual teeth.
- List the prominent characteristics of each permanent tooth.

Introduction

In this chapter each tooth in the permanent dentition will be described and illustrated. It is well to remember that teeth show considerable variations in size, shape, and other characteristics. Certain teeth show a greater tendency to deviate from the normal. The descriptions that follow are of normal teeth.

To make it easier for the dental assistant to relate these descriptions to his or her work in assisting the doctor to chart the mouth of the patient, detailed sketches of all aspects of the teeth are included.

Maxillary Central Incisor

The maxillary central incisor looks like a wedge when viewed mesially or distally with the point of the wedge at the incisal (cutting) edge of the tooth (Figure 27-1).

The labial surface resembles a thumbnail in outline. The mesial margin is nearly straight and meets the incisal edge at almost a 90° angle, but the distal margin meets the incisal edge in a curve. The incisal edge is straight, but the cervical margin is curved in the shape of a half moon. There are two developmental grooves on the labial surface.

The lingual surface is quite similar to the labial surface in outline, but it is smaller in all dimensions. There are marginal ridges at the mesial and distal margins. Generally, there is a cingulum at the junction of the lingual surface and the cervical line. Sometimes a deep

pit (the lingual pit) is found in conjunction with the cingulum. As the dental assistant assists the doctor in a root canal procedure (which includes removing the pulp tissue and refilling the hollow length of the root), the dental assistant may see the doctor make an external opening through this pit into the root canal.

As with all anterior teeth, the root of the maxillary central incisor is single. This root is from one and one-

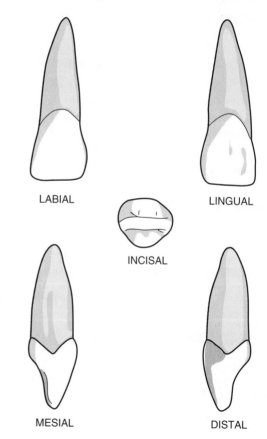

Figure 27-1 Maxillary central incisor.

fourth to one and one-half times the length of the crown. Usually, the apex of the root is inclined distally to a slight degree. The line angles of this tooth are well rounded.

Maxillary Lateral Incisor

The maxillary lateral incisor is much like the maxillary central incisor, but it is shorter, narrower, and thinner (Figure 27-2).

The developmental grooves on the labial surface are not so evident as those of the central incisor. More significant, however, is the distoincisal edge, which is well rounded with the curvature continuing to the cervical line. The mesiolabial angle is nearly straight, paralleling the long axis of the tooth for half its length. Then it turns inward as it approaches the cervical line.

The shape of the lingual surface varies with the individual. In some persons it is markedly **concave** (having an inward curvature, almost spoonlike in appearance), and in others it is flat. The lingual surface is the same width as the facial surface. The root is cone shaped but sometimes flattened mesiodistally.

Maxillary Cuspid

The maxillary cuspid is said to be the longest and strongest tooth in human dentition (Figure 27-3).

The labial surface of the crown differs considerably from that of the maxillary central or lateral incisors. By comparison, the incisal edges of the central and lateral incisors are nearly straight, and the cuspid has a definite point, or cusp. The distoincisal cutting edge is the longer of the two. Therefore, the tip of the cusp is closer to the mesial surface than to the distal surface. The curvature of the labial surface is more prominent by the **labial ridge** (a ridge which extends from the tip of the cusp to the cervical line). The developmental grooves, which are so prominent on the labial surface of the central incisor, are present here, extending two-thirds of the distance from the tip of the cusp to the cervical line.

The lingual surface has the same general outline as the labial surface but is somewhat smaller because the mesial and distal surfaces of the crown tend to move toward each other as they meet the lingual surface. The lingual surface is concave, with very prominent mesial and distal marginal ridges and a **lingual ridge** (a ridge that, like the labial ridge, extends from the tip of the cusp toward the cervical line). There is generally a cingulum in the cervical portion of the lingual surface of the crown.

The root is single and is the longest root in the arch. It is usually twice the length of the crown because the cuspid is designed for seizing and holding.

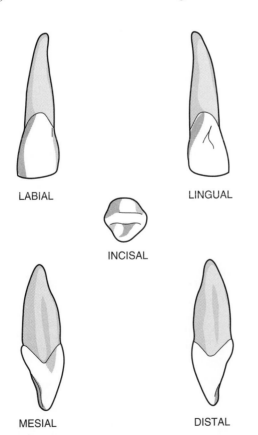

Figure 27-2 Maxillary lateral incisor.

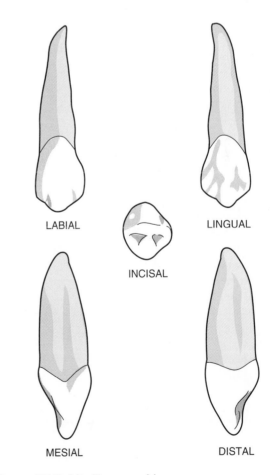

Figure 27-3 Maxillary cuspid.

Progressing into a dental health career, the dental assistant will notice the frequent use of cuspids as **abutment teeth** (teeth that anchor a bridge).

Maxillary First Bicuspid (Premolar)

The maxillary first bicuspid (premolar) is the fourth tooth from the median line. It is considered to be the typical bicuspid ("bicuspid" means having two cusps). However, as has been mentioned before, they are currently called premolars because they are just in front of or mesially to the molar teeth (Figure 27-4).

The buccal surface is somewhat similar to the labial surface of the cuspid. In the case of the bicuspid (premolar), however, the tip of the buccal cusp is located in the center of the "biting" edge; this is called the occlusal edge, or **occlusal margin**. Therefore, the mesioocclusal and disto-occlusal edges appear to be of equal length. From the cusp tip to the cervical margin there is a slight ridge, the **buccal ridge** (a ridge on the buccal surface which extends from the tip of the cusp to the cervical margin) which is similar to the labial ridge found in cuspid teeth.

The lingual surface is narrower and shorter than the buccal surface and is smoothly convex in all directions. The cusp tip is in the middle of the occlusal edge.

The contact areas are normally located in the occlusal third or at the junction of the occlusal and middle thirds (refer back to Figure 26-5).

The occlusal surface has a buccal cusp and a lingual cusp (Figure 27-5). There is also a mesial marginal ridge and a distal marginal ridge. These correspond to the marginal ridge on the lingual surfaces of anterior teeth. There are two fossae on the occlusal surface. The one near the mesial marginal ridge is called the **mesial fossa**, and the one near the distal marginal ridge is called the **distal fossa**. The two cusps are separated by a groove, known as the central groove, and a triangular ridge extends downward from the tip of each cusp toward the **central groove** (a groove found on the central portion of the occlusal surface that separates the buccal from the lingual cusp). One is called the buccal triangular ridge and the other the lingual triangular ridge.

The root is quite flat on the mesial and distal surfaces. In approximately half of the maxillary first bicuspids, the root is divided at the apical third. When it is so divided, the tips are slender and finely tapered.

Maxillary Second Bicuspid (Premolar)

The maxillary second bicuspid (premolar) resembles the first bicuspid (premolar) very closely, but it is smaller in all dimensions. It has a single root ((Figure 27-6).

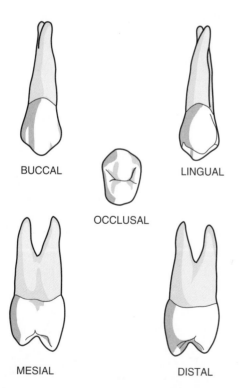

Figure 27-4 Maxillary first bicuspid (premolar).

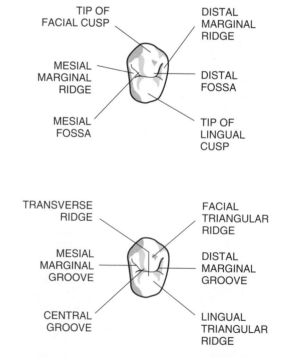

Figure 27-5 Occlusal surface of maxillary first bicuspid (premolar).

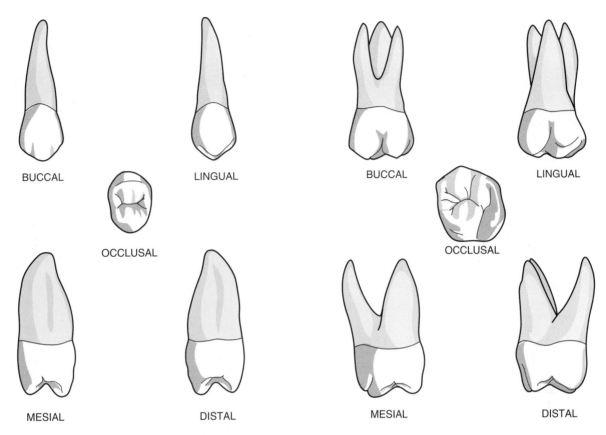

Figure 27-6 Maxillary second bicuspid (premolar).

Figure 27-7 Maxillary first molar.

Maxillary First Molar

The maxillary first molar is the sixth tooth from the median line (Figure 27-7). The first molars are often called "six-year molars," because they erupt when the child is about six years of age.

The buccal surface is **convex** (having an outward curvature) in all directions. The **buccal groove**, which continues over from the occlusal surface, is quite prominent and terminates in the middle third of the buccal surface.

The lingual surface resembles the buccal surface but is somewhat smaller. The **distolingual groove** of the occlusal surface continues over onto the lingual surface, where it fades out in the middle third. In a great many instances there is a prominent lobe, or cusp, on the lingual surface of the mesiolingual cusp. There is a fifth cusp in addition to the four cusps on the occlusal surface. This is called the cusp of Carabelli.

In all molars the pattern of the occlusal surface is quite different from that of the bicuspids (Figure 27-8). The cusps are large and prominent, and the broad grinding surfaces are broken up into rugged-appearing ridges and well-defined grooves. By the nature of these physical characteristics of the occlusal surfaces, it can be seen why most **mastication** (chewing and grinding) takes place on the molar teeth. The occlusal surface has four cusps—the mesiobuccal, the mesiolingual, the distobuccal, and the distolingual. The cusp of Carabelli can be seen when the tooth is viewed occlusally, but it does not form part of the occlusal surface. All the cusps are prominent, the mesiolingual being the highest. The mesial and distal margins differ from those of the bicuspids in that they are broader and appear stronger. An oblique ridge, which is not present on the bicuspids (premolars), appears here. (It should be noted that it also appears on the maxillary second and third molars but often is not so pronounced.) The oblique ridge runs from the mesiolingual cusp to the distobuccal cusp and is marked in its midsection by the passage of the distal groove. On the mesial side of the oblique ridge is the central fossa: on the distal side is the distal fossa, which is smaller than the central fossa. In the distal fossa the most prominent feature is the distolingual groove; it parallels the course of the oblique ridge.

The roots of the first molar are widespread, which tend to give the tooth strength and firm anchorage. The maxillary first molar has three roots, which are named according to their location—mesiobuccal, distobuccal, and lingual. The lingual root is the largest.

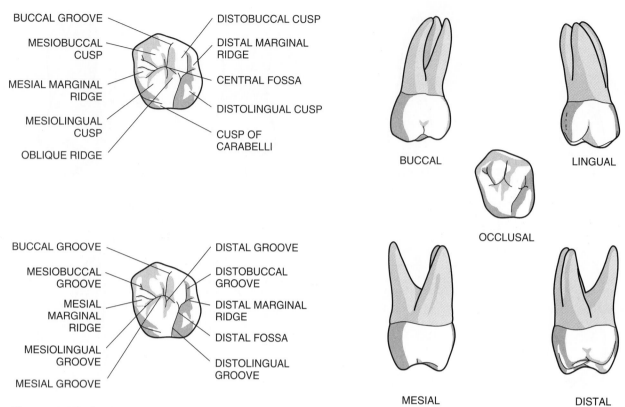

Figure 27-8 Occlusal surface of maxillary first molar.

Figure 27-9 Maxillary second molar.

Maxillary Second Molar

The maxillary second molar is the seventh from the median line (Figure 27-9). The second molars are often called "12-year molars," because they erupt when the child is about 12 years of age.

Because it has the same function as the maxillary first molar, its physical characteristics are the same, except that it is smaller, and the cusp of Carabelli does not appear. There is a marked reduction in the size of the distolingual cusp.

Maxillary Third Molar

The maxillary third molar is the eighth tooth from the median line (Figure 27-10). Third molars are often called "wisdom teeth," because they erupt when the young adult is passing into manhood or womanhood. This tooth is much smaller than either the maxillary first or second molar, and the occlusal outline is almost circular, owing to the nearly complete disappearance of the distolingual cusp.

The occlusal surface is generally covered with numerous fissures and grooves.

The root may have from one to as many as eight divisions. These divisions are usually fused and are often curved distally.

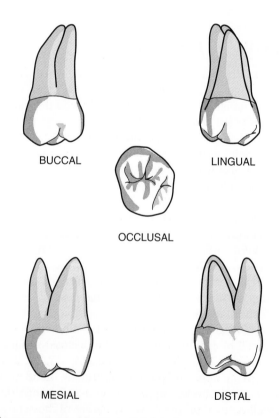

Figure 27-10 Maxillary third molar.

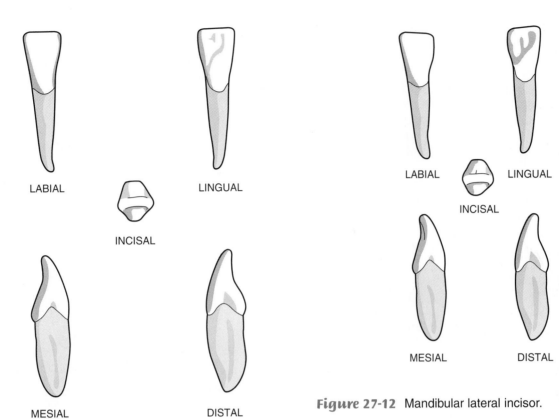

Figure 27-11 Mandibular central incisor.

Figure 27-12 Mandibular lateral incisor.

Mandibular Central Incisor

The mandibular central incisors are, as a general rule, the first permanent (succedaneous) teeth to erupt, replacing deciduous teeth (Figure 27-11). They are the smallest teeth in either arch.

The labial surface of the mandibular central incisor is widest at the incisal edge. Both the mesial and the distal surfaces join the incisal surface at almost a 90° angle. Although these two surfaces are nearly parallel at the incisal edge, they move toward one another at the cervical margin. The developmental grooves may or may not be apparent. When present, they appear as very faint furrows.

The lingual surface is concave from the incisal edge to the cervical margin.

The root is slender and much flattened on its mesial and distal surfaces.

Mandibular Lateral Incisor

The mandibular lateral incisor is a little wider mesiodistally than the mandibular central incisor, and the crown is slightly longer from the incisal edge to the cervical line (Figure 27-12).

The incisal edge is not at right angles to the mesial and distal edges as it is in the mandibular central incisor.

The root is single and much flattened on its mesial and distal surfaces.

Mandibular Cuspid

The mandibular cuspids, like the mandibular incisors, are smaller and more slender than the opposing teeth in the maxillary arch (Figure 27-13).

The labial surface of a mandibular cuspid is much the same as that of a maxillary cuspid, except that the distoincisal cutting edge is almost twice the length of the mesioincisal edge.

The lingual surface, as a rule, is very smooth, and a cingulum is rarely present.

The root is not so long as the maxillary cuspid root and is flatter mesiodistally

Mandibular First Bicuspid (Premolar)

A mandibular first bicuspid (premolar) is the fourth tooth from the median line. It is the smallest of the four bicuspids (Figure 27-14). Viewed from its buccal aspect, it shows a marked constriction at the cervical line; the term "bellcrowned" is used to describe this characteristic appearance. The mandibular first bicuspid differs greatly from the maxillary first bicuspid. Although there are two cusps—a buccal and a lingual—the latter has little prominence (in most cases) and might be compared to the cingulum on the lingual surface of the maxillary cuspid. The buccal cusp is long and sharp and resembles the cusp of the mandibular cuspid.

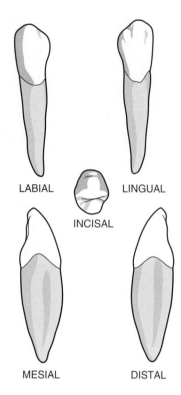

LABIAL   LINGUAL

INCISAL

MESIAL   DISTAL

Figure 27-13 Mandibular cuspid.

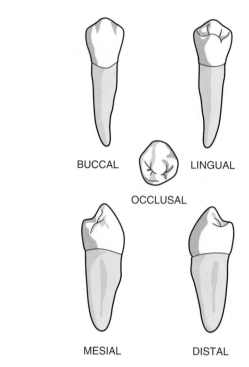

BUCCAL   LINGUAL

OCCLUSAL

MESIAL   DISTAL

Figure 27-14 Mandibular first bicuspid (premolar).

The buccal surface is very convex in all directions.

The mesial surface is distinctly convex in the occlusal third but is concave in the other two-thirds.

The distal surface is shaped like the mesial surface.

The lingual surface is small and very convex and appears to overhang the lingual surface of the root.

Mandibular Second Bicuspid (Premolar)

The mandibular second bicuspid (premolar) is the fifth tooth from the median line (Figure 27-15).

Its buccal surface characteristics are the same as the first bicuspid (premolar), with a prominent buccal ridge.

The lingual surface is similar to that of the mandibular first bicuspid (premolar), with the exception that there may be two lingual cusps.

The occlusal surface of the tooth occurs in different patterns. The first is the three-cusp type, in which the lingual groove divides the lingual marginal ridge into two distinct parts. This type of occlusal surface takes the shape of a Y. In the Y-form the buccal, the mesiolingual, and the distolingual cusps are evident. A less common two-cusp type has no lingual groove, but the central groove forms a half circle; there are only two prominent cusps—the buccal and the lingual.

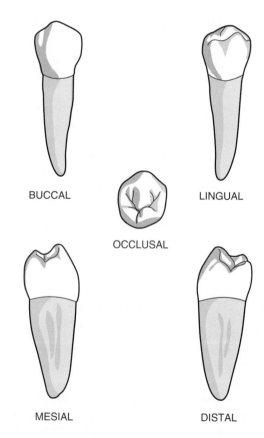

BUCCAL   LINGUAL

OCCLUSAL

MESIAL   DISTAL

Figure 27-15 Mandibular second bicuspid (premolar).

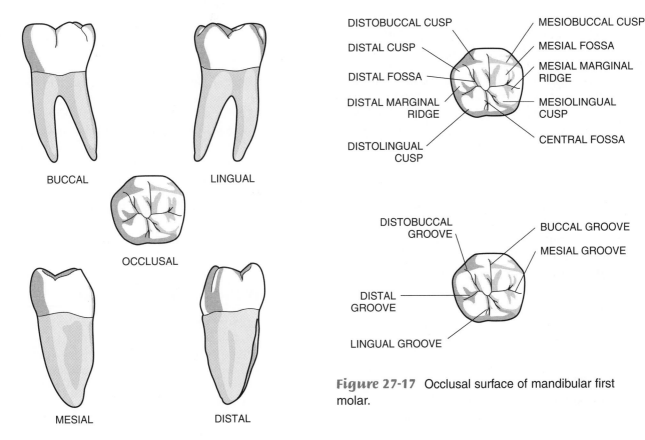

Figure 27-17 Occlusal surface of mandibular first molar.

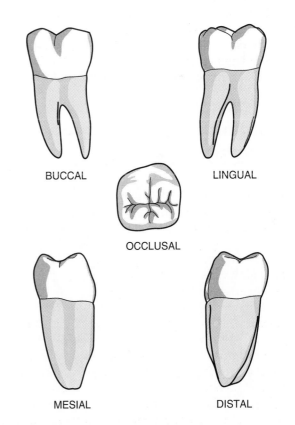

The root of the tooth is single, and in many instances the apical region is quite curved.

Mandibular First Molar

The mandibular first molar is the sixth tooth from the median line. It is the first permanent tooth to erupt (Figure 27-16).

The buccal surface of this tooth is more convex than its counterpart in the maxillary arch. There are two grooves on the buccal surface: the buccal groove, which is an extension of the buccal groove from the occlusal surface, and the distobuccal groove, an extension of the distobuccal groove from the occlusal surface.

The lingual surface is smaller in area than the buccal surface and is marked by an occlusal margin. The margin shows two distinct cusps created by a sharply defined lingual groove that ends in the middle third of the surface.

There are five cusps on the occlusal surface (Figure 27-17). This is in contrast to the maxillary first molar, in which the fifth cusp is on the lingual surface of the mesiolingual cusp (Figure 27-18). On the mandibular first molar, this fifth cusp is called the distal cusp. It is between the distobuccal and the distolingual cusps but nearer to the buccal surface than to the distal surface.

Figure 27-16 Mandibular first molar.

Figure 27-18 Mandibular second molar.

The other two cusps are the mesiobuccal and mesiolingual. The mesiolingual cusp is the highest cusp.

Three main grooves on the occlusal surface have already been mentioned: the buccal groove, which helps to distinguish the mesiobuccal and the distobuccal cusps; the distobuccal groove, which likewise extends over the facial margin and separates the distobuccal cusp from the distal cusp; and the **lingual groove**, which divides the lingual margin into two portions and thus creates the distolingual cusp and the mesiolingual cusp. The remaining two grooves that should be noted are the mesial groove and the distal groove. The mesial groove runs from the central fossa over the mesial marginal ridge. The distal groove also originates in the central fossa and runs over the distal marginal ridge, where it separates the distal cusp from the distolingual cusp.

The tooth has two roots, a mesial and a distal.

Mandibular Second Molar

The mandibular second molar is the seventh tooth from the median line.

The buccal surface has only one groove, the buccal groove, which originates in the occlusal surface and extends over the buccal margin onto the buccal surface; it usually ends in a deep fossa, the buccal fossa.

The lingual surface resembles that of the mandibular first molar in that it has a lingual groove. However, in this tooth the area of this surface is almost as great as that of the buccal surface.

The mesial and distal surfaces are more convex than those of the first molar.

The greatest difference between the occlusal surfaces of the mandibular first and second molars is that the occlusal surface of the second molar has no fifth cusp. Four cusps—the mesiobuccal, the mesiolingual, the distobuccal, and the distolingual—are outlined by the buccal, lingual, mesial, and distal grooves. A central fossa is present and appears in the geometric center of this surface.

There are two roots and they are smaller than those of the first molar.

Mandibular Third Molar

The mandibular third molar appears in many shapes, forms, and sizes (Figure 27-19). Its general appearance is similar to the two other mandibular molars, but it has smaller surfaces, more supplemental grooves, and four or five cusps, which are not so sharply differentiated as those of the first two molars.

The roots, usually two in number, often show a distinct distal curvature.

All third molars, whether maxillary or mandibular, often vary widely from the usual pattern.

SUGGESTED ACTIVITIES

- Using a typodont, study similarities and differences of the teeth. For example, compare sizes of all maxillary molars to one another and determine the number of cusps each tooth has. Also determine which teeth have buccal grooves, distolingual grooves, cusp of Carabelli, oblique ridges, mesial fossae, distal fossae, and central fossae.

- Using the drawings of teeth, label the following on pertaining teeth: labial ridge, lingual ridge, buccal ridge, occlusal, incisal edge, and developmental grooves.

- Using extracted, disinfected teeth, identify the anatomy of each tooth to include the roots. Determine which teeth have one root, two roots, or three roots.

- Placing all the extracted teeth in one grouping, identify and select individual teeth, starting with the maxillary central incisor through the mandibular third molar.

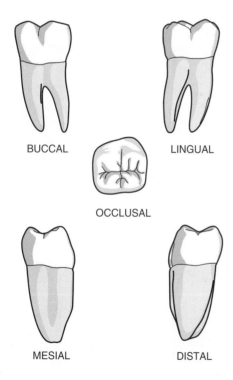

BUCCAL LINGUAL

OCCLUSAL

MESIAL DISTAL

Figure 27-19 Mandibular third molar.

REVIEW

1. Which tooth is usually the longest in the human dentition?
   a. Maxillary first molar
   b. Maxillary cuspid
   c. Maxillary central incisor
   d. Mandibular first molar

2. Which of the bicuspids (premolars) may have two roots? Which bicuspid may have two lingual cusps?
   a. Maxillary first bicuspid, mandibular second bicuspid
   b. Maxillary second bicuspid, mandibular first bicuspid
   c. Mandibular first bicuspid, maxillary second bicuspid
   d. Mandibular second bicuspid, maxillary second bicuspid

3. How many cusps and roots does the mandibular first molar have?
   a. Three roots, four cusps
   b. Three roots, five cusps
   c. Two roots, four cusps
   d. Two roots, five cusps

4. Name the longest root of the maxillary first molar.
   a. Mesiobuccal root
   b. Lingual root
   c. Distobuccal root

5. Where is the cusp of Carabelli located?
   a. On the lingual of the mandibular first molar
   b. On the lingual of the mandibular second molar
   c. On the lingual of the maxillary first molar
   d. On the lingual of the maxillary lateral incisor

Oral Exam

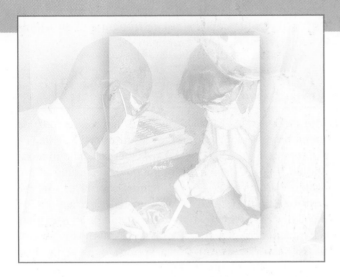

assistant sees a suspicious lesion, it is that person's responsibility to bring awareness to the dentist about the findings, who in turn relates the concern to the patient. The dental assistant must remain attentive to the sequencing of events and keep all information confidential. It should be established that the oral cavity is used as an indicator of the overall general health of the patient. Thus, if visual changes in tissues exist, they should be noted in the patient's chart and evaluated by the dentist. Blood pressure is taken and vital signs are recorded; see Chapter 10. Depending on the date of the last radiographs, the patient may need a more recent series at this time, to become part of the current oral examination.

Taking a Medical History

The complete assessment of a patient's overall health is necessary in providing optimum dental care. In many dental offices the patient is usually given the medical history form and asked to fill it out as completely as possible using a pen; see Chapter 10, Figure 10-1. When it is returned, the dental assistant should seat the patient in the treatment room and the information reviewed there. The patient's signature should indicate that the content is reliable and thereby is considered a legal document. Any dialog should not take place in the reception room where other patients may be within listening distance of confidential information. When reviewing the medical history with the patient, it is wise to follow up on certain conditions that were answered in the affirmative.

Conditions Requiring Further Information

- Adverse reactions to treatment or medications
- Alcohol use—amount and frequency
- Allergies—type and substances
- Asthma—severity
- Bleeding (hemophilia)—prolonged bleeding, history of coagulation problem

OBJECTIVES

After studying this chapter, the student will be able to:

- Recognize, locate, and describe normal structures in the oral cavity.
- Recognize conditions that require further information when recording a medical history.
- Recognize deviations from normal structures in the oral cavity.
- Describe the procedure for an oral exam.
- Use several examination methods to achieve a competent examination.
- Identify extraoral deviations from the normal.
- Locate predominant areas where oral cancerous lesions may develop.
- Identify the appearance of oral cancer.
- Explain how to document pertinent findings on the patient's chart.

Introduction

The purpose of intraoral and extraoral head and neck examinations is to help prevent further development of possible life-threatening diseases such as leukemia, human immunodeficiency virus (HIV), diabetes, or cancer that may manifest in the oral cavity. When the dental

- Breathing difficulties—persistent cough, caused by asthma
- Cancer or tumor—radiation therapy, blood count
- Diabetes—severity, vision, kidney, cardiovascular complications
- Epilepsy—type, frequency of seizures, medication
- Heart diseases—medication, pacemaker, transplant (should consult physician)
- Heart murmur—valvular involvement, antibiotic pre-medication
- Hospitalization—operations, illnesses
- Immune system disorder—as HIV or acquired immunodeficiency syndrome (AIDS)
- Joint replacement—antibiotic premedication
- Pregnant—due date, history of other pregnancies
- Radiation therapy—head and neck area, amount of radiation received (should consult physician)
- Rheumatic fever/heart disease—antibiotic premedication
- Sexually transmitted disease—may not acknowledge, however, may have oral manifestations
- Stroke (CVA)—how long ago, resulting disabilities
- Tobacco use—form, amount per day/week
- Tuberculosis—active or passive, cough, medication
- Weight gain/loss—how much gained or lost within a length of time, on a diet program

Following completion of the medical history, the dental assistant should sign and date it as being the person responsible for recording its content. If the patient is a minor, the parent or legal guardian should have input in supplying medical history information and sign it accordingly.

At this time the dental assistant would begin to evaluate the extraoral and intraoral structures. It is essential that the dental assistant recognize all structures when performing these examinations.

Structures in the Oral Cavity

The oral cavity is lined by the oral mucosa or mucous membrane, which is covered by **squamous** (scalelike or flat) epithelium. The general appearance of the mucosa should be pink or may be pigmented, according to the patient's skin color. The structures should exhibit no **lesions** (injury, wound, or white patches), irritations, or swellings. The gingiva should appear pink, **stippled** (orange peel appearance), with knife-edge papillae, not glossy, soft, swollen, or of a spongy consistency that bleeds readily (Figure 28-1).

For the purpose of orientation to structures in the oral cavity, a list with anatomic descriptions is provided.

Maxillary Arch

- *Hard palate.* Also known as the roof of the mouth.
- *Rugae.* Numerous tissue ridges located in the anterior region of the palate.

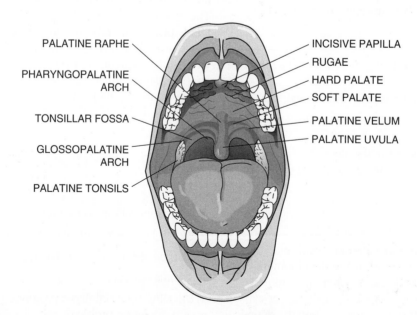

Figure 28-1 Oral cavity (hard palate, rugae, incisive papillae, palatine raphe, soft palate, palatine velum, glossopalatine arch, palatine uvula, pharyngopalatine arch, palatine tonsils, tonsillar fossa).

- *Incisive papillae.* Prominence of tissue located behind maxillary central teeth.
- *Palatine raphe.* Narrow ridge which extends from the incisive papillae along the entire length of the hard palate.
- *Soft palate.* Located behind the hard palate and lacks the bony quality of the hard palate. The posterior portion hangs down as a curtain and is referred to as the palatine velum (veillike structure).
- *Glossopalatine arch* or *Palatoglossal arch.* Also known as anterior tonsilar pillar arch, located within the palatine velum anterior to palatal tonsils.
- *Palatine uvula.* A small conical extension at the midline of the soft palate.
- *Pharyngopalatine arch.* Also known as posterior tonsilar pillar, located at the most posterior arch dividing the oral cavity and pharynx.
- *Palatine tonsils.* Glandular tissue located between the glossopalatine and the pharyngopalatine arches.
- *Tonsilar Fossa.* Shallow depression which contains the palatine tonsil.

Mandibular Arch and Tongue

- *Pterygomandibular Fold.* Linear elevation extending from pterygoid process to the retromolar pad at posterior end of mandibular process.
- *Sublingual ducts.* There are 10–15 on each side, along the base of the tongue.
- *Lingual veins.* Parallel to lingual frenum. Bilateral on ventral surface of tongue.
- *Lingual frenum.* Fold of mucous membrane which attaches the tongue to the floor of the mouth.
- *Fimbriated fold.* Fold of mucous membrane under tongue on either side of lingual frenum.

Tongue

- *Papillae.* Fingerlike projections of tissue on the tongue, not the actual taste bud.
  a. *Filliform.* Slender, taper point papillae which cover the anterior two-thirds of the tongue.
  b. *Fungiform.* Mushroom-shaped papillae, bright red, scattered among the filliform along sides, middle, and tip of tongue.
  c. *Vallate/circumvallate.* There are between 8–12 positioned in a "V" form in the posterior area of tongue.

- *Fissures.* Median sulcus or major groove along midline of tongue
- *Lingual tonsilar tissue.* Located at the lateral and posterior part of the base of the tongue.

Buccal Mucosa

- *Parotid papilla.* Raised mass of tissue on cheek opposite maxillary second molar at the opening of Stensen's duct.
- *Linea alba buccalis.* Whitish linear fold at line of occlusion. Occurs from closely adapted cheeks.
- *Fordyce's spots (granules).* Sebaceous glands occurring lateral to the corner of the mouth, often opposite molars.
- *Mucobuccal fold.* Reflection of the mucous membrane onto the alveolar process.
- *Vestibule.* Space bound by walls of the cheek and teeth and alveolar process.
- *Vestibular fornix.* Base of the fold within the vestibule.
- *Labial frenum.* Maxillary and mandibular fold of mucous membrane which connects the inner surface of the lip to the midline of the gingiva.
- *Buccal frenum.* Fold of mucous membrane which attaches the buccal mucosa to the gingiva around the bicuspid area.

Gingiva (Figure 28-2)

- *Free gingiva.* Sleevelike portion of gingiva, which encircles the coronal portion of the tooth.
- *Sulcus.* Space between the tooth and free gingiva.
- *Gingival margin.* Crest of the free gingiva.
- *Interdental Papillae.* The free gingiva that lies bucally and lingually between two teeth.
- *Col.* The "valley" between the buccal and lingual papillae.
- *Free gingival groove.* The dividing line between free and attached gingiva.
- *Attached gingiva.* Portion of gingiva that is attached to the alveolar bone, exhibiting an "orange peel" appearance (stippling).
- *Interdental groove.* Formed by depression of alveolar bone between teeth.
- *Retromolar pad.* Area of thickened gingiva behind mandibular molars.

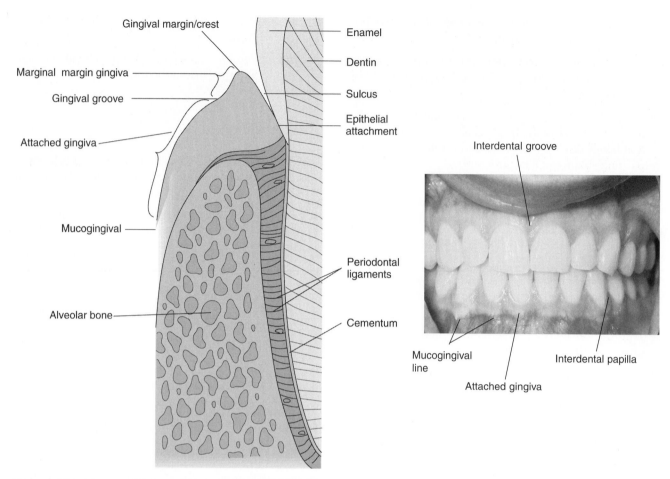

Figure 28-2 Parts of the gingiva (free gingiva, sulcus, gingival margin, interdental papillae, free gingival groove, attached gingiva, interdental groove, mucogingival line divides attached and alveolar mucosa).

- *Maxillary tuberosity.* Area of thickened gingiva behind maxillary molars.
- *Mucogingival line (junction).* Scalloped line dividing the attached gingiva and the alveolar mucosa.

Lips (Figure 28-3)

- *Nasolabial sulcus.* The sulcus which runs from the ala (wing) of the nose to the corner of the mouth.
- *Labial commisure.* Thin fold which connects the upper lip with the lower lip.
- *Philtrum.* Shallow depression from the center of the upper lip to the base of the nose.
- *Vermillion border.* Reddish border of lip.
- *Labial mucosa.* Mucous membrane lining the inside of the lip.
- *Orbicularis oris.* Musculature of lip.
- *Minor salivary glands.* Provide mucous secretion within the lining of the lips.

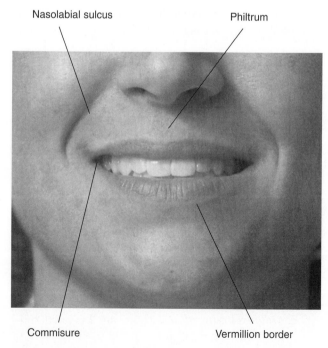

Figure 28-3 Parts of the lips.

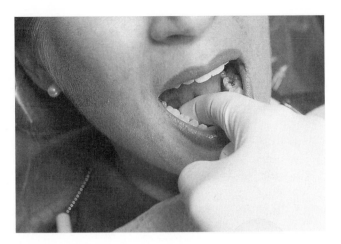

Figure 28-4 Digital exam.

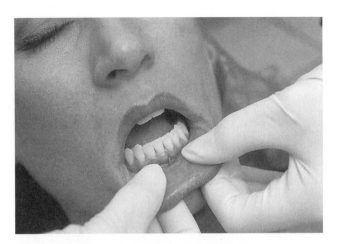

Figure 28-5 Bidigital exam.

Examination Methods

When performing an examination, the dental assistant uses all senses except for taste to effectively assess conditions that may be present. Visual, tactile, sense of smell, listening, and others such as percussion, electrical pulp test, and instrumentation may be used during the exam.

Visual

A visual assessment of the patient takes place the first time the dental assistant sees the patient. The dental assistant observes the **gait** (the manner in which the patient carries himself or herself), any evidence of **asymmetry** (right and left sides are not the same), skin color being pale or flushed, or **jaundiced** (yellow appearance overall, including the sclera or white portion of eyes).

Feeling/Palpation

Using one's hands or the sense of touch to feel the consistency of the area being palpated is useful to detect swelling or lumps. The following palpatory methods may be used:

- *Digital.* Using a single finger to detect abnormalities such as tori (bone outgrowth) on the mandible or midline of maxilla (Figure 28-4).

- *Bidigital.* Using two digits such as the thumb and index finger on one hand to detect abnormalities on the lips or tongue (Figure 28-5).

- *Bimanual.* Using two hands at the same time in the same location pressing the tissue from either side to detect abnormalities, as on the floor of the mouth (Figure 28-6).

- *Bilateral.* Using two hands on similar structures on contralateral sides to simultaneously detect TMJ (temporomandibular joint) abnormalities (Figure 28-7).

Sense of Smell/Olfactory

Using the sense of smell is one way to detect foul breath that may be indicative of poor oral hygiene or periodontal involvement; it could also lead to the possibility of stomach ailments or other systemic disorders. Alcohol consumption can also be detected in this manner.

Auscultation/Listening

When the patient is asked to move his or her jaw up and down or side to side, the operator must **auscultate** (listen) for abnormal clicking or grinding noises that may take place as the result of movement.

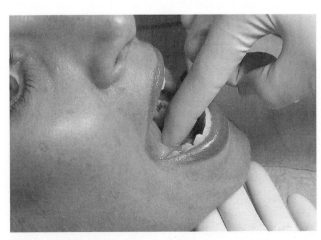

Figure 28-6 Bimanual exam.

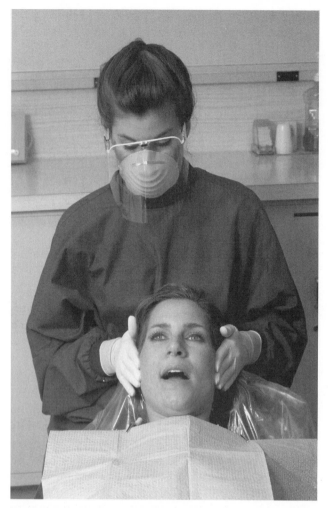

Figure 28-7 Bilateral exam (examining the TMJ using both hands contralaterally).

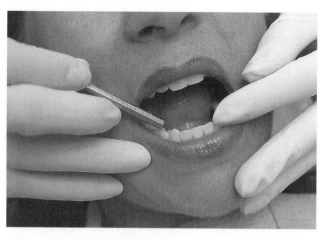

Figure 28-8 Percussion.

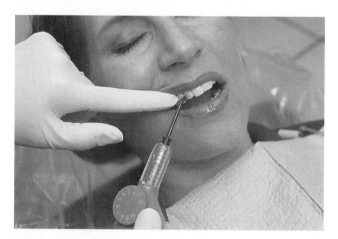

Figure 28-9 Pulp tester.

Percussion

When percussion is applied, the dentist performs it. The handle of an instrument is used to tap on teeth in question, compared with the sensation of the same tap on healthy teeth (Figure 28-8). The patient responds accordingly. However, if a tooth is painful when pressure is applied, percussion should be avoided.

Pulp Tester

The pulp tester, also called vitalometer, may be used by the dental assistant in some states. The purpose for its use is to determine if a tooth is **vital** (alive) or nonvital (Figure 28-9).

Instrumentation

Use of a periodontal probe to determine sulcular and pocket depths or the explorer to assess presence of caries is the responsibility of the dentist or dental hygienist.

Extraoral Examination

After taking the medical history and vital signs and while the patient is still in an upright position, the dental assistant, who is fully protected by face mask, eyewear/face shield, and gloves, begins an **extraoral** (outside-the-mouth) examination. The dental assistant would have already made an overall assessment of the patient's gait, skin color, asymmetry of the face (possibly due to swelling or presence of tumors), disabilities, and breathing problems at the time the patient walked into the treatment room. The procedure begins with bilateral palpation of the following:

● Parotid gland located in front of the ear.
● The TMJ by having patient open and close the jaw, moving it forward, back, and from side to side to

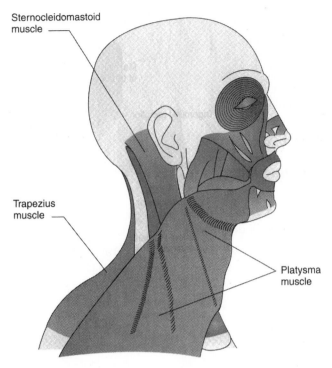

Figure 28-10 Lymph nodes in the sternocleidomastoid muscle area.

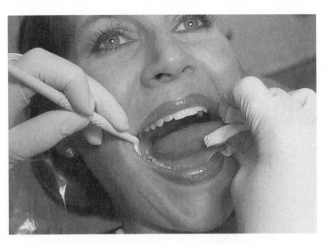

Figure 28-11 Examination of the tongue.

detect clicking, popping, or **crepitus** (grinding sounds).

- Lymph nodes located in front and behind the **sternocleidomastoid muscle** (muscle that arises from the sternum and clavicle and attaches to the mastoid process of the skull), just inside the clavicle, and under the lower jaw should also be palpated (Figure 28-10).

- In the same area, the dental assistant should also palpate the **submandibular** (below-the-mandible) and **submental** (below-the-chin) salivary glands.

    If any lumps, tenderness, and mobility of lymph nodes or glands are detected, they should be noted in the chart and brought to the attention of the dentist.

Intraoral Examination

The patient should be reclined in a supine position for better access and visibility. The dental assistant should have a routine when performing examinations to avoid missing any areas. A good place to start may be the upper right and end with the lower right.

- The lips are palpated bidigitally. The dental assistant should place the index finger inside the mouth and the thumb outside the mouth; otherwise, it may be uncomfortable for the patient if the dental assistant alternates between the "wet" finger and the dry

thumb palpating the skin with wet fingers. The vermilion border and the **commissure** (angle of the mouth) are observed for color and texture changes. The lips should be rolled upward (for maxillary) or downward (for mandibular) to inspect the labial **frena** (frenum is singular) for tightness and length.

- The **buccal mucosa** (inside cheek area) is visually inspected and should exhibit a pinkish color. It is also palpated bimanually using one hand on the outside of the cheek and the other inside on the mucosa. The Stensen's duct opening is inspected and "milked" by sliding the finger along the length of the salivary duct while pushing the saliva through the duct opening to detect the presence of salivary stones. It is possible that the dental assistant may see a **linea alba buccalis** (a white-line demarcation of the area where maxillary and mandibular teeth occlude) and **fordyces granules** (sebaceous glands) that are normal. On the other hand, the operator may see white patches in this area, possibly **leukoplakia** (precancerous condition exhibiting white patchy lesions).

- The tongue is grasped with a gauze square and extended out. It is moved from side to side while the operator visually inspects the lateral borders, the ventral/dorsal surfaces of the tongue, and the floor of the mouth (Figure 28-11). The lingual frenum is observed for tightness and length. The tongue is also palpated bidigitally for possible tumors. It is conceivable to encounter a geographic tongue in which there is uneven distribution of the filiform papilla. Another **atypical** (not typical) occurrence is the fissured tongue that appears to have deep grooves on the dorsal side of the tongue.

- The floor of the mouth is examined and palpated using a bimanual technique by placing one hand under the jaw and fingers of the other hand on the floor of the mouth (Figure 28-6).

- Using a mouth mirror, the facial and lingual gingiva of the maxillary and mandibular arches are inspected for inflammation and bleeding. With the mouth mirror, the soft palate and oral pharynx are also inspected for any deviations.

Oral Cancer

While performing the oral inspection, it is essential to look for lesions that may manifest the presence of oral cancer, keeping in mind that when oral cancer is discovered early, there is a 90% cure rate. The predominant areas to look for cancerous lesions include:

- The floor of the mouth
- The lateral borders of the tongue
- The oropharynx to include the soft and hard palates
- The lower lip

The appearance of oral cancer takes many forms. They could range from white patches to ulcerated lesions. However, it is wise to be on the alert for any of the following:

- White patches on the mucosa could be a precancerous condition, namely, leukoplakia.
- Redness similar to an inflammation may appear. It may be of any shape or size.
- A sore that does not heal within a normal period, usually two weeks.
- A lesion that appears ulcerated, manifesting a gray to yellow center surrounded by red, inflamed tissue.
- Hardened tissue, similar to a wartlike appearance.
- A lesion with any of the above characteristics that is nonmobile or fixed, having embedded itself into muscle or bone.
- Inflammation of the lymph nodes resulting in their enlargement and hardening. Patient may complain of a lump in the neck.

Introducing the topic of oral cancer here is to encourage the dental assistant to be aware of oral cancer while performing an oral exam. See Chapter 59.

Charting the Teeth

All findings of the teeth are recorded on a chart to include existing restorations, possible caries, fixed and removable prosthetics, and missing, mobile, and malpositioned teeth. The dental assistant may use the air and water syringe to aid in locating **supragingival** (above-the-gingival-line) calculus. See Chapter 30 for charting symbols.

- A multicolor pen should be used to determine existing restorations, charted in blue, vs. required treatment, charted in red.

- A mouth mirror is used to examine the teeth.
- A system for charting should be developed to avoid missing areas. For example, when using the universal charting system, one would begin with tooth 1, the maxillary right third molar, and conclude with tooth 32, the mandibular right third molar. See Chapter 30.

SUGGESTED ACTIVITIES

- Study all anatomic parts of the oral cavity and verbally point them out on a fellow classmate.
- Using Universal Precautions, perform an extraoral and intraoral inspection on a fellow classmate and include charting of the teeth.

REVIEW

1. Name three general characteristics of inflammation of gingival tissue: (1) glossy, (2) swollen, (3) stippled, and/or (4) spongy.
   a. 1, 2, 3   c. 1, 2, 4
   b. 2, 3, 4   d. 1, 3, 4

2. Match the following terms with their corresponding definitions:

   ___ a. Bimanual   1. Listening for abnormal sounds during examination

   ___ b. Bilateral   2. Grinding sounds coming from a joint

   ___ c. Bidigital   3. The manner in which the patient carries himself or herself

   ___ d. Percussion   4. Using the sense of smell during examination

   ___ e. Auscultation 5. Tapping a part of the body during examination

   ___ f. Olfaction   6. Using two hands on similar structures contralaterally

   ___ g. Gait   7. Right and left sides are not the same

   ___ h. Crepitus   8. Using two hands simultaneously in the same location

   ___ i. Jaundice   9. Yellow appearance on the skin including sclera of eyes

   ___ j. Asymmetry   10. Using a finger and thumb simultaneously in the same location

3. Fordyce's granules are also known as:
   a. Sebaceous glands   c. Leukoplakia
   b. Fatty tissues   d. Precancerous lesions

4. To touch or feel using the hands or fingers describes this term:
   a. Bimanual   c. Auscultation
   b. Bidigital   d. Palpation

5. Name the three conditions observed when assessing the patient visually: (1) patient's five senses, (2) patient's gait, (3) evidence of asymmetry, and/or (4) skin color, including sclera of the eyes.
   a. 1, 2, 3   c. 1, 2, 4
   b. 2, 3, 4   d. 1, 3, 4

Basic Dental Charting

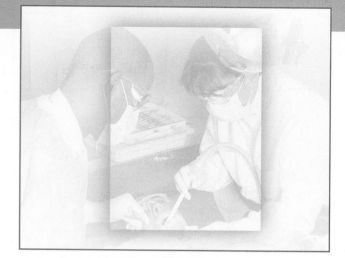

After studying this chapter, the student will be able to:

- Describe the three systems used to chart permanent and primary teeth.
- Chart the correct tooth number or letter for permanent and primary teeth for the Universal, Palmer, and International systems.
- Define the six standard classifications of cavities.
- Name the tooth surfaces and their abbreviations.

Introduction

One of the many duties delegated to the dental assistant is the charting of the teeth. This is an exact recording of the dental conditions present and the dental services to be rendered and serves as a legal record of the patient. It includes the types of dental restorations, treatment of periodontal tissues, extractions, replacement of missing teeth, and other information regarding the oral condition of the patient.

General Anatomy of Mouth

- A full complement of deciduous, or primary, teeth numbers 20; a full set of permanent teeth numbers 32.
- Teeth are classified as those of either the maxillary arch or the mandibular arch.
- Each arch is divided by an imaginary line between the two central incisors, creating a right half and a left half.
- Each half arch constitutes one-fourth of the teeth, and each half-arch is referred to as a **quadrant**. Thus, there are four quadrants of teeth in the mouth.
- In referring to position, the teeth on the *patient's* right side are indicated as right; those on the *patient's* left side are indicated as left.
- If an adult has all 32 teeth, there are 8 teeth in each quadrant. A child would have 5 deciduous teeth in each quadrant.

Identification of Teeth

Identification of teeth may be made through the use of numbers and letters. Several systems have been developed that are used by dentists; the specific system used is, of course, a matter of preference.

Universal System

The American Dental Association (ADA) officially adopted the **Universal System** for charting teeth in 1968. In this system each tooth has its own number (permanent teeth) or letter (primary teeth), and this particular number or letter refers only to that one specific tooth.

The permanent teeth are numbered from 1 to 32, and the letters A–T are used for primary teeth.

Permanent Teeth (Figure 29-1)

1. Begin with tooth number 1, maxillary right third molar, and work around the arch to number 16, maxillary left third molar.
2. On the mandibular arch, start with tooth number 17, mandibular left third molar, and work around to number 32, mandibular right third molar.

Primary Teeth (Figure 29-2)

1. Begin with the letter A, maxillary right second molar, and work around the arch to the letter J, maxillary left second molar.
2. On the mandibular arch, start with the letter K, mandibular left second molar, and work around the arch to the letter T, mandibular right second molar.

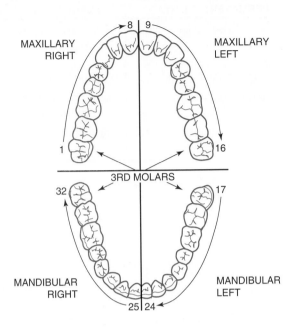

Figure 29-1 Permanent teeth—Universal System.

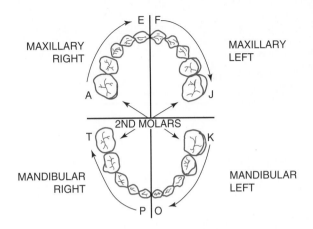

Figure 29-2 Primary teeth—Universal System.

Palmer System

In the **Palmer System** the teeth are numbered the same for each quadrant, 1–8 for permanent teeth and letters A–E for primary teeth. To distinguish which quadrant and tooth is to be recorded, a symbol, or "bracket," is used to denote the maxillary and mandibular arch, as well as the right and left side of the patient.

To determine the correct arch and quadrant, Figure 29-3 may be used as a guide.

MAXILLARY RIGHT	MAXILLARY LEFT
MANDIBULAR RIGHT	MANDIBULAR LEFT

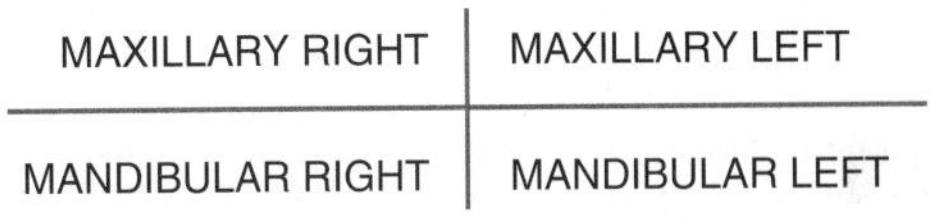

Figure 29-3 Arch and quadrant guide for Palmer System.

Permanent Teeth (Figure 29-4)

1. In each quadrant the teeth are numbered from 1 to 8, beginning with the central incisors as 1 and working toward the third molar, number 8.

2. Use the quadrant bracket to denote the maxillary and mandibular arch and right or left side.

3. *Caution:* The correct bracket must be used with the tooth number for proper identification of tooth and quadrant.

   Examples: Maxillary right second molar   7⌋

   Mandibular left lateral   ⌐2

Primary Teeth (Figure 29-5)

1. In each quadrant, the teeth are lettered A–E, beginning with the central incisors as A and working toward the second molar, E.

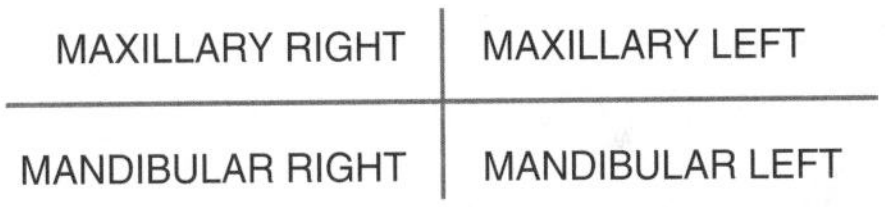

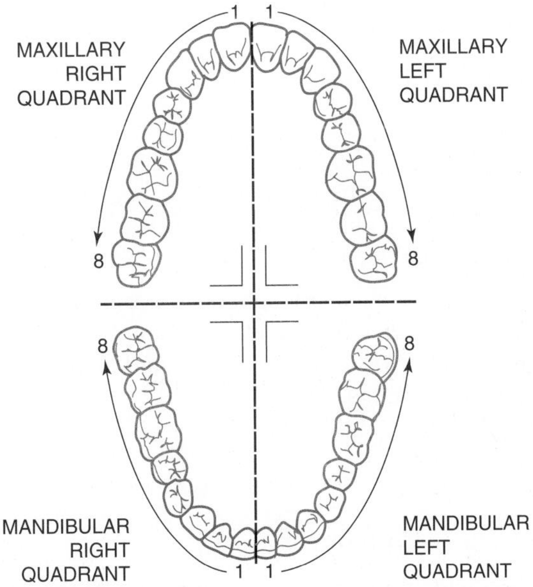

MAXILLARY RIGHT	MAXILLARY LEFT
MANDIBULAR RIGHT	MANDIBULAR LEFT

Figure 29-4 Permanent teeth—Palmer System.

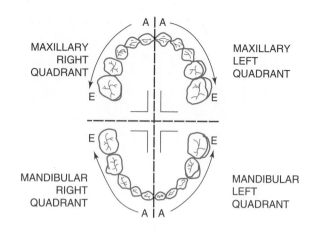

Figure 29-5 Primary teeth—Palmer System.

2. Use the quadrant bracket to denote the maxillary or mandibular arch and right or left side.

3. *Caution:* The correct bracket must be used with the tooth letter for proper identification of tooth and quadrant.

Examples: Maxillary left central ⌐A

Mandibular right second molar E⌐

Fédération Dentaire International System

The Fédération Dentaire **International System** was designed to be used with the computer. The system uses a two-digit number to identify each tooth. The first number denotes the quadrant and the second number identifies the specific tooth in that quadrant. The quadrant numbers are 1–4 for the permanent teeth and 5–8 for the primary teeth (Figure 29-6).

Permanent Teeth (Figure 29-7)

1. Teeth are numbered 1–8, beginning with the central incisors as 1 and third molars as 8.

2. The quadrants are numbered 1–4, beginning with the maxillary right as 1, maxillary left as 2, mandibular left as 3, and mandibular right as 4.

3. Teeth in the maxillary right quadrant are recorded as 11–18; the maxillary left quadrant, 21–28; mandibular left quadrant, 31–38; and mandibular right quadrant, 41–48.

Examples: Maxillary right lateral: 12

Mandibular left cuspid: 33

Primary Teeth (Figure 29-8)

1. Teeth are numbered 1–5, beginning with the central incisors as 1 and second molars as 5.

PERMANENT TEETH		PRIMARY TEETH	
MAXILLARY RIGHT QUADRANT	1	MAXILLARY RIGHT QUADRANT	5
MAXILLARY LEFT QUADRANT	2	MAXILLARY LEFT QUADRANT	6
MANDIBULAR LEFT QUADRANT	3	MANDIBULAR LEFT QUADRANT	7
MANDIBULAR RIGHT QUADRANT	4	MANDIBULAR RIGHT QUADRANT	8

Figure 29-6 Quadrant numbering for International System.

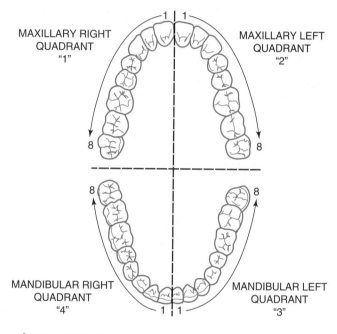

Figure 29-7 Permanent teeth—International System.

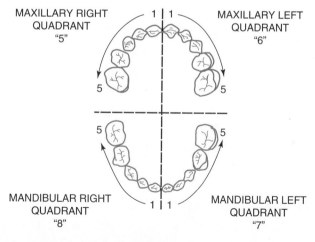

Figure 29-8 Primary teeth—International System.

2. The quadrants are numbered 5–8, beginning with the maxillary right quadrant as 5, maxillary left quadrant as 6, mandibular left quadrant as 7, and mandibular right quadrant as 8.

3. Teeth in the maxillary right quadrant are recorded as 51–55; maxillary left quadrant, 61–65; mandibular left quadrant, 71–75; and mandibular right, 81–85.

   Examples: Maxillary right first molar: 54

   Mandibular left central incisor: 71

Cavity Classifications

A system for identifying tooth surfaces and teeth is used when recording dental conditions on a patient's dental chart.

G. V. Black (father of modern dentistry) developed the Standard Classification of Cavities. There are six Classes: I, II, III, IV, V, and VI. Each class represents a particular type of caries (dental cavity) or restoration.

Class I, Anterior and Posterior Teeth

Class I caries occur in the developmental areas of the teeth, grooves, and fossae. When a developmental groove becomes faulty because of decay, it is called a fissure, and a defective fossa is called a pit. Pit and fissure caries are found on the following teeth:

1. On the occlusal surfaces of premolars and molars (Figure 29-9)

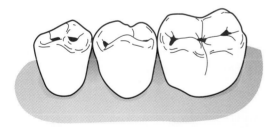

Figure 29-9 Caries—occlusal surfaces of premolars and molars.

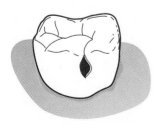

Figure 29-10 Caries—facial and lingual surfaces of molars.

2. On the facial (buccal) groove and pit of mandibular molars; on the lingual groove and pit surfaces of maxillary molars (Figure 29-10)

3. On the lingual pits of maxillary incisors, at the cingulum (Figure 29-11)

Class II, Posterior Teeth

Class II caries occur on the proximal surfaces (mesial or distal) of premolars and molars and involve two or more surfaces (Figure 29-12).

Class III, Anterior Teeth

Class III caries occur on the proximal surfaces (mesial or distal) of incisors and cuspids (Figure 29-13).

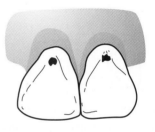

Figure 29-11 Caries—lingual surface (cingulum) of maxillary incisors.

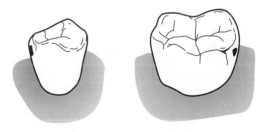

Figure 29-12 Caries—proximal surfaces of premolars and molars.

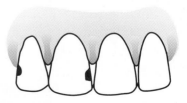

Figure 29-13 Caries—proximal surfaces of incisors and cuspids.

Class IV, Anterior Teeth

Class IV caries occur on the proximal surfaces (mesial or distal) of incisors and cuspids and involve the incisal edge/angle (Figure 29-14).

Class V, Anterior and Posterior Teeth

Class V caries occur on the gingival or cervical third of a tooth, facial or lingual surfaces (Figure 29-15).

Class VI, Anterior and Posterior Teeth

Class VI caries or defects that occur on the incisal edge of anterior teeth or cusp tips of posterior teeth (Figure 29-16).

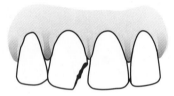

Figure 29-14 Caries—proximal surfaces of incisors and cuspids involving incisal edge or angle.

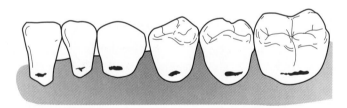

Figure 29-15 Caries—gingival or cervical third of teeth.

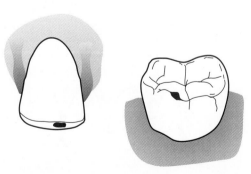

Figure 29-16 Caries—defect on incisal edge or cusp tip of teeth.

Abbreviations of Tooth Surfaces

In the charting of teeth and dental condition, the surfaces of the teeth are abbreviated in order to aid in the recording of information.

The abbreviations for single tooth surfaces are as follows:

Abbreviation of Single Tooth Surfaces

- Mesial = M
- Distal = D
- Labial = La
- Lingual = L or Li
- Buccal = B or Bu
- Incisal = I
- Occlusal = O or Occ
- Facial (buccal surfaces) = F

When two or more surface names are combined, such as mesial and occlusal, the combined two surfaces are referred to as mesio-occlusal, or MO. In combining surfaces names the *-al* ending of the first surface is dropped and the letter *o* is substituted. If three surfaces are combined, the same rule applies to the second surface, and it is referred to as mesio-occluso-distal, or MOD. When two or three surfaces involve the mesial, *M* is used first, as in MI, MO, and MOD. When two surfaces involve the distal, *D* is used first, as in DI, DO, or DL. When neither mesial nor distal are used, buccal or lingual are used first, as in BO or LO.

Common abbreviations for combining surface names include the following:

Abbreviations for Combining Surfaces

- Mesio-occlusal = MO
- Disto-occlusal = DO
- Mesio-occluso-distal = MOD
- Mesioincisal = MI
- Distoincisal = DI
- Distolingual = DL
- Bucco-occlusal = BO
- Linguo-occlusal = LO

Completed restorations using abbreviations are illustrated in Figure 29-17.

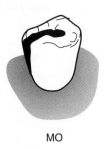
MO

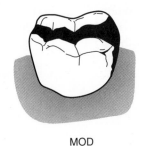
MOD

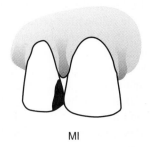
MI

Figure 29-17 Completed restorations.

SUGGESTED ACTIVITIES

● Study the Universal System of charting. Use Figures 29-1 and 29-2 as guides to complete Review 1 and 2 of this chapter.
● Study the Palmer System. Use Figures 29-4 and 29-5 as guides to complete Review 3 of this chapter.
● Study the International System. Use Figures 29-7 and 29-8 as guides to complete Review 4 of this chapter.

REVIEW

1. Using the Universal System, identify the following permanent teeth by placing the corresponding number for the correct tooth number beside the tooth:

Permanent Teeth
___ a. Maxillary right first molar
___ b. Maxillary right lateral
___ c. Maxillary left central
___ d. Maxillary left cuspid
___ e. Maxillary left third molar
___ f. Mandibular left second molar
___ g. Mandibular left central incisor
___ h. Mandibular right central incisor
___ i. Mandibular right first molar
___ j. Mandibular right third molar

1. Tooth #9
2. Tooth #16
3. Tooth #18
4. Tooth #3
5. Tooth #11
6. Tooth #32
7. Tooth #7
8. Tooth #24
9. Tooth #30
10. Tooth #25

2. Using the Universal System, identify the following primary teeth by placing the corresponding number for the correct tooth letter beside the tooth:

Primary Teeth
___ a. Maxillary right first molar
___ b. Maxillary right central incisor
___ c. Maxillary left lateral
___ d. Maxillary left second molar
___ e. Mandibular left first molar
___ f. Mandibular left central incisor
___ g. Mandibular right central incisor
___ h. Mandibular right second molar

1. Tooth #J
2. Tooth #B
3. Tooth #O
4. Tooth #E
5. Tooth #T
6. Tooth #G
7. Tooth #L
8. Tooth #P

3. Using the Palmer method, identify the following permanent teeth by placing the corresponding number for the correct tooth number beside the tooth:

___ a. Maxillary right first molar
___ b. Maxillary right lateral
___ c. Maxillary left central incisor
___ d. Maxillary left second molar
___ e. Mandibular left cuspid
___ f. Mandibular left second molar
___ g. Mandibular right central incisor
___ h. Mandibular right first molar

1. Tooth # $\overline{7}$
2. Tooth # $\overline{6|}$
3. Tooth # $\underline{2|}$
4. Tooth # $\overline{|3}$
5. Tooth # $\underline{|1}$
6. Tooth # $\underline{6|}$
7. Tooth # $\overline{1|}$
8. Tooth # $\underline{|7}$

4. Using the Fédération Dentaire International System, identify the following permanent teeth by placing the corresponding number for the correct tooth number beside the tooth:

___ a. Maxillary right first molar

___ b. Maxillary right lateral

___ c. Maxillary left central incisor

___ d. Maxillary left second molar

___ e. Mandibular left cuspid

___ f. Mandibular left second molar

___ g. Mandibular right central incisor

___ h. Mandibular right first molar

1. Tooth #41
2. Tooth #27
3. Tooth #46
4. Tooth #37
5. Tooth #16
6. Tooth #21
7. Tooth #12
8. Tooth #33

5. Match the following classification of cavities with their definitions:

___ a. Class I

___ b. Class II

___ c. Class III

___ d. Class IV

___ e. Class V

1. Mesial or distal proximal surfaces on premolars and molars

2. Mesial or distal proximal surfaces of incisors and cuspids

3. Occlusal surfaces of premolars and molars, buccal occlusal surfaces of mandibular molars, lingual occlusal surfaces of maxillary molars, and lingual pits of maxillary anterior teeth

4. Facial or lingual surfaces on gingival or cervical third of any tooth

5. Mesial or distal proximal surfaces of incisors and cuspids involving incisal edge

Interpretive Charting

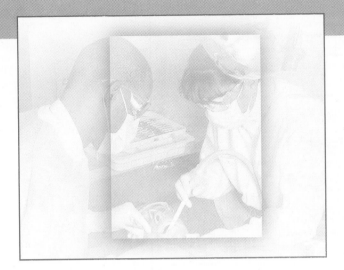

OBJECTIVES

After studying this chapter, the student will be able to:

- Identify the tooth surfaces on an anatomic and geometric diagram.
- Chart conditions present using appropriate charting symbols, abbreviations, and code.
- Interpret the charted dental conditions from an anatomic and geometric diagram.
- Record services rendered in proper sequence on a dental chart.

Introduction

A patient's dental chart is a legal record of dental services. As with all legal records, any information must be current, accurate, complete, and concise. Care must be taken to ensure that they are properly filed and stored to prevent loss or damage.

There are many designs and types of dental charts; selection of a particular dental chart is based on the dentist's preference.

Dental Charts

Dental charts are used for recording clinical data obtained from the patient during an oral examination and radiographic diagnosis (Figures 30-1 and 30-2).

The dental chart includes conditions present and dental treatment rendered while under the care of a particular dentist.

A system for recording this information must be one that is consistently practiced and can be completed in a minimal amount of time.

Documentation of information becomes a legal record and, as such, should be done with extreme care. The importance of accuracy cannot be stressed enough. Dental health care workers (DHCW) must be knowledgeable and use proper identifiable charting abbreviations. Should change on information already documented become necessary, a single line should be drawn and the person's name making the change should be recorded next to it. Whiteout or erasures are not acceptable.

A dental chart may have several specific sections where patient information is recorded, indicated by letters in the list below and shown in Figure 30-3:

A. *Patient personal information.* Full name of patient, age, home address and telephone number, billing address, employment, personal physician's name and address, and financial information.

B. *Charting area.* Representation of the maxillary and mandibular teeth.

C. *Medical precautions.* Patient's medical conditions of specific concerns must be noted and updated on subsequent visits.

D. *Anesthesia.* Consent, other pertinent remarks.

E. *Radiographic history.* Patient's radiographic history record.

F. *Remarks.* Reserved for the dentist's personal notations.

G. *Fee estimate.* Date, treatment plan, and fee.

Detailed description of services rendered, charges, payment received, and balance due are shown in Figure 30-4.

Anterior/Posterior Relationship of Teeth

To accurately record dental conditions on a patient's chart, one must understand the anterior/posterior relationship of the teeth as they relate to the maxillary and mandibular arches. View of the maxillary and mandibular teeth with the mouth open is shown in Figure 30-5. *Note:* The anterior/posterior relationship of the teeth remains the same whether viewed in the arches or on a straight line. For a view of the same teeth in a straight line, see Figure 30-6.

231

Figure 30-1 Dental chart. (Courtesy of Professional Publishers, Cupertino, CA.)

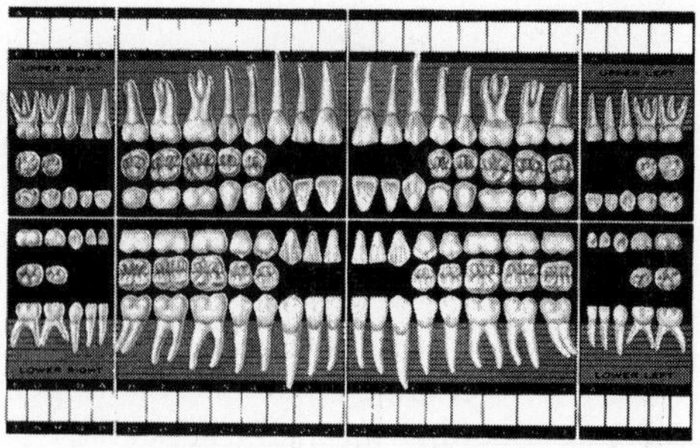

Figure 30-2 Reverse side of dental chart. (Courtesy of Professional Publishers, Cupertino, CA.)

A. PATIENT PERSONAL INFORMATION

Name _White Ryan J._ Home Phone _(818)123-0000_ Business Phone _(818)541-0000_ Date_ May 14, 2001_
Home Address _1000 E. Green Street_ City _Pasadena_ Date of Birth _July 4, 1952_ Age _48_ Referred by _M. Lamb_
Occupation _Engineer_ Empoyer _City Engineering_ Employer Address _000 E. Walnut_ City _Pasadena, CA 91101_
Marital Status_Single_ Spouse's Name —— Spouse's Occupation ——
Employer —— Employer's Address —— City —— Credit Rating _Good_
Person Financially Responsible_Self_ Relationship to You —— Recall____
Billing Address_1000 E. Green Street_ City _Pasadena_ Zip _91101_ Dental Insurance _Delta Plan_____
Physician _John V. Martin, M.D._ Phone _(818)300-0000_ Former Dentist _Deceased_ Address ——

B. CHARTING AREA

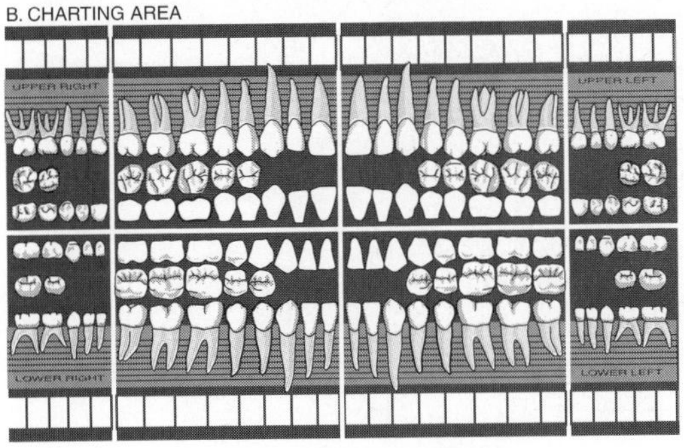

C. MEDICAL PRECAUTIONS
MEDICAL PRECAUTIONS:

D. ANESTHESIA
ANESTHESIA: YES [ ] NO [ ]
REMARKS_____

E. RADIOGRAPHIC HISTORY
RADIOGRAPHIC HISTORY:
DATE   SURVEY   DATE   SURVEY

F. REMARKS

REMARKS

G. FEE ESTIMATES
FEE ESTIMATES
DATE   TREATMENT   FEE

Figure 30-3 Parts of a dental chart. (Courtesy of Professional Publishers, Cupertino, CA.)

PATIENT'S NAME _Ryan J. White_
BILLING NAME _same_
ADDRESS _1000 E. Green Street_
Pasadena, CA 91101

FINANCIAL ARRANGEMENT _____
Delta Plan

1 • 2 • 3 • 4 • 5

DATE	SERVICES	CHARGES		PAID		BALANCE	
5-14-01	FM X-rays	65	00			65	00
5-14-01	FM Prophy	60	00			125	00
5-26-01	Radiogr Diag and Est	—	—			125	00
	CK 90-0012			125	00	—	—
						—	—
6-10-01	14 MOD Dycal, ZOE base Amal Anes Lido						
	plain 1 cart	80	00			80	00
6-17-01	8 M Dycal, Sealer Composite Anes Lido					80	00
	plain 1 cart	75	00			155	00
6-24-01	19 FGCr prep and Imp Temp Cr seat ZOE					155	00
	Anes Lido plain 1 cart	—	—			155	00
7-01-01	19 FGCr seat ZnP	350	00			505	00

FORM C • 103 • C

Figure 30-4 Area for recording services rendered. (Courtesy of Professional Publishers, Cupertino, CA.)

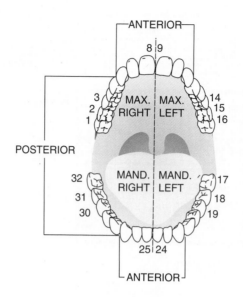

Figure 30-5 View of teeth with mouth open.

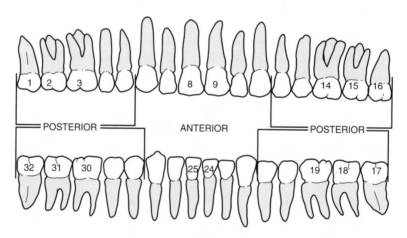

Figure 30-6 View of teeth in a straight line.

Tooth Diagrams

The most commonly used tooth diagrams on dental charts are anatomic and geometric representations.

Anatomic Diagram

The *anatomic diagram* may show only the crowns of the teeth (Figure 30-7), crown and a small portion of the root, or crowns and all of the root(s) (Figure 30-8).

Tooth surfaces on the anatomic diagram may be difficult to identify. Figure 30-9 represents the facial, occlusal, and lingual tooth surfaces:

- Rows 1 and 5 represent facial surfaces, posterior, and anterior teeth.
- Rows 2 and 4 represent occlusal surfaces, posterior teeth.
- Row 3 represents lingual surfaces, posterior, and anterior teeth.

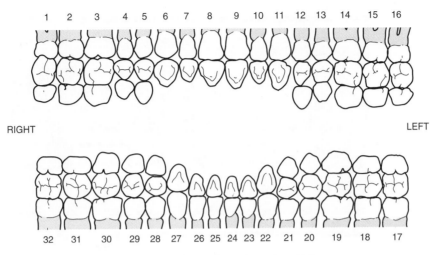

Figure 30-7 Anatomic diagram—tooth crowns and small portion of root(s).

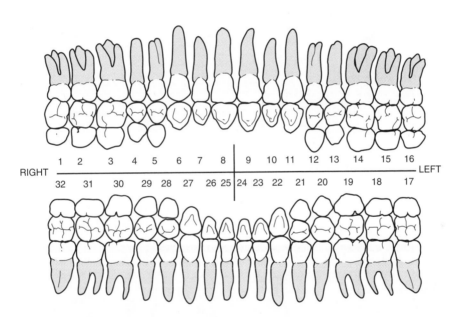

Figure 30-8 Anatomic diagram—tooth crowns and roots.

Figure 30-10 represents the mesial and distal interproximal surfaces (anterior and posterior) as indicated by vertical lines on the chart.

Geometric Diagram

The *geometric diagram* represents teeth using the circle or circles. The coronal or crown surfaces of the teeth are shown in Figures 30-11 and 30-12.

The geometric diagram shows only the crowns of the teeth of permanent dentition numbered 1–32 (Figure 30-13). The middle two rows represent primary dentition and are lettered A–T.

Tooth surfaces on the geometric diagram are less difficult to identify, because all five surfaces are represented within the circle. Figure 30-14 represents the different tooth surfaces with the geometric diagram method.

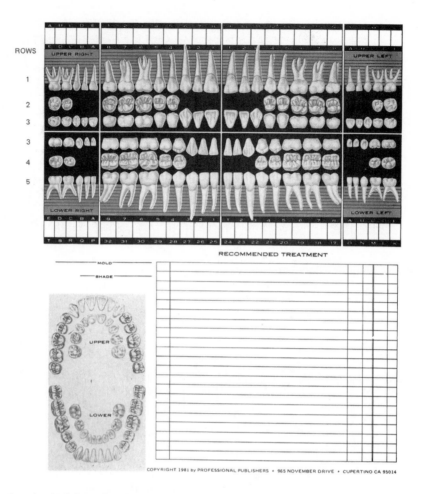

Figure 30-9 Chart showing the facial, occlusal, and lingual surfaces. (Courtesy of Professional Publishers, Cupertino, CA.)

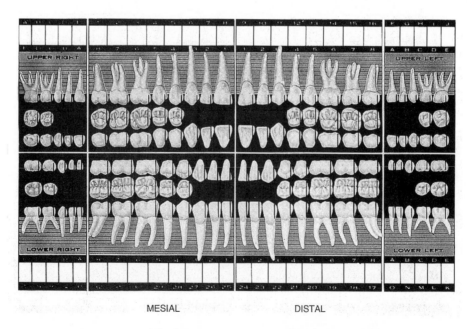

MESIAL   DISTAL

Figure 30-10 Mesial and distal surfaces of teeth. (Courtesy of Professional Publishers, Cupertino, CA.)

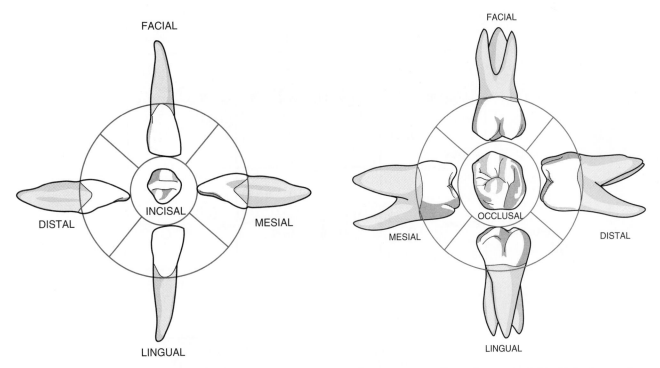

Figure 30-11 Anterior tooth divided into five surfaces.

Figure 30-12 Posterior tooth divided into five surfaces.

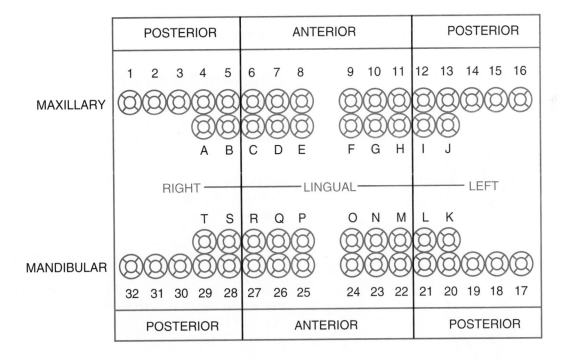

Figure 30-13 Geometric diagram—representation of teeth surfaces.

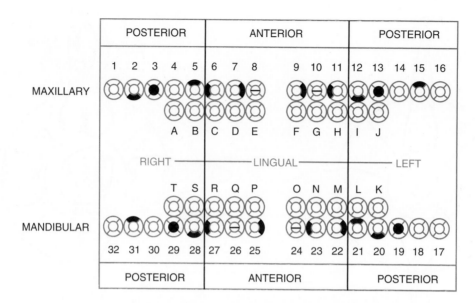

Figure 30-14 Geometric representation of teeth with occlusal, incisal, facial, linqual, mesial, and distal surfaces.

TOOTH NO.	TOOTH NO.
2 LINGUAL	19 OCCLUSAL
3 OCCLUSAL	20 FACIAL (BUCCAL)
5 FACIAL (BUCCAL)	21 LINGUAL
6 DISTAL	22 DISTAL
7 MESIAL	23 MESIAL
8 INCISAL	24 INCISAL
9 DISTAL	25 MESIAL
10 INCISAL	26 INCISAL
11 MESIAL	27 DISTAL
12 LINGUAL	28 FACIAL (BUCCAL)
13 OCCLUSAL	29 OCCLUSAL
15 FACIAL (BUCCAL)	31 LINGUAL

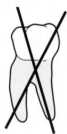

Figure 30-15 Missing tooth.

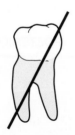

Figure 30-16 Tooth to be extracted.

Charting Symbols

Missing Teeth. Refers to a tooth that has been surgically removed or to a tooth that has never formed. An X is drawn through the tooth (Figure 30-15).

To be Extracted. A tooth that is to be surgically removed. A diagonal line is drawn through the tooth (Figure 30-16).

Unerupted or Impacted Tooth. Tooth that has not erupted and is encased in tissue or bone. Circle the tooth. An arrow is used to indicate the direction of an **impaction** (an embedded tooth that has not erupted; Figure 30-17).

Drifting Teeth. After teeth are removed and not replaced, opposing and surrounding teeth often drift into space created by the extraction. A maxillary tooth will drift downward, and a mandibular tooth will move upward. This is indicated with vertical arrows (Figure 30-18).

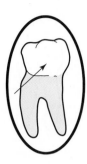

Figure 30-17 Unerupted or impacted tooth.

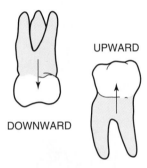

Figure 30-18 Drifting teeth.

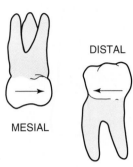

Figure 30-19 Mesial or distal drift.

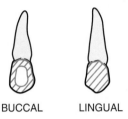

Figure 30-20 Three-quarter crown.

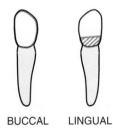

Figure 30-21 Full metal crown.

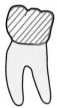

Figure 30-22 Porcelain crown fused to metal.

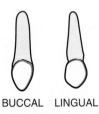

Figure 30-23 Full porcelain crown.

Mesial or Distal Drift. A tooth may drift from mesial to distal or visa versa, and horizontal arrows are used to indicate direction (Figure 30-19).

Three-Quarter Crown. Covers the mesial, distal, lingual, and incisal or occlusal surfaces of a tooth. The facial surface of the tooth is *not* involved. This type of restoration is used on anterior teeth or maxillary premolars. The clinical crown is outlined and diagonal lines drawn on the lingual surface and around the edges of the facial surface (Figure 30-20).

Full Metal Crown. The clinical crown is outlined and diagonal lines drawn through the crown (Figure 30-21).

Porcelain Crown Fused to Metal. Outline facial and lingual surface of crown. On lingual surface a moon-shaped line with slash marks is drawn at cervical third of tooth (Figure 30-22).

Full Porcelain Crown. Outline the full surface of the crown (Figure 30-23).

Porcelain Veneer. Outline the facial portion of the crown (Figure 30-24).

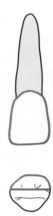

Figure 30-24 Porcelain veneer.

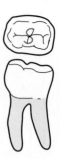

Figure 30-25 Sealant.

Sealant. Place the letter S on the occlusal surface (Figure 30-25).

Implant. Draw horizontal lines on the root portion of the tooth (Figure 30-26).

Figure 30-26 Implant.

Fixed Bridge. Indicate abutment teeth by outlining surface of restoration whether full or three-quarter crown(s). Draw an X through missing teeth. Draw two horizontal lines through the crowns of **abutments** (anchor teeth for the **bridge**). Extend the lines through the **pontic** (suspended portion or tooth replacement; Figure 30-27).

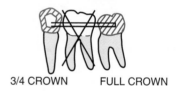

3/4 CROWN   FULL CROWN

Figure 30-27 Fixed bridge.

Fractured Tooth. Draw a jagged line in area of fracture (Figure 30-28).

Abscessed Tooth. To indicate an **abscess** (localized collection of pus) at apex of the root(s), draw a small circle over the end of the root(s) involved (Figure 30-29).

Figure 30-28 Fractured tooth.

Root Canal. Record **endodontic** (*endo-* = within; *donto-* = tooth) treatment by drawing a vertical line through the root canal(s) (Figure 30-30).

Post and Core. Draw the core on the crown portion and the post on the root portion of the tooth (Figure 30-31).

Figure 30-29 Abscessed tooth.

Periodontal Pocket(s). The pocket depth is recorded by using one or more diagonal lines in pocket area(s). The depth of pocket is recorded in millimeters (mm) (Figure 30-32).

Periodontal Abscess. Draw a circle in area of the abscess (Figure 30-33).

Figure 30-30 Root canal.

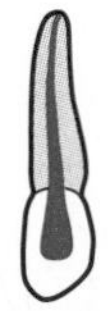

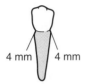

Figure 30-31 Post and core.

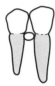

4 mm | 4 mm

Figure 30-32 Periodontal pocket(s).

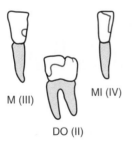

Figure 30-33 Periodontal abscess.

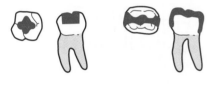

OCC   MOD

Figure 30-34 Amalgam restoration.

M (III)   MI (IV)

DO (II)

Figure 30-35 Composite restoration.

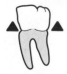

Figure 30-36 Overhanging margin on restoration.

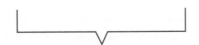

Figure 30-37 Brackets.

Amalgam Restoration. Outline restoration and shade in surfaces involved, such as MO, DO, DLG, occ., or buccal pit (Figure 30-34).

Composite Restoration. Outline tooth colored restoration. For Class III restoration, outline with a half-moon in the area of involvement. For a Class IV, include the incisal edge (Figure 30-35).

Overhanging Margin on Restoration. An overhanging margin on a restoration is indicated by placing a shaded triangle in the area of involvement, mesial or distal surface (Figure 30-36).

Brackets. Brackets are used to indicate a partial or full denture (Figure 30-37).

Partial Denture. Draw an X through the missing teeth and a bracket along the lingual surface of the arch (Figure 30-38).

Full Denture. Draw an X through the entire arch and a bracket along the lingual surface (Figure 30-39).

Suggested Abbreviations for Dental Terms

Abscess	Abs
Adjustment	Adj
Amalgam	Amal
Anesthetic	Anes
Bitewing	BW
Composite	Com
Crown	Cr
Denture	Dent
Diagnosis	Diag
Examination	Exam
Extraction	Ext
Estimate	Est
Fixed bridge	Fix Br
Full gold crown	FGCr
Full mouth	FM
Full upper	FU
Gold inlay	GI
Gold onlay	GO
Impression	Imp
Partial upper	PU
Porcelain fused to metal	PFM
Preparation	Prep
Prophylaxis	Prophy
Radiographs	Radiogr
Removable	Rem
Root canal	RC
Study models	SM
Temporary	Temp
Zinc-oxide-eugenol	ZOE
Zinc phosphate	ZnP

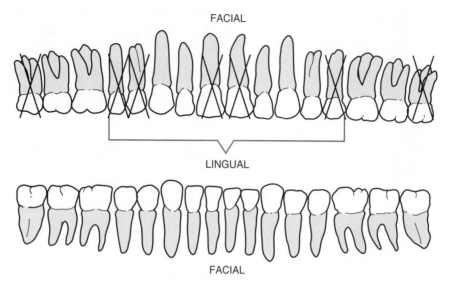

Figure 30-38 Partial denture.

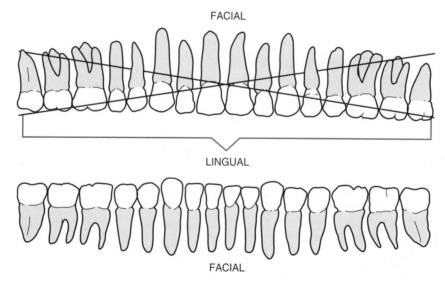

Figure 30-39 Full denture.

Anesthetics

Lidocaine	Lido
Xylocaine	Xylo
Carbocaine	Carbo

Charting Conditions Present

Chart conditions present using the appropriate charting symbols, abbreviations, and the following code:

● Blue represents work completed or conditions not requiring treatment.

  1. Outline, then shade in *blue* amalgam restorations in good condition.

  2. Outline in *blue* tooth colored restorations.

  3. Outline and place diagonal lines in *blue* gold restorations.

  4. Indicate in *blue* missing teeth, root canal(s).

● Red indicates that treatment is required.

  1. Outline in *red* dental caries, fractures.

  2. Indicate in *red* impactions, extractions, abscesses, periodontal pockets, overhanging margins.

  3. *Solid blue, outlined in red* restoration present to be replaced.

Note: Because this text is only two color, it has only the green charting color; blue charting symbols are rendered in black. Your charting exercises, however, should be done correctly in red and blue.

Charting Anatomic Diagram

Posterior Teeth. Chart dental caries by outlining the occlusal and proximal (mesial and/or distal) surfaces. *Outline* occlusal (A), facial (B), and lingual (C) surfaces in *red* (Figures 30-40, MO, and 30-41, MOD).

Anterior Teeth. Chart dental caries by drawing a half-moon on the proximal surface (mesial or distal) in the area of involvement (contact area) (Figures 30-42, Mesial, and 30-43, Distal).

Restorations in *good condition* are *shaded* (amalgam) in *blue* (Figure 30-44) or *outlined* (tooth colored) (Figure 30-45). Indicate type of restorative material using appropriate abbreviations.

Charting Geometric Diagram

Posterior Teeth. Chart dental caries by *outlining* occlusal and proximal (mesial and/or distal) surfaces in *red* (Figures 30-46, Mesial, and 30-47, Mesial and Distal).

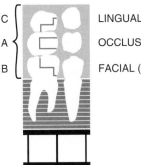

Figure 30-40 Mesial caries—posterior teeth (lingual, occlusal, and facial views).

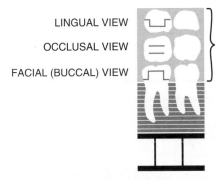

Figure 30-41 Mesial and distal caries—posterior teeth (lingual, occlusal, and facial views).

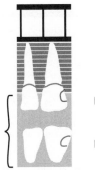

Figure 30-42 Mesial caries—anterior teeth (facial and lingual views).

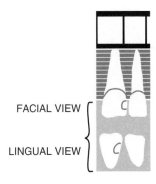

Figure 30-43 Distal caries—anterior teeth (facial and lingual views).

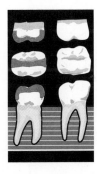

Figure 30-44 MOD amalgam—posterior tooth.

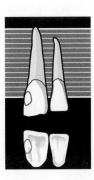

Figure 30-45 M composite—anterior tooth.

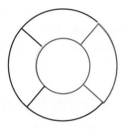

Figure 30-46 Mesial caries—posterior tooth.

Anterior Teeth. *Outline* proximal (mesial or distal)

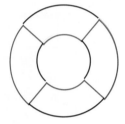

Figure 30-47 Mesial and distal caries—posterior tooth.

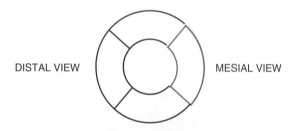

Figure 30-48 Mesial caries—anterior tooth.

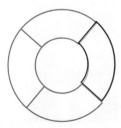

Figure 30-49 Distal caries—anterior tooth.

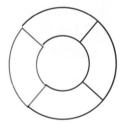

Figure 30-50 Mesial composite—anterior tooth.

surface in *red* (Figures 30-48, Mesial, and 30-49, Distal).

Restorations in *good condition* are *outlined* (tooth colored) or *shaded* (amalgam) in *blue* (Figures 30-50, Mesial, and 30-51, MOD). Indicate type of restorative material using appropriate abbreviations.

Charted anatomic and geometric diagrams are shown in Figures 30-52 and 30-53, respectively. These figures represent the same charted conditions present.

Recording Services Rendered

Whenever a patient receives dental treatment, information regarding the treatment must be entered on the patient's chart under "services rendered." Other pertinent information, such as instructions to the patient, must also be recorded on the patient's chart. *Remember:*

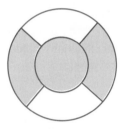

Figure 30-51 MOD amalgam—posterior tooth.

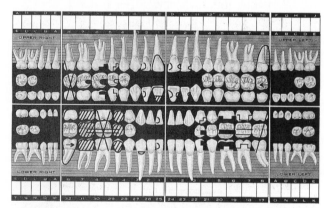

Tooth No.		Tooth No.	
1	Missing	18	Mesial and Distal Caries
2	Occlusal (mesial pit) amalgam	19	MOD Amal
3	MO Amal	21	DO Amal
4	Mesial Caries	25	Distal Com
7	Distal Com	27	Facial V Com
8	PFM	29	FGCr – Pontic
9	Mesial and Distal Caries	30	Missing
10	Distal Com	31	FGCr – Pontic
16	Impacted (mesially)	32	Impacted (mesially)
17	To Be Extracted		

Figure 30-52 Anatomic chart with charted conditions present. (Courtesy of Professional Publishers, Cupertino, CA.)

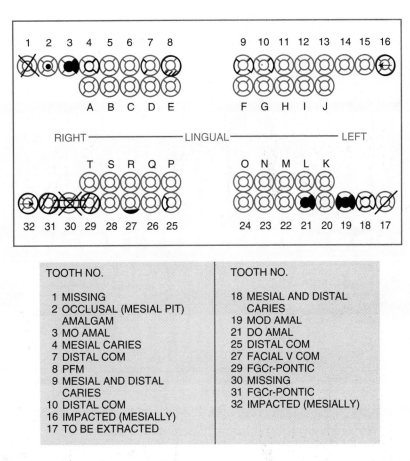

Figure 30-53 Geometric chart with charted conditions present.

TOOTH NO.	TOOTH NO.
1 MISSING	18 MESIAL AND DISTAL
2 OCCLUSAL (MESIAL PIT)	CARIES
AMALGAM	19 MOD AMAL
3 MO AMAL	21 DO AMAL
4 MESIAL CARIES	25 DISTAL COM
7 DISTAL COM	27 FACIAL V COM
8 PFM	29 FGCr-PONTIC
9 MESIAL AND DISTAL	30 MISSING
CARIES	31 FGCr-PONTIC
10 DISTAL COM	32 IMPACTED (MESIALLY)
16 IMPACTED (MESIALLY)	
17 TO BE EXTRACTED	

This information must be in ink or typewritten, accurate, complete, and concise.

A shorthand for recording dental treatment has been established that identifies the tooth by number or letter, the tooth surfaces by abbreviations, and other charting symbols.

Recording Services

1. All entries are to be printed in ink or typed.
2. Record only one transaction per line.
3. Date each entry. Use numbers for date (2-17-05).
4. Use abbreviations to save time and space.
5. List entries in a given sequence.

Sequence in Recording Entries

Entries to be recorded must follow a particular sequence; refer to Figure 30-4:

1. Date treatment was rendered.
2. Tooth/teeth, to be identified by a specific tooth number or letter and surface(s) involved.

3. Dental procedure that involves the entire mouth, such as a prophylaxis and examination.
4. Protective and restorative materials. List the type or protective material (Dycal, ZOE, Copalite) and restorative (composite, amalgam, gold) material.
5. Anesthetic: type used: Indicate generic (lidocaine) or brand name (Xylocaine) without vasoconstrictor (plain), number of cartridges (1.8 ml). With vasoconstrictor (epinephrine), record ratio (1:100,000) and number of cartridges.
6. Fee, cost of restoration or dental treatment.
7. Payment, amount received.
8. Balance, after payment

SUGGESTED ACTIVITIES

● Using infection control practices, look inside a classmate's mouth to find and chart all class I, II, III, IV, and V restorations.

● Practice making entries on the dental chart, with the instructor's guidance.

REVIEW

Using the accompanying anatomic chart and Universal System, identify the following:

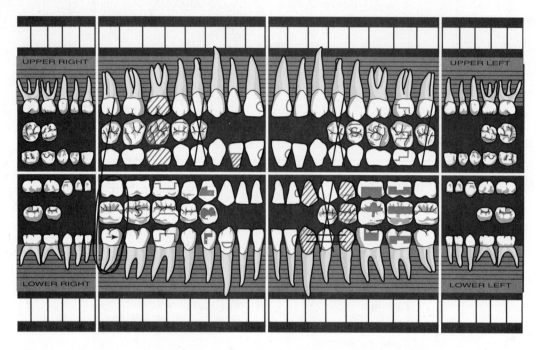

UPPER RIGHT   UPPER LEFT

LOWER RIGHT   LOWER LEFT

Anatomic diagram for charting symbols. (Courtesy of Professional Publishers, Cupertino, CA.)

1. How many teeth are extracted or missing?
   a. 3
   b. 5
   c. 2
   d. 6

2. Of those extracted teeth, how many are replaced by a bridge?
   a. 2
   b. 3
   c. 1
   d. none

3. Indicate the tooth number(s) where a full gold crown exists.
   a. 3, 20, 22
   b. 3, 7, 21
   c. 3, 20, 21
   d. 7, 20, 21, 22

4. Which teeth are restored with amalgam restorations?
   a. 9, 15, 30
   b. 8, 27, 23
   c. 18, 19, 28
   d. 23, 27, 30

5. Which tooth has a Class V composite restoration?
   a. 9
   b. 27
   c. 7
   d. none

6. Indicate which posterior teeth have sealants.
   a. 12, 13, 30
   b. 3, 4, 18
   c. 3, 4, 19
   d. 13, 14, 31

Dental Handpieces

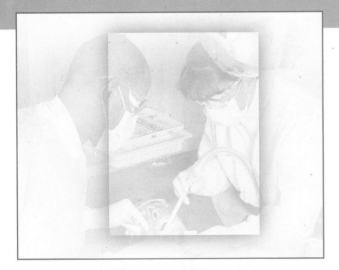

The dental handpiece is used:

- In operative and restorative dentistry to:
  1. Cut tooth structure for various types of preparations.
  2. Remove old metal restorations.
  3. Polish teeth and finish various types of restorative materials.
- In oral surgery and for implant procedures.

Dental handpieces are classified according to the design, speed, mode of operation, and method by which the rotary instrument is held in the handpiece.

OBJECTIVES

After studying this chapter, the student will be able to:

- Identify the three basic parts of a dental handpiece.
- Identify dental handpieces according to design, mode of operation, and method by which the rotary instrument is held in the handpiece.
- Discuss the purpose of the dental chuck.
- Discuss the use of a fiberoptic system.
- Explain the importance of sterilizing handpieces.

Parts of the Dental Handpiece

The basic parts of a dental handpiece are the following (Figure 31-1):

- *Head.* The end of the handpiece that holds the rotary instruments, such as burs, mandrels, polishing stones, and the like.
- *Shank.* The handle portion of the handpiece.
- *Connecting end.* Where the handpiece attaches to the power source of the motor or unit.

Introduction

Dental handpieces are specifically designed to be used with various types of rotary instruments, such as burs, stones, and finishing discs. Most dental handpieces are used in the oral cavity. However, some are specifically designed for use in the dental laboratory.

Basic Handpiece Design

There are three basic handpiece designs:

- The straight handpiece
- The contra-angle handpiece
- The right-angle handpiece.

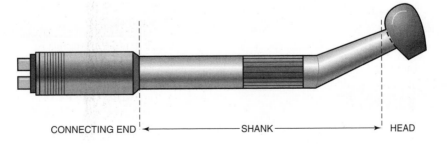

CONNECTING END ◄——————— SHANK ———————► HEAD

Figure 31-1 Parts of a dental handpiece.

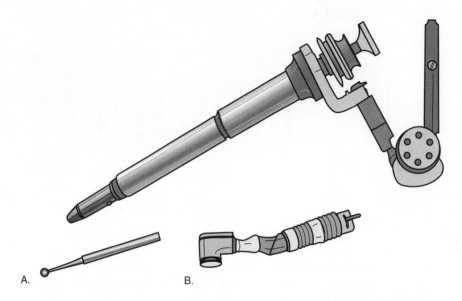

Figure 31-2 Belt-driven straight handpiece with (A) straight-shanked bur and (B) contra-angle handpiece.

The Straight Handpiece

The straight handpiece is straight shanked and therefore can be used to hold a *contra-angle* or *right-angle* handpiece (Figure 31-2). The straight handpiece may also be used with a straight-shanked rotary instrument on anterior teeth or where a direct approach to the teeth is possible.

A straight handpiece may be a low-speed, belt-driven type that is attached to an arm assembly made up of a series of pulleys and a belt that is mounted on an electric motor used in the laboratory. One end of the belt is mounted over the pulley end of the handpiece and carried over the arm assembly pulleys to the dental motor pulley.

The straight handpiece may also be operated by compressed air or by electric power (Figure 31-3). Handpieces that are operated by compressed air are attached to the dental unit by means of a flexible tubing with a "quick" connect-disconnect or threaded adaptor (Figure 31-4). The connecting end of the handpiece is attached to the tubing adaptor (Figure 31-5). The tubing adaptor may have two to four holes or input-output openings. The number of input-output holes is dependent on the handpiece. The connecting end of the handpiece is designed with the same number of tubes as there are input-output holes. The input-output holes provide the handpiece with air and water from the dental unit.

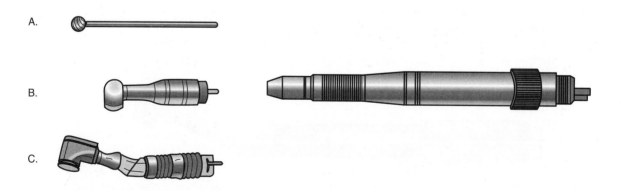

Figure 31-3 Air-driven straight handpiece with (A) straight-shanked bur, (B) right-angle, and (C) contra-angle handpieces.

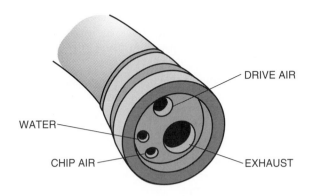

Figure 31-4 Adaptor end of tubing.

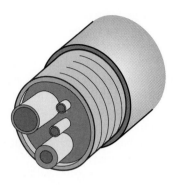

Figure 31-5 Connecting end of the handpiece.

The Contra-Angle Handpiece

The contra-angle handpiece is designed to provide the operator with greater visibility and accessibility to the oral cavity during operative dentistry. It may be a friction grip type (Figure 31-6) or latch-type (Figure 31-7).

The head of the contra-angle handpiece is offset from the shank portion of the handpiece (Figure 31-6). The contra-angle handpiece is available for use with the straight handpiece (Figures 31-2 and 31-3) or as a single-unit friction grip handpiece (Figure 31-1).

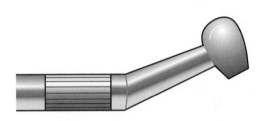

Figure 31-6 High-speed contra-angle handpiece.

The Right-Angle Handpiece

The term right angle refers to the way in which the head of the handpiece forms a 90° degree angle to the shank. The most popular right-angle handpiece is the prophy-angle (Figure 31-8). The right-angle handpiece with a rubber cup is attached to the straight handpiece and is used for polishing teeth. Disposable prophy angles are supplied with rubber cup or brush already attached.

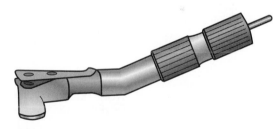

Figure 31-7 Latch-type (low-speed) contra-angle handpiece.

Dental Handpiece Speeds

Handpieces may be classified as low speed, slow speed, or high speed, also referred to as *air-turbine* handpieces. Speed may be defined as the number of *revolutions per minute* (rpm) or the number of times a rotating instrument, such as a bur, will make during 1 minute. The higher the rpm, the faster the speed of the handpiece.

Low-speed handpieces operate at a very low rpm, below 10,000, and are generally used with the dental laboratory engine.

The slow-speed handpieces may operate at speeds up to 150,000 rpm. The slow-speed handpiece generally produces less friction heat (the rubbing or touching of one object against another). Frictional heat is the result of the rotary instrument coming in contact with the tooth structure or restorative material during the dental procedure.

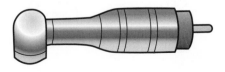

Figure 31-8 Prophy-angle (right-angle) handpiece.

Frictional heat is generated regardless of the operating speed of the handpiece or the tooth structure or dental material the rotary instrument comes in contact with.

The high-speed, or air-turbine, handpieces operate at speeds of 500,000 rpm or more. Because high-speed, or air-turbine, handpieces operate at such high speeds, they produce a great deal of frictional heat. However, they are more efficient in cutting hard tooth structures. To minimize frictional heat, a coolant, such as air, water, or an air-water spray, must be used. If frictional heat is not controlled, the pulp may be seriously traumatized, resulting in permanent injury or damage to the tooth.

Power Source for the Dental Handpiece

A source of energy (power) is needed to operate all dental handpieces. The flow of power may be activated by the use of a *foot control* or a **rheostat** (a device used to regulate an electric current without interrupting the circuit of flow). A rheostat is used with the belt-driven handpiece and is operated by electricity. A foot control is used with the air-turbine handpiece and is operated by compressed air.

Methods for Holding Rotary Instruments in Handpieces

The rotary instrument (*bur*) may be held in place by tightening a bur-rod knob at the end of the handpiece (straight handpiece) or by using a special bur tool provided by the manufacturer. Newer handpieces may have either a button or release lever that is used to secure and release the rotary instrument.

Inside the head of the handpiece is a small metal cylinder called a **chuck**. The chuck is designed to hold the shank portion of the rotary instrument in the handpiece.

Rotary instruments, such as burs, stone, and mandrels, are inserted into the chuck and are held in position by either a *latch-type* or *friction-grip* system. Refer to Chapter 32.

A latch-type handpiece uses a special notched-shank rotary instrument. The rotary instrument is inserted into the chuck and is held in the handpiece by a movable latch (Figure 31-7).

Friction-grip rotary instruments are used with the air-turbine handpiece. The rotary instrument (bur) is inserted into a special metal chuck in the head of the handpiece and may be secured by a wrench-tightening system (Figure 31-9). To secure the rotary instrument, either a control knob on the handpiece or a special tool is provided by the manufacturer for use with their handpiece.

The newer friction-grip/air-turbine handpiece may have an automatic button or release lever that allows the operator to secure and remove the rotary instrument instantly.

The head of a friction-grip or air-turbine handpiece is designed to hold a short, round-shanked, small-diameter, friction-grip rotary instrument.

Fiberoptic System for Handpieces

Fiberoptic refers to a light system that uses special glass fibers called optical (vision) bundles (bound together) to carry a source of light to the dental handpiece. Fiber optics may also be used with other diagnostic accessories or tools for use within the mouth. Fiberoptic systems can

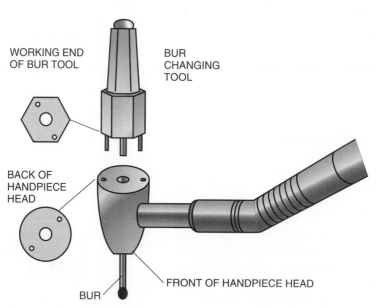

Figure 31-9 Bur-changing tool.

be used with both slow-speed and high-speed handpieces to provide an additional source of light to the oral cavity in addition to the dental light from the unit.

Two fiberoptic systems are available: One system carries the light via the optical bundles to the handpiece from a remote source, such as a control box. The second system, a bulb, is attached to the rear of the handpiece and the light is carried through the optical bundles within the tubing of the handpiece and from the dental unit.

An advantage of using the fiberoptic system is the improved visibility for the operator during tooth preparation.

Sterilization of Dental Handpieces

It is no longer acceptable to merely wipe the handpiece with a disinfectant. Dental handpieces are exposed to and contaminated with many microorganisms during use. Because of the variety of dental handpieces available today, a single specific procedure for the sterilization, care, and maintenance of a handpiece is impossible.

According to the Centers for Disease Control and Prevention (1987),

Handpieces should be sterilized after use with each patient, since blood, saliva or gingival fluid of patients may be aspirated into the handpieces or waterline. Handpieces should be flushed at the beginning of the day and after the use with each patient. Manufacturers' recommendations should be followed for use and maintenance of waterlines and check valves and for flushing of handpieces. The same precautions should be used for ultrasonic scalers and air/water syringes. (p. 47)

Maintenance of Handpieces

Maximum effectiveness with minimum damage to the handpieces can be accomplished by using the following precautions:

1. Carefully follow the manufacturer's printed instructions, and do not vary from these instructions. If there is a doubt about any step, call the manufacturer.

2. After dismissing the patient, put on utility gloves and PPE (personal protective equipment).

3. Depress the foot control (rheostat) and direct the handpiece toward a disposable paper towel inside the sink for at least 15 seconds to remove as many contaminants (saliva, blood, other debris) as possible from the internal tubings of the handpiece or take the handpiece to the laboratory or sterilizing room to use the handpiece maintenance air station and lubricating unit also available for the same purpose; these units should be shielded to prevent cross-contamination or aerosolization (Figure 31-10).

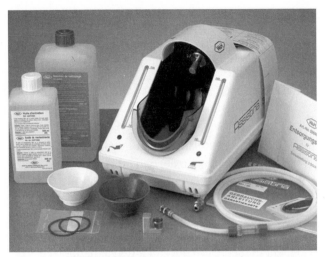

Figure 31-10 Handpiece maintenance air station and lubricating unit. (Courtesy of A-dec, Inc., Newberg, OR.)

4. In the treatment room, stretch the tubing of the handpiece to the sink and hand scrub the handpiece and tubing with soap and water. It is preferable to leave the bur in the handpiece to prevent any soap from entering the chuck.

5. Rinse and dry the handpiece. Remove the bur and set aside for future sterilization.

6. Remove the handpiece from the tubing and place in an appropriate pouch or bag for sterilization.

7. Spray the handpiece tubing with a recommended surface disinfectant and allow to dry for the prescribed time.

8. Wash, dry, and remove utility gloves.

9. Sterilize the handpiece in either a steam autoclave or a chemical vapor sterilizer. DO NOT USE DRY HEAT. *Note:* Various manufacturers furnish instructions on the care and maintenance of their handpieces, such as lubricating or oiling. These instructions must be followed in each individual case.

SUGGESTED ACTIVITIES

- Identify the various types of handpieces and give uses for each.
- Practice attaching rotary instruments and/or other handpieces to the straight handpiece.
- Practice attaching rubber cups and brushes to the right-angle handpiece.
- Practice attaching rotary instruments to the friction-grip handpiece.
- Read the manufacturer's recommendations to sterilize and lubricate each type of handpiece.

REVIEW

1. Name the three basic parts of a dental handpiece.
   a. Shank, head, neck
   b. Head, neck, connecting end
   c. Head, shank, connecting end
   d. Shank, neck, connecting end

2. List the three basic designs for dental handpieces.
   a. Straight, contra-angle, right angle
   b. Contra-angle, air turbine, friction grip
   c. Air turbine, straight, contra-angle
   d. Right angle, air turbine, contra-angle

3. Name the two systems used to hold a rotary instrument in the head/chuck of a dental handpiece.
   a. Burs, latch type
   b. Snap-on, latch type
   c. Friction grip, latch type
   d. Right angle, latch type

4. Give the advantage of using the contra-angle handpiece over the straight handpiece.
   a. Provides greater comfort to the operator
   b. Provides greater access and visibility within the oral cavity
   c. Provides better handpiece control
   d. Provides faster tooth reduction

5. When is frictional heat created?
   a. When the handpiece is activated
   b. When a rotary instrument comes in contact with water
   c. When the handpiece uses a fiberoptic system
   d. When a rotary instrument contacts the tooth structure

Rotary Instruments

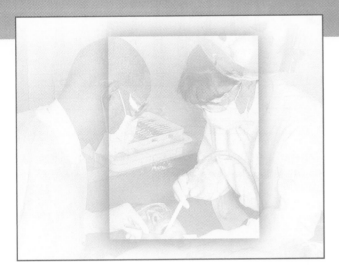

OBJECTIVES

After studying this chapter, the student will be able to:

- Identify the parts of a cutting bur.
- Discuss the advantages of using tungsten carbide burs.
- Discuss the uses of the basic cutting burs.
- Discuss the advantages of using diamond rotary instruments.
- Recognize the various stones and discs used in dentistry.
- Discuss the procedure for sterilizing the various rotary instruments.

Introduction

Rotary instruments such as burs, stones, and discs are used with the dental handpiece. The different types of rotary instruments are classified according to how they are used within the oral cavity.

Burs

Cutting Burs

The most common rotary instruments are the *cutting burs*. The cutting burs are small rotary instruments that are inserted and held in the head/chuck of the dental handpiece. Cutting burs are used to cut and shape tooth structure for various types of restorations and for removing old restorations from the teeth.

Parts of a Cutting Bur

- *Head.* The cutting portion of the bur.
- *Neck.* The portion of the bur that joins the head to the shank.
- *Shank.* That part of the bur that is inserted and held in the head of the handpiece (Figure 32-1).

    The head of the dental handpiece will determine the type of bur shank that can be used, *straight, latch-type,* or *friction-grip* (see Figures 31-1 and 31-2).

- The straight handpiece will require a straight long-shanked bur (Figure 32-2).

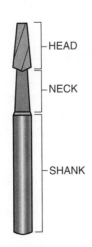

Figure 32-1 Parts of the cutting bur.

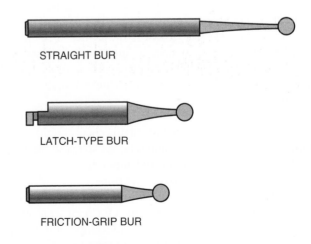

STRAIGHT BUR

LATCH-TYPE BUR

FRICTION-GRIP BUR

Figure 32-2 Types of bur shanks.

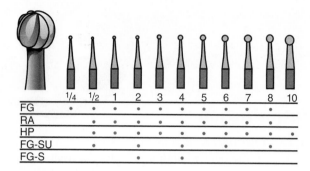

	1/4	1/2	1	2	3	4	5	6	7	8	10
FG	•	•	•	•	•	•	•	•	•	•	•
RA		•	•	•	•	•	•	•	•	•	
HP		•	•	•	•	•	•	•	•	•	•
FG-SU	•		•		•		•		•		
FG-S				•		•					

Figure 32-3 Round bur. (FG= Friction grip; RA = right angle; HP = hard-piece; FG-SLU = surgical; FG-S = short shank; • indicates available). (Courtesy of Miltex Instruments Co., Lake Success, NY.)

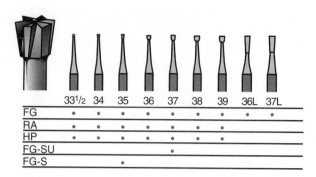

	33½	34	35	36	37	38	39	36L	37L
FG	•	•	•	•	•	•	•	•	•
RA	•	•	•	•	•	•	•		
HP	•	•	•	•	•	•	•		
FG-SU								•	
FG-S			•						

Figure 32-4 Inverted cone bur. (Courtesy of Miltex Instruments Co., Lake Success, NY.)

- The contra-angle handpiece will use a latch-type.
- The air turbine handpiece will use a friction-grip bur.
- Short-shanked burs ordinarily used in pediatric (children's) dentistry are available in both latch type and friction grip.

Types of Cutting Burs

Cutting burs are made of either steel or tungsten carbide. *Tungsten carbide burs* are extremely hard and can be used many times for cutting hard tooth structures. Tungsten carbide burs are manufactured for use with the high-speed, or air-turbine, handpieces. The use of *steel burs* in operative dentistry is limited. Steel burs are not as hard as tungsten carbide and may become dull after one use when cutting hard tooth tissue such as enamel. Under this situation, the bur must then be discarded.

Cutting burs are named according to the shape of the bur head and the angle of the cutting blades. The name of the bur denotes the shape of the bur head, and the bur number indicates the size of the bur head. The lower the bur number in a series, the smaller the head of the bur. The numbers that are assigned to the individual bur groups may vary according to the manufacturer. The letter *L* following a number indicates a longer length cutting head.

The basic bur shapes are round, inverted cone, straight and tapered fissure plain cut, straight and tapered crosscut, end cut, and wheel. The pear-shaped and rounded-head straight and taper fissure burs are new additions to the list of cutting burs.

The *round bur* (Nos. 1/4, 1/2, 1–10) is used for opening pit and fissure cavities and for removing other dental caries. The round bur is ideal for opening pulpal chamber(s) in endodontic treatment (Figure 32-3).

The *inverted cone* (Nos. 33 1/2-39, 36L, 37L) is designed for shaping **undercuts** (type of cavity design

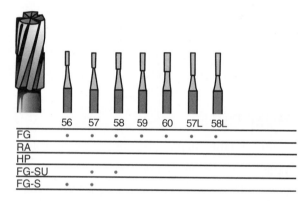

	56	57	58	59	60	57L	58L
FG	•	•	•	•	•	•	•
RA							
HP							
FG-SU	•	•					
FG-S	•	•					

Figure 32-5 Plain fissure straight bur. (Courtesy of Miltex Instruments Co., Lake Success, NY.)

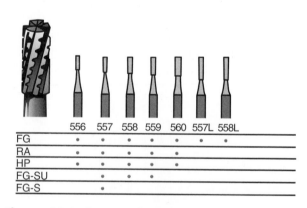

	556	557	558	559	560	557L	558L
FG		•	•	•	•	•	•
RA		•	•	•	•		
HP		•	•	•	•		
FG-SU		•	•	•			
FG-S	•						

Figure 32-6 Crosscut fissure straight bur. (Courtesy of Miltex Instruments Co., Lake Success, NY.)

whereby the pulpal wall itself is slanted to lock in the restoration in place) of the pulpal wall of the tooth, to help retain the restorative material (Figure 32-4).

The *plain fissure straight* (Nos. 56–60, 57L, 58L; Figure 32-5), and the *crosscut fissure straight* (Nos. 556–560, 557L, 558L; Figure 32-6) are used to form parallel walls and flat floors in preparations.

The *plain fissure taper* (Nos. 169–172, 169L, 170L, 171L; Figure 32-7) and *crosscut fissure taper* (Nos. 699–703, 699L, 700L, 701L; Figure 32-8) are used to create **divergent** (slightly narrowed at the pulpal floor) walls of the preparation and to avoid undercuts.

The *end cutting bur* (Nos. 957, 958) is used to prepare the shoulder for crown preparations (Figure 32-9).

The *wheel bur* (Nos. 12, 14) is used for cutting slots in preparations for crowns and inlays retention and making undercuts in Class V restorations (Figure 32-10).

The burs used for opening, shaping, and extending the internal line angles of occlusal restorations are the *pear-shaped burs* (Nos. 329–332, 331L; Figure 32-11); the *plain fissure straight-rounded* head (Nos. 56R–59R; Figure 32-12); the *plain fissure taper-rounded head*

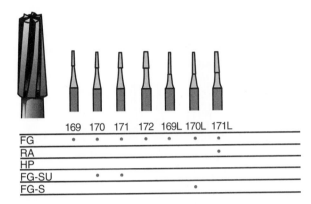

Figure 32-7 Plain fissure taper bur. (Courtesy of Miltex Instruments Co., Lake Success, NY.)

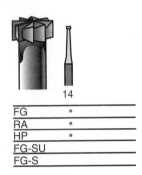

Figure 32-10 Wheel bur. (Courtesy of Miltex Instruments Co., Lake Success, NY.)

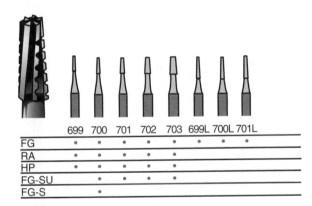

Figure 32-8 Crosscut fissure taper bur. (Courtesy of Miltex Instruments Co., Lake Success, NY.)

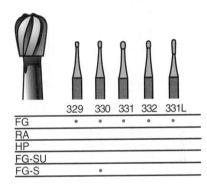

Figure 32-11 Pear bur. (Courtesy of Miltex Instruments Co., Lake Success, NY.)

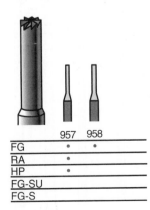

Figure 32-9 End-cutting bur. (Courtesy of Miltex Instruments Co., Lake Success, NY.)

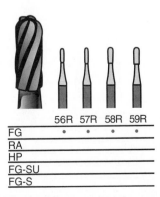

Figure 32-12 Plain fissure straight—round head bur. (Courtesy of Miltex Instruments Co., Lake Success, NY.)

(Nos. 1170, 1171; Figure 32-13); and the *crosscut fissure straight-rounded* head (Nos. 1557–1559, Figure 32-14).

Special burs include No. 245 (Figure 32-15), and Nos. 1931 and 1958 (Figure 32-16); they are used for preparation and bulk removal of gold, amalgam, and other metals.

Surgical Burs

Surgical burs are available in various sizes and shapes and may be made of either steel or tungsten carbide. They are designed for use with varied shank lengths (Figure 32-17). Surgical burs are used to cut through the bone of an impacted tooth or to split the crown or root(s) during an extraction. Surgical burs are also used for implant procedures (Figure 32-18).

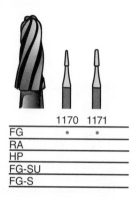

	1170	1171
FG	•	•
RA		
HP		
FG-SU		
FG-S		

Figure 32-13 Plain fissure taper—round head bur. (Courtesy of Miltex Instruments Co., Lake Success, NY.)

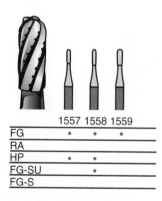

	1557	1558	1559
FG	•	•	•
RA			
HP	•	•	
FG-SU		•	
FG-S			

Figure 32-14 Crosscut fissure straight—round head bur. (Courtesy of Miltex Instruments Co., Lake Success, NY.)

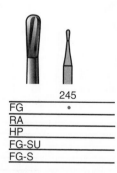

	245
FG	•
RA	
HP	
FG-SU	
FG-S	

Figure 32-15 Special bur for amalgam preparation. (Courtesy of Miltex Instruments Co., Lake Success, NY.)

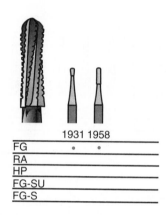

	1931	1958
FG	•	•
RA		
HP		
FG-SU		
FG-S		

Figure 32-16 Special bur used for removal of metals. (Courtesy of Miltex Instruments Co., Lake Success, NY.)

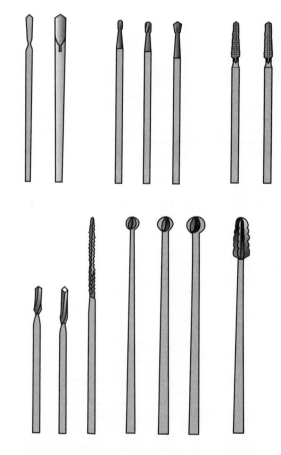

Figure 32-17 Surgical burs.

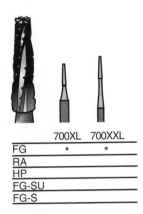

	700XL	700XXL
FG	•	•
RA		
HP		
FG-SU		
FG-S		

Figure 32-18 Specialty burs for implants. (Courtesy of Miltex Instruments Co., Lake Success, NY.)

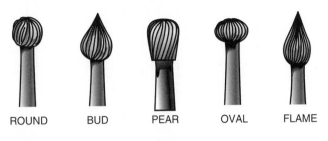

ROUND   BUD   PEAR   OVAL   FLAME

Figure 32-19 Finishing burs.

Acrylic Burs

Burs that are used for quick removal of marginal excess or occlusal adjustments of partial and full dentures are the *acrylic burs* (Figure 32-20).

Mandrels

A *mandrel* is a metal-shanked rotary instrument that is designed to hold (mount) stones, discs, and wheels. The mandrel has a bur-type shank. The head of the mandrel may have a notched center or a screw to hold the disc or wheel on the mandrel. Mandrels are used with straight, contra-angle or friction-grip handpieces (Figure 32-21).

Finishing Burs

Finishing burs are available in various sizes, shapes, and lengths (Figure 32-19). Finishing burs are made of either steel or carbide. The head of the bur may have as few as 6 or as many as 40 cutting blades. The number of cutting blades will determine the final smoothness or finish. The burs with the higher number of blades are used for ultrafine finishing of restorative materials, such as composites and glass ionomers.

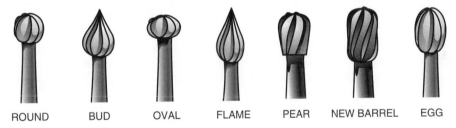

ROUND   BUD   OVAL   FLAME   PEAR   NEW BARREL   EGG

Figure 32-20 Acrylic burs.

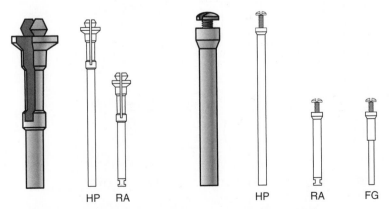

HP   RA   HP   RA   FG

Figure 32-21 Mandrels. (Courtesy of Miltex Instruments Co., Lake Success, NY.)

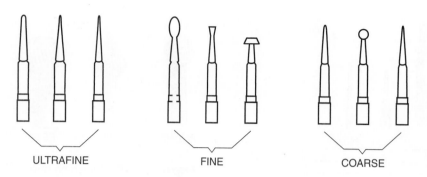

ULTRAFINE   FINE   COARSE

Figure 32-22 Diamond stones.

Stones

Stones used in dentistry are available in a full range of sizes, shapes, and grits. The **grit** (particle size of the abrasive that controls the cutting action) of a stone depends on the type of abrasive material that is used. Examples of abrasive materials include diamond, silicon carbide, and aluminum oxide.

The abrasive particles may be glued onto a backing material or mixed with a binding agent (matrix) that bonds the particles to one another. Some stones are molded onto a mandrel before the binder is allowed to harden; these stones are referred to as *mounted stones*.

Diamond Instruments/Stones

The cutting portion of a diamond stone is composed of minute crystals of natural or man-made diamonds. The diamond crystals are either electroplated or bonded directly to a one-piece hardened stainless steel shank. Diamond stones are used because of their excellent abrasive or cutting action and are available in various grits from ultrafine to coarse. The grit determines the size and number of diamond crystals; the smaller the crystal, the finer the grit. Diamond stones vary in sizes, shapes, length, and function (Figure 32-22). To help

identify the various grits of a diamond stone, the manufacturer may notch or color code the shank of the diamond stones.

Although carbide burs have basically six to eight cutting surfaces, diamond stones have thousands of cutting edges.

Larger-size heads of diamond stones are used for gross reduction of tooth structure; other diamonds are used for cutting and shaping the tooth preparation. Diamond stones with an ultrafine grit may be used to finish and polish the surfaces of composite and glass ionomer restorative materials.

Abrasive Stones

Abrasive stones may be used within the oral cavity or in the dental laboratory. Although some abrasive stones are mounted directly on a mandrel, other stones are unmounted and require a mandrel.

Stones are available in a variety of colors and shapes. The color of the stone denotes the type of abrasive material and the grit.

One of the abrasives used for stones is *silicon carbide* and is generally recommended for working on ceramics, tooth structure, and plastics (Figure 32-23).

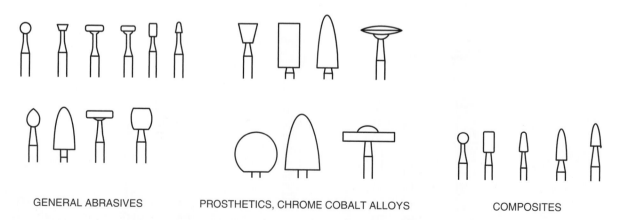

GENERAL ABRASIVES   PROSTHETICS, CHROME COBALT ALLOYS   COMPOSITES

Figure 32-23 Mounted abrasive stones.

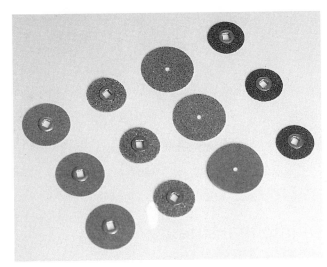

Figure 32-24 Sandpaper discs vary in sizes, types, and grits.

Additional stones made of either *garnet* or *aluminum oxide* may also be used for polishing metals. These stones are used in the laboratory.

Some abrasive stones are said to be **heatless** (creating less heat) and are composed of silicon carbide and rubber. During the finishing process the matrix material is weakened, causing the abrasive to be worn away as the stone comes in contact with the tooth structure or the restoration.

Discs

Discs form a group of abrasive rotary instruments and are used for various operative and laboratory procedures. Discs may be rigid or flexible, paper, or with water-resistant plastic backing. The discs are available in a large variety of grits and sizes (Figure 32-24). The abrasive coating can be one of several materials, such as diamond, garnet, quartz, sand, and aluminum oxide. The shape of a disc may be flat, concave, or convex and must be mounted on a suitable mandrel.

Discs are classified according to their grit—coarse to extra fine. When ordering discs, the size, shape, abrasive material, grit, and type of mandrel to be used must be specified.

Sandpaper Discs

The abrasive materials that are used for *sandpaper discs* may include sand, garnet, emery, and cuttlefish bone. The grit of the material will vary according to the abrasive material. Sandpaper discs must be mounted on a mandrel and may be snap-on discs with either a metal or plastic centered notch or a pinhole to accommodate the screw-head mandrel (Figure 32-24). Sandpaper discs are not reusable and should be removed from the mandrel before the mandrel is sterilized.

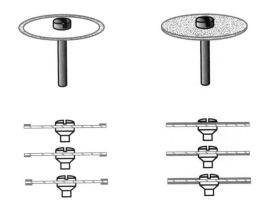

Figure 32-25 Diamond discs.

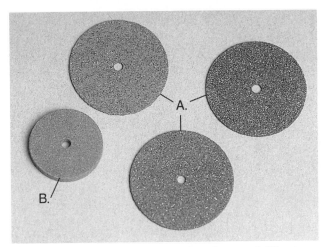

Figure 32-26 (A) silicone carbide discs and (B) rubber disc.

Diamond Discs

Diamond crystals or particles are bonded to a metal disc, some to the outer edge of the disc, and others to the entire surface of the disc on one or both sides (Figure 32-25). *Diamond disc* shapes vary from flat to concave to convex and are used for contouring and shaping tooth preparations.

Silicon Carbide (Carborundum) Discs

Silicon carbide discs are thin and very brittle and are used primarily in the laboratory; however, they can be used in the oral cavity in selective procedures. The disc may be used several times, but once damaged, it should be discarded (Figure 32-26A).

Rubber Discs

Rubber discs are molded in the shape of wheels. These abrasive rotary instruments may be soft or hard with the abrasive particles embedded in the rubber. Two types of abrasives found in the rubber are silicon carbide and aluminum oxide. Rubber wheels are available in various grits—fine, medium, and coarse—and may be mounted or unmounted (Figure 32-26B). They are used for finishing and polishing metal restorations.

Sterilization of Rotary Instruments

Because rotary instruments are used within the oral cavity, they must be cleaned and sterilized or disposed of after each patient use.

Carbide and Steel Burs

The following methods are recommended for the care of carbide and steel burs. *Caution:* Heavy utility gloves should always be worn when handling contaminated instruments.

1. Wearing utility gloves, place burs in a container with a solution of water and a neutral pH detergent or a recommended cleaner to loosen dried debris. *Note:* An ultrasonic unit may be used to clean the burs. To prevent damage to the cutting blades of the bur, place burs in a heat-resistant bur block. This will keep the burs from touching one another during the cleaning (vibrating) process, because corrosion can occur when two different metals in a solution come in contact with each other during the cleaning cycle.

2. Remove burs from solution with appropriate instrument.

3. With a nylon or stainless wire bur brush, remove any remaining debris from the burs. Rinse burs under running water.

4. Thoroughly dry burs by placing them on an absorbent towel.

5. Place burs in a bur block, and prepare for sterilization. *Always* follow the manufacturer's instructions regarding sterilization procedures.

Recommended methods for sterilizing carbide and steel burs include the following:

1. Dry heat (170°C, 340°F) for 1 hour.

2. Chemiclave (unsaturated) with chemical vapor (132°C, 270°F) 20 minutes at 20 psi (pounds per square inch).

3. Steam autoclave (121°C, 250°F) for 20 minutes at 15 psi. DO NOT USE COLD sterilizing solutions for the sterilization of carbide burs. The agents used in these solutions often contain strong oxidizing chemicals that may dull and weaken the carbide burs.

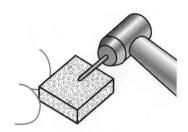

Figure 32-27 Clean-a-diamond square.

Diamond Instruments

The cleaning and sterilization of diamond instruments, stones, and discs are accomplished in the same manner as for the burs. Diamond stones and discs become clogged with hard and soft debris during use. This debris must be removed in order to clean and sterilize the diamond stones.

One may use disposable or nondisposable chips of aluminum oxide for cleaning clogged diamond stones and discs (Figure 32-27). The use of disposable chips is recommended to prevent cross-contamination. Disposable chips should be discarded after use. Aluminum oxide chips can extend the life of diamond stones.

Stones

The various stones used within the oral cavity must be cleaned and sterilized according to the manufacturer's instructions.

Discs

The type of abrasive material used for the discs will determine whether they are to be discarded or sterilized. Sandpaper discs are always discarded. Rubber discs are cleaned and sterilized according to the manufacturer's instructions.

SUGGESTED ACTIVITIES

- Identify the various cutting burs and give uses of each.
- Form a study group to review each type of bur.
- Practice drawing each bur and identify the corresponding numbers.
- Identify other rotary disc-type instruments and give uses of each.

REVIEW

1. Name the parts of a cutting bur: (1) head, (2) shank, (3) shaft, and/or (4) neck.
   a. 1, 2, 3
   b. 2, 3, 4
   c. 1, 2, 4
   d. 1, 3, 4

2. What are the advantages of using tungsten carbide burs?
   a. Easier to sterilize without losing sharpness
   b. Cut tooth structure faster
   c. Do not rust or corrode
   d. Extremely hard and can be used many times for cutting tooth structures

3. Match the type of bur with its corresponding numbers.
   ___ a. Round bur
   ___ b. Inverted cone
   ___ c. Plain fissure straight
   ___ d. Crosscut fissure straight
   ___ e. Plain fissure taper
   ___ f. Crosscut fissure taper
   ___ g. End cutting
   ___ h. Wheel

   1. 556-560, 557L, 558L
   2. 699-703, 699L, 700L, 701L
   3. 1/4, 1/2, 1-10
   4. 14
   5. 33 1/2 -39, 36L, 37L
   6. 56-60, 57L, 58L
   7. 169-172, 170L, 171L
   8. 957, 958

4. Name the bur most commonly used for excavating caries from teeth.
   a. Inverted cone
   b. Round
   c. End cutting
   d. Plain fissure taper

5. What is the function of a mandrel?
   a. To create undercuts
   b. To finish a restoration
   c. To hold unmounted stones, discs, and wheels
   d. To polish acrylic dentures and partial dentures

6. Give the advantage of using diamond stones.
   a. Have excellent abrasive or cutting action
   b. Are supplied in many shapes
   c. Are easily cleaned
   d. Are excellent finishing burs

Hand Instruments for Operative Dentistry

OBJECTIVES

After studying this chapter, the student will be able to:

- Select the basic examining instruments.
- Discuss the uses of the basic examining instruments.
- Name the parts of a cutting instrument.
- Identify the various cutting instruments.
- Discuss the uses of the various cutting instruments.
- Discuss the formula numbers of the cutting instruments.
- Identify the other hand instruments.

Introduction

Some hand instruments may be used for selected operative procedures within the oral cavity. Others may be used in a variety of procedures.

Hand instruments are classified into several groups. They include the basic examining instruments: mouth mirror, explorer, periodontal probe, and cotton pliers (forceps). In addition, there are cutting instruments, amalgam instruments, plastic instruments, and scalers.

Basic Examining Instruments

Explorers

The *explorer* is a slender, pointed instrument that is used primarily to examine the various tooth surfaces. The working portion, or tip (point), of the explorer is very sharp and allows the operator to check the natural surface(s) of a tooth/teeth, the grooves, and fossae for any defects and other unusual conditions.

There are several styles of explorers with a variety of tips and angles; some, generally made of steel, are **single ended** (having one working end) or **double ended** (having two working ends using the same handle) (Figure 33-1). Selection is determined by a specific need.

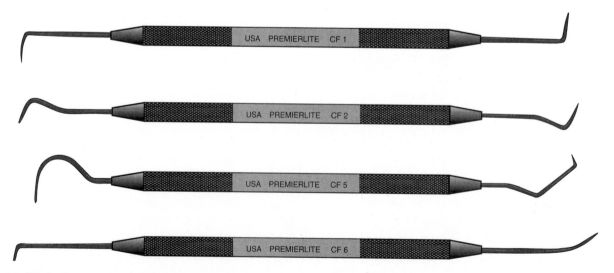

Figure 33-1 Explorers. (Courtesy of Premier Dental Products/ESPE-Premier Sales Co., King of Prussia, PA 19406)

REGULAR MIRROR   FRONT SURFACE MIRROR

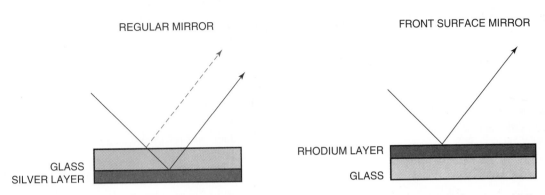

GLASS
SILVER LAYER

RHODIUM LAYER
GLASS

Figure 33-2 Regular and front-surface mirrors. (Courtesy of Miltex Instrument Co., Lake Success, NY.)

Uses of Explorers

- To examine the tooth for any developmental defects or faulty groove or fossa
- To check for faulty margins of a restoration
- To remove excess cement from around the margins of a restoration during cementation
- To remove excess restorative material from around the matrix band before the band is removed
- To place A gingival retraction cord prior to taking an impression

Mouth Mirror

The primary function of the *mouth mirror* is to allow the operator to see the various areas of the mouth that are impossible to see with direct vision. **Indirect vision** is a term employed when the operator uses the mouth mirror to view an area within the mouth. This allows the operator to view the area as it is reflected in the mirror.

Dental mirrors are available with plane (regular) or magnifying surfaces. Regular mirrors are made with a silver coating on the back of the glass. This results in light being reflected from the surface of the glass as well as from the silver layer. This creates a "ghost image" and may cause considerable eye strain. The reflecting layer of a front-surface mirror is made with **rhodium** (a reflective metal) on the surface of the glass. The rhodium surface reflects a clear vision, free from all distortion, thereby eliminating the so-called ghost image (Figure 33–2).

The stem portion of a mouth mirror may have either a simple- or a cone-socket stem (Figure 33-3). This type of stem allows the mirror to be replaced without having to purchase a new mirror handle when its surface becomes scratched or damaged.

Uses of Mouth Mirrors

- To view various areas within the oral cavity
- To retract the cheek and/or tongue for better access and visibility

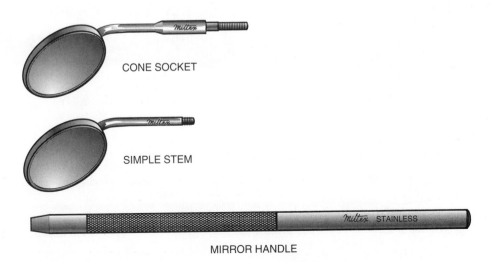

CONE SOCKET

SIMPLE STEM

MIRROR HANDLE

Figure 33-3 Mirror stem styles. (Courtesy of Miltex Instrument Co., Lake Success, NY.)

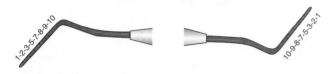

Figure 33-4 Periodontal probe (Courtesy of Miltex Instrument Co., Lake Success, NY.)

- To reflect light into an area that is being examined or treated

Periodontal Probe

The periodontal probe has a round, tapered blade with a blunt tip. The blade is marked in millimeters (mm) and is used to measure the depth of the gingival sulcus. (Figure 33-4).

Cotton Pliers (Forceps)

Cotton pliers are a standard instrument used in most operative and restorative procedures. They allow the operator more flexibility in the manipulation of various materials that are used within the oral cavity.

Cotton pliers are a two-bladed or beaked instrument and are available with either a locking or nonlocking handle. The beak may be straight or at an angle (Figure 33-5).

Uses of Cotton Pliers

- To grasp or transfer materials from within or out of the mouth
- To retrieve other instruments or materials from sterile storage areas and to avoid contamination with the fingers
- To place and remove wedges used with matrix bands
- To place and remove cotton rolls from the oral cavity
- To aid in the placement of gingival retraction cord

Cutting Instruments

Cutting instruments are used primarily to refine the walls and margins of cavity preparation. They are available in single-ended or double-ended styles. Double-ended instruments are more practical, because they reduce the number of instruments required for a given procedure.

Some cutting instruments are referred to as right and left and come in pairs (spoon excavators, enamel hatchets). Other cutting instruments may be classified according to their use on the mesial or distal surfaces of a tooth (binangle chisels, special hoes, and gingival margin trimmers).

Parts of the Cutting Instrument (Figure 33-6)

- Blade—cutting portion
- Shank—turned portion connecting shaft with blade; may be either straight or angled
- Shaft—handle of the instrument

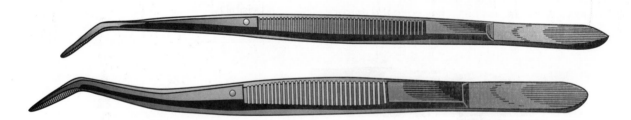

Figure 33-5   Cotton pliers (forceps) (Courtesy of Miltex Instrument Co., Lake Success, NY.)

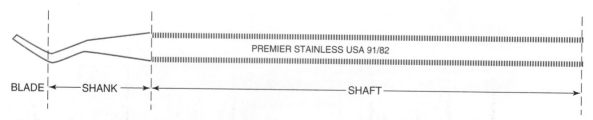

PREMIER STAINLESS USA 91/82

BLADE — SHANK — SHAFT

Figure 33-6 Parts of a cutting instrument (Courtesy of Miltex Instrument Co., Lake Success, NY.)

Description of Cutting Instruments

Straight Chisel. An instrument with a straight blade, **beveled** on one side (beveled or having a slanted portion on the cutting edge of the blade; Figure 33-7).

● The longest side of the beveled blade is always toward the bulk of the tooth.

● It is used on maxillary or mandibular anterior teeth in Class III or IV preparations.

● It can be used for planing down the enamel surface in cavity preparations.

Wedelstaedt Chisel. The *Wedelstaedt* chisel is an instrument with a curved blade beveled on one side. Similar to the straight chisel. It is used in the same manner as the straight chisel (Figure 33-8).

Bin-Angle Chisel. The bin-angle chisel has a chisel blade placed at an angle to the shaft in the form of a hoe, i.e., two angles (Figure 33-9).

● The longest side of the beveled blade is always toward the bulk of the tooth.

● It is used on the maxillary posterior teeth in Class II preparations.

● It is used for smoothing or forming line angles of the buccal and lingual axial wall, either mesial or distal.

Enamel Hatchet. An enamel hatchet has a chisel blade placed at an angle to the shaft in the form of a hatchet (Figure 33-10).

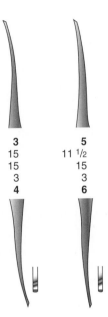

Figure 33-8 Wedelstaedt chisels (Courtesy of Miltex Instrument Co., Lake Success, NY.)

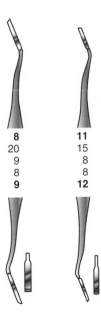

Figure 33-9 Bin-angle chisels (Courtesy of Miltex Instrument Co., Lake Success, NY.)

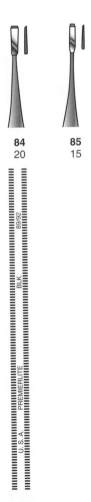

Figure 33-7 Straight chisels (Courtesy of Miltex Instrument Co., Lake Success, NY.)

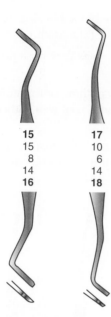

Figure 33-10 Enamel hatchets (Courtesy of Miltex Instrument Co., Lake Success, NY.)

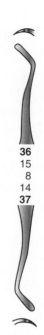

Figure 33-11 Spoon excavators (Courtesy of Miltex Instrument Co., Lake Success, NY.)

- The longest side of the beveled blade is always toward the bulk of the tooth.
- It is used on the mandibular posterior teeth in Class II preparations.
- It is used for smoothing or forming line angles of the buccal or lingual axial wall of the mesial or distal surfaces of the tooth.
- It is available in pairs, right and left. (When right and left are indicated, this refers to the patient's right and left.)

Spoon Excavator. This instrument is similar to a gingival margin trimmer in its angles and curve of blade but with the convex side of the blade beveled to form a cutting edge entirely around the periphery of the blade. This is a true lateral cutting instrument (Figure 33-11).

- Used on all maxillary and mandibular teeth
- Used to excavate decay; should be used instead of burs to remove decayed dentin, especially when close to the pulp
- May also be used as an amalgam carver
- Double ended, in pairs, right and left

Gingival Margin Trimmer. This instrument has a chisel blade placed at an angle to the shaft in the form of a hatchet, with the blade curved to buccal or lingual. The cutting edge is at a definite angle to the shaft of the instrument (Figure 33-12).

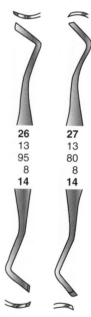

Figure 33-12 Gingival margin trimmers (Courtesy of Miltex Instrument Co., Lake Success, NY.)

- The beveled blade with the longest point toward, or away from, the shaft of the instrument will determine mesial or distal cutting.
- The short pointed end of the bevel is placed toward the floor of the gingival margin wall.
- It is used on the maxillary and mandibular posterior teeth in Class II preparations.
- It is a mesial and distal cutting, double-ended instrument.

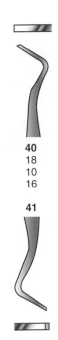

40
18
10
16
41

Figure 33-13 Special hoe (Courtesy of Miltex Instrument Co., Lake Success, NY.)

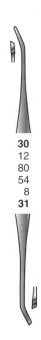

30
12
80
54
8
31

Figure 33-14 Angle formers (Courtesy of Miltex Instrument Co., Lake Success, NY.)

● It is used for placing the bevel on the gingival margin wall. One end of the instrument (short pointed end of the bevel) is placed on the buccal wall, and, in a lateral motion, the gingival margin floor is planed starting from the buccal to the lingual wall; then the instrument is reversed, and the same operation is performed, only from the lingual to the buccal wall.

● It is sometimes used in reverse position to form line angles and point angles in Class II preparations.

Special Hoe. This instrument has a bin-angle blade placed at an angle to the shaft (Figure 33-13).

● Used on the maxillary posterior teeth

● Used to plane the mesial and distal axial walls

Angle Former. The *angle former* is similar to a hoe with the cutting edge placed at a definite angle to the long axis of the instrument (Figure 33-14).

● The definite angle of the beveled blade (the longest point) is placed toward the mesial or distal surface of the tooth.

● It is used on the maxillary and mandibular teeth in Class III and V preparations.

● It is used to make definite point angles and to sharpen line angles.

● It may be used to establish **cavosurface** (junction of the cavity and the exterior tooth surface) bevels.

Formula Numbers of Instruments

Formula numbers on the handle are descriptive of the size of the blade and the angle at which it is set to the shaft. Some consist of three numbers and others four.

1. Three numbers in the formula (Figure 33-15):

   ● The *first* number represents the width of the blade in tenths of a millimeter (A).

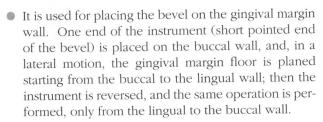

PREMIER STAINLESS USA 13/14   20 9 14

Figure 33-15 Three-unit instrument formula (A) Width of blade in tenths of mm. (B) Length of blade in mm. (C) Angle blade forms with shaft (Courtesy of Miltex Instrument Co., Lake Success, NY.)

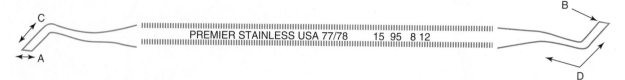

Figure 33-16 Four-unit instrument formula (A) Width of blade in tenths of mm. (B) Angle of cutting edge of blade with shaft (C) Length of blade in mm. (D) Angle blade forms with shaft (Courtesy of Miltex Instrument Co., Lake Success, NY.)

- The *second* number designates the length of the blade in millimeters (B).

- The *third* number shows in degrees the angle that the blade forms with the shaft (C).

2. Four numbers in the formula (Figure 33-16):

- The *first* number represents the width of the blade in tenths of a millimeter (A).

- The *second* number represents in degrees the angle that the cutting edge of the blade makes with the shaft (B).

- The *third* number designates the length of the blade in millimeters (C).

- The *fourth* number shows in degrees the angle that the blade forms with the shaft (D).

Amalgam Instruments

Amalgam instruments include the amalgam carrier, well, condensers, carvers, and burnishers.

Amalgam Carrier

The *amalgam carrier* is used to carry and dispense a pliable mix of silver amalgam into the tooth preparation.

The carrier may be single ended or double ended with both a large and small end and is made of metal or plastic. The carrier may have either a lever-action or plunger-type release (Figure 33-17).

Amalgam Well

The *amalgam well* is made of stainless steel and is used to hold the triturated amalgam while loading the amalgam carrier (Figure 33-18).

Amalgam Condensers

Amalgam condensers (pluggers) are used to condense (pack) restorative material into the cavity preparation. The working end, or **nib**, of the condensers is available

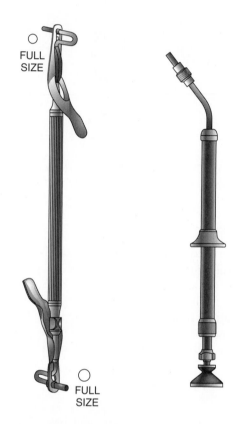

Figure 33-17 Amalgam carriers. (Courtesy of Miltex Instrument Co., Lake Success, NY.)

Figure 33-18 Amalgam well. (Courtesy of Miltex Instrument Co., Lake Success, NY.)

in a variety of sizes and shapes—round, oval, rectangular, and diamond—and may be single or double ended.

The face of the nib may be smooth or serrated. The angle of the shaft of a condenser may vary. The variation in the angle of the shaft and the shape of the nib allows the operator access to specific areas within the tooth preparation (Figure 33-19).

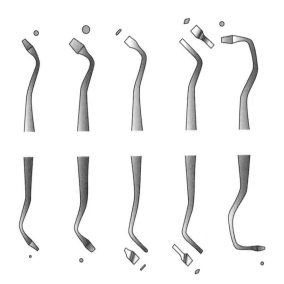

Figure 33-19 Amalgam condensers .

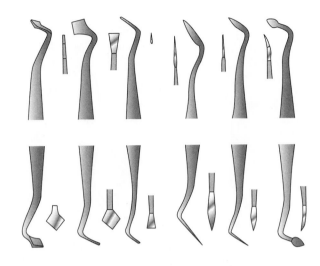

Figure 33-20 Carvers.

Carvers

Carvers are used to re-create the anatomy of the tooth before the amalgam restorative material has hardened. The working end of a carver may vary in design and size, from a pointed working end to an oval (disc) or rounded one. The angle of the blade may be shaped like a hoe or a hatchet blade (Figure 33-20).

Cleoid-Discoid.

The *cleoid-discoid* is an instrument with pointed or disk-shaped blades placed at an angle to the shaft with a cutting edge around the entire periphery. At one end is the cleoid (claw-shaped) blade and at the opposite end is the discoid (disc-shaped) blade (Figure 33-21).

● Used primarily as a carver

● Usually a double-ended instrument (the combination of both the cleoid and discoid)

Gold Knives.

Gold knives are specific types of carvers that are used to remove excess restorative material. The cutting edge is a thin, sharp, single- or double-ended, knife-type blade. It can be used on the interproximal surfaces of a tooth to eliminate improperly contoured or overhanging amalgam restorations which extend from the occlusal to the gingival margins (Figure 33-22).

Burnishers

Burnishers are used to smooth the surface and margins of an amalgam restoration while the material is still workable. A burnisher may have a working end that is

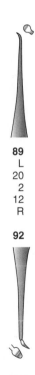

Figure 33-21 Cleoid-discoid carver. (Courtesy of Miltex Instrument Co., Lake Success, NY.)

smooth in the shape of a ball, egg or a combination of a ball and blade (Figure 33-23).

Plastic Instruments

Plastic instruments are a group of instruments used to place and condense restorative materials. They may be

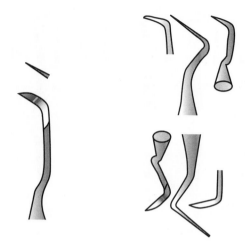

Figure 33-22 Gold knives.

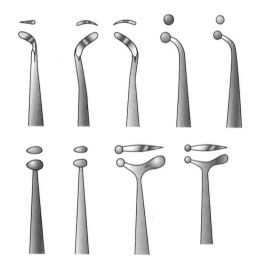

Figure 33-23 Burnishers.

made of either metal or plastic and are single or double ended. The working end can vary (Figure 33-24).

Plastic instruments should be used when placing tooth colored restorations; otherwise, the material may become discolored if a metal instrument is used. Plastic instruments are available in several designs.

Recently developed plastic carriers may be used in conjunction with the plastic instruments to place composite and glass ionomer restorative material (Figure 33-25).

Scalers

Scalers are designed to remove calculus deposits from tooth surfaces above and below the gingiva. The blades have cutting edges on the inner surface (face) of the blade. Scalers are paired instruments with various angled shanks and blades to allow access to all tooth

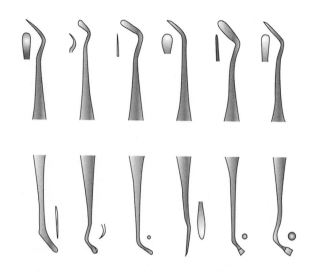

Figure 33-24 Plastic instruments. (Courtesy of Miltex Instrument Co., Lake Success, NY.)

surfaces of teeth. They may be purchased in a variety of blade sizes and shanks (Figure 33-26).

Crown and Bridge Scissors

Crown and bridge scissors have small cutting blades designed to shape and trim temporary crowns (metal or plastic). The blades may be either curved or straight (Figure 33-27). The handles may vary in length and size.

Cement Spatulas

Cement spatulas are designed with a variety of blade lengths and widths. Cement spatulas are usually single-ended, metal instruments with a flat blade and a rounded end. They are used primarily for mixing dental cements (Figure 33-28).

Sterilization of Hand Instruments

Refer to Chapter 8.

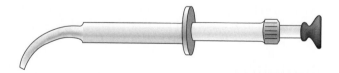

Figure 33-25 Plastic syringe used for placing tooth restorative materials.

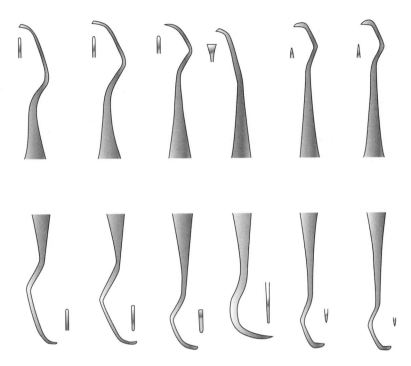

Figure 33-26 Assorted scalers. (Courtesy of Miltex Instrument Co., Lake Success, NY.)

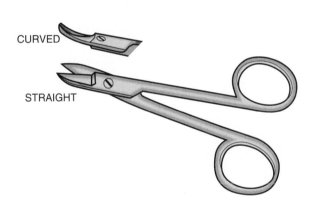

CURVED

STRAIGHT

Figure 33-27 Crown and bridge scissors. (Courtesy of Miltex Instrument Co., Lake Success, NY.)

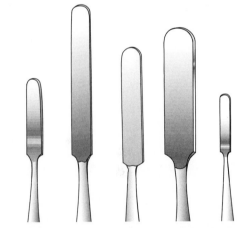

Figure 33-28 Cement spatulas. (Courtesy of Miltex Instrument Co., Lake Success, NY.)

SUGGESTED ACTIVITIES

● Identify the cutting instruments and give the uses of each.

● Identify amalgam condensers, carvers, and burnishers.

● Recognize other hand instruments used in dentistry and explain the use of each.

REVIEW

1. Name the four basic examining instruments used in dentistry.
   a. Mouth mirror, explorer, cotton pliers, spoon excavator
   b. Mouth mirror, explorer, cotton pliers, straight chisel
   c. Mouth mirror, cotton pliers, spoon excavator, periodontal probe
   d. Mouth mirror, explorer, cotton pliers, periodontal probe

2. Refining the walls and margins of cavity preparations is the primary function of which of the following instruments:
   a. Plastic instruments
   b. Cutting instruments
   c. Carving instruments
   d. Examining instruments

3. Bin-angle chisels, special hoe, gingival margin trimmers, and spoon excavators are used for which of the following cavity classification:
   a. Maxillary Class II
   b. Maxillary Class III
   c. Mandibular Class II
   d. Mandibular Class IV

4. Enamel hatchets, gingival margin trimmers, and spoon excavators are used for which of the following cavity classification:
   a. Maxillary Class IV
   b. Maxillary Class I
   c. Mandibular Class II
   d. Mandibular Class I

5. The function of a gold knife is to:
   a. Remove excess amalgam from the occlusal surface
   b. Re-create the anatomy of the tooth before the amalgam restorative material has hardened
   c. Remove excess amalgam from the interproximal surfaces to prevent overhanging margins
   d. Remove calculus deposits from tooth surfaces above and below the gingival surface

Dental Equipment in the Treatment Room

CHAPTER

34

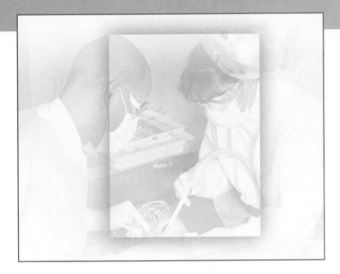

- Discuss the function of the oral vacuum system.
- State the requirements for a properly designed dental assistant's stool.
- State the requirements for a properly designed dentist's operating stool.
- Explain the function of the intraoral camera.
- Identify parts of the intraoral camera.
- Discuss the procedure for intraoral camera use.

Introduction

The *dental treatment room* (operatory) is the primary work area of the dentist and of the chairside dental assistant. The size of the treatment room and the floor plan and equipment should be designed and organized to offer comfort and convenience for the operator and dental assistant (Figure 34-1).

The primary equipment in a dental treatment room includes the dental chair, dental unit, dental operating

OBJECTIVES

After studying this chapter, the student will be able to:

- Identify the parts of the dental chair.
- Identify the parts of the dental unit.
- Explain the function of the dental lamp.

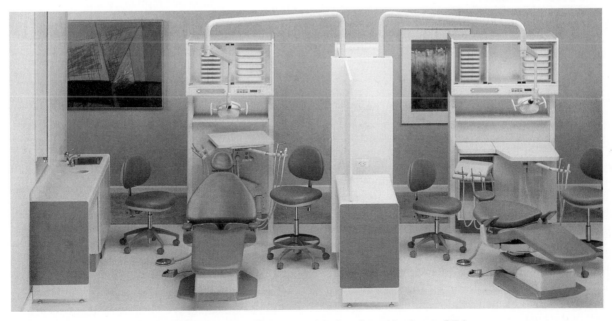

Figure 34-1 Equipment in the treatment room. (Courtesy of A-dec, Inc., Newberg, OR.)

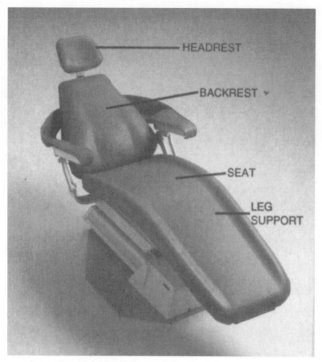

Figure 34-2 The dental chair. (Courtesy of A-dec, Inc., Newberg, OR.)

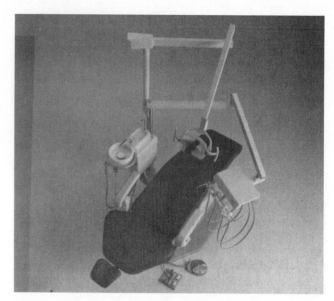

Figure 34-3 Cuspidor on floor-mounted unit. (Courtesy of A-dec, Inc., Newberg, OR.)

light, operating stools, and mobile cart(s) or cabinet. In addition, the x-ray machine, intraoral camera, and air-brasive system may also be considered part of the equipment.

The Dental Chair

Most dental chairs used today are a contour-type and are designed for use in four-handed sit-down dentistry. The dental chair supports the patient's head and body.

Parts of the Dental Chair

● *Body of chair.* This includes the backrest, seat, and leg supports (Figure 34-2).

● *Armrest.* Usually movable by lifting or sliding backward to allow easy access when seating the patient, the armrest may have a sling to support and secure the patient's elbows.

● *Headrest.* Supports the patient's head (Figure 34-2).

● *Control panel.* Has controls that allow the body of the chair to be moved from the upright to the supine position and to raise and lower the height of the chair. Controls may be located either on the side or on the back of the backrest.

● *Swiveled lever.* Allows the base of the chair to be rotated from side to side.

The Dental Unit

The dental unit is controlled by master on/off switches. The function of the dental unit is to supply water, air, electricity, and a system for oral evacuation.

Dental units are available in several designs. Some are mounted to the floor (Figure 34-3); others are mobile (Figure 34-4). The basic features of a dental unit include the dental handpieces, air-water syringe, and oral evacuation system, and the unit may or may not have a **cuspidor** (a bowl with circulating water, used by the patient for spitting or emptying the mouth).

Today, with four-handed, sit-down dentistry the operator has greater flexibility with the use of either a mobile unit or cart.

The same features are available on the floor-mounted unit. However, the oral evacuation system may be a part of the dental assistant's cart (Figure 34-5).

Parts of the Dental Unit

● *Dental handpiece(s).* These are a part of the dental unit. The type of unit employed in the treatment room will determine the dental handpiece arrangement.

● *Foot control.* The foot control (rheostat) is positioned on the floor close to the chair and activates the dental handpiece(s). The disc-shaped foot control is attached to the unit with flexible tubing (Figure 34-6).

● *Air-water syringe.* Air is used to dry the surfaces of the teeth. Water is used to rinse the oral cavity. Most air-water syringes will deliver (1) a stream of water, (2) a stream of air, and (3) a combination spray of air and water (Figure 34-7).

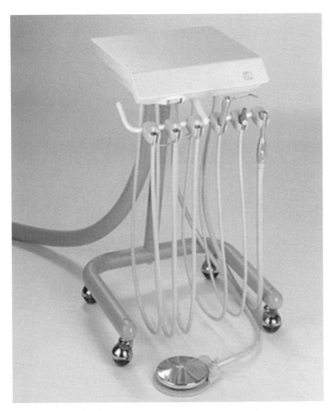

Figure 34-4 Mobile dental unit. (Courtesy of A-dec, Inc., Newberg, OR.)

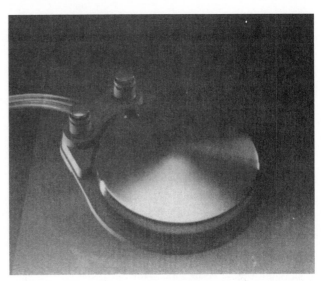

Figure 34-6 Foot control/rheostat. (Courtesy of A-dec, Inc., Newberg, OR.)

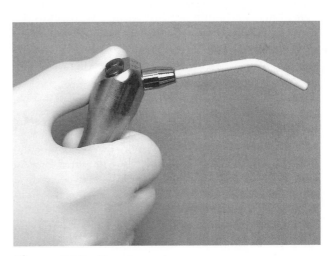

Figure 34-7 Air-water syringe.

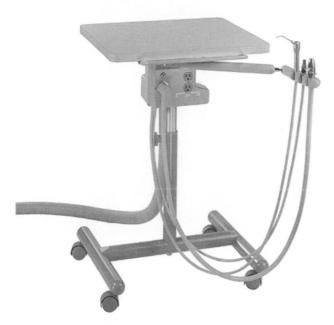

Figure 34-5 Assistant's cart. (Courtesy of A-dec, Inc., Newberg, OR.)

- *Oral vacuum.* An oral vacuum is used to suction water and debris from the patient's oral cavity. With the use of the high-volume oral vacuum (evacuation) system, the unit cuspidor has virtually been eliminated. The placement of the oral vacuum tip during

selected operative procedures aids in the retraction of the tongue and cheek, thereby keeping the field of operation free of water and debris while providing optimum visibility for the operator. In the **washed-field technique**, the dental handpiece provides a fine jet of air/water spray during the preparation of a tooth. The oral vacuum system has proven to be the most efficient method to control and remove the water from the patient's oral cavity.

- *Saliva ejector.* The function of the saliva ejector is to remove and control the saliva level and to hold the tongue away from the field of operation. A saliva ejector may also be used to maintain a dry environment during placement of restorative materials.

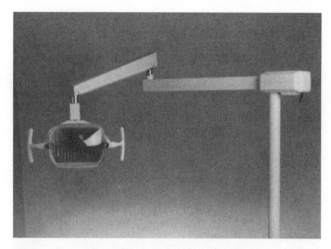

Figure 34-8 Dental operating light attached to dental unit. (Courtesy of A-dec, Inc., Newberg, OR.)

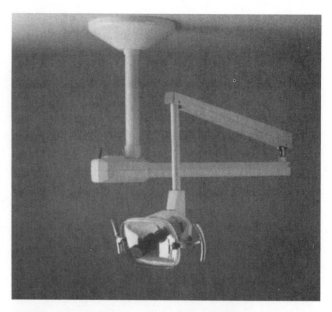

Figure 34-9 Ceiling-mounted dental operating light. (Courtesy of A-dec, Inc., Newberg, OR.)

● *Cuspidor.* A cuspidor is used by the patient to empty the mouth of oral debris. A dental unit may or may not have a cuspidor. Cuspidors may be fixed to the dental unit or be a part of the oral evacuation system of a portable unit (Figure 34-3).

The Operating Light

The dental operating light provides the bright light necessary for viewing the oral cavity.

The dental operating light may be attached to the dental unit (Figure 34-8), or be ceiling mounted (Figure 34-9). The dental light is designed with two handles, one on either side. The handles allow the dental light to be adjusted according to the procedure.

Care and cleaning of the dental light should be conducted according to manufacturer's recommendations.

The Dental Cabinet

Dental cabinets may be fixed to the wall or be free-standing and provide storage space for sterile instruments, tray setups, and any other supplies needed for the various dental procedures (Figure 34-1). When a mobile cabinet is part of the treatment room furnishings, it provides additional storage space as well as a working surface for the chairside dental assistant (Figure 34-10). Generally, storage space in a mobile cabinet is limited to those materials and supplies needed immediately at the chair.

Operating Stools

Operating stools are used in four-handed, sit-down dentistry and allow the operator and chairside dental assistant to be seated. The stools used by the operator and

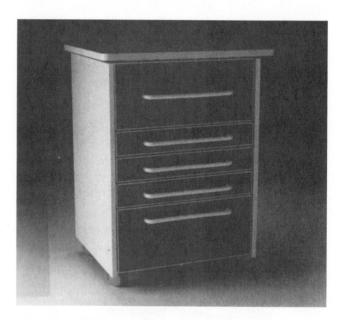

Figure 34-10 Assistant's mobile cabinet. (Courtesy of A-dec, Inc., Newberg, OR.)

dental assistant will vary in design. Features of a well-designed treatment room should include an operator stool and a dental assistant stool (Figure 34-11).

Operator's Stool

1. The seat of stool should be padded and may be flat surfaced or contoured.

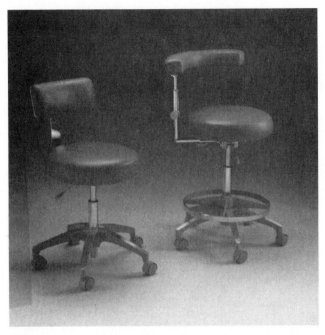

Figure 34-11 Left: Operator's stool. Right: Dental assistant's stool. (Courtesy of A-dec, Inc., Newberg, OR.)

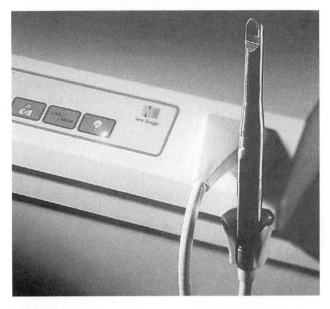

Figure 34-12 Intraoral camera system. (Courtesy of Air Techniques, Inc.)

2. The stool base should have four to five casters to prevent tipping.

3. The stool must have an adjustable lever, beneath the seat, to adjust the height of the seat from the floor.

4. The stool must have an adjustable back support.

Dental Assistant's Stool

1. The seat of the stool should be padded for the comfort of the dental assistant.

2. The stool should have five casters and be broad enough to prevent tipping.

3. The stool should have a foot ring to support the feet.

4. The stool must have a lever that can adjust leg length and for correct height.

5. The stool may have an adjustable support arm. The purpose of the arm is to provide the dental assistant with needed support to the upper body (torso).

X-Ray Machine

The x-ray machine may be a part of the operating or treatment room or housed in a separate area of the dental office. Refer to Chapters 62 and 68.

Intraoral Camera

The intraoral camera is a powerful and valuable diagnostic tool that makes use of the computer to **digitize** its images. Visualizing structures within the oral cavity is, no doubt, one of the best methods to enlighten patients with their dental conditions and to use as a marketing tool for cosmetic dentistry. Modern technology advances have designed a camera that can interface with a computer system or other imaging systems such as digital radiography. Today's intraoral camera is much smaller than its predecessor; thus it can be easily moved from place to place (Figure 34-12).

Cameras should have convenient features such as focusing with ease; ability to produce sharp, clean, and true color images; and capability of being protected from cross-contamination. They should also be adaptable in producing an image of a full arch vs. a single tooth. Cameras range in size from cart-based systems to hand-held wireless portable systems with self-contained monitor for focusing.

Component Parts

The component parts of an intraoral camera consist of the following:

● A camera unit that includes the handpiece, which when inserted into the oral cavity takes intraoral photos. To capture the picture either a foot pedal connected to some cameras or a button located on the handpiece and maneuvered by the touch of a finger is connected to other cameras. A light source for visibility is attached to the handpiece. The lens on the camera may be designed to produce either intra- or extraoral photos, eliminating the need for changing lenses. Some cameras support the fact that the handpiece is designed with an autofocus lens for easier use.

- A color printer with a footswitch.
- A color TV monitor with built-in VCR.
- A docking station fiberoptic illumination system (eliminates wires to the camera) may be set up in each treatment room, permitting the camera to be moved from room to room.

    It readily integrates with a personal computer. If the dental practice is computerized, digital images may be saved on the hard drive, floppy disk, or zip drive. An optional component is a sound system which enhances the operating procedure, either by recording comments that can be played back while doing treatment planning or by using the voice-activated commands to capture, display, edit, format, annotate, and store images, thus freeing the hands for easier control.

Camera Utilization

To utilize the intraoral camera, the operator turns on and prepares the camera unit by placing a disposable sleeve on the handpiece to prevent cross contamination; then inserts it into the mouth. When inserted into the mouth, the operator locates the area of interest and uses a pedal to select either a single image or quad (four images on one screen) screen images (Figure 34-13). Another pedal or a handpiece button captures the image on the screen. To print a copy, a footswitch is used to activate the printer.

Airbrasive Cavity Preparation System

Mechanical abrasion, also known as airbrasion, is produced by fine particles of aluminum oxide or sodium bicarbonate under controlled compressed air at 65–100 psi (pounds per square inch) and water pressure of 20–60 psi. Airbrasion is used on the tooth surface for polishing, stain removal, and cavity preparation (refer to Figure 13-8).

Benefits

Although lacking in some dental offices, this system is fast becoming integrated in daily office routine. There are several benefits for making it a part of the dental office equipment:

- It removes enamel, dentin, and restorative material gently without compromising other healthy tissues if they are protected.

- The patient rarely needs to be anesthetized.
- Less tooth structure is removed.
- It does not generate heat or vibration, as does the dental handpiece.
- It increases patient comfort due to less vibration and reduced anesthesia needle use.

Precautions

Though there are numerous benefits in using an airbrasion system, the operator should be aware of some precautions in the method of use. Some areas of concern include:

- There is a high level of aerosol production that should warrant the use of high-volume evacuation.
- High levels of contamination of infectious diseases are more prevalent due to aerosol production.
- Pitting of adjacent teeth or restorations may occur if airbrasion is misdirected.
- Patients need eyewear protection and overall hair and body coverall, and lips should be lubricated to prevent drying effect of the sodium bicarbonate.
- When using airbrasion for polishing or stain removal, it should not contact cementum as it can be readily removed.
- Free gingival tissue may become traumatized when subjected to airbrasion.

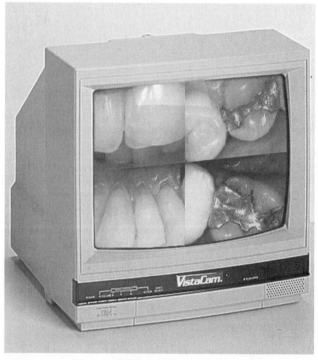

Figure 34-13 Quad images revealed on the monitor. (Courtesy of Air Techniques, Inc.)

Equipment Disinfection

It is advisable to always follow the manufacturer's recommendation when disinfecting dental equipment. However, because of the variation in design, materials used, and technical aspects of the dental equipment, any procedure of disinfection must be systematic and thorough. Also, it is imperative that barriers be used whenever possible. Refer to Chapter 36.

SUGGESTED ACTIVITIES

● Become familiar with each type of equipment in a dental office.

● Practice seating a fellow classmate on the dental chair and learn the function of each control button.

● Experience operating the dental unit. Practice running the dental handpiece using the foot control or rheostat. Take the air-water syringe and practice delivering a spray of water, then air, and lastly a combination spray of water and air.

● Learn to use the oral vacuum; practice holding it as if it were in the mouth of a patient.

● Check the dental cabinet and locate where materials and supplies are kept.

● Learn to sit at the dental assistant's stool. Practice adjusting the lever to the proper height.

● Understand how to turn on the x-ray unit and how to adjust the milliamperes and kilovoltage peak.

● Practice using the intraoral camera. Learn how to hold the handpiece and how to operate the pedal or handpiece button to capture the image on the monitor.

REVIEW

1. Indicate the features of the control panel on the dental chair: (1) it rotates the base of the chair, (2) it moves the body of the chair from the upright position, to a supine position, (3) it raises the height of the chair, and/or (4) it lowers the chair.
   a. 1, 2, 3
   b. 2, 3, 4
   c. 1, 2, 4
   d. 1, 3, 4

2. Indicate the features of dental units: (1) oral evacuation system, (2) curing light, (3) dental handpieces, and or (4) air-water syringe.
   a. 1, 2, 3
   b. 2, 3, 4
   c. 1, 2, 4
   d. 1, 3, 4

3. The rheostat:
   a. Controls the dental light
   b. Activates the oral vacuum
   c. Controls the saliva ejector
   d. Activates the dental handpieces

4. In the washed-field technique:
   a. The dental handpiece provides air and water spray during the preparation of the tooth.
   b. The air and water syringe is used to spray the tooth during preparation.
   c. The cuspidor is used to empty the mouth.
   d. A cup of water is used for the patient to rinse the mouth.

5. Indicate the features of the dental assistant's operating stool. It should have (1) five casters to prevent tipping, (2) a foot ring to support the feet, (3) an arm rest to provide support for the wrists, and/or (4) a lever that adjusts leg length for the correct height.
   a. 1, 2, 3
   b. 2, 3, 4
   c. 1, 2, 4
   d. 1, 3, 4

6. The lens of the intraoral camera is located:
   a. On the mouth mirror
   b. Separately from the apparatus
   c. On the handpiece

7. What does the airbrasive unit use to remove particles from teeth?
   a. Aluminum oxide
   b. Cement
   c. Sodium chloride
   d. Potassium sulfate

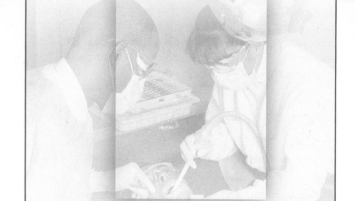

OBJECTIVES

After studying this chapter, the student will be able to:

- Discuss the four operating zones as they relate to the dental team.
- Identify the three basic systems for instrument delivery.
- Explain the optimum seating position of the operator during operative dentistry.
- Explain the optimum seating position of the chairside dental assistant during operative dentistry.
- Explain the correct seating and head position of the patient for operative dentistry.

Introduction

The proper positioning of the patient and dental team may improve the delivery of dental care. The manner in which the operator and chairside dental assistant are positioned in relationship to the patient is important for efficiency and increased productivity.

Four-handed, sit-down dentistry provides the dental team with the opportunity to function as a coordinated and organized unit.

The system of four-handed, sit-down dentistry allows the operator and chairside dental assistant to work while seated. The chairside assistant provides a second pair of hands for the operator.

The patient is placed in the **supine** (lying on back with face up) position in the dental chair, while the operator and chairside dental assistant are seated on either side of the chair.

Operating Zones for Dental Team

The working zones in which the dental team must operate can best be described by the hours on the face of a clock. With the patient seated and placed into a supine position, the patient's oral cavity represents the center of the clock (Figure 35-1).

The operator and chairside dental assistant are positioned according to the hours on the face of a clock.

The clock may be divided into four working zones (Figure 35-2):

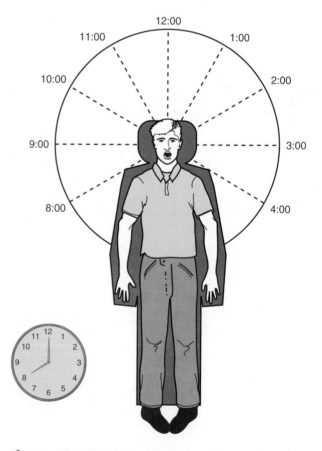

Figure 35-1 Patient's oral cavity represented as the center of the clock.

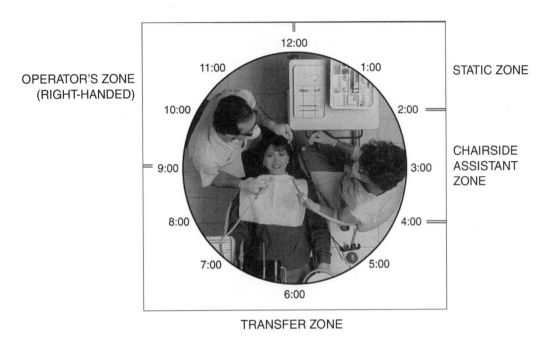

Figure 35-2 Working zones. (Photo courtesy of A-dec, Inc., Newberg, OR.)

1. Operator's zone—8 to 12 o'clock if the operator is right handed or 12 to 4 o'clock if left handed. The operator's zone is the working area in which the operator is positioned to have access to all areas of the patient's oral cavity.

2. Dental assistant's zone—2 to 4 o'clock if the operator is right handed or 8 to 10 o'clock if left handed. The dental assistant's working zone is generally limited to either the 3 o'clock (right-handed operator) or 9 o'clock position (left-handed operator) throughout the dental procedure, regardless of the operator's position.

3. Transfer zone—4 to 8 o'clock position. The transfer zone is the area where the operator and dental assistant will exchange instruments and materials for delivery to and from the oral cavity during the dental procedure. This is also referred to as **transthorax** delivery (across the chest).

4. Static zone—12 to 2 o'clock or 10 to 12 o'clock position is regarded as a nonactive zone. Equipment such as a mobile cabinet or cart may be placed in this zone.

Basic Systems for Instrument Delivery

Over-the-Patient Delivery

The majority of dentists use the *over-the-patient delivery system*. In this delivery system, the so-called dental unit is mounted on a post with an arm system that brings the controls to the operator (Figure 35-3).

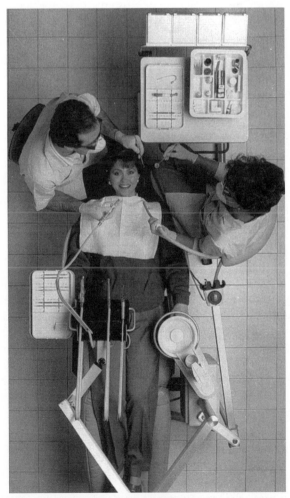

Figure 35-3 Over-the-patient delivery system for instrumentation. (Courtesy of A-dec, Inc., Newberg, OR.)

The over-the-patient delivery system is highly flexible in terms of positioning equipment and exchange of instruments. Instruments may be presented from across the patient's chest (transthorax delivery) or from either side of the patient. This system is ideal for either two- or four-handed dentistry and may be used by the operator while in the seated or standing position. Instruments will be in full view of the patient at all times with this delivery system.

Advantages of the Over-the-Patient System

- Offers suitable instrumentation in the location and exchange of dental instruments.
- Allows for two- or four-handed, stand-up or sit-down dentistry.
- Allows the operator direct access to the lower quadrants.
- Requires minimal movement by the operator and chairside dental assistant during operative dentistry.
- Minimizes eye fatigue, because the operator does not need to constantly adjust his or her eyes to oral-cavity distance.
- Minimal operatory floor space is required for equipment.

Disadvantages of Over-the-Patient Delivery

- Reduces dental assistant's access to chair controls positioned on the operator's side of the chair.
- Tubing from the unit to the handpiece(s) may drag over the patient's chest during the operative procedure.

Side Delivery

The *side-delivery system* is developed specifically for four-handed, sit-down dentistry. Instrument exchange is best achieved through the use of separate cart(s) for the operator and chairside dental assistant. In addition, the operator may use a wall- or cabinet-mounted unit along with the dental assistant's cart. With the side-delivery system, operative instruments are exchanged peripheral to the patient's view, i.e., outside his or her normal center of vision.

Advantages of the Side-Delivery System

- Offers the operator and chairside dental assistant increased ability to view the oral cavity during all sit-down dental procedures.
- Offers flexible seating and instrument location.
- Offers the dental team mobility with the use of cart or mobile cabinets. Operator and chairside dental assistant are able to move more freely at the chair with the use of a cart or mobile cabinet.
- Tubing from the unit to handpiece(s) may be straight or coiled. Coiled tubing has less chance to drag across the patient.
- Provides operator and chairside dental assistant better access to the patient and chair.
- Instruments are kept out of view of the patient.
- If wall-mounted units are used, minimal floor space is required.

Disadvantages of Side-Delivery System

- Requires more operatory floor space when split-cart systems are used.
- A poorly located umbilical tubing arrangement may interfere with the ability of operator and chairside dental assistant to move freely within the working zone(s).
- Reduces dental assistant's access to operator's instruments.

Rear-Delivery System

In the *rear-delivery system*, the instruments are located behind the chair. A single cart or a cabinet- or wall-mounted unit can be used. The instruments are always at the rear of the chair and are generally out of the view of the patient (Figure 35-4). Rear delivery is most effective in sit-down, four-handed dentistry.

Advantages of the Rear-Delivery System

- Operative instruments are out of the patient's view.
- Provides excellent dental assistant access to operative instruments.
- Provides the dental assistant with a stable work surface when a dual-purpose cart or cabinet is used.
- Allows the patient easy access to chair and efficient movement within the working zone(s) of the operator and chairside dental assistant.
- Requires minimal operator space.

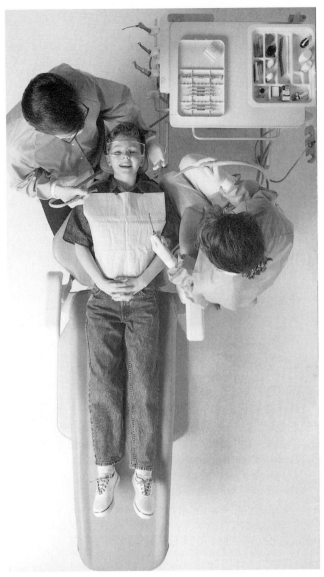

Figure 35-4 Rear delivery system for instrumentation. (Courtesy of A-dec, Inc., Newberg, OR.)

Disadvantage of the Rear-Delivery System

● Limited to sit-down dentistry.

Positioning of Operator and Chairside Dental Assistant

Position of Operator

The position of the operator is critical to the fixed environment of the dental team. The entire system is based on the operator's position during the dental procedure. The operator must assume a desirable seated position. The patient, chairside dental assistant, and equipment are arranged according to this position.

The objectives for proper positioning of the operator should include the following criteria:

1. The operator must be seated so that the entire surface of the operator's stool is supporting his or her weight.

2. The height of the stool should be adjusted so that the operator's thighs are parallel to the floor with both feet on the floor.

3. The operator's elbows should be at the height of the patient's mouth, close to the body.

4. The operator is seated in a relaxed and unstrained position with the back and neck upright and with the top of the shoulders parallel to the floor.

5. The distance from the operator's eyes to the patient's oral cavity should be approximately 14–18 inches.

Position of Chairside Dental Assistant

The dental assistant must have easy access and visibility to the oral cavity during the treatment procedure. This can be accomplished when the dental team is seated and properly positioned.

For the dental assistant to function in an efficient manner the following criteria should be followed:

1. The dental assistant should be seated in the 3 o'clock position for a right-handed operator or the 9 o'clock position for a left-handed operator.

2. The dental assistant's stool should be 4–6 inches higher than the operator's. This will allow the dental assistant greater visibility for most areas of the oral cavity.

3. The dental assistant should be seated as close to the dental chair as possible.

4. The dental assistant should be seated well back onto the seat of the stool. The stool back support must be properly adjusted in order to provide needed back support.

5. The dental assistant's back should be straight (erect) with the body-support arm adjusted to support the upper body just under the rib cage.

6. The dental assistant's legs should be directed toward the patient's head, with the dental assistant's thighs parallel to the seat of the chair.

7. The dental assistant's feet should rest on the foot support at the base of the stool.

SUGGESTED ACTIVITY

● Working with a group of three individuals, practice positioning each person as the operator, the dental assistant, and the patient. Use a rotation system whereby each person experiences all three positions. Use guidelines outlined for each position and practice them.

REVIEW

1. Match the column on the left with the column on the right. The operating positions below are for a right-handed operator.

   ___a. Operator's zone   1. 12 to 2 o'clock

   ___b. Dental assistant's zone   2. 2 to 4 o'clock

   ___c. Transfer zone   3. 8 to 12 o'clock

   ___d. Static zone   4. 4 to 8 o'clock

2. Four-handed, sit-down dentistry is a system that:
   1. Allows the operator and chairside dental assistant to work in a seated position
   2. Places the chairside dental assistant at the 10 to 2 o'clock position
   3. Allows the chairside dental assistant to provide a second pair of hands
   4. Allows the operator to reach for needed instruments during operative procedures

   a. 1, 2
   b. 2, 3
   c. 3, 4
   d. 1, 3

3. Advantages of over-the-patient delivery system include:
   1. Keeping the instruments out of the patient's view
   2. Needing minimal floor space for equipment
   3. Requiring minimal movement by the operator and chairside dental assistant during operative dentistry
   4. Minimizing operator's eye fatigue

   a. 1, 2, 3
   b. 2, 3, 4
   c. 1, 2, 4
   d. 1, 3, 4

4. Proper operator positioning include (1) placing the height of the stool so that operator's thighs are parallel to the floor with feet on floor, (2) operator's elbows should be at the height of the patient's mouth, close to the body, (3) operator's wrists should be at the height of the patient's oral cavity, and/or (4) the distance from operator's eyes to patient's mouth should be 14–18 inches.

   a. 1, 2, 3
   b. 2, 3, 4
   c. 1, 2, 4
   d. 1, 3, 4

5. Proper chairside dental assistant's position include: (1) placing the dental assistant's stool at 2–3 inches higher than the operator's, (2) placing the dental assistant's feet on the foot support at the base of the stool, (3) positioning the dental assistant's legs directed toward the patient's head, and/or (4) sitting as close to the dental chair as possible.

   a. 1, 2, 3
   b. 2, 3, 4
   c. 1, 2, 4
   d. 1, 3, 4

Preparing the Treatment Room and Seating the Dental Patient

OBJECTIVES

After studying this chapter, the student will be able to:

- Discuss the correct procedure for using the spray-wipe-spray method for disinfecting the dental operatory.
- Prepare the dental operatory using the appropriate barriers.
- Discuss the proper position of the patient's oral cavity in relationship to the operator.
- Discuss the role of the chairside dental assistant in seating the patient for operative dentistry.
- Discuss the supine position as it pertains to the dental patient.

Introduction

Preparation of the treatment room requires meticulous care. The primary area of concern lies in the fact that cross-contamination of infectious germs may occur if proper guidelines are not followed. The phrase "Do unto others as you would have them do unto you" should play an important role here. The dental assistant should put herself or himself in the place of the patient when preparing the room and exercise strict measures of infection control.

Preparing the Treatment Room

Materials needed include:

- 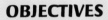 Antimicrobial soap
- Disposable towels
- Utility gloves
- Surface disinfectant
- Sponge
- Barrier materials

Preparing the dental operatory or treatment room requires that all work surfaces and equipment be either disinfected or protected with appropriate barriers.

Surfaces that cannot be barriered must be disinfected with an appropriate surface disinfectant, such as iodophors or other disinfectants approved by the Environmental Protection Agency (EPA).

The daily routine requires that the operatory be cleaned, disinfected, and ready for the placement of the barriers. It is recommended that at the beginning and end of each day, the surfaces of the dental chair, unit, and countertop/cabinet(s) be sprayed with the surface disinfectant. However, only those surfaces that can withstand the application of a surface disinfectant should be sprayed. The technique of spray-wipe-spray is recommended. *Note:* Extreme care must be taken during the spray-wipe-spray procedure to avoid directing the spray onto the control panel of the chair, unit, and face of the dental light. Should the spray accidentally come in contact with the electrical system, it may permanently damage the dental equipment.

To prepare for the spray-wipe-spray procedure, the dental assistant should:

1. Wash hands with antimicrobial soap in cool water for 15 seconds, rinse, and dry.

2. Put on utility gloves.

3. Apply appropriate surface disinfectant to all working surfaces that can safely withstand the surface disinfectant. First spray, then wipe surfaces with sponge or disposable towel using a frictional wiping action. Spray a second time, and allow surfaces to dry for 10 minutes.

4. Wash and dry utility gloves once equipment and working surfaces have been disinfected.

5. Spray outer surface of gloves with disinfectant and hang to dry.

6. Wash hands in cool water and dry.

Placing Barriers

The routine spray-wipe-spray procedure between patients will depend on the extent to which *barriers* are

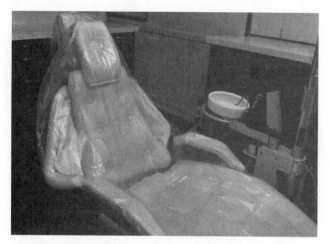

Figure 36-1 Full chair drape. (Courtesy of Perio Support Products, East Irvine, CA.)

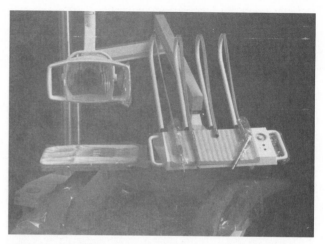

Figure 36-2 Disposable sleeves for handpiece and water syringe. (Courtesy of Perio Support Products, East Irvine, CA.)

used. The placement of barriers will save time between patients in disinfecting the treatment room.

Many barriers are available for use and include disposable plastic covers, Baggies, plastic perforated self-sticking sheet wrap, and aluminum foil. For barriers to be effective, they must be **impervious** (resist passage) to moisture and the penetration of microorganisms.

Dental Chair

- Headrest and body of chair should be covered with a disposable plastic full-chair drape (Figure 36-1).

Dental Unit

- Dental handpieces must be autoclaved.
- Handpiece hoses/tubing should be covered with disposable plastic sleeve (Figure 36-2).

Air-water Syringe

- Handle and tubing should be covered with disposable plastic sleeve (Figure 36-3).
- Syringe tip should be autoclaved or, if disposable, discarded.

Oral Vacuum

- Suction hose or tubing should be covered with disposable plastic sleeve (Figure 36-3).
- Vacuum tip should be autoclaved or, if disposable, discarded.

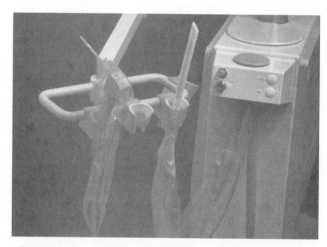

Figure 36-3 Disposable tubing cover for air-water syringe and oral vacuum. (Courtesy of Perio Support Products, East Irvine, CA.)

Saliva Ejector

- Hose/tubing should be covered with disposable plastic sleeve.
- Ejector tip should be disposable and therefore discarded.

Dental Operating Light

- On handles, plastic bags or perforated plastic sheet wrap should be used (Figure 36-4).
- On the light switch, perforated plastic sheet wrap should be used.

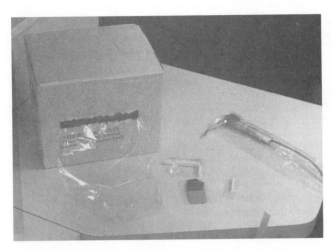

Figure 36–4 Disposable wrap or perforated sheets for various applications. (Courtesy of Perio Support Products, East Irvine, CA.)

X-ray Machine

● On tubehead/arms, disposable plastic bag or perforated plastic sheet wraps should be used.

● Exposure button/handle should be covered with disposable tube-shaped plastic bag.

● Cone/cylinder should be covered with a disposable tube-shaped plastic bag. *Note:* Perforated sheet wrap should be used to adjust exposure dial when exposing x-ray films.

Bracket and Instrument Trays

● Disposable tray covers or liners should be used on unit bracket tray and instrument tray(s). Instruments and tray should be covered with plastic wrap until ready to use. All metal and/or plastic instrument trays should be sterilized after each patient.

Completion of Dental Treatment

When the dental procedure has been completed, services rendered must be entered on the patient's chart. The operator will direct the dental assistant to record these; then, the dental assistant will:

1. Remove gloves and wash hands. Refer to Chapter 7.

2. Make an entry of services rendered on the patient's chart using a pen. If the computer is used, the key-

board should be barriered with plastic wrap and changed after every patient.

3. Record all instructions given the patient on the patient's chart.

The operator will:

1. Return patient to upright position.

2. Excuse himself or herself, remove gloves and place in appropriate waste receptacle, and wash hands.

3. Thank the patient and leave the operatory.

Dismissing the Patient

The dental assistant will:

1. Remove drape or bib and set aside.

2. Lower the chair to a height that will enable the patient to comfortably leave the chair.

3. Raise arm of chair and assist the patient out of the chair and check to make certain the patient has gathered all personal items.

4. Escort patient to the reception desk.

Cleaning the Treatment Room

After each patient the dental assistant will remove barriers, disinfect needed surfaces, then replace barriers. Surfaces that are not barriered must be disinfected.

The dental assistant will:

1. Put on utility gloves.

2. Remove all barriers and place in appropriate waste receptacle. Blood- and/or saliva-contaminated items must be placed in a suitably labeled BIOHAZARD receptacle.

3. Remove dental instruments from treatment room to the sterilization area for further care. Refer to Chapter 8.

4. Spray surface disinfectant on those surfaces that were not barriered and wipe with sponge or disposable paper towel using a frictional wiping action to remove debris.

5. Once the disinfection process is completed, remove utility gloves; wash, rinse, and dry the hands; spray gloves with an approved disinfectant; and hang to dry.

6. Replace barriers. Treatment room is now ready for the next patient.

Procedure 27 Seating the Dental Patient for Operative Dentistry

Materials Needed

Antimicrobial (controls or destroys microorganisms) soap
Disposable towel(s)
Patient chart
Pen
Drape/neckchain/bib
Disposable oral vacuum tip
Disposable saliva ejector
Sterile handpiece(s) in pouch
Sterile basic instrument setup in pouch
Stethoscope/aneroid, mercury-type manometer
Appropriate tray setup
Protective eyewear
Face mask
Disposable gloves/gowns

Instructions

Seating the Patient

The dental assistant's and operator's personal protective equipment, consisting of eyewear, face mask, gloves, and disposable gowns should be available for immediate use.

Once the treatment room has been disinfected and the appropriate barriers placed, the patient is escorted from the reception/waiting room to the treatment room by the dental assistant. When the patient is in the treatment room, the dental assistant will:

1 Adjust the height of the chair so that the patient can easily be seated.

2 Invite the patient to be seated and adjust the headrest. Note: It is suggested that an area be set aside for the patient's coat or wrap. Do not allow the patient to leave personal articles in the reception or waiting room. There should be a designated area/place in the treatment room, in view of the patient, for his or her handbag or other valuables.

3 The patient is in an upright position for placement of drape and/or bib and should remain in this position until the operator is seated. If the patient is wearing lipstick, offer a tissue, and ask the patient to remove lipstick.

4 At this time, the patient's health history is reviewed, and any changes should be recorded on the patient's chart. Refer to Chapter 10.

5 Vital signs are taken and recorded on the patient's chart.

6 Next, the dental assistant will wash hands for 15 seconds using antimicrobial soap and cool water. Then rinse hands in cold water, and dry with disposable paper towel.

7 Don gloves and slightly rinse in cool water. Dry.

8 With gloved hands, sterile items such as the saliva ejector, air/water syringe, and oral vacuum tip are placed. The dental handpiece(s) is (are) removed from the sterilizing pouch and attached to the appropriate hose(s)/tubing.

9 Sterile instruments or tray setup are selected and placed according to the system used for instrumentation.

10 Should the basic setup of the mouth mirror, explorer, periodontal probe, and cotton pliers be sterilized in a separate pouch, they may be removed and placed on the tray at this time.

Positioning the Patient

Generally, it will be the operator who will place the patient in the supine position.

Dental chairs that are automatically programmed for positioning the chair tend to place the patient into the supine position too quickly. This could frighten the patient. Therefore, the patient should be slowly lowered into the supine position.

In the supine position, the patient's legs and head should be at the same level. The patient should be positioned in the chair with little bending at the waist. Patients who are placed with their legs higher than their head are not considered to be in a supine position. Placing a patient for a long time in such a position is not recommended as it may cause numbness of the feet and legs.

Once the patient is seated and the instruments are in place, the operator is notified.

1 Upon entering the room the operator greets the patient.

continued

continued from previous page
Procedure 27 *Seating the Dental Patient for Operative Dentistry*

2 The operator reviews the patient's chart, and checks any notation made on the chart by the dental assistant.

3 The operator discusses the procedure to be done.

4 The operator washes and dries hands.

5 The operator dons protective eyewear, face mask, and gloves (protective gown/jacket should already be on).

6 The operator positions himself or herself on the stool.

7 The operator places the patient in the supine position. It is important that the dental patient be in the proper position with the patient's oral cavity centered in the vicinity of the operator's lap and at the height of the operator's elbows. The operator must have access and visibility in order to work in all areas within the oral cavity.

8 Once the patient and dental team are properly seated, the dental operating light is brought into position. *Note:* When turning the dental light on, the beam of light is first directed toward the patient's chest, then toward the patient's oral cavity. Care must be taken to avoid directing the light beam into the patient's eyes.

9 The dental team starts the dental treatment.

SUGGESTED ACTIVITIES

● Practice preparing dental treatment room, dental chair, and unit using appropriate disinfection procedures.

● Practice placing appropriate barriers on dental chair, dental light, and unit.

● Practice seating and draping another student, adjusting the height of the chair and the headrest.

REVIEW

1. The routine in preparing the dental treatment room includes (1) cleaning, (2) disinfecting, (3) sterilizing, and/or (4) getting it ready for barriers placement.
   a. 1, 2, 3
   b. 2, 3, 4
   c. 1, 2, 4
   d. 1, 3, 4

2. Barriers placed on equipment must _____ to be effective.
   a. Be impervious
   b. Inhibit bacterial growth
   c. Be used on counter tops
   d. Be sterilized

3. In what position is the patient when his or her head and legs are at the same level?
   a. Trendelenburg
   b. Semisupine
   c. Supine
   d. Upright

4. What procedure should be followed when turning on the dental light?
   a. The beam of light is directed to the patient's face.
   b. The beam of light is directed to the patient's head and then to the oral cavity.
   c. The beam of light is directed to the patient's oral cavity.
   d. The beam of light is directed to the patient's chest and then to the oral cavity.

5. Indicate the procedure the chairside dental assistant follows when recording services rendered on the patient's chart: (1) uses a tissue to hold the pen and enters services rendered; (2) removes exam gloves, washes hands, and enters services rendered; (3) if a computer is used, the keyboard is barriered with plastic wrap and services rendered is entered; and/or (4) uses a plastic barrier on the pen and enters services rendered.
   a. 1, 2
   b. 2, 3
   c. 3, 4
   d. 1, 4

6. The procedure for cleaning the treatment room includes (1) using utility gloves to remove all barriers and placing them in the appropriate waste receptacle, (2) removing and preparing dental instruments for sterilization, (3) spraying surface disinfectant on nonbarriered surfaces, and/or (4) removing utility gloves and disposing them.
   a. 1, 2, 3
   b. 2, 3, 4
   c. 1, 2, 4
   d. 1, 3, 4

Principles and Applications of Oral Evacuation

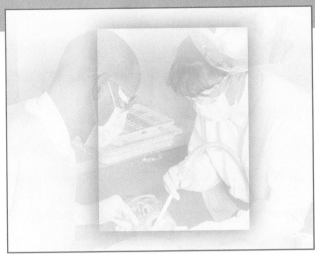

OBJECTIVES

After studying this chapter, the student will be able to:

● Discuss the washed-field technique.
● State the advantages for using oral vacuum/high-velocity suction.
● List the parts of the oral vacuum system.
● Demonstrate the correct thumb-to-nose and modified pen grasp hand positions.
● Discuss the basic rules for oral vacuum tip placement.
● Demonstrate the correct oral vacuum tip placement for maxillary and mandibular posterior teeth.
● Demonstrate the correct oral vacuum tip placement for maxillary and mandibular anterior teeth.

Introduction

Today, most dental handpieces operate at speeds higher than 150,000 rpm (revolutions per minute) and require the use of a water coolant to reduce the frictional heat that is produced during the cutting and shaping of tooth tissues. The use of water as a coolant in operative dentistry is called the **washed-field technique**.

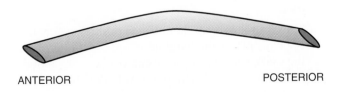

ANTERIOR   POSTERIOR

Figure 37-1 Oral vacuum tip.

Because a considerable amount of water is released from the handpiece during this procedure, a *high-volume evacuator (HVE)* or *oral vacuum system* is needed. This system provides a quick and efficient method for the removal of water and debris from the oral cavity.

The Oral Vacuum System

Parts of the Oral Vacuum System

● *Removable oral vacuum tip.* Plastic or metal, open-ended cylinder (Figure 37-1).
● *Handle.* Where tip is inserted and the on/off control dial or button is located (Figure 37-2).
● *Hose.* Flexible tubing that connects the handle to the suction or vacuum source of the unit (Figure 37-3).

The universal oral vacuum (OV) tip is slightly curved in the middle, and the tip ends are beveled. One end of the beveled tip is for use on the anterior maxillary and mandibular teeth, whereas the opposite end is used for the maxillary and mandibular posterior teeth.

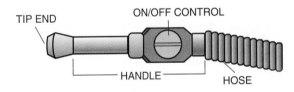

TIP END   ON/OFF CONTROL

HANDLE   HOSE

Figure 37-2 Parts of the oral vacuum system.

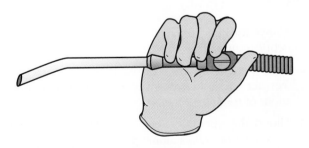

Figure 37-3 Thumb-to-nose grasp for holding oral vacuum with tip in place.

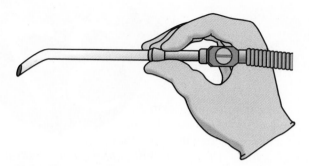

Figure 37-4 Modified pen grasp for holding oral vacuum with tip in place.

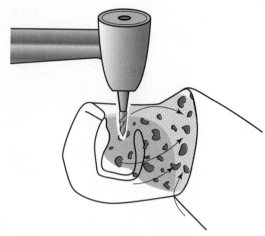

Figure 37-5 Correct placement of oral vacuum tip.

To identify which end of the oral vacuum tip is anterior or posterior, the bend in the tip may be used as a guide. If the beveled end of the tip faces toward the floor, the tip is used for the maxillary and mandibular anterior teeth, designated as A (anterior) (Figure 37-1). For the maxillary and mandibular posterior teeth, the bevel will be directed upward, designated as P (posterior) (Figure 37-1).

The hose/tubing must be flexible and long enough to allow access to each quadrant or area within the oral cavity.

Hand Grasp for Oral Vacuum Tip

The two methods for holding the oral vacuum tip/handle/hose include the **thumb-to-nose grasp** (Figure 37-3), and the **modified pen grasp** (Figure 37-4). The thumb-to-nose grasp is used for the maxillary and mandibular posterior teeth. The thumb-to-nose grasp is very effective in controlling the oral vacuum tip when used for retracting the patient's cheek and tongue. The modified pen grasp is used when working on the anterior maxillary and mandibular teeth.

Advantages of the High-Volume Evacuator (HVE)

1. Allows for rapid removal of oral fluids, water, and debris from oral cavity.
2. Oral vacuum tip may be used in the retraction (**retract** = to hold back away from the area of operation) of tongue or cheek.
3. Allows the operator greater visibility with proper placement of oral vacuum tip.
4. Reduces chair time, because patient can remain in the supine position without having to be placed in an upright position for rinsing and emptying mouth.

Disadvantages of the High-Volume Evacuator (HVE)

1. The oral vacuum may be noisy when on.
2. If oral vacuum tip is too close to oral tissues, it may accidentally grab them and cause some trauma.
3. May trigger gag reflex should the tip touch the soft palate.
4. Improper placement of tip may interfere with operator's access and visibility.

Basic Rules for Oral Vacuum Tip Placement

A dental assistant working with a right-handed operator will hold the oral vacuum tip/handle with the right hand, while the left hand is free to hold the air/water syringe or transfer instruments. (The procedure is reversed when working with a left-handed operator.)

1. The beveled portion of the oral vacuum tip should be parallel to either the buccal or lingual surfaces of the teeth.
2. The tip should be as close to the tooth as possible and slightly distal of the tooth being prepared.
3. The middle of the tip opening should be even with the occlusal surface (Figure 37-5). Care must be taken not to draw the water coolant away from the bur or handpiece before it has a chance to cool the tooth.
4. The oral vacuum tip should be in position before the operator places the handpiece and mouth mirror in the oral cavity. The relationship between the mouth mirror and oral vacuum tip will depend on the quadrant or teeth being prepared.

See Table 37-1.

Table 37-1 Oral Vacuum Tip Placement Chart

Posterior Quadrant	OV Placement
Maxillary right	Adjacent to the lingual surfaces of posterior tooth being prepared (Figures 37-6A and B)

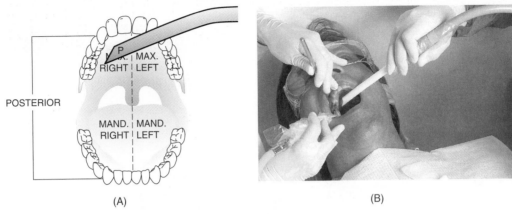

(A)   (B)

Figure 37-6 Oral vacuum placement for maxillary right quadrant.

Maxillary left Adjacent to the buccal or facial surfaces of the posterior tooth being prepared (Figures 37-7A and B)

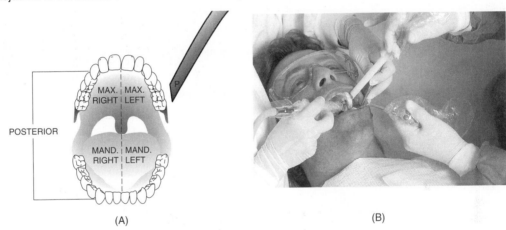

(A)   (B)

Figure 37-7 Oral vacuum placement for maxillary left quadrant.

Mandibular right Adjacent to the lingual surface and slightly posterior to the tooth being prepared (Figures 37-8A and B). Oral vacuum tip may aid in retraction of the tongue.

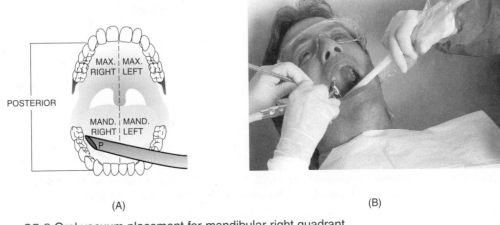

(A)   (B)

Figure 37-8 Oral vacuum placement for mandibular right quadrant.

Table 37-1	Oral Vacuum Tip Placement Chart (Continued)
Posterior Quadrant	**OV Placement**
Mandibular left	Placed along the buccal or facial surfaces of the teeth. The tip will aid in the retraction of the cheek (Figures 37-9A and B)

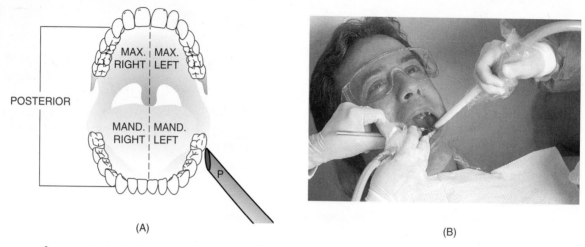

(A) (B)

Figure 37-9 Oral vacuum placement for mandibular left quadrant.

Anterior Maxillary and Mandibular	**OV Placement**
Maxillary anterior	
Facial/labial approach	Adjacent to the lingual surface near the incisal edge of tooth being prepared (Figures 37-10A and B)
Lingual approach	Adjacent to facial/labial surface near the incisal edge of tooth being prepared (Figures 3-10A and B)

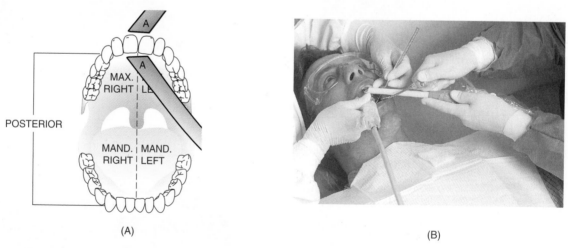

(A) (B)

Figure 37-10 Oral vacuum placement for maxillary anterior teeth, facial/labial and lingual approach.

Mandibular anterior

Facial/labial approach	Adjacent to the lingual surface of the tooth being prepared (Figures 37-11A and B)
Lingual approach	Adjacent to facial/labial surface of the tooth being prepared, with tip resting in the vestibule by the lower lip and surfaces of the anterior teeth (Figures 37-11A and B)

| **Table 37-1** | Oral Vacuum Tip Placement Chart (Continued) |

Mandibular anterior (Continued)

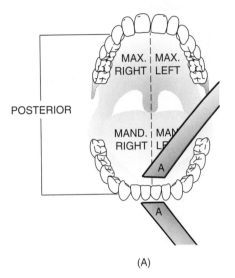

(A)

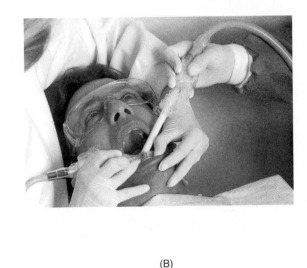

(B)

Figure 37-11 Oral vacuum placement for mandibular anterior teeth, facial/labial and lingual approach.

The general operating zone for the operator is the 9 to 11 o'clock position and the 2 to 3 o'clock for the dental assistant. Refer to Chapter 35.

Sterilization and Care of Oral Vacuum Tips

When the OV tip is removed from the hose, it should be placed in the ultrasonic cleaner or scrubbed carefully in a basin of water using a circular brush that fits within the lumen of the tip. One must always be careful not to produce bacterial aerosol when scrubbing instruments, and brushing the OV tip in a basin of water minimizes the problem. The OV tip is dried thoroughly and prepared for sterilization.

The material that the OV tip is made from dictates how it will be sterilized. If it is made of metal, it will be heat sterilized in an autoclave. If it is made of reusable plastic, it will need to be subjected to 10 hours of chemical liquid sterilization or placed in an ethylene oxide gas sterilizer, which does not use heat.

SUGGESTED ACTIVITIES

● Practice oral evacuation in groups of three. One serves as the patient, another as the operator, and the third as the chairside dental assistant.

● Using the air-water syringe, the operator will spray water on a selected tooth of the patient. The chairside dental assistant will evacuate the patient's mouth following the basic rules for oral vacuum tip placement.

REVIEW

1. A washed-field technique pertains to:
   a. Using the air/water syringe to wash the preparation
   b. Using a cup of water to have the patient rinse and wash the oral cavity
   c. Using a water coolant with a high-speed handpiece to reduce frictional heat during a cavity preparation

2. Match the column on the left with the one on the right. The oral vacuum positions are for each posterior quadrant.

___a. Maxillary right

___b. Mandibular left

___c. Mandibular right

___d. Maxillary left

1. Place OV tip adjacent to mandibular right lingual teeth
2. Place OV tip adjacent to maxillary left buccal teeth
3. Place OV tip adjacent to mandibular left buccal teeth
4. Place OV tip adjacent to maxillary right lingual teeth

3. State the basic rules for oral vacuum tip placement: (1) the middle of the tip opening should be even with the occlusal surface, (2) the OV tip should be in position before the operator places the handpiece and mouth mirror in the oral cavity, (3) the beveled portion of the OV tip should be parallel to either buccal or lingual surfaces of the teeth, and/or (4) the OV tip should be slightly mesial to the tooth being worked on.

a. 1, 2, 3
b. 2, 3, 4
c. 1, 2, 4
d. 1, 3, 4

4. Which hand grasp is used to hold the OV tip when working on posterior teeth?

a. Palm grasp
b. Thumb-to-nose grasp
c. Pen grasp
d. Overhand grasp

5. State the position of the oral vacuum tip for the maxillary anterior teeth, facial/labial approach.

a. Adjacent to the lingual surface near the incisal edge of the tooth being prepared
b. Adjacent to the facial surface near the cervical area of the tooth being prepared
c. Adjacent to the lingual surface near the cervical area of the tooth being prepared
d. Adjacent to the facial surface of the proximal tooth to the tooth being prepared

Instrument Transfer

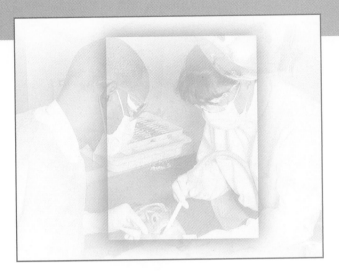

OBJECTIVES

After studying this chapter, the student will be able to:

- Discuss the chairside dental assistant's role in the retrieval and delivery of hand instruments.
- Cite the basic rules for instrument transfer.
- State the advantages for using a fulcrum when working in the oral cavity.
- Discuss the reasons for using the pen grasp, modified pen grasp, palm grasp and palm-thumb grasp.
- Demonstrate instrument transfer following the stated sequence: approach, retrieval, and delivery.

Introduction

There are several ways in which instruments may be transferred between dental assistant and operator. In four-handed, sit-down dentistry, the most frequently used instrument transfer involves the retrieval and delivery of instrument(s) into and out of the operator's hand during a dental procedure.

The transfer of instruments between operator and dental assistant takes place in the transfer zone near the patient's chin. Effective instrument transfer should involve little movement of the operator's fingers or eyes. A smooth transfer of instruments occurs when the chairside dental assistant is able to anticipate the operator's needs.

To aid the dental assistant in the delivery of the instruments, it is best to identify the fingers and thumb of the hand. The *thumb* is referred to by the letter *T*, and

the fingers are numbered: *index finger* (1), *middle finger* (2), *ring finger* (3), and *little finger* (4) (Figure 38-1).

If the operator is right-handed, the dental assistant's left hand is used to transfer and retrieve instruments. This frees the dental assistant's right hand to use the HVE or for retraction. For a left-handed operator the procedure is reversed.

In instrument transfer, the chairside assistant will select the correct instrument and hold it in his or her hand with the appropriate fingers until the operator signals the exchange. The dental assistant will remove the used instrument from the operator's hand and place the new instrument.

To hold the instrument to be delivered, the thumb, index (1), and middle (2) fingers work together to deliver the instrument, while the little finger (4) is used in the retrieval of the instrument from the operator's right hand. For greater stability in retrieval and delivery of an instrument, fingers 3 and 4 may be used.

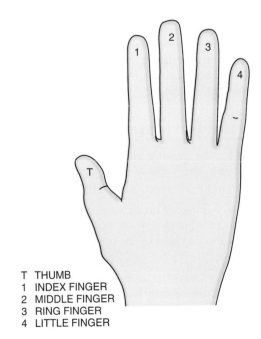

T   THUMB
1   INDEX FINGER
2   MIDDLE FINGER
3   RING FINGER
4   LITTLE FINGER

Figure 38-1 Hand with fingers identified by numbers.

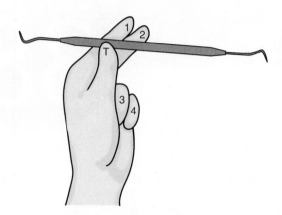

Figure 38-2 Hand position for instrument transfer.

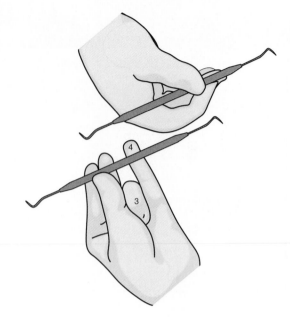

Figure 38-3 The approach with fingers in position.

Basic Rules for Instrument Transfer

1. Instrument should be held with thumb (T) and fingers 1 and 2 (Figure 38-2).

2. Instrument should be held close to the end opposite from the one that is to be used by the operator.

3. Instrument should be held with working end in proper operating position for the tooth being treated.

4. Working end of hand instrument or bur in handpiece should be directed downward for mandibular arch and upward for maxillary arch.

5. Instrument to be passed should be held in a position parallel to the instrument held by the operator. Instruments should be as close to one another as possible, but without becoming entangled during instrument exchange.

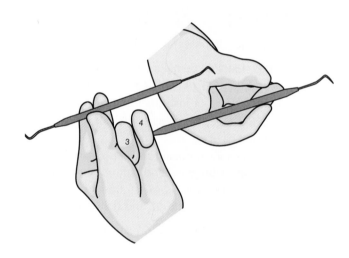

Figure 38-4 Position of fingers for removal of instrument.

Sequence for Instrument Transfer

A system for the passing and receiving of instruments may include the following movements: (1) the approach, (2) the retrieval, and (3) the delivery.

1. *Approach.* Finger 4 is extended (Figure 38-3), and the instrument is grasped by the handle (shaft) at the end opposite to that held by the operator (Figure 38-4).

2. *Retrieval.* Finger 4 is closed around the instrument handle and rests between fingers 3 and 4. As the unwanted instrument is lifted from the operator's hand, the dental assistant lifts the new instrument to a position slightly above the level of the operator's hand (Figure 38-5).

3. *Delivery.* The dental assistant lowers the new instrument into the operator's fingers; the delivery is complete when the operator grasps the instrument (Figure 38-6). *Note:* If the same two instruments are

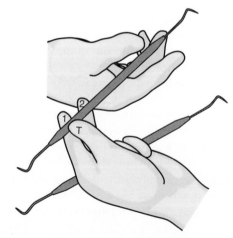

Figure 38-5 Delivery of new instrument into operator's hand.

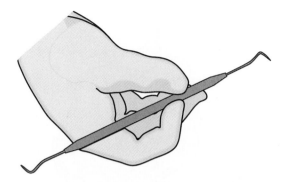

Figure 38-6 Instrument retained, fingers closed.

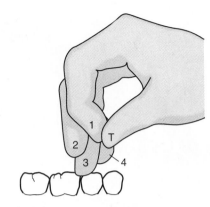

Figure 38-7 Finger rest position.

to be transferred a second time, the retrieved instrument is immediately repositioned from the little finger into the delivery finger position. One-handed instrument transfer is primarily used for hand instruments, the dental handpiece and the air-water syringe. In the transfer of the air-water syringe, the syringe is held by the nozzle tip, and the handle is delivered into the operator's hand.

Instrument Grasps

The first requirement when working within the oral cavity is to establish control of the dental instrument or handpiece. This is accomplished by the use of a **finger rest** that provides support or a point of rest for the fingers on the tooth surface (Figure 38-7).

The finger rest serves as a **fulcrum**, or base of support, for the fingers and allows the hand to move or rotate. The pad of the ring finger (3) is positioned on a given surface of a tooth, preferably in the same arch and as close to the tooth being treated as possible (Figure 38-7).

Finger rests and fulcrums, when used properly, will provide the needed stability to control the action of the instrument or dental handpiece, thereby preventing injury to the patient's oral tissues.

The most common instrument grasps used in operative dentistry are the modified pen grasp, palm grasp, and palm-thumb grasp.

Modified Pen Grasp

The conventional pen grasp is used as a foundation for the modified pen grasp. In the conventional pen grasp, the instrument is held with the thumb and index finger and the side of the middle finger.

With the modified pen grasp, the instrument is held with the same fingers, except that the pad of the middle finger (2) is held against the shank of the dental

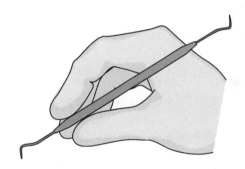

Figure 38-8 Modified pen grasp.

instrument. The ring finger acts as the finger rest and helps to hold and guide the movement of the instrument (Figure 38-8).

Palm Grasp

The handle of the instrument is held in the palm of the hand, and fingers grasp the handle of the instrument (Figure 38-9). The palm grasp is used with surgical and other types of forceps.

Palm-Thumb Grasp

The instrument is held firmly in the palm of the hand with the four fingers grasping the handle while the thumb is extended upward from the palm (Figure 38-10). This grasp is used with instruments having a straight shank and blade, such as the straight chisel or Wedelstaedt chisel.

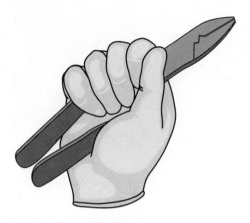

Figure 38-9 Palm grasp.

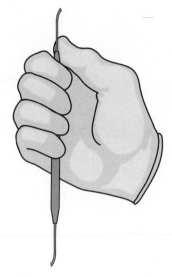

Figure 38-10 Palm-thumb grasp.

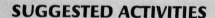

SUGGESTED ACTIVITIES

● Working in pairs; one will serve as the dental assistant, the other as the operator. Using the sequence of instrument transfer, each student will practice passing and receiving instruments.

● Practice placing a mouth mirror and explorer simultaneously into the operator's hands, assuming the operator is right handed.

● Practice exchanging forceps and the anesthetic syringe using the proper grasps.

REVIEW

1. Which finger is used in the retrieval of the instrument from the operator's hand?
   a. Index
   b. Middle
   c. Ring
   d. Little

2. Name the steps involved in passing and receiving instruments: (1) approach, (2) retrieval, (3) delivery, and/or (4) transfer.
   a. 1, 2, 3
   b. 2, 3, 4
   c. 1, 2, 4
   d. 1, 3, 4

3. Describe how the modified pen grasp is utilized.
   a. The instrument is held with the thumb, index, and middle finger pads.
   b. The instrument is held with the thumb and index finger pads and the side of the middle finger.
   c. The instrument is held with the thumb and middle finger pads.
   d. The instrument is held with the thumb and middle finger pads and the side of the index finger.

4. Identify the type of instrument whereby the palm grasp is utilized.
   a. Surgical curette
   b. Hand-cutting instrument
   c. Surgical forceps
   d. High-speed handpiece

5. What type of instrument is used with the palm-thumb grasp?
   a. Amalgam carvers
   b. Surgical scalpel
   c. Wedelstaedt chisel
   d. Hartzell instrument

Punching, Placing, and Removing a Dental Dam

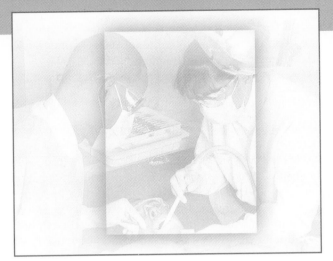

OBJECTIVES

After studying this chapter, the student will be able to:

- Select the armamentarium for both punching a dental dam and clamp placement.
- Prepare a precut square of dental dam for punching using a ruler and pen to mark the general guidelines.
- Punch a dental dam for the maxillary and mandibular arches, following the detailed instructions.

Introduction

A *dental dam* is a thin, flexible piece of latex rubber or non latex material used to isolate one or more teeth during various dental procedures. The purpose for using a dental dam is to provide an optimum working environment for the dentist and the dental assistant while protecting the patient during operative procedures.

Indications for Use

A dental dam is used in operative dentistry to maintain a clean, dry operating field while providing protection for the patient from inhaling debris and allowing the placement of various dental materials without fear of moisture contamination during a dental procedure. A dental dam aids in the retraction of the lips, tongue, and gingival tissues, allowing for better access to the field of operation during the preparation, placement, and finishing of a restoration. The use of a dental dam can be a positive step toward providing the dental patient with quality dentistry. In most recent years, the dental dam has been recognized in helping reduce transmission of infectious diseases due to **aerosolization** (infecting the atmosphere with airborne pathogens).

Contraindications

There are also contraindications, such as placing the dental dam on partially erupted teeth, **malaligned** (out of alignment) teeth, fixed bridge work, and patients who strongly resist the use of the dental dam, as might asthmatics or claustrophobics. If patients are highly sensitive or allergic to latex material, the nonlatex dental dam material should be used.

Selection of Dental Dam Materials

Dental Dam

Dental dam material may be purchased in rolls or precut sheets. The roll of dental dam is 6 inches wide and 18 feet long. It must be cut into the desired size. Precut dam is available in 5 X 5-inch sheets for children or 6 X 6-inch sheets for adults.

Dental dam may be purchased in different weights (thicknesses): (1) light, (2) medium, (3) heavy, (4) extra heavy, and (5) special heavy.

The heavier dental dam is more functional in that it is less likely to tear or be damaged by rotary instruments. It is also more effective in tissue retraction, but it is more difficult to place.

Dental dam is available in various shades. Dark gray or green dam is used because of the color contrast between the dam and tooth structure and because it reflects less light. It is available in latex rubber or nonlatex material.

Dental Dam Clamps

A *dental dam clamp* is used to anchor or secure the dental dam to a tooth, known as the **anchor tooth**. Clamps are available in various shapes and sizes and are classified according to their shape:

● *Winged clamp.* A clamp with engaging projections (Figure 39-1).

● *Wingless clamp.* A clamp without engaging projections. A W is used to identify the number of a wingless clamp, i.e., W8 (Figure 39-2).

● *Cervical clamp.* For Class V, facial restoration (Figure 39-3).

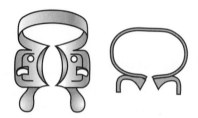

Figure 39-1 Winged clamp.

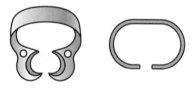

Figure 39-2 Wingless clamp.

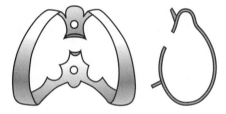

Figure 39-3 Cervical clamp.

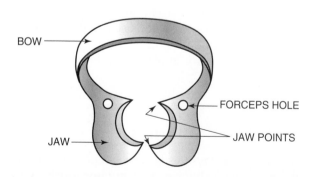

Figure 39-4 Parts of the dental dam clamp.

Parts of a wingless dental dam clamp are seen in Figure 39-4: (1) bow, (2) jaw(s), (3) forceps hole(s), and (4) jaw points.

Classification of clamps is also done according to the manufacturer, number, and use (Figure 39-5). Classification of clamps is outlined in Table 39–1.

Dental Dam Guides

The dental dam must be punched properly. Therefore, it is recommended that some type of guide be used as an aid in punching the dam. A plastic stencil or template with holes punched for the primary and permanent dentition can be used. The stencil is placed over the dam, and a pen is used for marking the holes on the dam (Figure 39-6).

In the case of a patient with malposed teeth, it is suggested that a wax bite or study model be used as a guide.

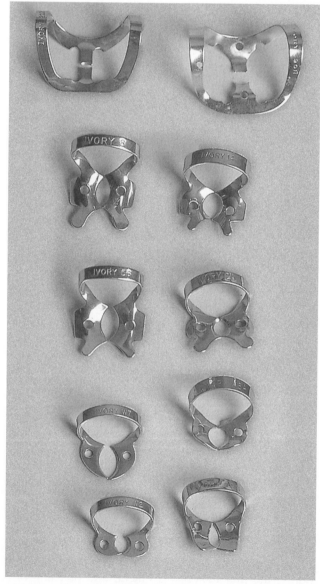

Figure 39-5 Cervical, molar, and bicuspid clamps.

Table 39-1 Assortment of Dental Clamps

Cervical Clamps	Molar Clamps
● Numbers 210, 211, 212: for Class V	● Number 2A: deciduous molars ● Number 26: molars ● Number 7: lower molars ● Number 8: upper molars

Premolar Clamps	Partially Erupted Molar Clamps
● Number 27: premolars and small third molars ● Number 00: premolar ● Number 0: small premolars ● Number 2: general purpose—premolars	● Number 8A: partially erupted molars ● Numbers 14, 14A: partially erupted molars, larger than 8A

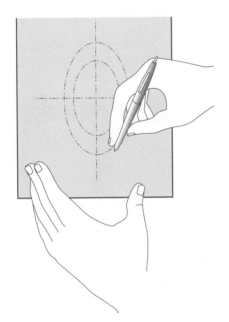

Figure 39-6 Marking holes on the dam.

The dental dam stamp has holes for the teeth embossed (raised) on the surface of the stamp and requires the use of an inked pad to transfer the pattern to the rubber dam (Figure 39-7).

Dental Dam Punch

The *dental dam punch* is designed with an adjustable wheel table or disc with five or six hole sizes. The punch must be adjusted to the proper hole size before the dam is punched. Care must be taken to align the punch point directly over the hole on the wheel table to be punched to prevent nicking the table holes and breaking or dulling the punch point (Figure 39-8).

Dental Dam Forceps

Dental dam forceps (Figure 39-9) carry the dental dam clamp to and from the tooth. The forceps beaks will spread the jaws of the dental dam clamp allowing the clamp to be positioned on the tooth. When in proper position, the handle lock is released and the forceps removed. In placing the clamp on the tooth, hold the forceps with a palm grasp (Figures 39-10 and 39-11).

Dental Dam Holders

The function of the *dental dam holder* is to maintain the position of the dam on the patient's face while holding

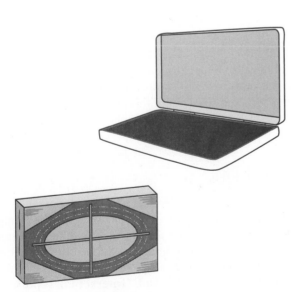

Figure 39-7 Dental dam stamp and inked pad.

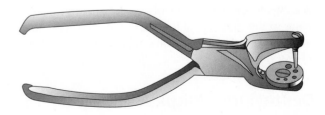

Figure 39-8 Dental dam punch.

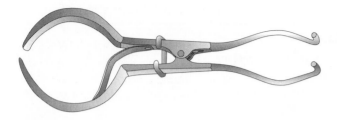

Figure 39-9 Dental dam forceps.

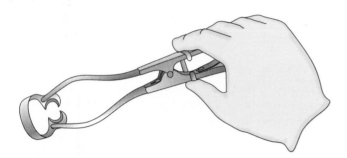

Figure 39-10 Position of forceps for mandibular arch.

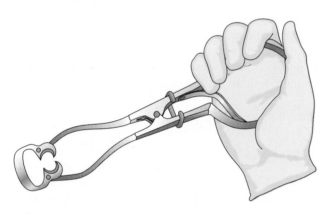

Figure 39-11 Position of forceps for maxillary arch.

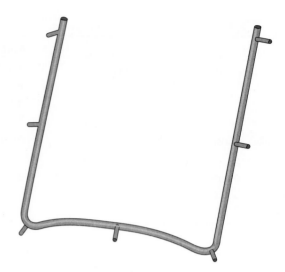

Figure 39-12 Young frame.

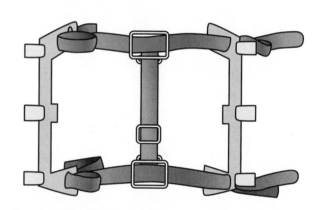

Figure 39-13 Woodbury holder.

for patient comfort and is placed underneath the dental dam to prevent the dam material from coming into contact with the patient's skin.

Inverting Instrument

Such an instrument is used to invert, or tuck, the dental dam around the teeth to prevent seepage of moisture. The instrument selected for this procedure must be dull, such as a Hartzell instrument, plastic instrument, or a beavertail burnisher

Dental Floss

At least four 18-inch lengths of waxed dental floss should be prepared. One length is placed on the clamp for ligation, another one is used to floss the teeth prior to dam placement, another one to wedge one end of the dam and a fourth one is used to aid in placement of the interseptal portion of the dam. (**interseptal/septum** is the portion of the dam located interproximally between two dental dam holes.)

the dam in place. There are basically three types of holders used to hold the dental dam in position: the Young Frame, the Ostby, and the Woodbury. The Ostby is used primarily for endodontics. The Young Frame is a metal frame that holds the rubber dam in place with projections that extend from the frame (Figure 39-12). The Woodbury uses two straps attached to two clip arms. One clip arm secures the rubber dam on one side of the face, while the straps are placed behind the patient's head, to the opposite side, where the other clip arm is fastened to the dam and the length is adjusted (Figure 39-13).

Dental Dam Napkin

The *dental dam napkin* is made from an absorbent material—paper, gauze, or flannel. The napkin is used

Scissors

The function of scissors is to cut the interseptals of the dam during removal and to cut floss used to wedge the opposing end of the dam.

Guidelines for Punching the Dental Dam

The rubber dam is prepared for punching; 6 X 6-inch precut squares are used. The dental dam is marked, using a stencil, a rubber stamp, or a pen and ruler as a guide. To mark the dental dam with a pen and ruler, the following guidelines are used as a reference:

1. The dam is divided into thirds vertically (Figure 39-14).

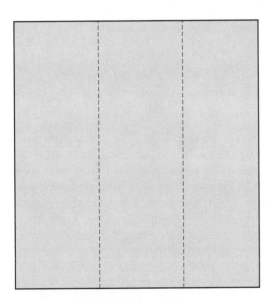

Figure 39-14 Dam is divided into thirds.

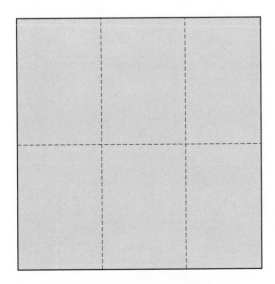

Figure 39-15 Dam is divided into half.

2. The dam is divided in half horizontally (Figure 39-15).

3. The center of the dam is marked. One inch from the upper edge of the dam is measured; this represents the upper lip line. Next, 2 inches from the lower center of the dam is measured; this represents the lower lip line (Figure 39-16).

4. Holes are punched equidistant from one another, approximately 3.5 mm. or 1/4 inch. The distance from one hole to the next should equal the distance from the middle of one tooth to the middle of the adjacent tooth. Work to be done on the maxillary arch requires that the central incisors be punched first (Figure 39-17).

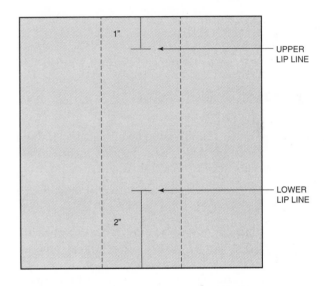

Figure 39-16 Center of the dam is marked.

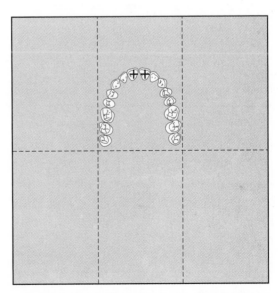

Figure 39-17 Central incisors (marked with plusses) are first to be punched in the arch.

Maxillary Arch

1. For standard positions, 1 inch from the center of the top edge of the dam is punched.
2. Variation in position:
   a. Distance from top edge of the dam should be increased for a patient with a moustache.
   b. Distance from top edge of the dam should be decreased for a patient with a very thin upper lip.
3. Remaining holes are punched following arch form.
4. Holes are punched to include cuspid on opposite side of arch.
5. For anterior tooth (teeth) being prepared, holes are punched from cuspid to cuspid.

Mandibular Arch

1. The first tooth to be punched is the clamped (anchor) tooth.
2. Mandibular first molar is positioned on the line where vertical and horizontal lines cross (Figure 39-18).
3. Hole is punched for tooth to receive clamp. If tooth other than first molar is to be the anchor tooth, adjustments must be made for clamp hole.
4. Remaining holes are punched to correspond to arch form.

Class V (Cervical Area) Restoration

1. Hole is punched for Class V restoration 1 mm facially from normal alignment (Figure 39-19). This compensates for the dam having to be stretched to fit the clamp.
2. One millimeter is allowed between the adjacent teeth in arch. *Note:* When punching the dam without the aid of a guide, care must be taken not to punch the width of the arch too shallow (flat) or too curved. In either case, the dam will not seat properly. Improper punching of the dam will result in puckering on the lingual or facial surface of the dam or in stretching the dam too taut, causing it to tear.

Guidelines for Selecting Hole Sizes

The dental dam punch has a wheel table with assorted size holes. The diameter of the hole increases with the number (Figure 39-20).

- Hole number 1—lower incisors
- Hole number 2—upper incisors
- Hole number 3—cuspids and premolars
- Hole number 4—molars
- Hole number 5—molars, and used for anchor tooth

The correct hole size on the punch plate should be selected for teeth to be isolated (Figure 39-21). Adjustment for missing or malpositioned teeth should be marked. Care should be taken in selecting the hole size. Too large a hole will result in leakage around the tooth; too small a hole will tear the dam. Clean-cut holes should be punched in the dam. There should be no dam material tags or frayed edges that would prevent the dam from properly sealing the area around the tooth from moisture or cause the dam to tear during placement.

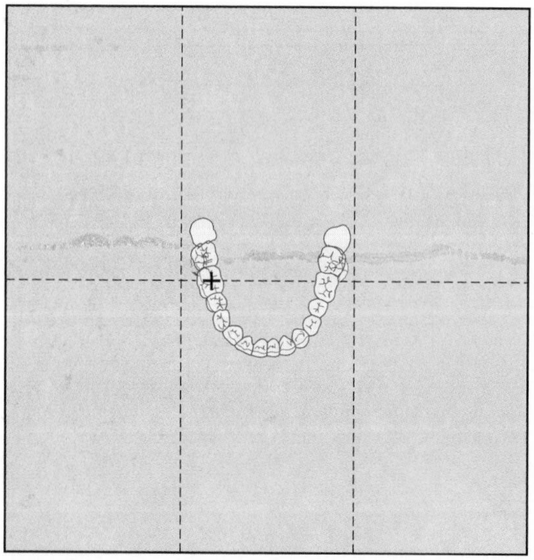

Figure 39-18 Position of mandibular first molar (marked with plus).

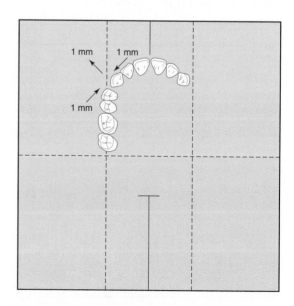

Figure 39-19 Punching a dam for a Class V.

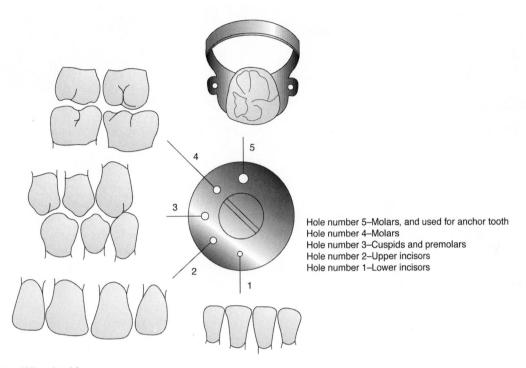

Hole number 5–Molars, and used for anchor tooth
Hole number 4–Molars
Hole number 3–Cuspids and premolars
Hole number 2–Upper incisors
Hole number 1–Lower incisors

Figure 39-20 Wheel table.

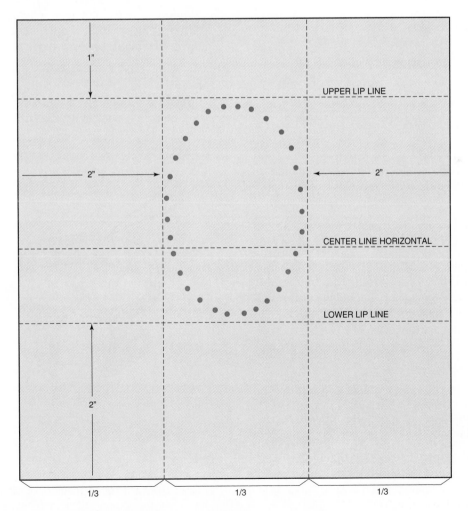

Figure 39-21 Diagram to facilitate punching the dental dam.

Procedure 28 Placing and Removing the Dental Dam

Materials Needed

Dental dam
Dental dam punch
Dental dam forceps
Dental dam clamp(s)
Dental dam holder—Woodbury, Ostby, or Young Frame
Dental dam napkin
Dental floss (ligature), four 18-inch lengths
Lubricant, water-soluble shaving cream or greaseless lubricant
Vaseline (patient's lips)
Cotton roll
Inversion instrument (beavertail, Hartzell, or plastic instrument)
Crown and collar scissors
Stick compound
Matches
Bunsen burner
Basic set (mouth mirror, explorer, cotton pliers)

Instructions

Placement

1 Explain the procedure to the patient. Examine the patient's mouth and check the position of the teeth; note any deviation in alignment and size of teeth.

2 Check contact or interproximal areas with dental floss (ligature). Teeth and soft tissue should be free of debris, plaque, and calculus.

3 Tie a piece of dental floss around the bow of the clamp as a safety precaution. Should the clamp slip off the tooth accidentally, the floss provides a means for retrieving it (Figure 39-22).

4 Select and try-in ligated clamp(s). The clamp jaws must rest securely on the tooth.

5 Punch a dental dam for teeth to be isolated.

6 Punch an identification hole in the upper right corner of the dam.

7 Lubricate the dam. Use a water-soluble shaving cream or a greaseless lubricant. The lubricant is applied to the undersurface of the dam. This aids in the placement of the dam.

8 Lubricate the patient's lips with vaseline.

9 Position clamp on anchor tooth with the bow of the clamp toward the distal surface of the tooth. When the clamp is placed on the tooth, position the lingual jaw of the clamp at the cervical surface (neck of tooth); then seat the facial jaw of clamp. Both points on each jaw must be in contact with the tooth to ensure its stability preventing it from rocking (Figure 39-22). Care should be taken not to impinge on the gingival tissue with the clamp.

10 Using forefingers of both hands, ease the punched dental dam by positioning the anchor hole over the bow of clamp, then under the jaws.

11 Slip the dam over the cuspid on the opposite side of the arch, and secure it with waxed dental floss. Fashion a loose knot in a length of dental floss. Slip over the cuspid. Tighten knot, making certain the floss remains on the topside of the dental dam.

12 When the holder is positioned, place the dam napkin as detailed earlier. Carefully pull dam material through the opening of the napkin. Arrange the napkin so it is flat against the patient's face (Figure 39-23).

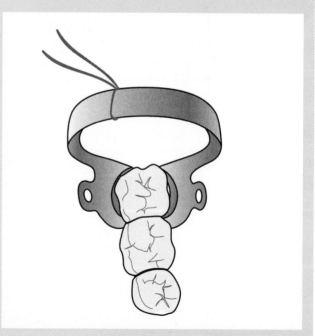

Figure 39-22 Proper position for clamp.

continued

continued from previous page
Procedure 28 Placing and Removing the Dental Dam

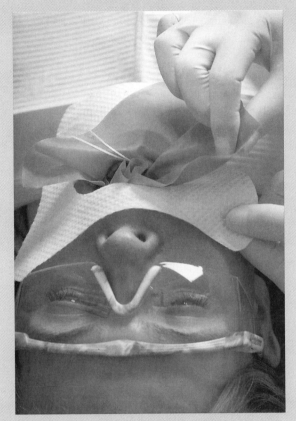

Figure 39-23 Dental dam napkin placement.

13 Fasten two clips on one side of the dental dam when using the Woodbury holder. Pass straps of holder around the back of patient's head and fasten the clips of the straps on the opposite side.

14 Complete dam placement.
 a. Stretch the remaining dam holes over the respective teeth to be isolated.
 b. Use a knifing action to pass the dam septa through the contact areas.
 c. With another piece of dental floss, pass the floss through the contact areas to help seat the dam. *Note:* If the Young Frame is used, secure dam to the frame by the projections on the frame.

15 **Invert/invaginate** ("tuck" or fold the raw edges of the dental dam holes that surround the isolated teeth to prevent moisture contamination) lingually and facially using a suitable inversion instrument, such as beavertail burnisher or a Hartzell instrument. A fulcrum is essential for better instrument control. Take the air syringe, and direct a stream of air on each tooth while the instrument inverts the edges of the dam.

16 Should the clamp require further stability, softened stick compound may be applied to the bow of the clamp and tooth. The compound is softened in an open flame until it bends, then placed in warm water and used.

17 Place saliva ejector. The saliva ejector may be placed under the dental dam in the floor of the mouth, on the opposite side of the arch from the working area. An alternative is to cut a small hole in the dam just behind the mandibular incisors and place the saliva ejector tip through the hole in the dam.

Note: Other techniques for placing a dental dam may be used, such as placing the bow of the clamp through the anchor hole in the dam first, then positioning the dam and clamp on the tooth as a unit. Once the clamp is securely placed on the tooth, the dam is slipped over the jaws of the clamp.

Removal

1 Remove saliva ejector.

2 To remove the dam, use scissors to cut the dental floss tie from opposing cuspid. Proceed to cut each septum of the dental dam. This is done by stretching the dam toward the facial surface and placing a finger under the dam by each septum (interseptal) as it is being cut. Tips of the scissors should be directed away fromthe arch. Cut each septum of the dental dam with one quick snip. Using this procedure protects the gingival tissue from being accidentally cut.

3 Remove the dental dam clamp with forceps.

4 Remove the dental dam holder.

5 Remove the dental dam and the napkin. With napkin, wipe area around the patient's mouth.

6 Inspect the dam to determineif all of its parts are intact. No tags of dental dam should be missing; no bits of dental dam should remain between teeth or in the sulcus; if so, check interproximal areas of teeth with dental floss. Remnants of a dental dam often cause periodontal problems.

7 Gently massage gingival tissue.

8 Rinse patient's mouth with warm water.

For better access and visibility, the dam should be punched two teeth distally from the tooth to be treated and across to the cuspid on the opposite side of the arch. A minimum of three teeth must be isolated, except in endodontic treatment, when a single tooth is isolated.

Care of Dental Dam Armamentarium

1. Dental floss tie should be removed from the bow of the clamp. The clamp, inverting instrument, and Young Frame should be washed with soap and water or placed in an ultrasonic unit to remove debris. Then they should be dried and prepared for the autoclave.

2. The dental dam punch, forceps, and scissors should be wiped with an antibacterial cleaner, dried thoroughly, and prepared for autoclave. (It is preferred to use a chemical autoclave to avoid rust formation on hinged instruments.)

SUGGESTED ACTIVITIES

- Prepare precut squares of dental dam for punching. Use ruler and pen to mark using general guidelines.

- Practice punching a dental dam for the maxillary and mandibular arch until you can punch a dam properly and with ease and confidence.

- Practice placing and removing a dental dam on a mannequin.

- Place and remove a dental dam from the following teeth to be treated: maxillary right first premolar, mandibular left first molar, mandibular left central incisor, and maxillary left lateral incisor.

- If state law permits, practice placing and removing a dental dam on classmate or patients.

REVIEW

1. Give the advantages for using a heavier dental dam material: (1) less likely to tear, (2) easier to place interproximally, (3) less likely to be damaged by rotary instruments, and/or (4) more effective in tissue retraction.
   a. 1, 2, 3
   b. 2, 3, 4
   c. 1, 2, 4
   d. 1, 3, 4

2. Give two reasons why the holes of the dam should be punched cleanly: (1) to prevent dam from tearing, (2) to ensure proper sealing of the area around the tooth, (3) to ensure proper size of hole, and/or (4) to ensure proper inverting of the dam.
   a. 1, 2
   b. 2, 3
   c. 3, 4
   d. 1, 4

3. Why is it advisable to punch a dental dam to include the opposing cuspid?
   a. To have adequate interproximal spacing
   b. To have better access and visibility
   c. To be able to work on more teeth
   d. To allow the holder to be better positioned

4. Why should dental floss be tied to the bow of the clamp?
   a. To provide a means of support to the clamp
   b. To ease the clamp on the tooth during its placement
   c. To provide a means for retrieving the clamp should it become dislodged
   d. To establish a means of locating the clamp at the time of removal of the dam

5. Indicate the purpose of directing a stream of air while inverting the dam.
   a. To cool the tooth down while inverting the dam
   b. To blow away debris that may accumulate during dam placement
   c. To dry the field of operation enabling the dam to stay inverted

6. In which direction should the bow of the clamp be positioned on a molar tooth?
   a. mesially
   b. distally

Assembling and Placing a Tofflemire Matrix Band and Retainer

OBJECTIVES

After studying this chapter, the student will be able to:

● Identify the parts of the Tofflemire matrix retainer.

● Prepare and assemble a Tofflemire retainer and matrix band for a designated maxillary and mandibular tooth.

● Apply the principles of wedging.

Introduction

The most common and generally accepted matrix retainer used today is the Tofflemire. The Tofflemire has two parts: the **retainer** and the **matrix band**. The retainer is a device used to hold and stabilize the matrix band. The matrix band is a contoured, thin strip of stainless steel and is used to form the missing wall(s) of a prepared tooth (Class II). It helps establish proper anatomic contour and restores correct proximal contact.

Parts of the Tofflemire Retainer

The parts of a Tofflemire retainer are as follows (Figure 40-1):

● *Frame.* The main body of the retainer to which the vise, spindle, and adjustment knobs are attached.

● *Vise.* Holds the ends of the matrix band in the diagonal slot.

● *Guide slots.* Enable the matrix band loop to be positioned to the right or left of the retainer.

● *Spindle.* A screwlike rod with a pointed tip used to lock the ends of the matrix band in the vise.

● *Outer knob or set screw.* Used to tighten or loosen the spindle against the matrix band in the vise.

● *Inner knob.* Used to slide the vise along the frame to either increase or decrease the size of the matrix band loop.

Tofflemire Matrix Bands

Matrix bands are supplied in assorted sizes for use with the Tofflemire retainer.

● *Universal band* (Figure 40-2)

● *Medium band* (Figure 40-3)

● *Medium mesio-occlusal-distal (MOD)* (Figure 40-4)

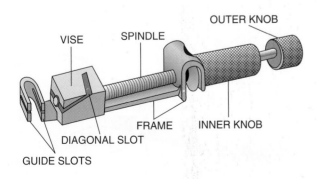

Figure 40-1 Parts of the Tofflemire retainer.

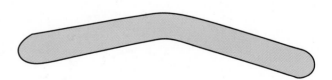

Figure 40-2 Universal band.

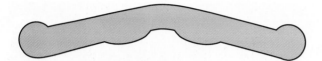

Figure 40-3 Medium band.

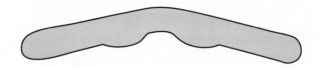

Figure 40-4 Medium MOD band.

The universal matrix band is used for premolars and molars with moderate gingival MOD extensions, and the medium and wide bands are used for deep MOD gingival extensions. Observe Figure 40-5 to determine the occlusal and gingival edge of the matrix band.

The highest curve of the matrix band is the occlusal edge and the inner curve is the gingival edge.

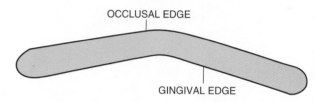

OCCLUSAL EDGE

GINGIVAL EDGE

Figure 40-5 Occlusal and gingival edges of band.

Procedure 29 Tofflemire Placement

Materials Needed

Tofflemire retainer
Matrix band(s)
Wedge(s) wood/plastic
Ball burnisher
Cotton or lab pliers
Mouth mirror

Instructions

Assembling the Tofflemire Retainer

1 Prepare the retainer to receive the matrix band. Hold the retainer so that the *diagonal slot* of the vise is visible (Figure 40-6).

2 Turn the *inner knob* (Figure 40-7), counterclockwise until the vise is positioned next to the guide slots. To accomplish this, the spindle tip must be inserted in the vise.

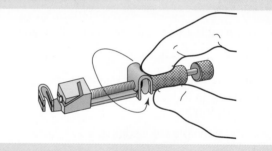

Figure 40-7 Inner knob of retainer.

3 Turn the *outer knob* (Figure 40-8), clockwise until the point of the spindle is barely visible in the diagonal slot.

4 With the opposite hand select the appropriate matrix band. The band should be determined according to the quadrant and before threading the band.

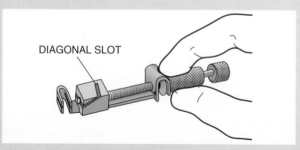

DIAGONAL SLOT

Figure 40-6 Diagonal slot of vise.

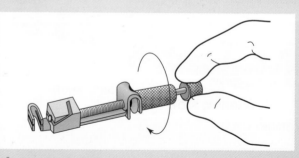

Figure 40-8 Outer knob of retainer.

continued

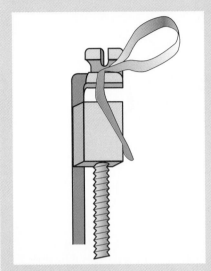

Figure 40-9 Loop in place for maxillary right.

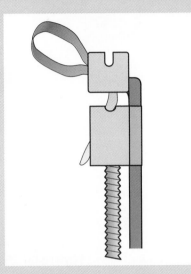

Figure 40-10 Loop in place for mandibular left.

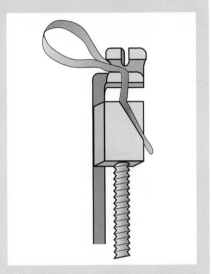

Figure 40-11 Loop in place for maxillary left.

In preparing the matrix, use the patient's maxillary arch and the operator's right and left hand as a reference guide. The retainer/band may be used interchangeably for the maxillary and mandibular quadrants. If the retainer/band is to be used for the maxillary right quadrant (Figure 40-9), it may also be used for the mandibular left quadrant by merely inverting the retainer (Figure 40-10). To load the retainer for the maxillary right and mandibular left quadrants, the loop of the matrix band will be directed toward the operator's right hand. To load the retainer for the maxillary left and mandibular right quadrants, the loop of the matrix band will be directed toward the operator's left hand. The retainer/band for the maxillary left quadrant (Figure 40-11), may be used for the mandibular right quadrant by inverting the retainer (Figure 40-12).

5 With opposite hand, hold the matrix band with the occlusal edge pointed toward the floor (Figure 40-13).

6 Loop the band end-to-end between thumb and forefinger. Hold joined ends together, allowing the band to remain in a tear-shaped loop and without a crease (Figure 40-14).

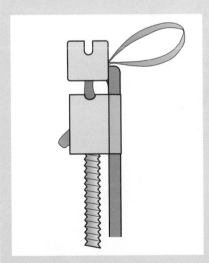

Figure 40-12 Loop in place for mandibular right.

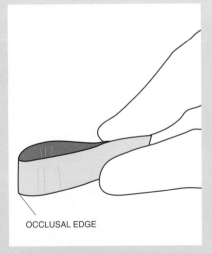

OCCLUSAL EDGE

Figure 40-13 Occlusal edge of band directed toward floor.

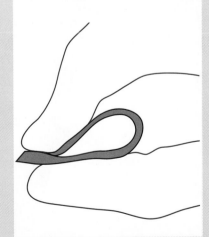

Figure 40-14 Folding ends of band to form loop.

continued

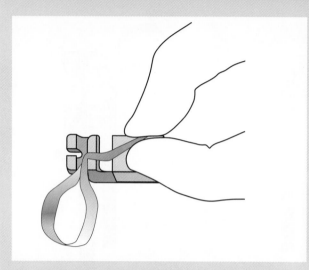

Figure 40-15 Band positioned in diagonal slot.

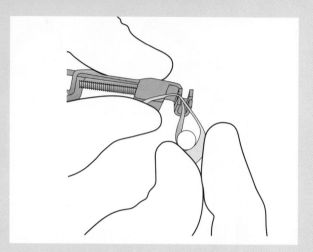

Figure 40-16 Contouring matrix band with instrument handle.

7 Slide the joined ends of the band into the diagonal slot of the vise (Figure 40-15). Continue threading the joined band so that it emerges from between the prongs of the guide slot according to Instructions.

8 Turn the outer knob clockwise until the tip of the spindle engages the matrix.

9 Use the handle of the mouth mirror to contour the band (Figure 40-16).

Placing the Retainer

1 Place the loop around the prepared tooth (gingival edge first), with the retainer frame parallel to the buccal surfaces of the teeth and with the slotted portion of the retainer facing the gingiva. This will place the loop lingually around the tooth (Figure 41-17).

2 Seat the loop into the interproximals, using one finger of one hand to stabilize the retainer. With the other hand, tighten the inner knob of the retainer by turning clockwise to close the band around the tooth (Figure 40-18). Sometimes jiggling the retainer

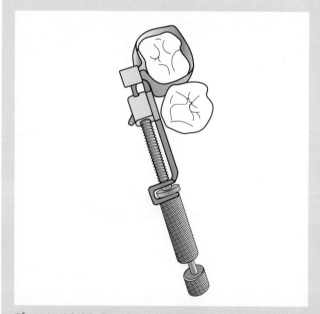

Figure 40-17 Positioning the loop on the tooth.

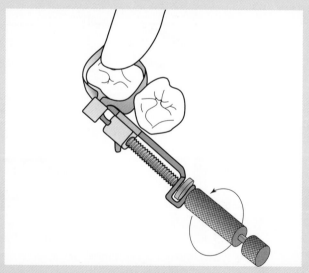

Figure 40-18 Stabilizing the loop.

continued

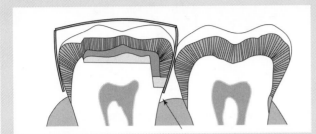

Figure 40-19 Cross section of matrix band, gingival margin.

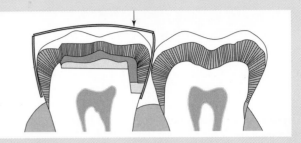

Figure 40-21 Cross section showing height of matrix band.

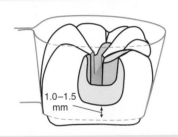

Figure 40-20 Distance between gingival margin of band and gingival step, 1.0–1.5 mm.

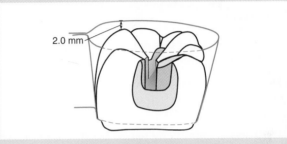

2.0 mm

Figure 40-22 Distance between highest cusp of tooth and occlusal border, 2.0 mm.

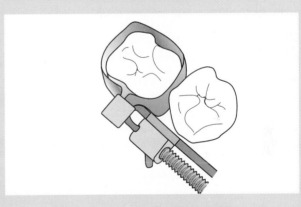

Figure 40-23 Band too tight, lacking contour.

is necessary to carry the gingival edge of the band past the gingival margin of the preparation.

3 Check to see that the guide slot is centered on the buccal of the tooth.

4 The matrix band should extend no more than 1.0–1.5 mm below the gingival margin of the preparation (Figures 40-19 and 40-20). The matrix band should extend no more than 2.0 mm above the highest cusp of the tooth (Figures 40-21 and 40-22).

5 Adapting the band is necessary to ensure contact with adjacent teeth. To adapt the band, use the ball burnisher, and contour the inner surface of the band so it is slightly concave at the contact area of the prepared tooth.

6 Check the band for tightness. A band drawn too tightly will produce a flat contour lacking in correct proximal contact (Figure 40-23). Too loose a band will cause an overcontoured restoration (Figure 40-24). Either may result in a change in anatomic contour and/or incorrect proximal contact.

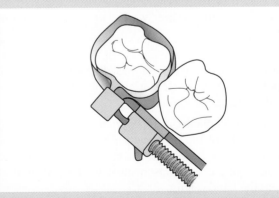

Figure 40-24 Band too loose, causing overcontoured band.

continued

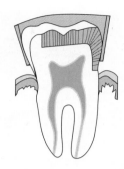

Figure 40-25 Band does not extend beyond tooth preparation.

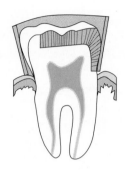

Figure 40-26 Band extends only to step of preparation.

Problems of Improper Band Placement

1. Band is not seated beyond the gingival step of the preparation (Figure 40-25).
2. The band width is too narrow and does not extend beyond the gingival step of the preparation (Figure 40-26).
3. The band is improperly seated because it impinges on the dental dam (Figure 40-27).
4. The band is improperly seated because it impinges on the gingival tissue (Figure 40-28).

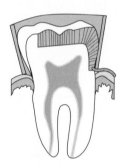

Figure 40-27 Band impinges on dental dam.

Wedging the Matrix Band

Once the matrix band has been placed on the tooth, a **wedge** is used to stabilize the matrix band. Wedges are wooden or plastic and triangular in shape and come in assorted sizes. Wedges are inserted between the teeth after the matrix band is placed around the tooth. Wedge(s) act as a brace to hold the matrix band against the tooth and prevent overhangs of restorative material. Wedge(s) separate the teeth slightly to compensate for the thickness of the matrix band.

1. The size of the embrasure(s) involved should be noted and the proper wedge(s) selected (Figure 40-29).
2. A wedge is generally placed in the lingual embrasure. Wedges are placed mesially (M), distally (D), or both if the restoration is MOD. Occasionally, buccal wedging is required.
3. With cotton pliers the appropriate wedge is chosen. The beaks of the instrument are used to grasp the wedge at the base. The wedge is inserted into the linguo-gingival embrasure next to the preparation and the band (Figure 40-30).
4. The base of the wedge should fit snugly on the gingival crest (Figure 40-31), with the point of the wedge directed into the lingual embrasure.

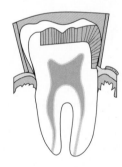

Figure 40-28 Band impinges on gingival tissue.

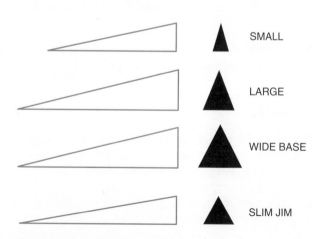

SMALL

LARGE

WIDE BASE

SLIM JIM

Figure 40-29 Wedge shapes and sizes.

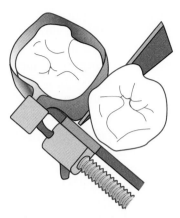

Figure 40-30 Wedge placed in lingual embrasure.

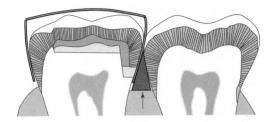

Figure 40-31 Cross section of tooth with band and wedge in proper position.

Problems with Improper Wedging

1. Improper placement of the wedge results in an overhang of the finished restoration.

2. If the matrix band is not wedged firmly enough to slightly separate the adjacent teeth, the restorative material will not provide a proper contact with the adjacent tooth.

3. When the matrix is not wedged properly, the restorative material will not provide the desired contact, contour, and protection of the interproximal gingiva.

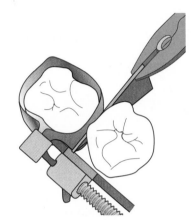

Figure 40-32 Removing wedge.

Removing the Wedge and Matrix

1. To remove the wedge, cotton or lab pliers are used to grasp the wedge at the base, and the wedge is removed from the lingual embrasure (Figure 40-32).

2. Holding the matrix firmly in place with the finger(s) of one hand (Figure 40-33), the *outer knob* of the retainer is slowly turned counterclockwise with the opposite hand.

3. The ends of the matrix band are loosened from the retainer.

4. The retainer is slowly removed toward the occlusal and away from the gingiva. Thus, the holder is removed, while the band remains in place.

5. Using cotton or lab pliers, the ends of the band are gently freed from around the tooth (Figure 40-34).

6. With fingers, either the mesial or distal portion of the band is grasped.

7. The matrix band is gently lifted from the proximal surface(s) of the restoration in an occluso-lingual direction using a rocking motion. *Note:* If possible, the side of the matrix band that is away from the restored proximal surface should be removed first.

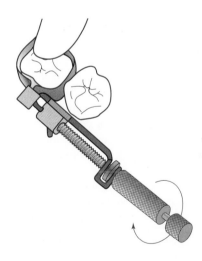

Figure 40-33 Removing retainer while stabilizing band.

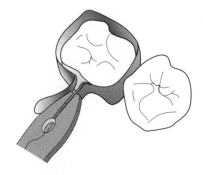

Figure 40-34 Removing band from tooth.

SUGGESTED ACTIVITIES

● Practice assembling the Tofflemire retainer and matrix band for maxillary and mandibular first molars.

● Use a typodont to practice placing a Tofflemire retainer/band on the following teeth: maxillary right first molar, mandibular left first molar, maxillary left first molar, and mandibular right first molar.

● Practice wedge placement with the Tofflemire retainer in place.

● Practice removal of wedge, retainer, and matrix band.

REVIEW

1. Match the parts of the matrix band retainer with their function.

   ___ a. Vise
   ___ b. Inner knob
   ___ c. Outer knob
   ___d. Spindle
   ___e. Guide slots
   ___f. Frame

1. A screwlike rod with a pointed tip used to lock the ends of the matrix band in the vise
2. Holds the ends of the matrix band in the diagonal slot
3. The main body of the retainer to which the vise, spindle, and adjustment knobs are attached
4. Used to slide the vise along the frame to either increase or decrease the size of the matrix band loop
5. Used to tighten or loosen the spindle against the matrix band in the vise
6. Slots that enable the matrix band loop to be positioned to the right or left of the retainer

2. What is the purpose of a matrix band?
   a. To provide a bevel at the gingival step
   b. To form the missing wall(s) of a prepared tooth
   c. To allow the placement of an amalgam restoration
   d. To stabilize the tooth during the placement of a restoration

3. When placing the Tofflemire, what should be the position of the retainer frame?
   a. Parallel to the lingual surfaces of the teeth with the slotted portion of the retainer facing occlusally
   b. Parallel to the facial surfaces of the teeth with the slotted portion of the retainer facing occlusally
   c. Parallel to the facial surfaces of the teeth with the slotted portion of the retainer facing gingivally
   d. Parallel to the lingual surfaces of the teeth with the slotted portion of the retainer facing gingivally

4. What is the purpose of using a wedge?
   a. To prevent an overcontoured restoration
   b. To prevent an undercontoured restoration
   c. To adapt the matrix band to the tooth
   d. To brace and hold the matrix band against the tooth to prevent overhangs

5. What outcome will a band drawn too tightly produce?
   a. An overcontoured restoration
   b. An undercontoured restoration
   c. An open proximal contact
   d. b, c
   e. a, c

Cavity Varnish, Liners, Calcium Hydroxide, and Dental Cements

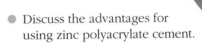

CHAPTER
41

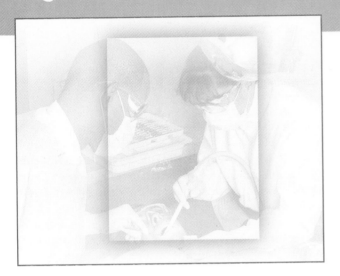

- Discuss the advantages for using zinc polyacrylate cement.
- Prepare a mix of zinc polyacrylate cement for cementation.
- Recognize the proper consistency of zinc polyacrylate for cementation.
- State the advantages for using zinc oxide eugenol cement.
- State the advantage for using reinforced zinc oxide cement over the conventional zinc oxide eugenol cement.
- Prepare zinc oxide eugenol cement for a base.
- Prepare zinc oxide eugenol cement for a temporary restoration.

OBJECTIVES

After studying this chapter, the student will be able to:

- Define the composition of a cavity varnish.
- Explain the difference between a cavity varnish and a cavity liner.
- Describe the basic technique for applying a cavity varnish.
- Select the materials needed to prepare calcium hydroxide for a base.
- Prepare calcium hydroxide for a base.
- Describe the technique for applying a cavity varnish to a prepared tooth.
- Describe the technique for applying a liner to a prepared tooth.
- Demonstrate the application of a varnish, base, and temporary restoration on a prepared stone model.
- Explain why water is the most critical ingredient in the zinc phosphate cement liquid.
- List the steps that can be used to reduce the exothermic reaction when spatulating zinc phosphate cement.
- Discuss the reason for using a cool glass slab when mixing zinc phosphate cement.
- State the purpose for using a thin-consistency mix when seating a permanent restoration.

Introduction

A *cavity varnish* is a special liquid used in conjunction with dental cements and restorative materials.

A *cavity liner* is used in the deepest portion and walls of the prepared cavity to seal dentinal tubules and also for pulp capping.

Calcium hydroxide is a cement-type material, considered to be a liner/base, used in deep cavities and for microscopic pulp exposures or near exposures. The benefit of calcium hydroxide is its therapeutic effect on the pulp, for it tends to stimulate the formation of secondary dentin—the most effective barrier to any further irritants.

Zinc phosphate is commonly referred to as a *crown* and *bridge cement*. Zinc phosphate can be used as an insulating base under restorations and for permanent **luting**, or cementation, of metallic restorations such as crowns, inlays, onlays, fixed bridges, and orthodontic appliances. However, it is noted for its irritating effect to the pulp.

Zinc polyacrylate (carboxylate or polycarboxylate) is used for cementation of permanent restorations, orthodontic bands, and bases under other types of restorations. The cement is manufactured with powder and liquid components.

Zinc oxide eugenol (ZOE) cement is noted for its sedative or soothing effect on the dental pulp. It is used as an insulating base to protect the pulp against mechanical

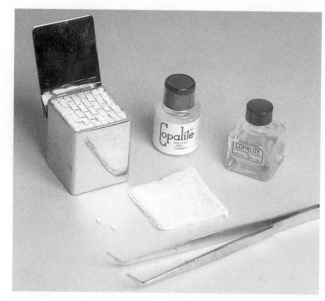

Figure 41-1A Cavity varnish, solvent, cotton pellets, and cotton pliers for placement.

and thermal trauma, for cementation of treatment restorations, for temporary restorations before permanent restorations are placed, and for root canal fillings.

Cavity Varnish

The varnish is composed either of a natural gum or resin (e.g., copal) or of a synthetic resin dissolved in an organic solvent of acetone, chloroform, or ether (Figure 41-1A).

After the varnish is applied to a cavity preparation, the solvent evaporates, leaving a thin film on the tooth surface that seals the exposed dentinal tubules against chemical irritants from certain cements and restorative materials. The varnish acts as a **semipermeable membrane**, preventing the passage of acids from the cements along the dentinal tubules to the pulp. A cavity varnish may also be applied when placing an amalgam restoration, because the varnish aids in reducing the number of metallic ions penetrating the tissues of the dentin and enamel, thus minimizing the discoloration of the tooth structure next to the restoration.

Therefore, cavity varnish is used for the following reasons:

- It prevents tooth sensitivity by sealing open dentinal tubuli.
- It acts as a semipermeable membrane, preventing acids from cements to enter dentinal tubuli.
- It aids in preventing tooth discoloration by impeding metallic ions from penetrating dentinal tissues.

The use of a cavity varnish depends on the type of cement or restorative material to be used. It is suggested

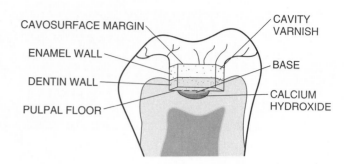

Figure 41-1B Cavity varnish applied after calcium hydroxide and base.

that the cavity varnish be applied prior to the placement of zinc phosphate cement, amalgams, and gold foil restorations. A cavity varnish is applied after calcium hydroxide—zinc oxide/carboxylate cement base (Figure 41-1B). A varnish is applied to the enamel and dentin walls up to the cavosurface margin.

A cavity varnish may be used with certain **composite restorations** (tooth colored resin restorative material), but as specified by the manufacturer; otherwise, it may interfere with the setting reaction of the material.

Varnishes that do not contain *copal* are selected to be used under composite restorations. Copal is known to interfere with the setting reaction of composite, glass ionomer, or resin restorations.

To be effective, a varnish must be thin, enabling it to flow over and seal the dentinal tubules. If the varnish becomes too thick to use, thinner may be added to the solvent, since a thick layer will not seal the tubules as well (see Table 42-1 for examples).

Cavity Liner

Another type of cavity sealant, called a *cavity liner*, is available. It is different from a cavity varnish in that it contains either calcium hydroxide or zinc oxide suspended in a solvent of natural or **synthetic** (man-made) resins. The liner is applied to the cavity preparation in the same manner as a cavity varnish. However, the liner must not go beyond the dentinoenamel junction of the preparation, because it will eventually dissolve and cause marginal leakage (Figure 41-2).

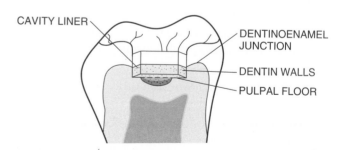

Figure 41-2 Application of a liner.

Procedure 30 Cavity Varnish Application

Materials Needed

Cavity varnish
Cotton pellet
Cotton pliers or disposable applicator pipette
Cotton roll

Instructions

1 Clean and dry the cavity preparation.

2 Select a cotton pellet for size of preparation.

3 Remove cap from varnish bottle. Quickly take cotton pliers with pellet and touch surface of varnish until pellet is moistened. Replace cap. Should pellet become saturated with excess varnish, press pellet against cotton roll to remove excess. *Note:* The cap of the bottle must be replaced immediately after each application; otherwise, the solvent will evaporate and the remaining solvent will become thick.

4 Apply varnish to the cavity preparation. Coat the entire surface of the preparation, dentin and enamel. It is not necessary to remove the varnish from the cavosurface margins of the tooth.

5 Dry with a gentle stream of air, using air syringe, for 15–20 seconds.

6 Apply second application of varnish. Two successive applications are necessary to provide a continuous layer without voids. A third application may be desired. To prevent cross-contamination when multiple applications are made, a clean disposable applicator pipette should be used each time. If an instrument is used, a clean uncontaminated instrument with a new cotton pellet must be used.

7 Dispose of cotton pellet in appropriate waste receptacle; clean and sterilize cotton pliers or applicator.

Cavity liners are supplied as zinc oxide type in which there are two pastes that are mixed into a homogenous mix that set up once placed in the cavity. They are also supplied as a single paste that is light cured after being placed in the cavity (see Table 42-1 for examples).

Calcium Hydroxide

Although classified as cement, calcium hydroxide is placed in the deepest portion of the cavity preparation where it stimulates the production of secondary dentin that aids in repairing dentin. It is supplied as a two-paste system, a *base* and a *catalyst* which are dispensed in equal amounts and mixed together to begin a setting reaction (Figure 41-3A). It is also supplied as a single paste that contains a polymer resin (similar to that of composites) that requires the blue light for a quick-setting reaction. It is considered to be more stable than the two-paste system and is not harmful to the pulp.

As a rule, the thicker the dentin, whether primary or secondary, between the surface of the cavity and the pulp, the better the protection from chemical and physical trauma. However, when a cavity penetrates the dentinoenamel junction more than 0.5 mm, calcium hydroxide is the ideal choice for a base (see Table 42-1 for examples).

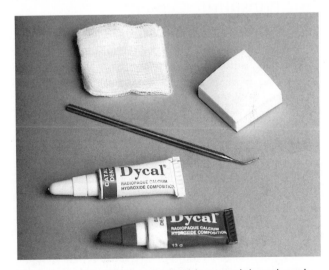

Figure 41-3A Calcium hydroxide material, pad, and small ball burnisher used for placement.

Calcium hydroxide is placed in the deepest portion of the preparation (Figure 41-3B), approximately 0.5–1.0 mm in thickness. With some calcium hydroxide–based cements (aqueous type), this layer does not provide sufficient hardness or strength to warrant its use alone as a base in a deep cavity. For this reason, it is usually overlaid with a stronger cement in order to provide protection against the forces of condensation and mastication.

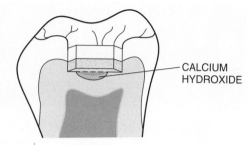

CALCIUM
HYDROXIDE

Figure 41-3B Application of calcium hydroxide.

Composition

Suspensions of calcium hydroxide are of two types: aqueous or nonaqueous. **Aqueous** (containing water) calcium hydroxide is formed when calcium hydroxide powder is mixed with distilled water. Nonaqueous calcium hydroxide contains calcium hydroxide and zinc oxide powder suspended in a chloroform solution of a natural or synthetic resin.

The light-cured calcium hydroxide is composed of urethane dimethacrylate that is activated by the visible blue light for a quick-setting reaction.

Dental Cements

Zinc Phosphate Cement

The cement is supplied as powder and liquid that must be mixed together by hand on a cool glass slab. The principal constituent of zinc phosphate powder is zinc oxide, plus a small amount of magnesium oxide. Zinc phosphate powders are available based on particle size, Type I and Type II.

Type I is a fine-grain cement powder that when spatulated with the liquid forms a thin-film thickness. **Film thickness** (thickness of cement) is an important factor in the seating of gold or porcelain restorations. The reason for this is that the thin layer of cement will flow into the minute internal surface irregularities of the cast restoration and the retentive features of the tooth preparation, resulting in greater retention.

Type II is a medium-grain powder that may be used as a posterior temporary restoration.

The liquid is principally orthophosphoric acid and water and, therefore, irritating to the pulp. The water content of the liquid is carefully established by the manufacturer; this must be maintained. When dispensing the liquid, the cap should not be left off the bottle, nor should the liquid be placed on the mixing slab for any period of time. Water content of the liquid may either evaporate or gain water if the relative **humidity** (amount of water in the air) is high. In either case, the setting time and properties of the cement will be affected.

The liquid may or may not contain zinc salts that act as a buffering agent. A buffer will counteract the effects of the acid in the liquid and improve its storage behavior.

When the powder and liquid are mixed, a chemical reaction occurs, and heat is released. This reaction is called **exothermic** (*exo-* = "outer", *thermos* = "heat"). As heat is produced, it speeds up the reaction even more. To reduce this reaction, and provide reasonable working time, any heat created must be **dissipated** (driven off) by spatulating over a large area.

To slow the exothermic reaction (to help dissipate the heat), the following steps may be taken during mixing:

- A cool glass slab is used.

- The mix is spread over a large area of the glass slab.

- **Increments** (small portions) of powder are added to the liquid.

These steps will affect to some degree the setting time.

Zinc phosphate cement must be mixed on a glass slab, never on a paper pad. The paper pad will not dissipate the heat of the mix. A thicker mix will set faster than a thin mix, with less powder.

The American Dental Association's (ADA) specifications for zinc phosphate cement state that the setting time is in the range of 5–9 minutes. Of all the mixing of cements used in dentistry, mixing of zinc phosphate cement is more critical, and each procedural step must be followed.

Procedure 32 Mixing Zinc Phosphate Cement

Materials Needed

Zinc phosphate powder
Zinc phosphate liquid
Spatula—metal
Dappen dish
Paper towels
Sodium bicarbonate solution

Instructions

1 Place clean spatula and cool glass slab on paper towel, along with the powder and liquid (Figure 41-4). The temperature of the glass the slab should be approximately 65–75°F (18–24°C). In selecting the powder and liquid, check to see that the brand of cement is the same for each bottle.

2 Shake powder before removing cap.

3 Place appropriate amount of powder onto the right end of the slab (left side if you are left-handed (Figure 41-5). The amount of powder to be used is determined by the liquid–powder ratio and the amount of cement required for the procedure.

4 Level powder with flat side of the spatula blade into a layer about 1 mm thick.

5 Divide powder into two equal portions with the spatula; divide each of these into quarters, then the first eighth into sixteenths, and the last quarter into eighths (Figure 41-6).

6 Shake liquid. Dispense liquid from dropper bottle according to powder–liquid ratio required for

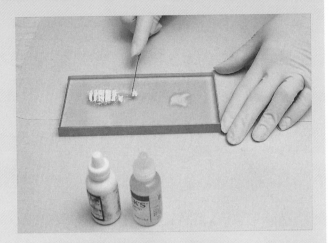
Figure 41-4 Assembling of materials.

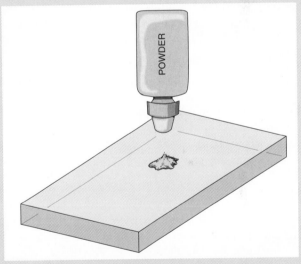
Figure 41-5 Dispensing powder onto glass slab.

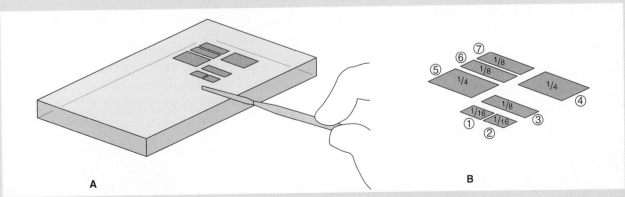
Figure 41-6 (A) Powder divided into increments. (B) Powder in incremental portions.

continued

continued from previous page
Procedure 32 Mixing Zinc Phosphate Cement

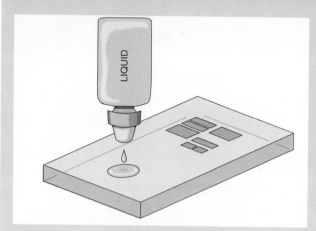

Figure 41-7 Dispensing the liquid.

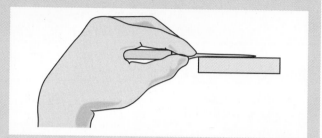

Figure 41-8 Spatula blade flat against glass slab.

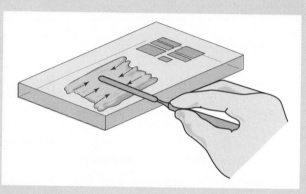

Figure 41-9 Spatulate mix over large area of glass slab.

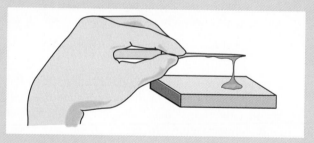

Figure 41-10 Consistency for cementation.

mix (Figure 41-7). To produce uniform drops, hold bottle vertically while dispensing the required numbers of drops on to the glass slab.

7 Place the correct number of drops (two for base and eight for cementation) onto the slab, approximately 1 1/2 to 2 inches away from the powder.

8 Replace cap immediately after dispensing liquid.

9 Hold spatula with an overhand grasp, with index finger resting near the neck of the spatula blade and your thumb along the side of the spatula handle.

10 Incorporate the first one-sixteenth of powder into the liquid. Use the flat side of the spatula blade to wet the powder particles.

11 Hold the spatula blade flat against the glass slab (Figure 41-8). Using a wide sweeping motion, spatulate the powder and liquid over a large area of the glass slab (Figure 41-9). The first increment (small portion) of powder will be spatulated for 15 seconds. Adding small amounts of powder will help neutralize the acid and achieve a smooth consistency of the mix. Each increment of powder must be thoroughly incorporated into the mix. The mix must be smooth, with no unmixed particles of powder or liquid remaining on the spatula or around the outer edge of mix.

12 Add the second increment; spatulate for 15 seconds; add the third increment, and spatulate for 15 seconds.

13 At this time, turn the spatula blade on edge, and gather the mass with two or three strokes to check the consistency.

14 Continue adding additional increments into the mix until the desired consistency is reached and within the prescribed time. The approximate time for each increment is 15, 15, 15, 20, 20, 15, and 20 seconds, for a total mixing time of 120 seconds (2 minutes).

15 Gather entire mass into one unit on the glass slab. The consistency for *cementation* is creamy and will follow the spatula for about 1 inch as it is lifted off the glass slab before breaking into a thin thread and flowing back into the mass (Figure 41-10). *Remember*: Zinc phosphate cement must

continued

be spatulated over a large area of the cool glass slab to help the heat dissipate. This will allow the maximum amount of powder to be incorporated into the mix, which will result in stronger cement. The consistency for a *base* should be puttylike (Figure 41-11) and can be rolled into a cylinder with the flat side of the spatula blade.

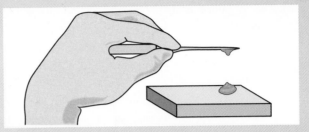

Figure 41-11 Puttylike consistency for insulating base.

Preparing the Cast Restoration for Cementation. The tooth is prepared with certain retentive features that provide the mechanical retention needed to hold the cemented cast restoration on the tooth. Also, the internal surface of the casting must be roughened, which helps in the retention of the cemented restoration.

Prior to cementation, the casting or restoration must be tried on the tooth to check for fit, occlusion, and the margins of the casting.

The cement for cementation must be thin enough to allow it to flow over the tooth and the surface irregularities of the casting. The function of the dental cement is to seal the margins of the restoration. If the cement is too thick, it will interfere with the seating of the restoration. In this case, the exposed layer of cement, the **cement line** (the layer of cement formed around the margin of the restoration), will gradually dissolve and disintegrate permitting the development of **microleakage** (a space between the tooth and the restoration) that may lead to recurrent dental caries.

Procedure 33 Cementing a Cast Restoration

Materials Needed

Basic set
Scaler
Cement powder and liquid
Cement spatula
Glass slab
High volume evacuator (HVE)
Saliva ejector
Cast restoration
Cotton rolls
Medarts crown seater
Bite sticks (orangewood sticks)
Cavity varnish
Dental floss
Polishing agent
Dappen dish
Right angle with prophy cup
Sandpaper discs on a mandrel or a finishing bur
Articulating paper and holder

Instructions

1 Wash the cast restoration in water using a brush to remove any debris. Dry the cast restoration and place in a clean dappen dish next to the glass slab.

2 When the operator is ready to seat the cast restoration, the teeth and surrounding area are isolated with cotton rolls and dried. *Note:* Varnish may be applied with cotton pliers and a small cotton pellet to diminish sensitivity to the tooth or teeth to receive the restoration.

3 Mix and apply the cement to the cast restoration, making sure the cement covers the entire internal surface of the casting.

4 Hold the glass slab closer while the operator removes a small amount of cement on an instrument to coat the tooth preparation.

5 Place the cast restoration in the palm of your hand with the internal portion of the cast facing up for the operator to remove and place on the tooth.

continued

continued from previous page
Procedure 33 Cementing a Cast Restoration

6 The operator seats the cast restoration on the tooth (teeth).

7 Pass the operator the Medarts crown seater to seat the cast restoration in its exact position while the patient bites on it.

8 Retrieve the Medarts crown seater and pass a bite stick to keep biting pressure until the cement begins to set. *Note:* While cement sets, a saliva ejector is placed in the mouth.

9 Retrieve the bite stick and saliva ejector and pass the operator a scaler to remove excess cement from the margins of the cast. Use the HVE to remove debris and moisture.

10 Retrieve the scaler and pass dental floss to the operator to remove excess cement from interproximal areas.

11 Retrieve the floss and pass articulating paper and holder to the operator to detect high spots on the cast.

12 If there are no high spots, retrieve the articulating paper and holder and pass the polishing agent in a dappen dish. Be sure that the right-angle prophy handpiece and prophy cup are already on the slow straight handpiece and ready to polish the new cast. If high spots exist, the operator will need to reduce them with sandpaper discs or a finishing bur.

13 Pass the air water syringe to rinse the mouth and use the HVE to evacuate the mouth.

Cleaning the Glass Slab and Spatula

1 Remove cement or excess powder from the glass slab with the spatula, and discard on a paper towel.

2 Wash spatula and glass slab in cool water.

3 Set particles may be removed with bicarbonate solution, baking soda, or by using the ultrasonic with a cement removal solution.

4 Thoroughly rinse glass slab and spatula. Dry.

Zinc Polyacrylate Cement

The composition of the powder is zinc oxide with a small amount of magnesium oxide. However, some manufacturers substitute magnesium oxide with stannous fluoride, which is added to the powder to increase strength and to reduce the film thickness. The liquid is polyacrylic acid and water.

When the powder and liquid are mixed together, the result is a cement that is extremely acid at the time of placement, pH of 1.7. However, the acid is rapidly neutralized during the setting reaction. Despite the acidity of the cement, zinc polyacrylate is less irritating to the pulpal tissue and is comparable to zinc oxide eugenol cement in that it is a soothing agent.

Zinc polyacrylate cement, also known as *carboxylate cement*, has an advantage over other dental cements in that it has the ability to adhere directly to the tooth structure. Through a process called **chelation** (a chemical reaction between two substances that join together to form an adhesive bond), the polyacrylic acid combines with the calcium in the tooth structure to form a primary adhesive bond. Because of this bonding action, when properly prepared, zinc polyacrylate cement can be used to attach orthodontic brackets directly to tooth enamel. A procedure called acid etching is used to prepare and roughen the enamel, which will allow the chelation or bonding to occur between the tooth enamel and orthodontic bracket. The same procedure may also be used when cementing crowns or fixed bridges.

However, gold or porcelain restorations must be thoroughly cleansed prior to cementation. Contaminants, such as chemical residue left from the acid pickling solution, will prevent the cement from adhering to the restoration. The underside of the gold restoration may be cleaned with an air abrasive or an abrasive bur, then washed and dried.

Zinc Oxide Eugenol Cement

The powder for the conventional zinc oxide eugenol cement is zinc oxide, resin, zinc acetate, and an accelerator. The liquid, eugenol, is found in clove oil. The improved or reinforced zinc oxide powder includes the addition of alumina and polymers (resins), and ethoxybenzoic acid (EBA) is added to the eugenol. The new additives to the powder and liquid increase the strength of the cement. Besides being distributed in the traditional standard package of powder and liquid, some forms are also available in capsule form, mixed in the amalgamator, and most recently, in the automix delivery system (Figure 41-12).

Procedure 34 Mixing Zinc Polyacrylate Cement

Materials Needed

Zinc polyacrylate powder
Zinc polyacrylate liquid or calibrated dispenser
Nonabsorbable paper mixing pad—or glass slab
Measuring scoop
Spatula

Instructions

Mixing Cement

1   Dispense one scoop of powder onto mixing pad or glass slab. Press measuring scoop firmly into powder. Withdraw measuring scoop from bottle, and remove excess powder with spatula. Powder should be flush with top of measuring scoop.

2   Place three drops of liquid on mixing pad near powder. Liquid should never be placed on the mixing pad or glass slab until just ready to be mixed. Exposure to air will cause loss of water and will result in the premature thickening of the mix. If liquid is dispensed from the plastic squeeze bottle, hold the bottle in a vertical position and squeeze. Release pressure when the drop separates from the nozzle tip. Should a calibrated liquid dispenser be used, push plunger rod to release three full calibrations, as marked on the plunger barrel.

3   Incorporate powder into the liquid in one increment. Begin spatulation. Spatulation should be rapid and be completed within 30 seconds. Do not overspatulate!

4   The consistency of polyacrylate cement for cementation is smooth and creamy, and the mass will flow from the spatula in a thin strand. The cement must be applied to the tooth and the object to be cemented while the mix is glossy. If the cement loses its sheen or becomes stringy, do not use it; it has started to set. For a base, the consistency should also be glossy. To facilitate the setting of the base, an instrument dipped in powder or in alcohol will cause the base to set faster.

5   The setting time for zinc polyacrylate is 3–4 minutes.

Cleaning the Spatula and Instrument

1   Immediately rinse spatula and instrument in cool water. If cement adheres to the spatula or instrument, it can be removed with a 10% solution of sodium hydroxide.

2   Dry and prepare instruments for sterilization.

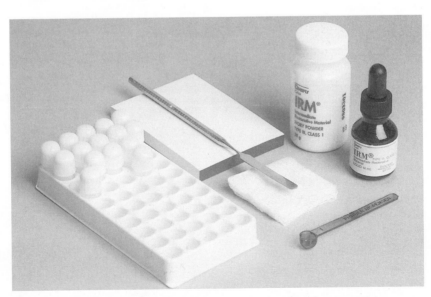

Figure 41-12 Encapsulated ZOE intermediate restorative material.

Procedure 35 Mixing Zinc Oxide Eugenol Cement

Materials Needed

Zinc oxide powder
Eugenol liquid
Parchment mixing pad
Metal spatula
Measuring device
Alcohol, 91% isopropyl or 70% ethyl alcohol
Sponge, 2 x 2 in.

Instructions

1 Place powder on mixing pad.
   a. Fluff powder before removing cap.
   b. Dispense one scoop of powder from large well with the measuring device, and place on mixing pad. A clean spatula may be used instead of the measuring device to dispense a portion of powder.
   c. Replace cap on powder bottle to avoid spilling and contamination.
   d. Divide powder into four equal portions.

2 Place liquid on mixing pad.
   a. Shake liquid.
   b. With pipette in liquid bottle, draw liquid into pipette; remove and hold pipette perpendicular (vertically) to the mixing pad.
   c. Dispense one drop of liquid onto pad, near powder, but not touching powder (Figure 41-13).

3 Spatulate cement.
   a. Draw first portion or quarter of powder into the liquid, and thoroughly spatulate.
   b. Draw next portion of powder into the mix, and continue to spatulate. Repeat procedure until desired consistency is reached.
   c. The spatulation time may vary with brand, generally between 30 seconds and 1 minute.
   d. The consistency for temporary cementation of a crown is a creamy consistency like a frosting (Figure 41-14).
   e. The consistency for an insulating base or temporary restoration is puttylike. It can be rolled into a cylinder, using the blade of the spatula (Figure 41-15).

4 Clean spatula.
   a. Wipe spatula with a 2 x 2 in. sponge moistened with alcohol.
   b. Wash, rinse, and dry.

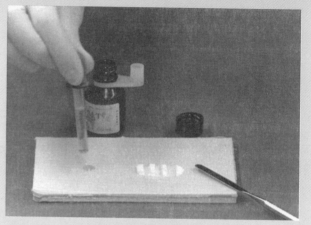

Figure 41-13 Liquid dispensed onto pad.

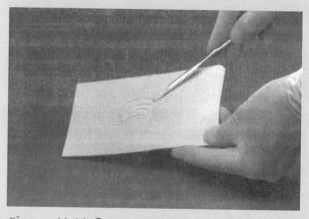

Figure 41-14 Creamy consistency for temporary cementation.

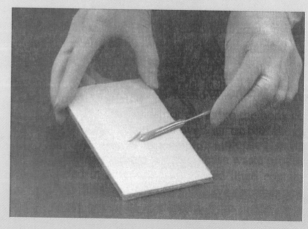

Figure 41-15 Puttylike consistency for base.

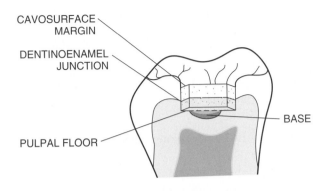

Figure 41-16 Applying base.

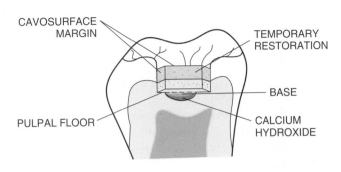

Figure 41-17 Double base and temporary restoration.

Applying Base and Temporary Restoration

Base. A base is applied to the cavity preparation, followed by the varnish (Figure 42-16).

A base may be one of the following: calcium hydroxide, zinc oxide eugenol, zinc phosphate, zinc polyacrylate, and glass ionomers cement.

Double Base and Temporary Restoration. A double base is used in deep cavity preparations for additional protection.

Calcium hydroxide is placed first, followed by another base material. Base material may serve as the temporary restoration or another type of temporary cement may be used (Figure 41-17).

Table 42-1 lists the dental cements and restorative materials in columns according to their function and use. The column heading states the use of the cement or restorative material. In each column the names and brands of the various cements or restorative materials that may be used are listed.

Surgical Cements and Periodontal Dressings

Surgical cements are applied to a surgical wound for protection, to aid in healing, and to diminish pain, hemorrhage, and trauma. Included in these are the eugenol-type, noneugenol and light-cured cements (see Table 42-2). Selection of the type used is based on the dentist's preference and whether the patient is sensitive to eugenol, which in certain individuals could cause inflammation or allergy.

The eugenol type is supplied in a two-paste system or a powder and liquid mixed to a putty consistency.

The noneugenol type is supplied as a two-paste system, a *base* and a *catalyst*, which are dispensed in equal amounts and mixed together to begin a setting reaction. When no longer tacky, it may be utilized; see

Chapter 57 for placement and removal of periodontal dressings.

The light-cured cement is supplied in a syringe dispenser that may be applied directly on the wound, where it is shaped and cured.

SUGGESTED ACTIVITIES

- Practice the application of cavity varnish on a prepared tooth on a stone model.
- Practice mixing calcium hydroxide base material and place it in the appropriate area of a prepared tooth on a stone model.
- Practice using the single-paste cavity liner by placing it in the appropriate area of a prepared tooth on a stone model and light curing it.
- Practice spatulating zinc phosphate to the correct consistency for permanent cementation.
- Practice spatulating zinc phosphate to the correct consistency for an insulating base.
- Practice mixing zinc polyacrylate for cementation.
- Practice spatulating zinc oxide eugenol cement for an insulating base or temporary restoration.
- Practice spatulating zinc oxide eugenol cement for cementation of a temporary crown.

REVIEW

1. What is the main purpose for applying a cavity varnish on a prepared tooth?
   a. To provide a sterile environment
   b. To prevent the restorative material from reaching the deepest portion of the prepared tooth
   c. To stimulate the formation of secondary dentin
   d. To seal exposed dentinal tubules against irritants

2. What takes place when a varnish is used with certain composite restorations?
   a. It causes the composite material to become grainy.
   b. It interferes with the setting reaction of the composite material.
   c. It adds gloss to the composite material.
   d. The copal in the varnish interferes with the setting reaction of the composite material.
   e. Both b and d.

3. Name the benefits calcium hydroxide offers when used as a base under deep restorations: (1) has a therapeutic effect on the pulp, (2) tends to stimulate the formation of secondary dentin, (3) is an effective barrier to irritants, and/or (4) seals dentinal tubules.
   a. 1, 2, 3
   b. 2, 3, 4
   c. 1, 2, 4
   d. 1, 3, 4

4. Name the order of placement of calcium hydroxide, cavity varnish, and zinc oxide carboxylate cement base in a cavity preparation.
   a. Cement base, calcium hydroxide, and cavity varnish
   b. Calcium hydroxide, cement base, and cavity varnish
   c. Cavity varnish, calcium hydroxide, and cement base
   d. Cement base, cavity varnish, and calcium hydroxide

5. In what area of the cavity preparation is a cavity liner placed?
   a. In the deepest portion of the cavity up to the pulpal floor
   b. In the deepest portion of the cavity up to the dentinoenamel junction
   c. In the whole cavity preparation that includes the enamel portion
   d. On the pulpal walls alone

6. What is the composition of zinc phosphate powder?
   a. Zinc acetate
   b. Zinc oxide
   c. Magnesium oxide
   d. Zinc phosphate
   e. Both b and c

7. What is the composition of zinc phosphate liquid?
   a. Water
   b. Eugenol
   c. Orthophosphoric acid
   d. Both a and c

8. Why is zinc phosphate cement mixed over a large area of the glass slab?
   a. To dissipate the heat caused by the reaction of the powder and liquid
   b. To break up the powder particles into finer ones
   c. To cause evaporation of the water content in the liquid
   d. To incorporate more liquid into the mix

9. What is another name for zinc polyacrylate cement?
   a. Crown and bridge cement
   b. Zinc phosphate
   c. Carboxylate cement
   d. Zinc oxide

10. Match the cements with their descriptions:
    ___a. Zinc phosphate
    ___b. Zinc oxide eugenol
    ___c. Zinc polyacrylate

    1. Combines with the calcium in the tooth structure for an adhesive bond
    2. Known for its exothermic reaction while being mixed
    3. Known for its sedative or soothing effect on the dental pulp

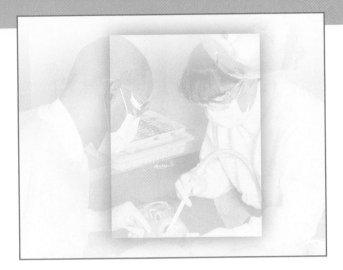

relatively "kind" to the pulp. However, in the case of a deep-cavity preparation or near-pulp exposure, a protective base such as calcium hydroxide is recommended. Glass ionomer cement also has the ability to release fluoride, which helps protect both the immediate and surrounding tooth structures from dental caries.

Composite restorations have a natural toothlike appearance and are used primarily in anterior teeth, Class III and V. However, stronger composites are available for posterior teeth.

Pit and fissure sealants are low-viscosity resin materials that are recommended to be placed on newly erupted deciduous or permanent teeth with defective fissures. The purpose is to seal the fissures for protection against the possibility of dental caries.

OBJECTIVES

After studying this chapter, the student will be able to:

● State the advantages of using glass ionomer cement.
● State four uses of glass ionomer cement.
● Discuss the bonding reaction of glass ionomer cement to enamel and dentin.
● Discuss the importance of removing the "smear layer" from the tooth preparation prior to placing a glass ionomer restoration.
● Prepare a glass ionomer for cementation by following the prescribed instructions.
● Name the two inorganic fillers used in a composite restoration.
● Name the polymer matrix material used in a composite restoration.
● State the two methods used in the polymerization of a composite restoration.
● State the advantage for using pit and fissure sealants.
● Select the materials needed for the preparation and placement of a pit and fissure sealant.
● Explain the procedure for preparing the tooth surfaces for receiving a sealant.

Introduction

Glass ionomer cements are used because of their high strength and low solubility and film thickness. They are

Glass Ionomers

Glass ionomer cement has the ability to bond to tooth structure (enamel and dentin). The bonding reaction occurs between the polyacrylic acid of the liquid and the calcium of the tooth. The powder contains fluoride aluminum and silicate (fluoroaluminosilicate glass). For bonding to occur, the tooth surface must be free of debris. After the tooth is prepared, a microscopic layer of mineralized tooth and bacterial debris known as the **smear layer** remains on the tooth. This smear layer must be removed before bonding can take place. To remove the smear layer, one must thoroughly cleanse the tooth structure with a conditioner composed of a 25% solution of polyacrylic acid. A blue coloring agent is added to the conditioner for visibility. The conditioner is applied directly over the dentin, including the dentinoenamel junction, for a minimum of 10 seconds. The tooth is rinsed with a steady flow of water for at least 30 seconds, then air dried with a gentle stream of air. Care must be taken to avoid dehydrating the tooth, as this may cause postoperative tooth sensitivity. This is particularly true when cementing crowns and bridges.

The conditioner is applied prior to placing the glass ionomer base or restorative material. The conditioner may be placed directly onto the tooth using the disposable applicator tip(s). The use of the conditioner is contraindicated when cementing crowns and bridges. In this case, the smear layer provides a protective layer for the tooth or abutment teeth.

331

Glass ionomer cement may be used as dentin replacement material (base) (Figure 42-1) and for the permanent cementation of crowns and bridges, orthodontic bands, cast posts, and core buildups (Figure 42-2). As a restorative material, glass ionomers may be used for anterior and posterior teeth (Figures 42-3 and 42-4) and are ideal for cervical or erosion lesions, root caries, and repair of crown margins.

Glass ionomer restorations pass through two setting stages and must be protected against moisture contamination and dehydration. A light-cure surface sealant or glaze is recommended to protect the restoration(s) during setting.

Glass ionomer cement is available as a powder and liquid and in capsules (Figure 42-5). The capsules require the use of a high-speed amalgamator to mix the cement.

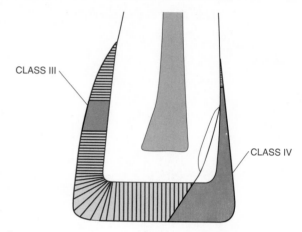

Figure 42-3 Anterior restorations, Class III and IV. (Courtesy of Premier Dental/ESPE-Premier Sales Co.)

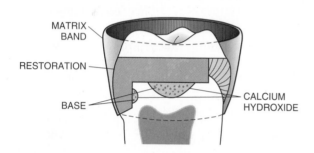

Figure 42-1 Placement of calcium hydroxide, dentin replacement base, and restoration.

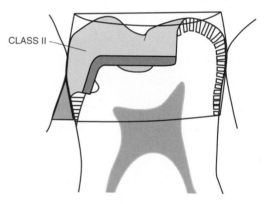

Figure 42-4 Posterior restoration, Class II. (Courtesy of Premier Dental/ESPE-Premier Sales Co.)

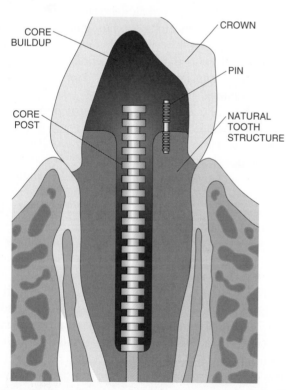

Figure 42-2 Cast post cemented in tooth with core buildup of glass ionomer cement.

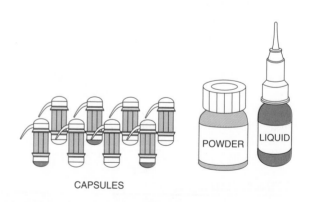

Figure 42-5 Systems for dispensing glass ionomer cements. (Courtesy of Premier Dental/ESPE-Premier Sales Co.)

Procedure 36 Applying Glass Ionomer

Materials Needed

High speed amalgamator
Glass ionomer capsule(s)
Capsule activator
Glass ionomer powder
Glass ionomer liquid
Scoop
Mixing pad
Spatula

Instructions

Preparing Ionomer Cement Using an Amalgamator

1 Activate the capsule with the activator (Figure 42-6).

2 Insert the activated capsule in the high-speed amalgamator.

3 Triturate for about 10 seconds. *Note:* The amount of time may vary depending on the make of the amalgamator (Figure 42-7).

4 Remove the capsule, insert it into an applier, and immediately remove the sealing pin. The nozzle tip of the capsule should be positioned for better access at 90° to the cavity preparation (Figure 42-8).

5 Express the material directly into the tooth preparation by squeezing the applier (Figure 42-9).

6 Working time will vary from 1 1/2 to 2 minutes depending on the glass ionomer.

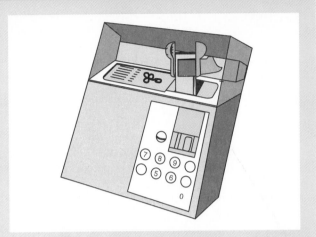

Figure 42-7 Trituration of capsule with amalgamator. (Courtesy of Premier Dental/ESPE-Premier Sales Co.)

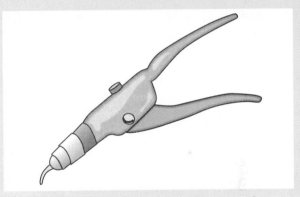

Figure 42-8 Capsule in applier. (Courtesy of Premier Dental/ESPE-Premier Sales Co.)

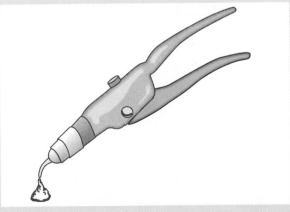

Figure 42-9 Applier used to express cement. (Courtesy of Premier Dental/ESPE-Premier Sales Co.)

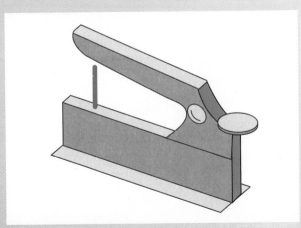

Figure 42-6 Capsule activator. (Courtesy of Premier Dental/ESPE-Premier Sales Co.)

continued

Preparing Glass Ionomer Cement (Powder and Liquid System)

Luting/Cementation

1 Shake powder to fluff material.

2 Dispense one level scoop of powder onto mixing pad (Figure 42-10).

3 Divide each scoop of powder into small increments (Figure 42-11).

4 Holding the liquid bottle vertically, dispense two drops of liquid onto mixing pad (Figure 42-11). Liquid should be placed on mixing pad just prior to mixing. Exposure to air will cause loss of water to the atmosphere. Keep bottles tightly sealed when not in use.

5 Draw the first increment of powder into the liquid. Spatulate each increment thoroughly before adding the next increment (Figure 42-12). Spatulation must be completed within 60 seconds, and the cement should have a glossy appearance. *Note:* Working time can be extended by mixing cement on a chilled, dry glass slab.

Dentin Replacement (Base)

1 Select the desired shade of powder to match or vary from the dentin shade.

2 Dispense one level scoop of powder onto the mixing pad (Figure 42-10).

3 Divide each scoop of powder into small increments (Figure 42-11).

4 Holding the liquid bottle vertically, dispense one drop of liquid onto the mixing pad (Figure 42-11).

5 Draw the first increment of powder into the liquid. Spatulate each increment thoroughly before adding the next increment (Figure 42-12). Spatulation must be completed within 30 seconds.

Placing Glass Ionomer Restoration

1 Place calcium hydroxide in deepest areas of preparation.

2 Apply conditioner to dentin for 10 seconds to remove smear layer.

3 Rinse tooth with a steady flow of water for 30 seconds.

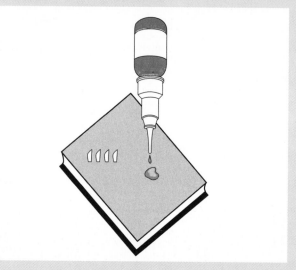

Figure 42-11 Dispensing liquid onto pad. (Courtesy of Premier Dental/ESPE-Premier Sales Co.)

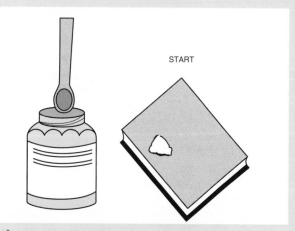

Figure 42-10 Measuring powder with scoop. (Courtesy of Premier Dental/ESPE-Premier Sales Co.)

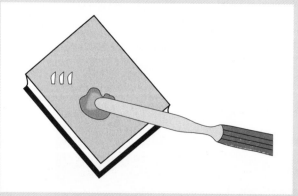

Figure 42-12 Adding increments of powder into liquid. (Courtesy of Premier Dental/ESPE-Premier Sales Co.)

continued

continued from previous page
Procedure 36 Applying Glass Ionomer

4 Dry tooth with a gentle stream of air. Do not dehydrate tooth.

5 Apply base to cover dentin, including dentinoenamel junction. Allow base to set for 2 minutes.

6 Etch enamel with etching gel/liquid for 30 seconds.

7 Rinse tooth with water for 60 seconds.

8 Dry tooth with a gentle stream of air. Do not dehydrate tooth.

9 Place glass ionomer restorative material. Place protective surface sealant when indicated.

Composites

Composite restorative material is composed of a polymer matrix, dimethacrylate (BIS-GMA), and inorganic filler particles such as quartz and lithium aluminum silicate. The inorganic filler particles are treated with an organic silane coupling agent that provides a bond between the inorganic fillers and the resin matrix. To make the material more **radiopaque** (whiter or lighter in appearance), composites may contain one of several elements such as barium, strontium, zinc, or zirconium.

The composites are classified according to particle size and the distribution of the inorganic fillers. Composites may contain fine irregularly shaped particle fillers or microfine particle fillers. The composites that are used today are a combination of the two particle sizes.

Commercial composites are available as *single-* (light-cured or photopolymerized) and *two-paste* (self-cured or autopolymerized) *systems.* The single-paste system (light-cured) is composed of a photoinitiator and an amine activator and is supplied in disposable light-proof syringes in various shades. The composite may be dispensed into a special composite syringe that is used to dispense the material into the cavity preparation. Once the composite material has been placed, **polymerization** of the composite is accomplished by shining a small beam of visible blue light onto the restoration for approximately 20–30 seconds. *Precaution:* The operator and chairside dental assistant should always wear light-filtering eye shields or use a light-screening safety tip when using visible blue light, refer to Figure 42-14.

Procedure 37 Applying Composite

Materials Needed

Composite base paste
Catalyst paste
Mixing pad
Disposable plastic spatula (supplied by manufacturer)

Instructions

1 Measure equal amounts of both base and catalyst paste on mixing pad.

2 Use one end of the spatula to remove a small amount of base paste, and place on the mixing pad.

3 With the other end of the spatula, remove an equal amount of catalyst paste, and place on the mixing pad. *Note:* Care must be taken not to cross-contaminate base paste with catalyst paste; otherwise, material will harden in jars.

4 With the same disposable spatula, spatulate base paste and catalyst together. Spatulation time is usually within 30 seconds. The mix will have a doughy consistency.

5 Throw used disposable spatula away after procedure.

In the two-paste system (self-cured), one paste is the base material and the second paste is the catalyst. The base contains an initiator, peroxide, and the second paste contains an activator, **amine** (an organic compound containing nitrogen), that serves as the catalyst when they are combined. The two pastes are spatulated together and packed into the tooth preparation with a plastic instrument. The mix will begin to harden within 1–2 minutes. Polymerization is the result of a chemical reaction that has occurred between the initiator (peroxide) and the activator (amine) that causes the material to harden. This reaction is called the amine-peroxide polymerization system.

Pit and Fissure Sealants

The anatomy of a tooth is important in the prevention of dental caries. During normal tooth development, the occlusal surface of posterior teeth form smooth-based depressions called *grooves*. These grooves are easily cleansed by the usual **excursion** (lateral or protrusive movement of the lower jaw) of food and the use of a toothbrush. However, if during the state of development the enamel fails to **coalesce** (grow together) properly, a faulty groove will result (Figure 42-13). This is called a *fissure.* The lack of enamel coalescence may only involve the enamel, or it may extend down to the dentinoenamel junction. The defective fissure becomes a potential trap for food debris, thereby increasing the chance of dental caries. The prevention of such caries may be controlled through the use of pit and fissure sealants.

There are three types of sealants: filled, unfilled, and fluoride-releasing filled. Filled sealants contain, in addition to BIS-GMA resins, microparticles such as glass, quartz, silica, and other fillers found in composite restorations that make them more resistant to abrasion. Although various types of resins have been used, the currently used commercial pit and fissure sealants are the bisphenol-A-glycidyl methacrylate (BIS-GMA) resins,

also known as unfilled sealants. The polymer is an epoxy resin with an acrylic monomer, bisphenol A, and glycidyl methacrylate. The BIS-GMA sealant may be polymerized by the conventional amine-peroxide system, whereby **autopolymerization** takes place, also known as chemically cured. With the light-cured system (Figure 42-14) also termed **photopolymerization**, the light, rather than a chemical, is the activator; the initiator is a light-sensitive chemical diketone that is activated by the visible light of a certain wavelength. By shining a small beam of visible blue light onto the resin surface, the light decomposes the initiator, causing polymerization to take place.

The success of the sealant technique depends on the ability of the resin to complete adaptation with the tooth surface. Therefore, the sealant should be of low **viscosity** (consistency of fluid that is sticky and thicker than water) in order for it to flow easily into the prepared pits or fissures, allowing the material to come in contact with all the small surface irregularities of the tooth. This requires special treatment to the tooth surface(s) prior to the placement of the sealant. The enamel surfaces must be cleaned thoroughly, then etched with an acid or conditioner, usually a concentrated solution of phosphoric acid (35–50%). This procedure produces a selective dissolution (dissolving) of the enamel surface, thereby providing the mechanical retention needed to hold the sealant. The open pores of the enamel will allow the resin to flow into the surface irregularities to form what are referred to as **resin tags**. This mechanical interlocking of the resin to the enamel surfaces increases the bond strength of the resin to the tooth structure.

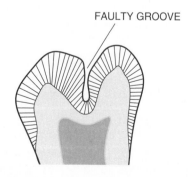

Figure 42-13 Occlusal fissures showing depth of fissure.

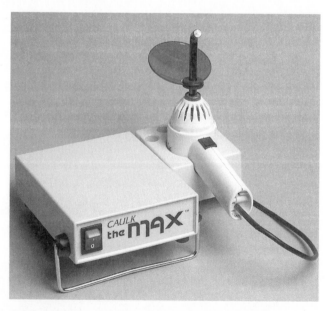

Figure 42-14 Visible blue-light curing device.

Procedure 38 Applying Pit and Fissure Sealants

Materials Needed

Basic setup (mouth mirror, explorer, and cotton pliers)
Prophy handpiece
Prophy brush/cup
Nonfluoride prophy paste
Dental dam setup or cotton rolls
Etching solution
Sealant
Cotton pellet
Applicator or syringe
Articulating paper
Small white or diamond stones
Light-cured system, depending on type of sealant

Instructions

1 The teeth are cleaned with a prophy brush and nonfluoride paste.

2 The teeth are rinsed and dried.

3 A dental dam is placed to isolate the teeth to be treated. Teeth are dried again.

4 A cotton pellet is moistened with the etching solution or conditioning agent, and applied to the occlusal surface(s) of the tooth or teeth.

5 The etching solution remains on the tooth surface(s) for approximately 30–60 seconds. Care must be taken not to apply the solution to other surfaces of the tooth or teeth.

6 The teeth are rinsed thoroughly (10–15 seconds) with water to remove the decalcified tooth debris from the etched surfaces.

7 The tooth surfaces are dried thoroughly with a stream of air for at least 15–30 seconds. This step is critical, because moisture contamination will interfere with the retention of the sealant. The prepared surface(s) should have a dull, slightly chalky appearance.

8 The sealant is applied with the applicator or syringe, depending on the brand of sealant to be used (Table 42-2). Air voids must be avoided when applying the sealant.

9 If the sealant is light cured, the tip of the gun is positioned about 2 mm from the sealant and exposed to the light for approximately 20 seconds.

10 Once the sealant has set, the occlusal surface(s) are examined with an explorer to determine whether the fissure or pit has been completely covered.

11 The occlusal surface(s) are checked with articulating paper. White or diamond stones may be used to adjust the contour of the sealant.

12 The dental dam is removed and the patient's mouth is rinsed with warm water.

Rationale for Placing Sealants

- To prevent bacteria from entering deep crevices such as pits and fissures of teeth in which initiation of dental caries may begin
- On children's primary molars
- On children with newly erupted permanent first molars
- On teenagers with newly erupted posterior teeth
- On women during pregnancy when caries rates are high

Helpful Suggestions

- Patient should wear eye protection during conditioning (etching) the tooth. Phosphoric acid can damage the eye if allowed to enter it.
- If a tooth needs to be etched again, the etchant should be left on for 10 seconds only.
- Fluoride treatment should be incorporated after sealant procedure to promote remineralization of etched area that was not covered by the sealant.

Table 42-1 lists the dental cements and restorative materials according to their function and use. Table 42-2 indicates the uses and lists the cements accordingly.

Table 42-1 Dental Cements and Restorative Materials

Cavity Varnishes and Liners	Bases Under Restorations	Temporary Restorations
Use: Seals the dentinal tubules, protects pulp from chemical irritants in certain cements and restorative materials.	**Use:** Protects pulp from mechanical, thermal or electrical stimuli.	**Use:** Protects tooth until permanent restoration is placed.
Cavity varnish: a solvent that, when applied to a cavity preparation, evaporates, leaving a resinous film on the surface. Applied to dentin and enamel walls. *Do not use with resins or composites.* • Copalite, Cavaseal, Caulk Varnish, Copaliner, Copa-Seal	**Calcium hydroxide:** stimulates the formation of secondary dentin. Used in deep cavities and for pulp capping. • Dycal, Pulpdent Paste, Hydrex, Pro Cal, ESPE AlkaLiner	**Zinc oxide eugenol:** placed into prepared cavity preparation. • Caulk ZOE B&T, Cadco ZOE
Cavity liner: a varnish-type material that contains calcium hydroxide, zinc oxide, or glass ionomer. • Ketac-Bond, Vitrebond-3M: glass ionomer used under composite, amalgam or porcelain. • GC Lining cement: used where a thin lining is indicated. • Pulpdent: a paste applied in a cavity preparation. • Cavitec: applied to the dentin walls *only*.	**Zinc oxide eugenol (ZOE):** soothing effect on irritated pulp. Adds bulk to cavity preparation when needed. • Cavitec, Cadco, ZOE, Caulk ZOE B&T	**Reinforced zinc oxide eugenol:** intermediate restoration, longer lasting temporary. • Caulk IRM, Zinroc
	Reinforced zinc oxide eugenol: stronger than regular ZOE but less soluble. • Caulk IRM, Pulpisol PR (Svedia)	**Noneugenol:** eugenol-free. • Freegenol, Nogenol, Tempbond NE, Zone Temporary Cement
Light-cured cavity liner: glass ionomer cement for lining. Used under composites, amalgams, inlays. Fluoride releasing. • Fuji Bond, Vitrebond—3M, Vivaglass liner, (Vivadent)	**Zinc phosphate:** stronger than ZOE, but acid in cement is irritating to pulp when used in deep cavity preparations. • Modern Tenacin, Mizzy, Fleck	**Automix temporary cement:** used with applicator gun and automix tips. No hand mixing. • Tempocem (eugenol or noneugenol), Direct Cem (noneugenol)
	Zinc Polyacrylate: mild effect on pulp comparable to zinc phosphate. • Durelon, PCA	**Zinc polyacrylate:** adheres to enamel and is stronger than zinc phosphate. • Durelon, PCA, Carboset, Poly-C
	Glass Ionomer: strong, kind to pulp, releases fluoride, anticariogenic property. • KETAC-BOND (Espe America), GC Dentin Cement, Vivaglass Base caps	**Zinc phosphate:** may be used as a temporary restoration. • Modern Tenacin, Mizzy, Fleck

Note: Bulleted items indicate trade names.

Table 42-2 Cements According to Uses

Cementation	Direct Esthetic Restorative Materials	Surgical Cements and Periodontal Dressings
Use: To cement "lute" (to seal) gold inlays, onlays, crowns, bridges, and orthodontic bands to permanent teeth.	**Use:** Restorations where esthetics are of primary importance.	**Use:** Applied to surgical wound to aid healing.
Zinc phosphate: cement applied to both the tooth/teeth and the gold casting(s) or orthodontic bands. • S.S. White Zinc Improved, Modern Tenacin, Mizzy, Fleck	**Composite resins:** used in anterior teeth and posterior teeth in *limited areas only*. Class III, IV, and I and II in limited conditions. • Prodigy, Concise, Prestige	**Surgical and periodontal dressings:** placed over a surgical wound to aid in the retention of medication. Reduces thermal shock.
Zinc polyacrylate (carboxylate cement) • Durelon, PCA	**Pit and fissure sealants:** used to prevent occlusal caries in newly erupted primary and permanent molars. • Delton, Epoxylite, Prisma Shield	**Eugenol:** placed over a surgical wound following periodontal surgery or gingival curettage. • Periocare, "PPC", Kirkland
Glass Ionomer: cementation of crowns and bridges, PJC; bonds to clean tooth structure enamel and dentin. • Ketac-Cem, Fuji Type I, Fuji Plus Capsules, Vitremer 3M	**Glass Ionomer:** used in small anterior restorations Class III, IV, posterior teeth Class I and II, Class V, and erosion or abrasion lesions. • Ketac Fil, Fuji Type II, Vitremer, Compoglass	**Noneugenol:** • Coe-Perio Pak (base and catalyst), Coe Perio Pak (automix), Zone **Light cured:** • Barricaid

Note: Bulleted items indicate trade names.

SUGGESTED ACTIVITIES

● Practice mixing glass ionomer cement for cementation. Using the powder and liquid system and a paper pad, determine the length of polymerization time. Next, practice mixing glass ionomer for cementation using a chilled glass slab and determine the length of polymerization time. Compare your results.

● Practice triturating glass ionomer cement according to manufacturer's directions and learn to load the capsule onto the applier.

● Practice mixing a composite restorative material using the two-paste system and determine the length of necessary setting time for complete polymerization to occur.

● Using a single-paste system, practice using the visible blue light and determine the length of setting time for complete polymerization to occur.

● Prepare a procedure for the application of a sealant.

● Using extracted and sterilized posterior teeth that are set in plaster, acid etch the teeth with phosphoric acid or conditioner; rinse thoroughly. Flow BIS-GMA mixed sealant onto one of the teeth. Allow to polymerize. On another tooth, flow the light-cured sealant and allow to polymerize using a visible blue light and eye protection. Test the results for polymerization.

REVIEW

1. Indicate the methods used in the polymerization of composite restorations: (1) methyl methacrylate, (2) polyacrylic acid, (3) amine-peroxide system, and/or (4) visible blue light.
   a. 1, 2
   b. 2, 3
   c. 3, 4
   d. 1, 4

2. Name the advantages for using glass ionomer cements: (1) release fluoride, (2) low solubility and film thickness, (3) slow setting reaction, and/or (4) kind to the pulp.
   a. 1, 2, 3
   b. 2, 3, 4
   c. 1, 2, 4
   d. 1, 3, 4

3. What is the meaning of the term smear layer?
   a. A layer of polymer on the tooth after the tooth is filled and finished
   b. A microscopic layer of mineralized tooth and bacteria debris remaining after the tooth is prepared
   c. A layer of cement that remains on the tooth after the tooth is restored
   d. A layer of etchant that is not rinsed off prior to restoring the tooth

4. Why is a low-viscosity resin used in pit and fissure sealants?
   a. Resin will flow easily into the prepared pit or fissure to contact those irregularities of the tooth.
   b. To cover the pits, fissures, and entire occlusal surface of the tooth
   c. To increase the strength of the sealant
   d. Both a and c

5. Why are pit and fissure sealants used?
   a. To seal defective pits and fissures of newly erupted teeth
   b. To seal beginning cavities preventing them from becoming larger
   c. To ensure that pits and fissures of posterior teeth in an adult are protected
   d. Both a and b

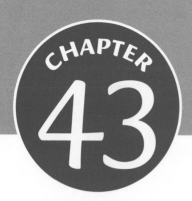
Dental Amalgam

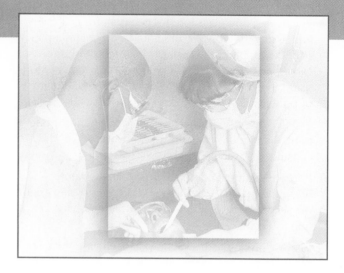

After studying this chapter, the student will be able to:

● Define the terms lathe-cut and spherical alloy.

● State the advantages for using a high-copper alloy.

● Discuss the chemical composition of a dental alloy.

● Discuss the hazards of mercury vapor.

● Discuss the principles of mercury hygiene as they apply to dental office personnel.

● Discuss the principles of mercury hygiene in the treatment room.

● Compare the types of capsules that can be used with a dental amalgamator.

● Discuss the advantages of using a premeasured sealed capsule over the traditional screw or friction-fit capsule.

● Explain the proper procedure for preparing a dental amalgam.

● Demonstrate the correct procedure for loading an amalgam carrier.

Introduction

Dental *amalgam* is one of the oldest restorative materials still in use today. A dental alloy is composed of two or more metals. Dental amalgam is a silver **alloy** that is combined with **mercury** (a metal that is liquid at room temperature). A dental alloy and mercury are placed in a capsule and mixed in a machine to form a pliable (plastic) mass capable of being packed into a cavity preparation. The dental assistant prepares the dental amalgam that will be used immediately by the dentist.

Types of Alloys

At present, available dental alloys consist of the conventional (traditional) low-copper (below 6% of copper) and high-copper (above 6% of copper) alloys. The con-

ventional low-copper alloys are composed of *lathe-cut* (filings) or *spherical* particles. High-copper alloys are a combination of lathe-cut and spherical particles or a single composition of spherical particles.

Lathe-Cut Alloy

Before 1961, lathe-cut (filings) alloy was the only type of alloy available. Lathe-cut alloy is produced by melting silver, tin, copper, and sometimes zinc together to form an **ingot** (metal cast into a bar). The ingot is then placed on either a lathe or a milling machine to produce **filings** (alloy particles) that are irregular in shape and have rough edges (Figure 43-1A). This type of alloy requires the use of more mercury when triturated.

Spherical Alloy

Spherical or spheroidal alloy particles are formed by **atomization** (to separate into atoms), a process in which the molten alloy is sprayed into a mist and the droplets cooled with either air or water. As the droplets solidify, **spherical** (round) particles of different sizes are formed (Figure 43-1B). This produces an alloy with a smoother surface that requires less mercury when triturated. Spherical alloys allow for improved carving and polishability of the amalgam restoration.

The American Dental Association's (ADA) specification No. 1 for dental alloys has been changed regarding the proportion of copper to other elements in the formula. Dental alloys that contain 6% or less copper are designated as low-copper, or conventional (traditional), alloys. Amalgam alloys that contain more than 6% copper are referred to as high-copper alloys.

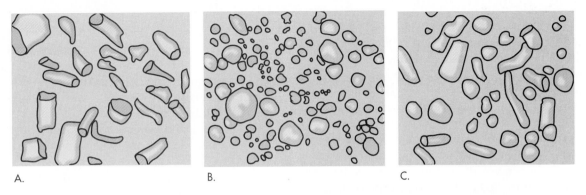

Figure 43-1 Photomicrograph of (A) lathe-cut alloy, (B) spherical alloy, and (C) admixed alloy. (Courtesy of Ferracane, *Materials in Dentistry: Principles and Applications*.)

Admixed Alloy

High-copper alloys are classified according to particle shape, such as lathe-cut (filings), spherical, or a combination of particles (admixed). **Admixed** alloy is a combination of the low-copper lathe-cut alloy and high-copper spherical alloy particles. Alloys with smaller particle sizes will usually produce amalgams with a smoother surface when carved and will result in a stronger restoration (Figure 43-1C).

Setting Reaction

During trituration of the conventional low-copper alloy, the silver-tin alloy particles will react with the mercury (Hg). This reaction will result in the combination of silver with mercury referred to as *gamma phase-1* and tin with mercury referred to as *gamma phase-2*. **Gamma** is a particular arrangement of atoms. **Phase** denotes a change in structure.

With the new high-copper alloy in gamma phase-2, copper will combine with tin, rather than tin with mercury. Both reactions form a matrix that holds the unreacted powder particles. The amalgam can be thought of as original alloy particles surrounded by a continuous matrix of silver-mercury and a little tin mercury in the conventional amalgam, or copper-tin in high-copper amalgams. The tin-mercury phase is the weakest phase in the conventional amalgam most likely to corrode. **Corrosion** is a chemical reaction of a nonmetallic substance with a metal. This phase is usually not present in the high-copper amalgams, which explains their superior properties.

Because high-copper alloys eliminate the weak tin-mercury phase, the result is an amalgam with improved strength, increased resistance to corrosion, and reduced marginal breakdown and failure. Over 90% of amalgams purchased today are high-copper alloys.

Composition

The chemical composition of a dental alloy may contain the following metals: silver (Ag), tin (Sn), copper (Cu), and zinc (Zn). *Note:* Not all alloys contain zinc.

Each metal used in a dental alloy has certain qualities that are needed to produce the desired restoration. The effects of each component are as follows:

Silver

- Used to form the metallic compound with mercury (Hg) that determines the dimensional changes that occur during hardening
- Increases strength of restoration
- Increases expansion
- Is slow to amalgamate
- Hardens rapidly
- Tarnishes easily
- Decreases setting time

Tin

- Aids in the **amalgamation** (chemical combining) of the alloy with the mercury because of its strong affinity for mercury
- Reduces expansion during setting
- Reduces strength
- Setting time is slower
- More susceptible to corrosion (conventional alloy)
- Tends to weaken the amalgam

Copper

- Increases strength and hardness
- Increases expansion of amalgam during hardening
- Reduces flow of finished restoration
- Resists corrosion (high-copper)
- Reduces marginal failure (high-copper)

Zinc

● Used to minimize the oxidation of the other metals present in alloy during manufacturing. Zinc is a scavenger and reacts with oxygen, preventing it from combining with silver, tin, or copper. *Note:* Should moisture contamination occur during manipulation or condensation of the amalgam, delayed expansion may occur. Zinc-containing dental amalgams are particularly sensitive to moisture. Zinc reacts with water to form the zinc oxide and hydrogen gas that may cause the unwanted and excessive expansion of the set amalgam restoration.

Mercury

The properties of mercury for use in the production of dental amalgams must meet the specification listed by the Council on Dental Materials, Instruments and Equipment of the ADA, Specification No. 6.

Dental mercury is one of the most commonly used metals in dentistry, and it is highly **toxic** (poisonous). It is the only metal that is liquid and **vaporizes** (particles of matter scatter and freely float in the air) at a relatively low room temperature. **Mercury vapor** (undetectable mercury molecules present in the air) has no color, odor, or taste and cannot be readily detected. Mercury may be absorbed into the body through inhalation or through the pores of the skin. Mercury vapor inhalation may occur during trituration, dispensing the amalgam mass from the capsule, and when polishing new amalgam restorations. Also, during the cutting and removal of amalgam restorations, mercury vapor and amalgam dust are created. The frictional heat created by grinding the amalgam causes the surface mercury to separate from the alloy, resulting in mercury vapor and **amalgam dust** (minute particles of alloy and mercury).

Mercury will penetrate the pores of the skin when touched with bare hands. Therefore, squeezing of the amalgam mass to express excess mercury should be avoided and is no longer an accepted technique.

Mercury plays an important role in the clinical behavior of the individual amalgam restoration. The average well-condensed amalgam should contain approximately 50% or less mercury.

Use of the Dental Amalgamator

A dental **amalgamator**, or *triturator*, is a specially designed machine used to **triturate** (the mechanical means of combining the dental alloy with mercury) a dental alloy with mercury to produce a silver amalgam restorative material (Figure 43-2).

Today several types of amalgamators are available. Although some amalgamators may operate at a single speed, others have variable speeds (low, medium, or high) and frequency levels (rate of speed and path in which the capsule moves during trituration).

The manufacturers of amalgamators provide information about which speed or frequency and trituration times are required for their particular type of amalgamator. Each amalgamator must be set for the type of dental alloy used—slow, medium, or fast.

Medium- and high-speed frequency amalgamators are recommended for use with improved high-copper alloys.

Generally the higher the speed or frequency, the shorter the trituration time. However, less than 6 seconds is not recommended, as it is insufficient to remove the alloy's oxide layer, a necessary step so that the particles can combine with mercury. Usually, trituration of the alloy or mercury for 10–15 seconds will produce a homogeneous and uniform mix.

Capsule

Amalgamators may be used with the traditional **capsule** and pestle or the premeasured sealed capsules containing both the alloy particles and mercury.

Traditional capsules are plastic or metal, screw type or friction fit. If the traditional capsule is to be used, the choice of a screw-type capsule over the friction-fit type is better, because the latter may release mercury vapor during the trituration process. Any type of capsule that releases mercury vapor is a health hazard to dental personnel.

Premeasured sealed capsules contain both dental alloy and mercury. The alloy powder particles and mercury are separated by a nonreactive thin foil that must be punctured by compressing or twisting the two parts of the capsule together. This releases the mercury into the alloy inside the capsule.

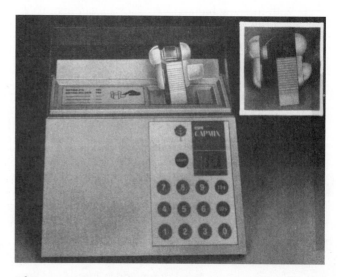

Figure 43-2 Dental amalgamator. (Courtesy of Premier Dental/ESPE Premier Sales Co.)

Another type of premeasured sealed capsule is electronically welded together. A plastic wafer inside the capsule contains the mercury and premeasured alloy. During the trituration cycle, the mercury is released from the plastic wafer, and the empty wafer is forced against the end of the capsule.

Some of the advantages of using premeasured sealed capsules are as follows:

● The portions of the alloy and mercury are consistent.

● They prevent any chance of mercury spill.

● They prevent the possibility that mercury vapor will be released during trituration.

Trituration

Trituration is the mechanical means of combining the dental alloy with mercury. *Amalgamation* is the actual chemical reaction that occurs between the alloy and mercury to form the silver amalgam.

To attain the maximum properties and desirable working characteristics of a dental amalgam, the manufacturer's instructions for trituration time must be followed.

Condensing the Amalgam

Dental amalgams do not adhere to the tooth structure. Therefore, adequate tooth structure must be present and the cavity preparation must offer sufficient retention.

An amalgam is placed into a cavity preparation by using an **amalgam carrier**, and condensing instruments, also known as pluggers, are used to **condense** (process of packing the amalgam into the prepared tooth) the amalgam. The dental amalgam must be placed rapidly and with enough force to ensure proper adaptation of the amalgam to the cavity walls of the preparation. Failure to condense the amalgam immediately after trituration can weaken the amalgam and may cause the amalgam to set before it is placed in the preparation. If the amalgam is not condensed within 3–4 minutes, a fresh mix should be prepared.

Procedure 39 Using the Amalgamator

Materials Needed

Gloves, mask, protective eyewear
Amalgamator
Premeasured sealed alloy and mercury capsule
Amalgam well, dappen dish, or possibly squeeze cloth
Amalgam carrier
Scrap container for amalgam

Instructions

Preparing the Amalgamator

1 Assemble materials (Figure 43-3). Select trituration time and speed for type of alloy and amalgamator used.

2 Prepare capsule according to type being used.

3 Insert capsule into prongs or clip of amalgamator (Figure 43-4). The capsule must be properly inserted; otherwise, it may become dislodged during trituration.

4 Close cover of amalgamator (Figure 43-5).

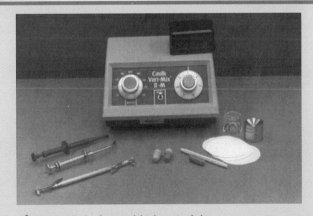

Figure 43-3 Assembled materials.

5 Triturate for prescribed time according to manufacturer's instructions (generally between 10–15 seconds depending on type of alloy used and whether the machine is set on slow, medium, or fast).

6 Activate timer (Figure 43-6). The timer will automatically switch off after the prescribed trituration time.

continued

continued from previous page
Procedure 39 Using the Amalgamator

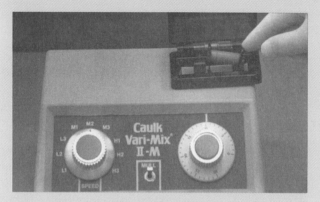

Figure 43-4 Capsule inserted into prongs or clip of amalgamator.

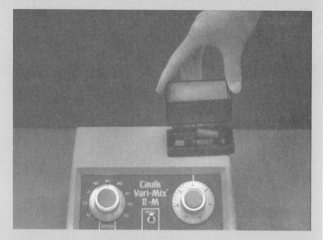

Figure 43-5 Cover closed over capsule.

7 Lift cover, and remove capsule from prongs or clip (Figure 43-7). If a traditional capsule with a **pestle** (a mechanical rod that breaks up the material within the capsule) is used, the pestle must be removed and the cap replaced on the capsule, then **mulled** (additional trituration given whereby the mixture is brought together after the pestle is removed) for 1 or 2 seconds.

8 Separate capsule, and empty contents into the amalgam well, into the dappen dish, or onto a squeeze cloth (Figure 43-8). Avoid touching the amalgam, even with gloved hands. *Note:* A well-mixed amalgam should have a glossy appearance with a smooth velvety consistency. An amalgam that crumbles when loading a carrier should be discarded, because it will be impossible to condense.

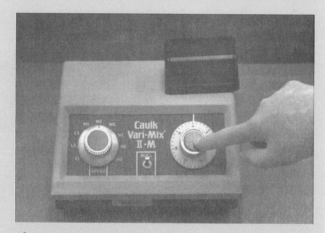

Figure 43-6 Timer activated.

9 Immediately recap capsule to reduce mercury vapor released during trituration.

Loading the Carrier

1 Hold amalgam carrier with an overhand grasp (Figures 43-9 and 43-10).

2 Begin loading carrier (Figure 43-11).

3 Pack carrier to form a compact cylinder (Figure 43-12). After carrier is packed, immediately pass to operator. Operator will dispense amalgam and return the carrier to the dental assistant. The dental assistant will exchange the carrier for a condenser. The operator now proceeds with condensing, while the dental assistant reloads the carrier. This procedure will be repeated until a sufficient amount of amalgam has been condensed into the tooth preparation.

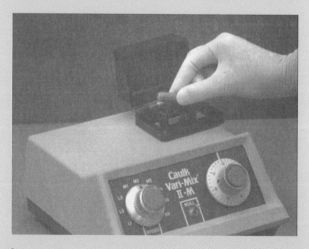

Figure 43-7 Capsule removed from amalgamator.

continued

continued from previous page
Procedure 39 Using the Amalgamator

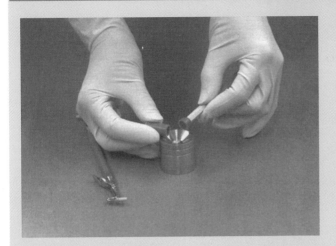

Figure 43-8 Amalgam placed in amalgam well.

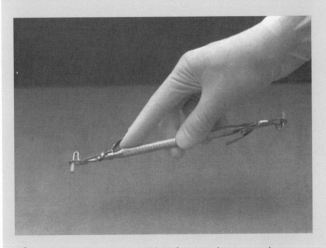

Figure 43-9 Hand position for amalgam carrier.

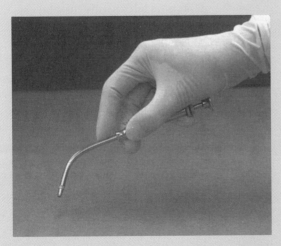

Figure 43-10 Hand position for amalgam carrier.

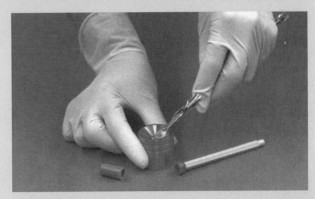

Figure 43-11 Beginning loading carrier.

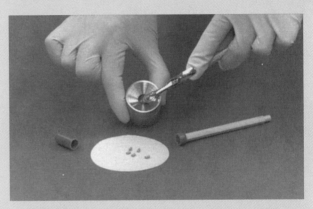

Figure 43-12 Amalgam carrier dispenses compact amalgam cylinders.

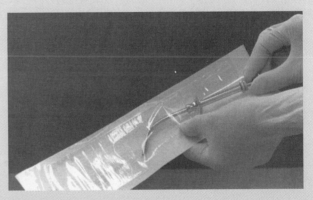

Figure 43-13 Carrier placed in sterilizing pouch.

Cleaning Up

1 Expel any excess amalgam into appropriate container.

2 Disinfect carrier with surface disinfectant. Place in Chemiclave pouch for sterilization (Figure 43-13).

Procedure 40 Amalgam Restoring

Materials Needed

Basic set-up

Anesthetic set-up

Dental dam set-up

Selection of cotton rolls, cotton pellets, 2 x 2 gauze sponges, and cotton-tipped applicators

Selection of burs for friction-grip and slow-speed hand pieces

Selection of hand cutting instruments

Matrix retainer, bands, and wedges

Condensers (pluggers)

Carving instruments

Amalgamator

Premeasured sealed alloy and mercury capsules

Amalgam well, dappen dish, or possibly squeeze cloth

Amalgam carrier

Articulating paper and holder

Floss

Instructions

Note: Dental personnel should always be attired using PPE (personal protective equipment), and the medical history should be taken prior to performing procedures intraorally.

1 Topical and local anesthetics are administered (refer to Chapter 51).

2 A dental dam is placed (refer to Chapter 39).

3 The dentist prepares the cavity using the high-speed handpiece while the dental assistant uses the HVE to remove water and debris and also maintains a clear vision for the dentist by using the air/water syringe on the mouth mirror to provide adequate visibility.

4 The dental assistant transfers necessary cutting instruments to shape the cavity preparation while maintaining visibility for the dentist.

5 Once the preparation is completed, it is cleaned and dried. If a base is required, it would be placed at this time. The dentist seals the dentinal tubules with cavity varnish (refer to Chapter 41 for bases, liners, and cavity varnish).

6 If the preparation is for a Class II restoration, a matrix band is placed (refer to Chapter 40).

7 The amalgam is prepared by the dental assistant following instructions on the procedure for using the amalgamator.

8 The dental assistant places the amalgam in the amalgam well and fills the carrier. If the carrier is double ended, both sides are loaded and passed to the dentist. While the dentist places the amalgam into the cavity preparation, the dental assistant picks up the smallest condenser and exchanges it for the carrier.

9 While the dentist condenses the amalgam, the dental assistant fills the carrier again and continues the exchange of instruments, gradually increasing the size of condensers until the preparation is filled. One must realize that the dental assistant is always one step ahead of the dentist.

10 As soon as the preparation is filled, the dental assistant exchanges the last condenser for an explorer. The dentist uses the explorer to loosen the amalgam from the matrix band and to begin contouring the marginal ridge. The dental assistant exchanges the explorer for cotton pliers.

11 The wedge is removed with cotton pliers and the matrix retainer loosened and removed. The dental assistant receives the matrix retainer while the dentist carefully removes the matrix band using cotton pliers.

12 The next step is the finishing phase. The dental assistant passes a burnisher to adapt the amalgam to the margins of the preparation on the occlusal aspect and begins to transfer carvers to restore tooth anatomy while evacuating and using the air syringe to keep the area free of debris. Scissors are exchanged for the last carving instrument.

13 The dentist removes the dental dam by cutting the interseptals of the dental dam with scissors. The dental assistant transfers the dental dam forceps to remove the clamp while retrieving the scissors. The forceps and clamp are retrieved, as are the dental dam frame, dam material, and napkin.

14 The dental assistant transfers articulating paper on a holder to check the height of the restoration. If the restoration is high, a carver will be transferred and the height of the restoration will be checked until it is of appropriate height. Floss is passed to the dentist to check the interproximal area and to remove debris. The oral cavity is rinsed and evacuated and the patient is dismissed. *Note:* The patient should be cautioned to avoid chewing on the new restoration for a few hours.

Advantages of Dental Amalgams

1. They can be triturated into a smooth plastic mass within seconds and remain this way for approximately 3 minutes, allowing for proper placement and condensation.
2. They can be placed, condensed, and readily adapted to the cavity walls.
3. They can receive and retain a polish 24 hours after the restoration has been placed.
4. When correctly manipulated, the restoration will have limited dimensional changes (expansion and contraction).

Disadvantages of Amalgams

1. They lack edge strength and will fracture if not supported by the presence of adequate tooth structure.
2. They lack esthetic appeal because of their silver color; therefore, they are used in posterior teeth for Class I, II, and V.
3. They have a tendency to **tarnish** (simple surface discoloration of a silver alloy).

Recommendations for Mercury Hygiene

The ADA recommends that a program of mercury hygiene be established within each dental practice. The dentist has a dual responsibility to the dental staff and himself or herself to control mercury vapor in the dental office.

In 1984, the Occupational Safety and Health Administration (OSHA) Act mandated that the dentist provide a workplace that is free from any occupational hazards.

Potential office hazards involving mercury can be eliminated by practicing appropriate mercury hygiene. A great deal of concern has been directed toward the biological effects of mercury. To inform the dental profession of the potential dangers of mercury, the Council on Dental Materials, Instruments and Equipment of the ADA, has established the following guidelines:

Dental Office Personnel Responsibilities

1. Disposable gloves, face mask, and glasses or shield should be worn when working with dental amalgam.
2. A no-touch technique should be used when handling mercury. Skin that is exposed to mercury should be cleansed with soap and water and rinsed thoroughly under running water.
3. Premeasured capsules should be used to achieve exact ratio of alloy and mercury, rather than the traditional capsule that must be loaded with dental alloy and mercury before trituration.
4. An amalgamator that has a protective hood should be used to reduce the chance of any mercury vapor being released into the atmosphere. Screw-type or frictional-fit capsules that must be pressed together may leak during trituration. Both can be checked for leakage by wrapping adhesive tape around the point where the two parts of the capsule join. Leakage will show up as small drops of mercury on the adhesive tape. Leaking capsules should be discarded.
5. All used capsules should be reassembled immediately after dispensing the amalgam. The used dental amalgam capsule is highly contaminated with mercury vapor.
6. Office personnel should have periodic urine analyses to check for any mercury in the body. The ADA suggests that mercury testing be a part of all dental office personnel on a regular health evaluation basis. More information concerning a mercury testing service is offered by the ADA Council on Dental Therapeutics, 211 East Chicago Avenue, Chicago, IL 60611. Request pamphlet 3-005-3.

Treatment Room

1. Unwanted mercury and amalgam scraps should be stored in a tightly sealed, unbreakable jar containing used x-ray fixer, glycerin, or mineral oil. Storing scrap amalgam under water is not an effective means of controlling mercury vapor.
2. Carpeted floors in treatment rooms are not recommended. Mercury in carpeting is impossible to retrieve and significantly increases mercury hazard. A household vacuum should never be used to clean up mercury spills, as it tends to vaporize the mercury rather than collect it.
3. Water spray and high-volume evacuation should be used when cutting old amalgams or finishing new restorations, because the heat created will release some mercury vapor. A face mask should be worn to reduce mercury vapor and amalgam dust inhalation.
4. Working with mercury or amalgam near a heat source should be avoided.
5. All operations involving mercury should be performed over areas that have an impervious and suitable lipped surface. This will allow easier recovery of unwanted mercury or amalgam scraps.
6. Treatment rooms should have proper ventilation to reduce the possibility of mercury vapor inhalation. Frequent changes in the office air filter system is of utmost importance.

7. Mercury-contaminated items such as gloves, mask, used capsules, squeeze cloths, and the like should be disposed of in a labeled polyethylene bag and sealed.

Suggestions for Controlling Mercury Spills

1. Mercury spills should be cleaned up immediately regardless of amount. Small droplets may be recovered by using a fresh mix of amalgam or lead foil from an x-ray film packet. Spills of mercury should be cleaned up, because small droplets of mercury have a high vapor potential as atmospheric temperature increases. That is to say, the higher the room temperature, the more likely it is that mercury will vaporize.

2. Dental offices that use large quantities of mercury should be equipped with a mercury-spill kit. The kit should include disposable rubber gloves, a mercury vapor respirator, a hypodermic needle with a large lumen, a syringe, adhesive tape for picking up droplets, polyethylene bags for disposal, and a sulfur solution for coating droplets prior to retrieval and disposal.

3. The Council on Dental Materials, Instruments and Equipment specifically advises against the use of ultrasonic condensers when condensing amalgam, because mercury vapor is released from the amalgam.

SUGGESTED ACTIVITIES

- Practice using the amalgamator and prepare a mix of amalgam.
- Practice loading both types of amalgam carriers from an amalgam well, dappen dish, or squeeze cloth.

REVIEW

1. What is the purpose of including zinc in a dental amalgam?
   a. It gives strength.
   b. It acts as a scavenger and reacts with oxygen, preventing it from combining with other metals.
   c. It aids in the amalgamation of the alloy with the mercury because of its strong affinity with mercury.
   d. It determines the dimensional changes that occur during the hardening process.

2. Which is the only metal that is liquid and vaporizes at a relatively low room temperature?
   a. Silver   c. Mercury
   b. Copper   d. Tin

3. What is the purpose of using copper in a dental amalgam?
   a. It gives strength, hardness, and expansion of the amalgam during hardening.
   b. It tarnishes easily.
   c. It minimizes oxidation of other metals present in the alloy during manufacturing.
   d. It is more susceptible to corrosion and tends to weaken the amalgam.

4. Name the two means by which mercury can enter the body system: (1) through the digestive system, (2) by direct contact through the pores of the skin, (3) through inhalation of mercury vapor, and/or (4) through the eyes.
   a. 1, 2   c. 3, 4
   b. 2, 3   d. 1, 4

5. Name the best precautionary measures that may be used by office personnel to reduce potential hazards of mercury vapor: (1) using premeasured capsules, (2) using threaded capsules, (3) using an amalgamator that has an ultra-high-speed setting, and/or (4) using an amalgamator that has a protective hood.
   a. 1, 2   c. 3, 4
   b. 2, 3   d. 1, 4

6. For the following statements, indicate if the statement is true or false.
   ____ a. Trituration is the mechanical means of combining the dental alloy with mercury.
   ____ b. Mercury products are disposed directly into the trash can.
   ____ c. The average well-condensed amalgam should contain approximately 70% or less mercury.
   ____ d. An alloy is composed of two or more metals.
   ____ e. It is necessary to have adequate tooth structure to support an amalgam restoration.
   ____ f. It is necessary for the dental assistant to wear disposable gloves, a face mask, and eyewear while handling a dental amalgam.
   ____ g. When cutting or removing old amalgam restorations, water spray and high-volume evacuation are used.
   ____ h. The maximum approximate working time for condensing an amalgam is 2 minutes.

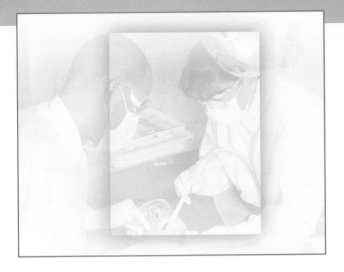

OBJECTIVES

After studying this chapter, the student will be able to:

- Discuss the basic composition of an irreversible colloid.
- Discuss the physical and chemical properties of alginate.
- Discuss the factors that influence the stability of alginate.
- Select the armamentarium needed to mix alginate impression material.
- Measure correct water-to-powder ratio.
- Spatulate mix to a creamy, smooth homogenous mass.
- Select a tray for full-arch maxillary and mandibular alginate impressions.
- Spatulate alginate material and load the trays.
- Select and prepare the appropriate maxillary and mandibular tray for an alginate impression.
- Take a maxillary and mandibular alginate impression, to include the accurate reproduction of all teeth, and supporting tissues (soft tissue, muscle attachments, tuberosities, or retromolar pads).
- Prepare wax and take a wax bite for centric occlusion.
- Discuss the basic composition, advantages, and failures of a reversible hydrocolloid impression material.

Introduction

Hydrocolloid materials were the first elastic impression materials to be developed. However, other types of elastic impression materials are currently available. Hydrocolloids are known as irreversible and reversible.

Alginate material falls under the category of irreversible hydrocolloids and, once in a plastic state, cannot return to its original state. Alginate is used for making study models, for primary impressions of edentulous mouths, and for making impressions in areas in which partial dentures are to be fabricated.

Reversible hydrocolloids have the ability to change from a solid state to a liquid state and back again to a solid state. They are capable of producing extremely accurate **dies** (a replica of a single prepared tooth or several teeth on which a restoration is fabricated) with excellent reproduction of detail well suited for the constructions of **wax patterns** (re-creation of the tooth or portion of the tooth using wax) for cast restorations.

Irreversible Hydrocolloid (Alginate)

Composition

Alginates are salts of **alginic acid** (crystalline compounds that are typically water soluble and are extracted from seaweed). However, alginate is insoluble until potassium or sodium salts are added to make it soluble. When alginate is mixed with water, it has the ability to set or gel.

Dental alginates are called **irreversible colloids** (have the ability to change from a liquid state (sol) to a semisolid state (gel) but do not have the ability to change from a semisolid to a liquid state). A **colloid** is a gelatinous substance with large inorganic molecules that remain suspended and do not diffuse or spread once the chemical change occurs. The material is supplied as flourlike powder and consists essentially of soluble potassium alginate and calcium sulfate. The exact proportion of each chemical may vary with the manufacturer, but in general, percentages of alginate composition are as follows:

- Potassium alginate   15%
- Calcium sulfate   16%

- Trisodium phosphate   1%
- Diatomaceous earth   60%
- Zinc oxide   4%
- Potassium titanium fluoride   3%

When mixed with *calcium sulfate*, a **reactor** (causes a chemical change), *potassium alginate* produces an insoluble calcium alginate. This chemical reaction must be delayed until the impression material has been mixed with water, placed on the impression tray, and carried to the mouth. A third soluble salt, *trisodium phosphate*, is added as a retarder.

Calcium sulfate will react first with the trisodium phosphate before reacting with the soluble potassium alginate. As long as trisodium phosphate is present, the **gelation** (a process by which a colloid changes from a sol to a gel state) reaction between the potassium alginate and calcium sulfate will be prevented. Therefore, when the trisodium phosphate is exhausted, the calcium ions will begin to react with the potassium alginate.

The purpose of *diatomaceous earth* (a finely ground silicate filler) is to act as a filler. Proper amounts of filler can increase the strength and stiffness of the mix and ensure a firm surface that is not tacky. Fillers also help to form the sol by dispersing the alginate powder particle in the water. Zinc oxide is also added as filler and has some influence on the setting time.

Potassium titanium fluoride is added to ensure a hard, dense stone cast surface.

Alginate powder contains about 60% diatomaceous earth. When fluffed, these particles can be inhaled and may prove to be a health hazard. (Recent studies have shown dental alginate to be a health hazard). A new dustless alginate has been introduced to eliminate the presence of these fine airborne particles. Jeltrate Plus is coated with a glycol (an alcohol derived from a carbohydrate) to make it dustless. Jeltrate Plus has a strength 50% higher than standard Jeltrate. The powder is more easily wetted by the water when mixed.

Currently, a two-paste dust-free alginate substitute system, *Ultrafine*, is available. Ultrafine is supplied as two pastes (base and catalyst) that contain water and silicone oil. Ultrafine is similar to standard alginate in strength but is easier to mix because of the two-paste system.

Gel Structure

The gelation of a hydrocolloid is the changing of a sol to a gel. The **sol** is the colloidal solution, and the semisolid state is termed colloidal **gel**. During this phase of changing from a sol to a gel, fibrils will branch and intermesh to form a brush heap structure. These fibrils are composed of chains, sometimes called *micelles*. The structure resembles the intermeshing of twigs in a brush pile. The final structure can be envisioned as a brush heap of calcium alginate fibrils in a network of filler particles and excess water.

Gel Strength

Manipulation of alginate material will affect the wet strength. For example, if too much or too little water is used in mixing, the gel will be weakened. Proper water-to-powder ratio is specified by the manufacturer. When an insufficient amount of time is used for mixing, the strength of the final gel will be radically reduced. When there is insufficient spatulation (undermixing), the ingredients do not dissolve enough to permit the chemical reactions to proceed uniformly throughout the mass. Overmixing also produces poor results, because any calcium alginate gel formed during prolonged spatulation will be broken up. The strength of the mix depends on exact measurements of powder and water, as well as correct spatulation to obtain a smooth, creamy mix within the specified time.

Gelation Time

Manufacturers make dental alginates that have different properties. Some, for instance, are made to set faster than others (Type I, fast set); some set slower for additional working time (Type II, regular or normal set):

Type I, Fast Set

Working Time	Setting Time
68°F (20°C), 1 min, 45 sec	1 min, 45 sec
72°F (22°C), 1 min, 45 sec	1 min, 45 sec
75°F (24°C), 1 min, 30 sec	1 min, 45 sec

Type II, Regular Set

Working Time	Setting Time
68°F (20°C), 2 min, 15 sec	2 min, 15 sec
72°F (22°C), 2 min	2 min, 15 sec
75°F (24°C), 2 min	2 min

Temperature Change

Cool water will delay gelation time, and warm water will hasten it. It is of the utmost importance to read and carefully follow the manufacturer's directions.

It is always wise to use alginate that has been certified by the Council on Dental Materials, Instruments and Devices.

Dimensional Stability

Alginate impressions should be poured as soon as possible, because the material undergoes dimensional changes as time elapses. Such changes in dimensions are termed syneresis or imbibition. **Syneresis** refers to a loss of water by evaporation due to exposure to the air; the result is a shrinkage in dimension. **Imbibition** may occur when a substance takes on additional water, causing a swelling of the material. Consequently, alginate impressions should not be stored in water. Either of these dimensional changes produce an inaccurate impression in the poured model or cast.

Alginate gels currently used in dentistry exhibit reasonably good dimensional stability in an atmosphere of 100% humidity. If the alginate impression has to be preserved for a short time, it should be placed in an airtight container with a moistened paper towel to produce an atmosphere of 100% humidity. However, for the most accurate and satisfactory results, impressions should be poured immediately after being taken. There is no adequate method for storage of any of the hydrocolloid impression materials.

Mixing Alginate Impression Material

The major physical and chemical properties of alginate have been described. Alginate impressions are taken by:

● Inserting impression trays loaded with alginate impression material onto one arch of the dental patient

● Allowing the material to gel or set

● Removing the impression from the mouth

● Pouring the impression in plaster

Mixing or spatulation of alginate impression material requires practice to obtain the smooth, homogenous mass needed to take an accurate impression of the dental arch.

Procedure 41 Mixing Alginate

Materials Needed

Protective glasses
Face mask
Alginate impression material
Water measure
Powder scoop
Paper cup or paper towel
Room temperature water
Plaster flexible bowl
Alginate spatula

Instructions

Assemble all materials needed for the procedure (Figure 44-1).

1 Measure required amount of room temperature water (70–72°F). Carefully read meniscus (the concave surface of a column of liquid with its lowest point in the center) on measuring gauge (Figure 44-2).

2 Pour water into mixing bowl (Figure 44-3).

3 Fluff alginate powder when using powder from a vacuum-sealed container. Do not shake, but roll the container from side to side several times (Figure 44-4). Otherwise a hazardous aerosol cloud (aerosol—fine particles that float in the air)

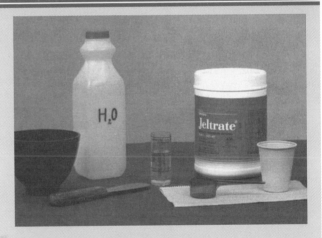
Figure 44-1 Materials assembled.

will form inside the container. Therefore, it is best to allow the container to be left unopened for about 2 minutes. After opening the container, disturb the contents as little as possible. If the alginate powder is inhaled, it can become a health hazard; wearing a face mask can reduce this risk.

4 Fill powder scoop. Gently tap handle of scoop against rim of container. Cut powder with spatula inside scoop to avoid air pockets (Figure 44-5). Level powder with spatula (Figure 44-6). Place powder in paper cup or on paper towel.

continued

continued from previous page
Procedure 41 *Making Alginate*

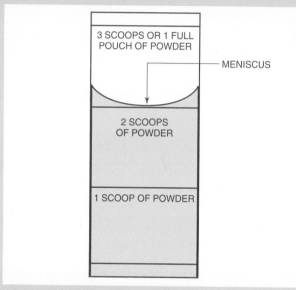

Figure 44-2 Reading meniscus.

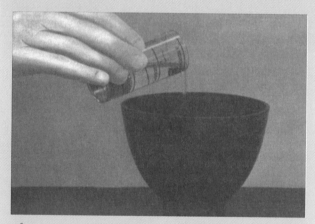

Figure 44-3 Placing water into bowl.

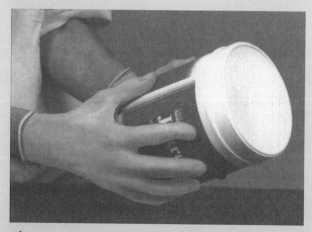

Figure 44-4 Rotating alginate container.

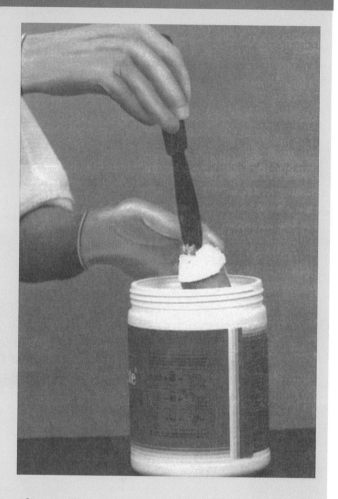

Figure 44-5 Eliminating air pockets.

5 Replace alginate container cover immediately.

6 Carefully sift powder into water (Figure 44-7). If using premeasured packets, open with scissors and gently tap entire contents into water.

7 Stir the mix to wet all powder particles (Figure 44-8).

8 Begin spatulation in a stropping (back and forth) motion. Rotate bowl during spatulation, and, at the same time spread the mix against the side of the bowl to dissolve all the granules and to eliminate air voids (Figure 44-9). Do not allow alginate to spill out of the bowl.

9 Gather mix with spatula after approximately 20 seconds; replace mix in bottom of bowl (Figure 44-10). Continue spatulation until mix is creamy.

continued

continued from previous page
Procedure 41 *Making Alginate*

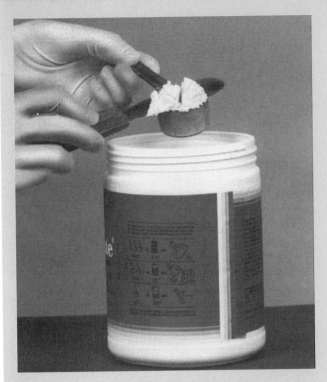

Figure 44-6 Leveling powder with spatula.

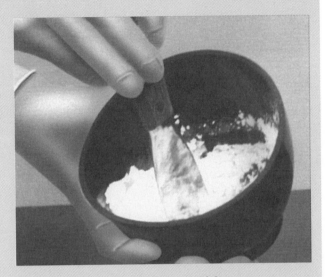

Figure 44-8 Wetting powder particles.

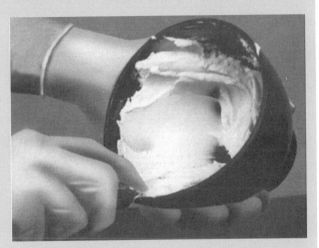

Figure 44-9 Spatulating material against side of bowl (stropping).

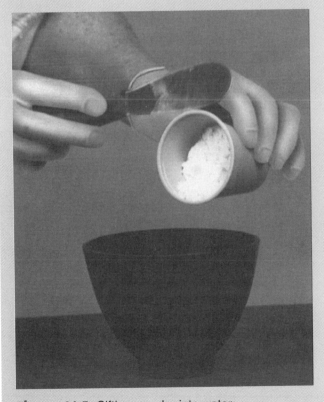

Figure 44-7 Sifting powder into water.

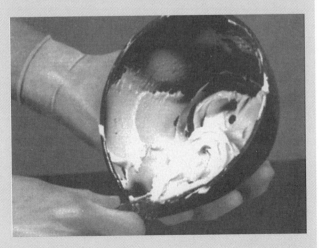

Figure 44-10 Gathering material.

continued

continued from previous page
Procedure 41 Making Alginate

Gather mass on spatula and load tray. Total mixing time of steps 6–9 is not to exceed 1 minute for regular set. *Note:* Alginate may be hand-mixed or mixed with a mechanical mixer (alginator) (Figure 44-11).

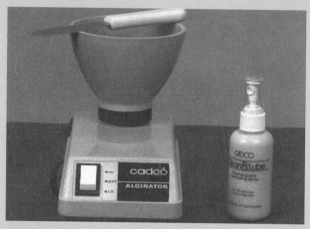

Figure 44-11 Mechanical mixer.

Loading Alginate Trays

The first consideration when taking an impression is the proper selection of the tray(s). The purpose of the tray is to control, carry, and confine the impression material in the patient's mouth. Trays may be made of disposable styrofoam, perforated or solid (rim lock) metal, or plastic. Trays may be full arch, anterior only, and right or left quadrant (Figure 44-12).

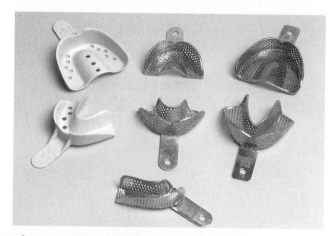

Figure 44-12 Tray assortment.

Procedure 42 Loading Alginate Trays Technique

Materials Needed

Impression trays
Alginate impression material
Measuring devices
Plaster flexible bowl
Small rubber bowl
Alginate spatula
Paper cup
Room temperature water
Paper towels

Instructions

Loading a Mandibular Impression Tray (2 scoops of powder)

Assemble all materials needed for the procedure:

1 Have a small bowl of water ready for smoothing tray alginate.

2 Spatulate alginate according to instructions.

continued

continued from previous page
Procedure 42 Loading Alginate Trays Technique

3 Remove half the alginate mix from bowl and load one side of tray (Figure 44-13).

4 With spatula, press alginate mix into tray (Figure 44-14).

5 Repeat procedure for opposite side of tray.

6 Wet fingers, and smooth the surface of the tray mix while gently pressing material to obtain retention (Figure 44-15).

7 Remove any unwanted material from border of the tray, especially the tongue area (Figure 44-16).

8 Loading time should approximate 30 seconds.

Loading a Maxillary Impression Tray (2–3 scoops of powder)

1 Have a small bowl of water ready for smoothing tray alginate.

2 Spatulate alginate according to instructions.

3 Remove alginate from bowl in one mass.

4 Place all of the alginate in the posterior area of the tray while holding spatula vertically to the plane of the tray (Figure 44-17).

5 With spatula, spread alginate evenly over entire tray, making certain that no open voids are created (Figure 44-18).

6 Wet fingers, and smooth the surface of the tray mix while gently pressing material to obtain retention.

7 Remove any unwanted material from border of the tray.

8 Loading time should approximate 30 seconds.

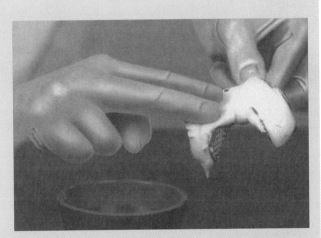
Figure 44-15 Smoothing surface of alginate with wet fingers.

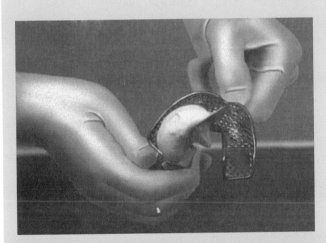
Figure 44-13 Loading half of mandibular tray.

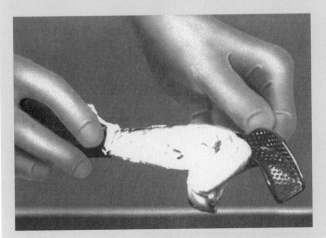
Figure 44-14 Pressing alginate mix into tray.

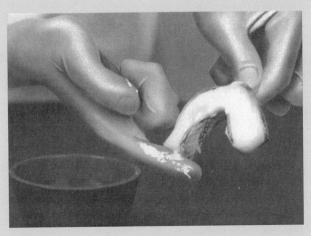
Figure 44-16 Removing unwanted material from border of tray.

continued

continued from previous page
Procedure 42 Loading Alginate Trays Technique

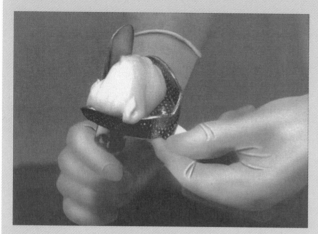

Figure 44-17 Loading maxillary tray.

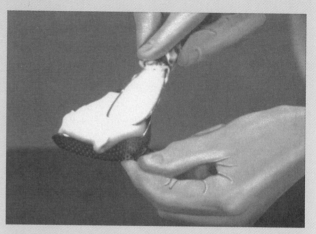

Figure 44-18 Pressing alginate mix over entire tray.

Cleaning Up

1 Remove impression material from tray(s) and place in ultrasonic unit with tray-cleaning solution (alginate remover). Rinse and dry tray(s).

2 Wash and dry bowls and spatula.

3 Return all items to proper place.

4 Clean the workstation.

Taking Alginate Impressions for Study Models

Through legislative measure, under their respective state Dental Practice Acts, some states have legally afforded additional duties and responsibilities to the dental assistant. Among these is taking alginate impressions for study models. For that reason, the object of this chapter will be to detail the essential steps in taking alginate impressions of the dental arches of patients.

Study models are made for several reasons. They are used in diagnosis and treatment planning, patient education, comparison for "before" and "after" models, recording tooth sizes and positions (in case of an accidental fracture or avulsion), rotated and malaligned teeth, height of the soft tissue, and occlusal relationship of maxillary and mandibular teeth.

Procedure 43 Taking Alginate Impressions

Materials Needed

Protective eyewear
Face mask
Disposable gloves
Maxillary and mandibular perforated trays
Beading wax
Lubricant for lips
Cotton rolls
Mouthwash

Plastic drape and/or patient napkin
Spatula, plaster
Laboratory knife
Alginate scoop
Alginate powder
Water vial
Room temperature water
Paper cup or paper towel
Mixing bowls, large and small

continued

continued from previous page
Procedure 43 Taking Alginate Impressions

Instructions

Seating and Preparing the Patient for Impressions

1 Seat patient upright in chair.

2 Drape and place patient napkin. *Note:* At this time the operator should wash and glove hands and don a face mask or shield.

3 Examine patient's mouth with mouth mirror.

4 Apply lubricant to patient's lips and corners of the mouth.

Selecting Impression Trays

1 The trays should cover the most distal teeth or the tuberosity/retromolar pads, whichever is most posterior.

2 The trays should allow about 3 mm (1/8 in.) of impression material on buccal, lingual, and facial surfaces of all teeth involved.

3 Incisors should set in the deepest anterior portion of the tray.

4 The tray should not impinge on the soft tissues.

Preparing Impression Trays

1 Try maxillary and mandibular trays in patient's mouth.

2 Slide tray in sideways and center in mouth as shown (Figures 44-19 and 44-20).

3 Observe trays, making certain that ample space is provided. Trays should NEVER impinge on soft tissues.

4 Adapt beading wax to peripheral edges of tray(s). This adds to patient comfort and prevents impinging on the tissues. Beading wax may be added to the length and dimension of tray(s) and helps to retain impression material in tray. For a high vault, a wax strip may be placed over the palatal area.

5 Retry prepared trays in patient's mouth.

6 Explain procedure to patient. The mandibular impression is taken first to accustom the patient to the taste, feel, and consistency of the impression material. Patients are less likely to gag on the lower impression.

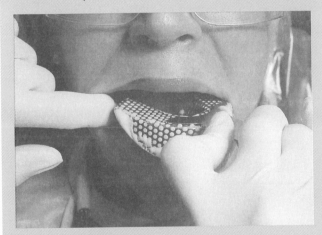

Figure 44-19 Inserting mandibular tray.

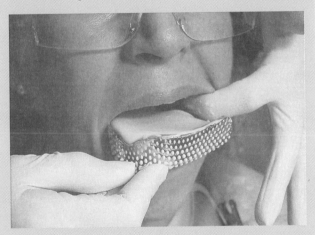

Figure 44-20 Inserting maxillary tray

The Gag Reflex

Should the gag reflex become a problem, the following instructions may be given:

1. Ask the patient to relax, pant, or breathe rapidly through mouth and or nose.

2. Direct the patient to extend one leg upward and concentrate on maintaining it in the same position until the impression is completed.

3. Place a small amount of imitation table salt on distal portion of tongue and instruct the patient to swallow. *Note: NoSalt* has a potassium chloride base, rather than the commonly used sodium chloride table salt.

4. Children may be given a mental chore, such as counting backward beginning with 100.

Procedure 44 Taking the Impression for Mandibular Arch

The position of the operator for the mandibular impression is between 8 and 9 o'clock, and for the maxillary impression between 9 and 12 o'clock.

The patient's shoulder should be positioned at about the same height as the elbow of the operator. Instruct the patient to rinse with mouthwash just prior to taking impression(s).

Instructions

1 Mix alginate and load tray.

2 Insert tray.

3 Hold tray in one hand and, with the other hand, retract cheek.

4 Slide tray in sideways until one-half of tray is inside the mouth; then rotate tray and seat (Figure 44-19). The handle of the tray should be centered (aligned with nose) and perpendicular to the anterior teeth. The anterior portion of the tray must be positioned over centrals or laterals to provide adequate impression material in the vestibular area. *Note:* Alginate impressions must provide detail of the facial surfaces of the anterior teeth and labial frenum and also of the mucobuccal attachment. The peripheral roll should be accurately duplicated in impression(s). Examine the impression(s) for detail. Large voids and lack of detail or completeness are reasons enough for retaking the impression(s).

5 Ask the patient to close his or her mouth slightly; this will relax the facial muscles and help the operator to seat the tray.

6 Depress heels of tray (posterior teeth) first (Figure 44-21).

7 Have the patient elevate tongue (toward roof of mouth); then depress tray downward, bringing it parallel to the occlusal plane (Figure 44-22).

8 Assist the patient in lifting the lip and cheek areas to allow complete seating of tray.

9 Position the tray by pressing firmly on the occlusal and incisal surfaces of the mandibular teeth using the index and middle fingers of each hand on top of the tray and resting the thumbs under the mandible.

10 Instruct patient to breathe deeply and slowly through the nose while the tray is in place.

11 When the impression material has set, lift cheek on one side with index finger and then on the other side to break atmospheric seal. Insert fingers over the handle portion of the tray to protect the opposing teeth.

12 Separate the impression from the teeth in one continuous vertical motion (upward for the mandibular arch).

13 Rinse impression in room temperature water following Centers for Disease Control and Prevention

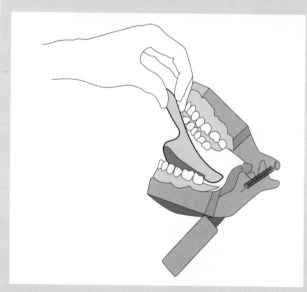

Figure 44-21 Shown on a typodont to demonstrate depressing heel of tray.

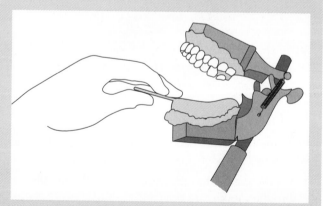

Figure 44-22 Shown on a typodont to demonstrate tray position, parallel to occlusal plane.

continued

continued from previous page
Procedure 44 Taking the Impression for Mandibular Arch

(CDC) guidelines. The CDC and the American Dental Association (ADA) guidelines on the care of hydrocolloid impression materials specify that blood and saliva should be thoroughly cleaned from the impression material that has been used in the mouth. Therefore, the dental assistant or auxiliary should rinse the impression(s) in room temperature water for 30 seconds, shake off excess water, then spray with 1 of 3 disinfectants: regular iodophor diluted according to the manufacturer's instructions, an acid glutaraldehyde (diluted 4 parts water to 1 part glutaraldehyde), or sodium hypochlorite (household bleach) diluted 10 parts water to 1 part bleach (Figure 44-23). Place impression(s) in a baggie for 10–30 minutes and label baggie with patient's name. After impression(s) have been disinfected, rinse, and pour immediately. Place in airtight container for 1 hour while plaster hardens.

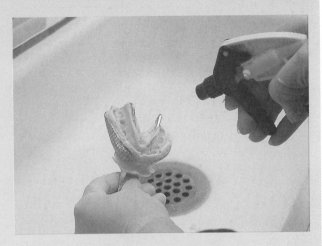

Figure 44-23 Disinfecting the impression.

Procedure 45 Taking the Impression for Maxillary Arch

Instructions

1 Mix alginate, and load tray with bulk of material toward the anterior portion of the tray.

2 Insert tray.

3 Hold tray in one hand and with the other hand retract cheek.

4 Slide tray in sideways until one-half of tray is inside the mouth; then rotate tray and seat (refer to Figure 44-20). The handle of the tray should be centered (aligned with nose) and perpendicular to the anterior teeth. The anterior portion of the tray must be positioned over centrals and laterals to provide adequate impression material in the vestibular area.

5 Seat posterior of tray first. This will expel material forward, instead of toward the throat (Figure 44-24).

6 Continue seating the anterior portion of the tray (Figure 44-25).

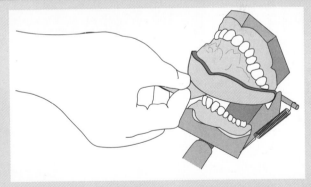

Figure 44-24 Shown on a typodont to demonstrate seating posterior of maxillary tray.

7 Lift upper lip to free it from the tray. Have patient relax cheeks and lips. Direct patient to use a "sucking on straw" technique to help bring lip over tray and obtain impression of muscle attachments.

continued

continued from previous page

Procedure 45 Taking the Impression for Maxillary Arch

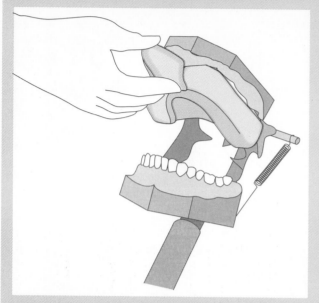

Figure 44-25 Shown on a typodont to demonstrate how to bring anterior of maxillary tray into position.

8 Patient's head should be tipped forward to prevent material from flowing into the throat, which could cause patient to gag.

9 Instruct patient to breathe deeply and slowly through the nose while tray is in place.

10 When impression material has set, lift cheek on one side with index finger, then on the other side, to break atmospheric seal. Insert fingers under the handle portion of the tray to protect the opposing teeth.

11 Separate the impression from the teeth in one continuous vertical motion (downward for the maxillary arch).

12 Follow the same procedure as directed for handling mandibular impression, step 13.

13 Shake excess water from impression, and wrap in wet paper towel and place in humidor. *Note:* After wax bite is taken, immediately pour impression in plaster. Refer to Chapter 48.

Procedure 46 Taking a Wax Bite

A wax bite provides occlusal relationship of the maxillary and mandibular teeth (Figure 44-26A–C).

Instructions

1 Place wax bite (horseshoe-shaped wax) in hot water to soften.

2 Take softened wax, and place over patient's mandibular teeth. Extend wax 1/4 in. beyond incisal edge of maxillary centrals, Figure 44-26A.

3 Have patient close firmly on wax until it has hardened. Patient must be in his or her true centric occlusion.

4 An air syringe may be used to hasten the cooling of wax bite, Figure 44-26B.

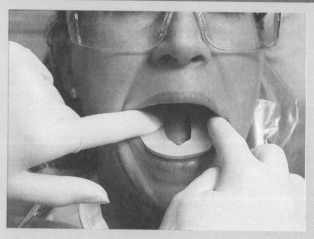

Figure 44-26A Taking a wax bite: positioning the wax bite on mandibular arch.

continued

5 Carefully remove wax bite and chill under cold water.

6 Remove wax bite from water and spray with appropriate disinfectant, Figure 44-26C.

7 Place patient's initials in upper right-hand corner of wax for identification purposes.

8 Retain wax bite. During model trimming, use to maintain centric occlusion. *Note:* Before dismissing the patient, remove any excess impression material from his or her face.

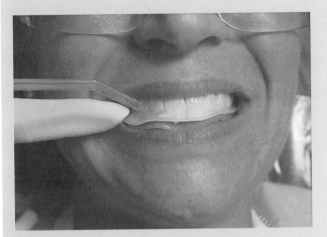

Figure 44-26B Cooling the wax bite using air syringe.

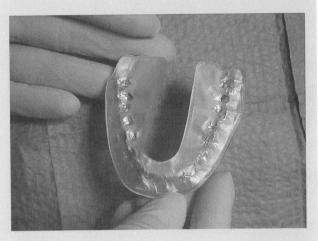

Figure 44-26C Wax bite.

Reversible Hydrocolloid

Reversible hydrocolloid (series of particles suspended in water), is considered to be **hydrophillic** (adapts to water), and it can be used repeatedly simply by heating and cooling. The term *reversible* indicates the capacity of the hydrocolloid to change from a liquid (sol) state to a semisolid (gel) state and vice versa under certain conditions. This physical effect is induced by a change in temperature. The temperature at which the change from the sol state to a semisolid material occurs is known as the **gelation temperature**. The final gel is composed of a brush-heap arrangement of fibrils of agar-agar enmeshed in water and is no different from the original fluid sol.

Reversible hydrocolloid is used for construction of crown and bridge work and partial dentures, not for study models. The principal use of this material is where accuracy and detail are demanded.

Hydrocolloid impression material is distributed by the manufacturer in a solid state and includes both tray and syringe material (Figure 44-27).

The tray material is supplied in tubes and in five different **viscosities** (having a fluid consistency with a tendency to resist flow) and colors. The type used may vary according to dentist preference.

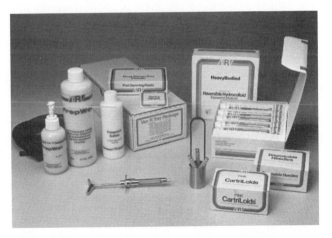

Figure 44-27 Hydrocolloid products. (Courtesy of Van R Dental Products, Inc., Los Angeles, CA.)

The syringe material is manufactured in various colors and three viscosities and forms (stick, backloading tubes, and preloaded cartridges). The color of the material denotes its viscosity. The difference of color between the tray and syringe material provides contrast and detail to the hydrocolloid impression. The composition of hydrocolloid is as follows:

- Agar-agar (seaweed), 8–15%
- Water by weight, 80–85%
- Borax, small amount
- Potassium sulfate, 2%
- Fillers, remaining portion

Agar-agar, extracted from a certain type of seaweed, provides a suitable colloid as a base for hydrocolloid impression materials. A colloid is a suspension of particles, or small groups of molecules, in some type of dispersing medium (i.e., distributed more or less evenly throughout the solution), which, in this case, is water.

Borax, in small amounts, is added by the manufacturer to increase the strength of the gel. Borax is a retarder for the setting of gypsum products. Thus, the presence of borax and the gel itself are detrimental to the impression material in that it retards the set of the gypsum die material that is poured into the impression. Therefore, to overcome the presence of borax in the impression material, potassium sulfate (approximately 2%) is currently added to commercial dental hydrocolloid impression materials. Potassium sulfate will harden the surface of the stone and will give a better model. Fillers, preservatives, and flavorings comprise the remaining components.

Gel Strength

Hydrocolloid gels are relatively weak elastic solids that are subject to tearing if the stress is applied rapidly and not maintained for a prolonged time. When a complete uniform gel is reached, the impression is removed with a quick "snap-out" action rather than a slow, teasing movement.

Gelation Time

Gelation of the hydrocolloid occurs when circulating cool water is drawn through the tray at approximately 60–70°F (16–21°C) for no less than 5 minutes. As gelation begins near the base of the tray, ice water should not be used, because it will promote rapid gelation and a concentration of stress in the hydrocolloid material. The minimum 5-minute gelling time is required to allow gelation to process until the gel is strong enough to resist distortion or fracture during removal.

Dimensional Stability

Because the large fraction of the volume of a hydrocolloid gel is occupied by water, the water content of such a gel has a considerable influence on the dimensional stability of the impression material. Loss of water results in shrinkage, and uptake of water produces swelling. Such changes in dimensions are termed syneresis or

imbibition. Syneresis refers to the loss of water by evaporation due to the exposure to the air; the result is a shrinkage in dimension. If a hydrocolloid gel is stored in contact with water, it will absorb additional water by the process of imbibition. Obviously, either circumstance will lead to a dimensionally unstable gel.

Advantages

- It is one of the most accurate of reproduction materials.
- It can be manipulated with comparative ease to get the impression.
- It allows the operator to take impressions of multiple preparations at one time.
- There is comparative ease in reproducing contour, anatomy, and detail.
- It is a relatively inexpensive material and convenient to use.
- The technique affords a clean and highly controlled procedure.

Failures

There are several common causes for failures in the use of reversible hydrocolloid materials:

Imperfection	Probable Causes
Grainy material	Inadequate boiling Conditioning temperature too low Conditioning time unduly long
Separation of tray and syringe material	Water-soaked layer of tray material not removed Undue gelation of either syringe or tray material
Tearing	Inadequate bulk Moisture contamination at gingiva Premature removal of impression tray from mouth Syringe material partially gelled when tray seated Improper removal of tray from the mouth
Irregularly shaped voids	Moisture or debris on tissue Material too cool or grainy
Rough or chalky stone cast	Inadequate cleansing of impression Excess water or potassium sulfate solution left in impression Premature removal of stone cast from impression Improper manipulation of stone; water-powder ratio

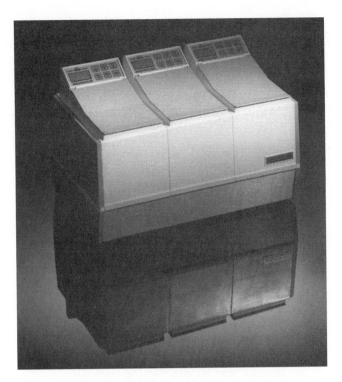

Figure 44-28 Hydrocolloid conditioner and accessories. (Courtesy of Van R Dental Products, Inc., Los Angeles, CA.)

Imperfection	Probable Causes
Distortion, inaccuracy	Impression not poured immediately
	Movement of tray during gelation
	Premature removal of tray from mouth
	Improper removal of tray from mouth
	Use of ice water during initial stages of gelation

The Hydrocolloid Conditioner

When the material is being liquefied, the temperature of the boiling compartment must reach 212°F (100°C), the storage compartment 150–155°F (66 to 68°C), and the tempering compartment 110–120°F (43 to 46°C). On the hydrocolloid conditioner, the temperatures are thermostatically regulated (Figure 44-28).

Types of Hydrocolloid Impression Trays

Trays used for hydrocolloid impressions are of the water-cooled type and include full upper and lower arches (Figure 44-29), full quadrant, and double-bite. All water-cooled trays require a tubing hose that is attached to the tray at one end; the water/vacuum source on the dental unit is attached at the opposite end.

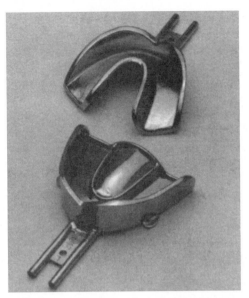

Figure 44-29 Full upper and lower water-cooled trays. (Courtesy of Van R Dental Products, Inc., Los Angeles, CA.)

3. The best method to alter the gelation time for alginate is to:
   a. Alter the amount of water in the mix
   b. Alter the temperature of the water
   c. Alter the mixing time
   d. Alter the manipulation time

4. What does the term syneresis mean?
   a. A substance takes on additional water, resulting in swelling of the material
   b. The gel strength when the material is overmixed
   c. The evaporation of water due to exposure to air resulting in shrinkage of dimension
   d. The gel strength when there is insufficient spatulation

5. Match each alginate material compound with the correct statement.

   ___ a. Potassium alginate
   ___ b. Calcium sulfate
   ___ c. Trisodium phosphate
   ___ d. Diatomaceous earth
   ___ e. Potassium titanium fluoride
   ___ f. Zinc oxide

   1. Ensures a hard, dense stone cast surface
   2. A filler that increases the strength and stiffness of the mix
   3. The retarder that delays the reaction
   4. The reactor that causes the material to set or gel
   5. A filler that has some influence on the setting time
   6. Mixed with calcium sulfate to produce insoluble calcium alginate

6. Why is beading wax added to the alginate impression tray?
   a. To add length to the tray
   b. To prevent impinging on the tissues
   c. To add height over the palatal area for individuals with a high vault
   d. For patient comfort
   e. All of the above

7. What is the best method to insert either the maxillary or mandibular impression tray into the mouth?
   a. Slide tray in sideways until one-half of tray is inside the mouth, then rotate tray and seat it.
   b. Carefully insert tray vertically and start seating the posterior portion.
   c. Insert the maxillary impression tray before the mandibular tray.
   d. Both b and c.

8. How can one determine that the tray is centered in the mouth?
   a. Align the tray handle with the nose.
   b. Align the tray handle with the central incisors.
   c. It should fit the arch in any position.
   d. Both a and b.

Custom Trays:
Acrylic and Silicone

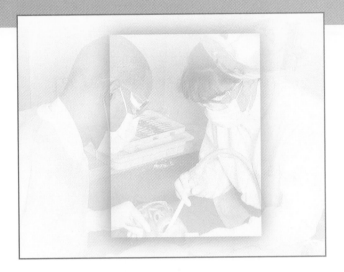

OBJECTIVES

After studying this chapter, the student will be able to:

● Discuss the two types of custom-made trays used for elastomeric impression material.

● Explain the function of a wax spacer.

● Make an acrylic custom-made tray using a plaster model.

● Prepare a custom-made tray using silicone putty.

Introduction

Custom-made trays are specifically designed to ensure adequate spacing between the teeth and tray, and the use of impression material with less bulk and uniform thickness in all areas of the tray, to produce the most accurate impressions.

Two types of custom-made trays may be fabricated for use with rubber-base (elastomeric) impression materials. One type is a self-cured acrylic resin, made in advance outside the patient's mouth using a **study cast** (a plaster replica of the patient's mouth). The second is a silicone putty, shaped within the patient's mouth using a rigid standard-stock tray and a moldable puttylike silicone paste material.

Self-Cured Acrylic Resin Tray

The self-cured acrylic resin tray is made on a study cast. It is constructed outside of the patient's mouth due to the **exothermic reaction** (producing heat due to a chemical reaction) that may reach up to 80°C, enough to burn the oral mucosa. A strong odor is also given off while curing. The recommended procedure for constructing an acrylic custom-made tray requires that an alginate impression of the individual's mouth be taken. The impression is poured in plaster and allowed to set and dry. The acrylic custom-made tray is then fabricated on this model.

An acrylic resin tray should be made at least 24 hours before needed because it undergoes **dimensional distortion** (continues to change its dimensions due to the relaxation of internal stresses). This property may also cause distortion of the elastic impression material if used prematurely.

The acrylic resin (methylmethacrylate) is available in powder and liquid form. The powder is known as a **polymer** (a long chain of many mers, or molecules of a compound capable of being chemically combined—*poly* means "many"). The liquid is termed a **monomer** (one mer—*mono* means "one"). When mixed together, a chemical reaction or polymerization begins to take place. The material will cure or polymerize (harden) in 5–7 minutes from the start of mixing.

Acrylic Manipulation Stages

1. It is fluid when monomer and polymer are first mixed.

2. It becomes thick, sticky, and shiny.

3. When it reaches a doughy consistency and is no longer shiny, it can be manipulated without sticking to the operator's fingers.

4. It reaches a rubbery form and begins to harden soon thereafter. At this stage it gives off tremendous heat, enough to melt wax.

5. When final hardness occurs, the material remains in this form.

Procedure 47 Constructing a Self-Cured Acrylic Resin Tray

Materials Needed

Plaster model
Glass jar or paper cup (not plastic)
Base plate wax
Vaseline
Bowl of hot water
Laboratory knife
Acrylic powder (polymer)
Acrylic liquid (monomer)
Measurers for resin
Small spatula or wooden tongue blade
Glass square or slab
Acrylic bur with straight handpiece
Pencil

Instructions

1 On the plaster model, outline with a pencil where the peripheral edge of the tray will be.

2 Apply a thin layer of Vaseline to the selected quadrant of plaster model.

3 Cut base plate wax to the width and length of the selected quadrant. One or two thicknesses of base plate wax may be used. The wax provides the necessary space needed for the elastomeric impression material. This wax is called a **spacer**.

4 Place wax in bowl of hot water to soften.

5 Remove softened wax from water and adapt to prepared quadrant. If necessary, trim excess wax with laboratory knife. Wax should cover crown portions of the teeth and extend approximately 4 mm beyond the gingival margin and the buccal and lingual surfaces (Figure 45-1). Cut out holes to serve as "stops." This will prevent overseating of tray. Do not place holes in the tray over a prepared tooth.

6 Coat the top surface of the wax spacer with Vaseline. Set aside.

7 Measure liquid and place in paper cup.

8 Measure powder and carry into liquid. *Note:* Follow manufacturer's instructions for proportions.

9 Spatulate for 30 seconds (Figure 45-2).

10 Allow acrylic to set for 2–3 minutes to doughy stage until gloss has disappeared and is nonsticky (Figure 45-3).

11 Lightly lubricate glass slab and hands with Vaseline.

12 Remove acrylic mix from paper cup with spatula or wooden tongue blade. With finger tips, form into a roll mass.

13 Place dough on glass slab, and flatten with hands to a uniform thickness (1/8 in.).

14 Carefully remove from glass slab, and adapt over wax spacer (Figure 45-4). Do not extend acrylic beyond wax spacer.

15 While material is pliable, form handle over anterior teeth. Handle should be parallel to the occlusal surfaces of the teeth. Should a separate handle be fashioned, place a drop of liquid where it will attach.

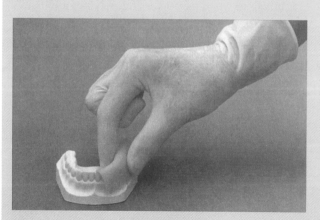

Figure 45-1 Placing a wax spacer.

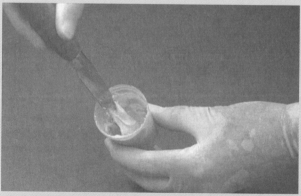

Figure 45-2 Monomer and polymer are spatulated in a paper cup.

continued

continued from previous page
Procedure 47 Constructing a Self-Cured Acrylic Resin Tray

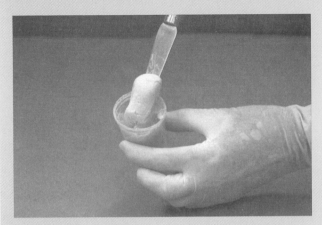

Figure 45-3 Resin set to doughy consistency.

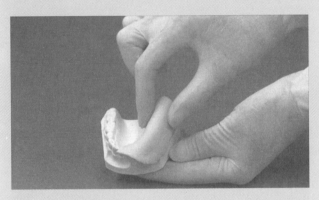

Figure 45-4 Acrylic resin adapted over wax spacer.

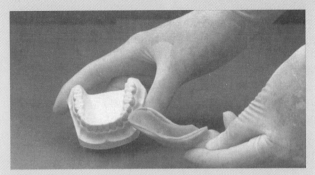

Figure 45-5 Tray and wax spacer removed from model.

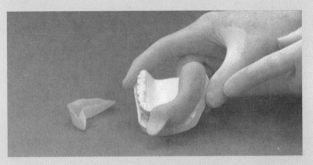

Figure 45-6 Wax spacer is removed and tray is repositioned on model for final curing.

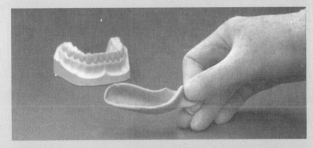

Figure 45-7 Completed acrylic quadrant tray.

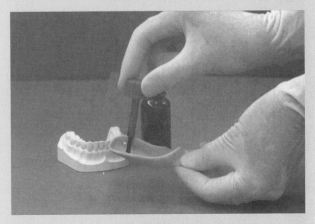

Figure 45-8 Tray adhesive applied to tray.

16 Remove acrylic tray from model before final curing has completed (Figure 45-5).

17 Remove wax spacer before wax melts. Reposition tray on the model for final curing, about 2 minutes (Figure 45-6). *Note:* As acrylic begins to cure, an exothermic reaction occurs (heat is given off).

18 Trim tray. Remove excess or rough areas on the tray with acrylic bur. The completed tray should be smooth in appearance, without undercuts, and uniform in thickness (Figure 45-7). The bur may also be used on the inside of the tray to remove excess tray material or undercuts. This will provide the necessary depth for the impression material. Rinse off powder particles and dry tray.

19 Prepare tray with tray adhesive. The adhesive must be applied to the tray so that the impression material will adhere to the acrylic tray. Two to three applications of the tray adhesive are required well in advance of the impression procedure (Figure 45-8).

Silicone Putty Tray

Silicone elastomeric impression materials are used for taking single-quadrant and full-mouth impressions. These materials use a moldable puttylike silicone paste material for making a custom-made tray. Standard stock-trays are used to help retain or hold the puttylike material. The custom-made tray is made directly in the mouth before the tooth or teeth are prepared.

The custom-made tray is set aside until the final impression is taken with the low-viscosity syringe impression material. A heavy-body or high-viscosity tray material may be used along with the syringe material. When ready, the syringe and tray materials are spatulated according to directions. The syringe material is placed in the syringe and injected onto the prepared tooth or teeth, and the tray material is placed into the putty tray. The custom-made tray is then repositioned over the teeth and allowed to set, between 6 and 8 minutes. This procedure may be referred to as the double- or multiple-mix technique.

The putty tray should remain in the rigid tray throughout the procedure of constructing and using it.

Procedure 48 Constructing a Silicone Putty Tray

Materials Needed

Measuring scoop
Perforated quadrant tray
Mixing pad, 1
Stiff spatula, 1
Plastic separator (polyethylene sheet)
Laboratory knife
Silicone putty paste
Catalyst liquid
Typodont to simulate patient's mouth

Instructions

1 Measure one level scoop of silicone putty and place on mixing pad (Figure 45-9).

2 Press putty into the shape of a thin wafer.

3 With spatula, cut shallow grooves (waffle pattern) into putty material.

4 Dispense four drops of catalyst liquid on top of putty material.

5 With spatula, carefully fold and knead the liquid into putty for approximately 20 seconds, until the liquid is completely incorporated in the putty and no trace of liquid is visible.

6 Immediately remove putty from mixing pad and vigorously knead with gloved (vinyl) hands for another 25 seconds. *Note:* Should any liquid remain on mixing pad, use putty to blot up remaining liquid from pad.

7 Shape putty into a roll and place into quadrant tray (Figure 45-10).

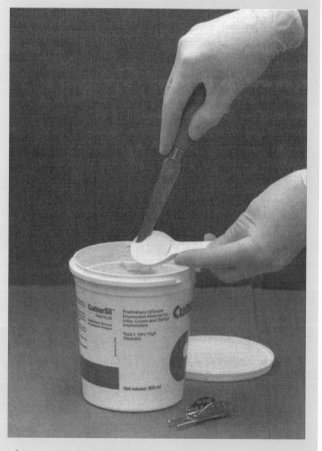

Figure 45-9 Silicone putty tray material.

continued

Continued from previous page
Procedure 48 Constructing a Silicone Putty Tray

8 Place plastic separator over top of putty/tray, and position tray over the area of the tooth to be prepared. Apply sufficient pressure to seat tray. The plastic separator prevents trapping undercuts on tray.

9 Remove putty tray impression from oral cavity, set aside to cure, approximately 2 minutes.

10 Remove plastic separator. Set aside until ready to take final impression (Figure 45-11).

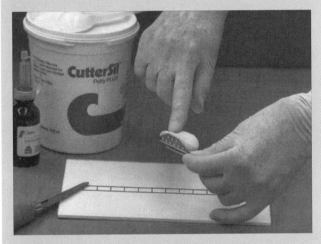

Figure 45-10 Rigid standard stock tray filled with putty material.

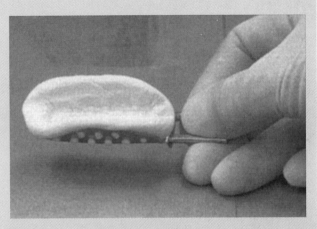

Figure 45-11 Silicone putty tray.

Other Custom Trays

Also available for fabrication of custom trays are a number of newer plastic materials. These include **thermoplastic** materials (having the ability to transform from a glassy, brittle solid to a softened, moldable plastic by the use of heat) in the form of wafers and beads that are heated, formed, and allowed to cool as well as a number of light-cured resin materials. While these materials can be quite convenient, few studies are available to document their effectiveness. As long as the basic criteria for custom trays are met, these materials should be acceptable. These criteria include rigidity, provision for bulk of impression material, and stability. These types of trays should also be made 24 hours in advance and the adhesive applied in a similar manner to the acrylic resin trays.

SUGGESTED ACTIVITIES

● Make an acrylic quadrant custom-made tray on a plaster model.

● Make a silicone putty tray using a typodont to simulate the patient's mouth.

REVIEW

1. Why are custom trays constructed?
   a. To ensure that there will be uniform space between the teeth and tray to produce accurate impressions
   b. To have a tight fit between tray and teeth
   c. To produce ample spacing between tray and teeth
   d. To control the bulk of the impression material
   e. Both a and d

2. Why is it necessary to construct self-cured acrylic resin trays outside the patient's mouth?
   a. It emits a strong odor.
   b. It produces exothermic reaction.
   c. The curing time is too lengthy.
   d. Both a and b
   e. Both b and c

3. What is the purpose for using baseplate wax when constructing a self-cured acrylic tray?
   a. To add dimension to the acrylic tray
   b. To increase acrylic tray length
   c. To provide necessary space for the impression material
   d. To minimize tissue impingement

4. How is the silicone putty tray material retained while constructing and using it?
   a. It is not necessary to have support due to the bulkiness of the material.
   b. A standard stock tray is used.
   c. Base plate wax is used temporarily.
   d. A plastic wafer is used.

5. What is the purpose of using a plastic separator while constructing a silicone putty tray?
   a. To separate the tray from the impression material
   b. To act as a spacer
   c. To prevent trapping undercuts on the tray
   d. To ensure that there will be adequate space for the impression material

Elastomeric Impression Materials

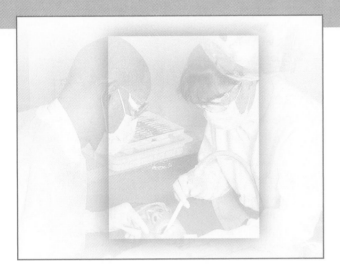

OBJECTIVES

After studying this chapter, the student will be able to:

- Discuss the advantages of using elastomeric impression materials over hydrocolloid impression material.
- Identify the four types of elastomeric impression materials.
- State the advantage(s) for using each type of elastomeric material.
- Discuss the disinfecting procedure used for each type of elastomeric impression.
- Select the materials needed to prepare polysulfide impression material.
- Prepare polysulfide rubber base impression material for both the syringe and tray.
- Prepare tray and syringe silicone impression material and take a quadrant impression of a typodont using the putty custom-made tray.
- Take an impression using a typodont.
- Assemble the automix cartridge unit.
- Prepare polyvinylsiloxane impression material using the automix cartridge unit.
- Discuss the technique of taking a bite registration.

Introduction

The rubberlike elastomeric impression materials polysulfide, silicones (condensation and addition), and polyether offer several advantages over hydrocolloid impression materials. The elastomer or rubberlike materials are stronger and more tear resistant than hydrocolloid. In other words, when the impression is removed from the mouth, the material will not tear. They also do not have the dimensional problems of syneresis or imbibition. With one exception, polyether is **hydrophilic** (capable of taking up water) and, if placed in water, will swell.

The elastomeric impression materials use a base and accelerator system. The base material is supplied in paste form, and the **accelerator** (a substance that speeds up a reaction) or **catalyst** (a substance capable of promoting or altering the speed of a chemical reaction but that does not take part in the reaction) may be a paste or a liquid. The materials are classified according to their **viscosity** (thickness of a fluid that causes it not to flow). The four classes are identified as:

1. Very high viscosity with puttylike consistency, used for custom trays
2. High viscosity, or heavy-bodied tray material
3. Medium or regular viscosity, used for full-arch impressions
4. Low viscosity, or light-bodied syringe material

Polysulfide Impression Material

The first rubber-base material introduced to dentistry was polysulfide, later changed to mercaptan for the chemical contained in the base paste. The terms *mercaptan* and *polysulfide* may be used interchangeably; however, it is more acceptable to refer to the spatulated material as mercaptan and the set rubberlike impression material as polysulfide. It is during **polymerization** (process of changing two or more like molecules to form a more complex molecule) that mercaptan reacts with the accelerator, lead dioxide. Examples of this material are Permlastic (Kerr Manufacturing Co.), Coe-Flex, Omniflex (Coe Laboratories), and Neoplex (Heraeus Kulzer). See Table 46-1.

Table 46-1 Properties of Elastomeric Materials

Material	Composition	Advantages	Disadvantages	Examples
Polysulfide	Mercaptan polymer	More working time Accuracy, detailed Tear resistant	Pour within 30 min Shrinkage Difficult to mix Stains clothing Odor objectionable Color objectionable	Permlastic (Kerr) Coe-Flex (Coe) Omniflex (Coe) Neoplex (Heraeus Kulzer)
Condensation "conventional" silicone	Dimethylsiloxane, silica Tin octoate Alky silicate	Easy to handle Odorless Patient acceptance	Pour within 30 min Poor tear strength Shorter shelf life	Accoe (GC America) Examix (GC America) Cuttersil (Heraeus Kulzer) Citricon (Kerr Manufacturing)
Polyvinylsiloxane/ addition silicone/ polysiloxane	Poly (vinyl) siloxane Platinum salt	Good dimensional stability Easy to handle Odorless Also available in automix Shorter working time	Prevent contact with latex gloves Some may produce hydrogen gas on setting that could affect pouring cast	Express (3M Co.) Extrude (Kerr Manufacturing) Imprint (3M Co) Reprosil (LD Caulk) Omnisil (Coe Laboratories) President (Coltene) Hydrosil (LD Caulk) Exaflex (GC International)
Polyether	Polyether polymer Alky aromatic sulfonate	Easy to handle Less dimensional change Very stable Not necessary to pour within 30 min	Not stored in humidity or water More difficult to remove from mouth due to stiffness Catalyst may cause skin irritation	Impregum (ESPE) Permadyne (ESPE) Polyiel NF (LD Caulk)

Composition

Polysulfide is supplied in a two-paste system. The base contains the mercaptan **polymer** (containing many parts or mers), and the accelerator contains lead dioxide, sulfur, and fillers added to form a paste. Lead dioxide is the substance that gives the final impression material its brown color. However, if the reactor is an organic peroxide, dyes may be added, making it possible to have many other colors of impression materials (see Table 46-1).

Uses

Polysulfide is used for single- or multiple-tooth preparations, quadrants, and full-arch impressions.

Advantages

Polysulfide material provides longer working time, accuracy, and a detailed impression of the margins of the tooth preparations. They offer excellent tear resistance as the impression is removed from the mouth (see Table 46-1).

Disadvantages

Polysulfide impressions should be poured within 30 minutes to minimize polymerization shrinkage and to ensure accuracy of the impression. Polysulfide is difficult to mix and handle. Care must be taken to avoid contact with the skin and clothing, as it will permanently stain fabrics. Patients often find the odor and color of the material objectionable (see Table 46-1).

Disinfecting Polysulfide Impressions

The American Dental Association (ADA) states that an impression should be rinsed as soon as it is removed from the mouth to remove saliva, blood, and debris prior to disinfection.

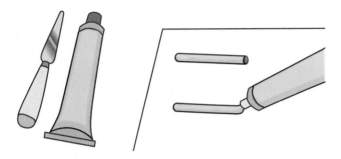

Figure 46-1 Dispensing material onto pad.

Polysulfide impressions may be immersed in an ADA-approved disinfectant. The ADA's list includes chlorine compounds, iodophors, combination synthetic phenolics, and various glutaraldehyde formulations. It is advisable to follow the manufacturer's recommended disinfectant for care of a particular elastomeric impression material.

The impression should be rinsed after it has been exposed to the disinfectant to remove any remaining solution that could affect the surface of the poured stone model.

Manipulation of Polysulfide Impression Material

Polysulfide products are dispensed as a two-paste impression system. The two pastes are spatulated together to form a rubberlike impression material (Figures 46-1, 46-2, and 46-3).

To take an impression with polysulfide, a custom-made tray should be used. The custom-made tray permits only enough space between the tray and teeth (or the part to be duplicated) for the impression material. As with all rubber-base impression materials, the less distance there is between the tray and the teeth, the more accurate the final impression. The thickness of the material between the teeth and sides of the tray should be approximately 2–4 mm.

Generally, a multiple mix of syringe and the tray material is used. In this procedure, the syringe material is mixed first (Figures 46-4 and 46-5). This enables the dentist to inject small amounts of the syringe material directly into the cavity preparation(s) and other areas where precise detail is needed. While the syringe material is being injected, the tray material is mixed and placed into the prepared custom tray.

Retention of the impression material in the tray is critical to the achievement of an accurate impression. Considerable force is generated when removing the impression from the patient's teeth. This force tends to pull it out of the tray. Therefore, tray adhesive is applied to prevent this from occurring.

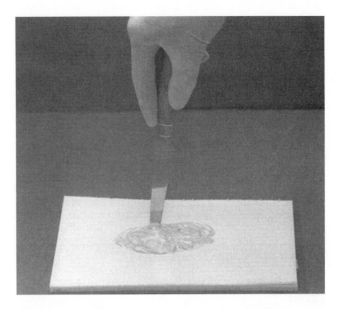

Figure 46-2 Mixing the accelerator into the base paste with tip of spatula.

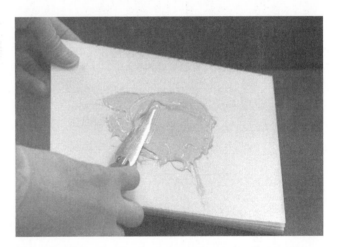

Figure 46-3 Continuing spatulation using flat portion of blade.

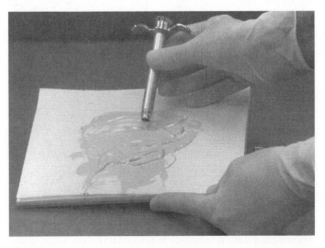

Figure 46-4 Loading syringe from nozzle end of barrel.

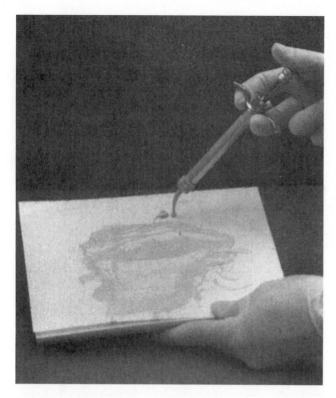

Figure 46-5 Expelling a small amount of syringe material to check the flow.

Advantages

Silicone is easy to spatulate and to handle. It is odorless and more pleasing in appearance. Patients accept it more readily, and the cost is lower than other elastomerics (see Table 46-1).

Disadvantages

Condensation silicone material must be poured within 30 minutes after removal from the patient's mouth. The set silicone impression has poor tear strength and tends to break when it is removed from the patient's mouth. It is expensive to purchase and generally is said to have a shorter **shelf life** (the stability of a dental material when it is stored). To extend the shelf life of a conventional silicone, it is recommended that it be stored in the refrigerator (see Table 46-1).

Disinfecting Silicone Impressions

As with polysulfide, the silicone impression should be rinsed immediately after removal from the mouth and prior to disinfection. Silicones can be disinfected in the same manner as polysulfide impressions using the immersion technique.

Condensation Silicone Impression Material

Condensation silicone rubber-base impression material, also known as "conventional" silicone was originally developed as a replacement for polysulfide because of the latter's objectionable odor, staining ability, and the difficulty encountered in spatulating it. Examples of this material are Accoe (GC America), Examix (GC America), Cuttersil (Heraeus Kulzer), and Citricon (Kerr Manufacturing Co.) (see Table 46-1).

Composition

Condensation silicone paste is composed of dimethylsiloxane and the reinforcing agent silica. Silica is added to control the viscosity of the paste and helps to reduce polymerization shrinkage. The catalyst is tin octoate, and the reactor is alky silicate. The manufacturer may supply the catalyst as either a liquid or a paste. As with polysulfide, it is spatulated with the accelerator to form the silicone rubber (see Table 46-1).

Uses

The condensation silicone impression materials are used for crown, bridge, and full-arch impressions.

Polyvinylsiloxane/Addition Silicone Impression Material

Polyvinylsiloxane or polysiloxane impression material, an improved silicone also known as "Addition Reaction Silicone," is more accurate than the conventional condensation silicone. It is available in a range of viscosities for various uses, including the two-phase, or **putty-wash**, technique (a technique whereby a putty tray and impression material are used together to get a final impression). With the putty-wash technique, the puttylike material is used to make a custom tray prior to the tooth being prepared. It is then set aside while the dentist prepares the tooth or teeth. The custom tray is used for the final impression (see Chapter 45).

A more recent hydrophilic polyvinylsiloxane impression material has been introduced. The stated advantage over the nonhydrophilic silicone is the improved marginal detail and the fact that it is not adversely affected by contact with the oral fluids. This allows the material to spread evenly over moist surfaces (tooth) without developing voids in the final impression.

Examples of this material are: Express (3M Co.), Extrude (Kerr Manufacturing Co.), Imprint (3M), Reprosil (L.D. Caulk), Omnisil (Coe Laboratories), President (Coltene/Whaledent), Hydrosil (Densply/Caulk), and Exaflex (G-C America) (see Table 46-1).

Procedure 49 Manipulating Condensation Silicone Impressions

Materials Needed

Mixing pads or measuring cup, 2
Spatulas, stiff, 2
Syringe, aluminum or plastic
Cleansing tissues
Plastic separator
Silicone tray material
Silicone syringe material
Catalyst liquid
Paper towels
Silicone putty tray

Instructions

Preparing Putty Tray

See Chapter 45.

Preparing Syringe and Tray Material

1 On one mixing pad, dispense the required number of graduations of syringe material as directed by the manufacturer (Figure 46-6).

2 On second mixing pad, dispense the required number of graduations of tray material as directed by manufacturer (Figure 46-7).

Spatulating Syringe and Tray Material

1 On mixing pad with tray material, dispense required amount of catalyst beside, but not touching, tray material.

2 On mixing pad with syringe material, dispense required amount of catalyst on top of syringe material.

3 Immediately begin spatulating syringe material to a homogeneous consistency. Spatulation time may vary from 30 seconds to 1 minute. There should be no trace of catalyst remaining on mixing pad.

4 Gather syringe material with spatula and prepare to load syringe (Figure 46-8). When using an aluminum syringe, remove plunger and nozzle end. Load barrel of syringe by taking nozzle end of barrel, with short rapid strokes, pulling the material into the syringe barrel. If a plastic syringe is used, remove plunger only. Load syringe from plunger end with the same technique as for the aluminum syringe (Figure 46-9).

5 For an aluminum syringe, wipe barrel end with cleansing tissue, replace nozzle tip, and insert plunger into barrel of syringe. With a plastic syringe, wipe plunger end of syringe, and insert plunger. Expel a small amount of syringe material through the plastic tip to check flow (Figure 46-10).

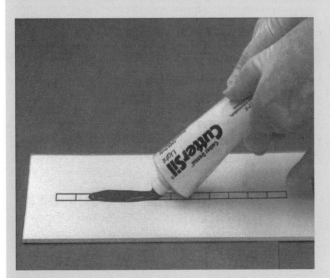

Figure 46-6 Dispensing syringe material.

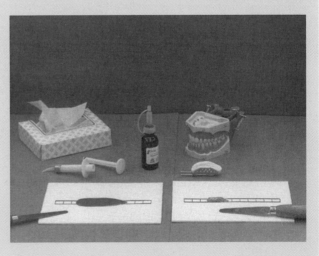

Figure 46-7 Materials prepared for mixing.

continued

continued from previous page

Procedure 49 *Manipulating Condensation Silicone Impressions*

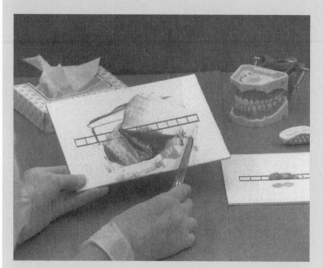

Figure 46-8 Gathering syringe material for loading.

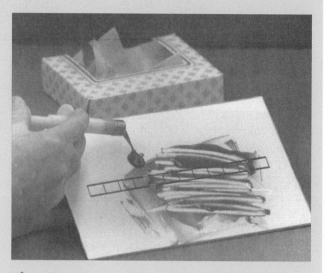

Figure 46-10 Checking flow of syringe material.

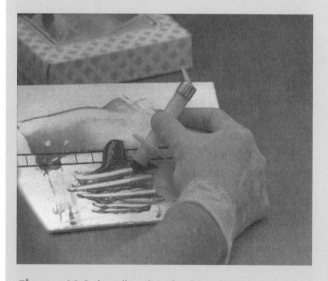

Figure 46-9 Loading the plastic syringe.

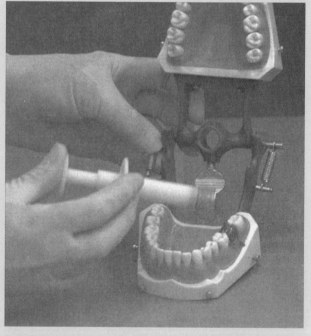

Figure 46-11 Shown on typodont to demonstrate injecting syringe material into prepared tooth.

6 Pass syringe to operator to inject material into prepared tooth (Figure 46-11).

7 While operator uses the syringe, immediately spatulate tray material. Gather tray material with spatula and line putty custom-made tray (Figure 46-12).

8 Retrieve syringe and pass tray to operator who will seat prepared putty tray over injected syringe material (Figure 46-13).

9 Material will cure a minimum of six minutes.

10 Operator will remove from patient's mouth with steady force and check impression for overall detail (Figure 46-14). Retrieve and rinse impression with cold water, dry, disinfect, and pour in stone. *Note:* Patient impressions must be disinfected prior to being poured in stones (refer to Disinfecting Silicone Impressions).

continued

continued from previous page
Procedure 49 *Manipulating Condensation Silicone Impressions*

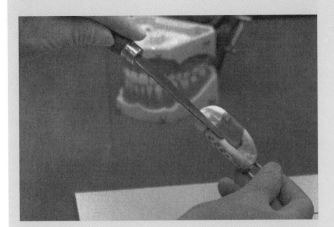

Figure 46-12 Lining putty custom-made tray.

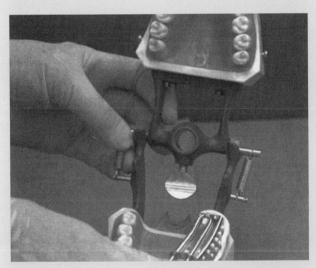

Figure 46-13 Shown on typodont to demonstrate seating the tray.

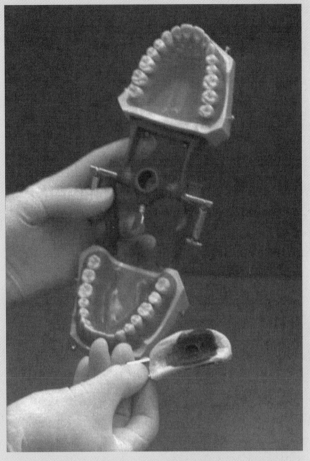

Figure 46-14 Impression of prepared tooth on a typodont.

Clean the Syringe

1 Disassemble syringe.

2 Remove excess material from nozzle tip and barrel of syringe.

3 Remove screw from plunger of aluminum syringe or O ring from plastic syringe. Clean excess material from screw or O ring. Replace screw; care must be taken not to overtighten screw. With plastic syringe, replace O ring.

4 Take brush, wash inside of barrel with water, and dry.

5 Reassemble syringe

Composition

Polyvinylsiloxane is supplied as a two-paste system. The base contains two polymers, polysiloxane and poly (vinyl) siloxane. The catalyst is a platinum salt. This system possesses incredible dimensional stability which allows for delayed pouring at the operator's convenience (see Table 46-1).

Uses

Polyvinylsiloxane impression material is used for crowns and **edentulous** (without teeth) impressions.

Advantages

Polyvinylsiloxane materials are highly accurate and exhibit long-term dimensional stability (the ability to retain their shape and size). The material has a shorter working and spatulation time. Polyvinylsiloxane is easy to spatulate, odor free, and clean to handle. These materials are also available in the automix devices (devices that mix the material) which greatly improve working time and mixing factors (see Table 46-1).

Disadvantages

Because polyvinylsiloxane has a shorter working and spatulation time, it tends to produce hydrogen gas (bubbles) on setting. For this reason, a waiting period is usually recommended before pouring the stone cast. However, newer hydrophilic polyvinylsiloxane materials have an additional additive, palladium, which absorbs the hydrogen bubbles and prevents the gassing effect. It should be noted that certain latex gloves may inhibit the setting of the puttylike impression material. Therefore, vinyl gloves must be worn when working with the material (see Table 46-1).

Disinfecting Polyvinylsiloxane Impressions

Care and disinfection of polysiloxane impression is the same as for other silicone impression materials.

Most elastomeric impression materials are spatulated on a paper mixing pad and with a stiff spatula. However, with the newer polyvinylsiloxane materials an automix hand gun may be used.

Automix Cartridge System

Silicone light- and medium-bodied impression materials and polyvinylsiloxane are available in a dual cartridge, or automix system (Figure 46-15). With the dual-car-

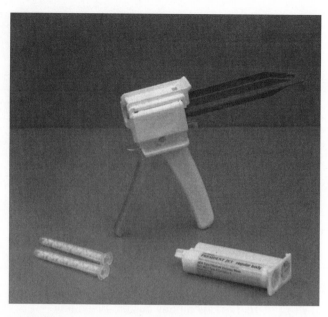

Figure 46-15 Component parts of automix system.

tridge system, the base paste is in one side of the cartridge, and the catalyst paste in the other. The cartridge is inserted into the automix unit with a trigger-type handle and movable plunger. By pressing the handle, the plunger forces the material through the cartridge. A mixing tip is attached to the cartridge. When the handle is firmly pressed, the plunger will apply pressure to the cartridge, forcing the material through the mixing tip. As the material is pushed through the mixing tip, the base and catalyst are folded over each other and mixed together, and an homogeneous mass is expelled from the mixing tip. At this time the impression material may be expelled directly into the syringe or into the prepared tooth or putty tray.

Procedure 50 Manipulating an Automix Cartridge System

Materials Needed

Automix unit
Dual cartridge, impression material
Mixing tip
Paper towel

Instructions

1 Assemble unit. Remove retainer plate (Figure 46-16).

2 Insert plunger by pushing up on the release lever (Figure 46-17).

continued

continued from previous page
Procedure 50 Manipulating an Automix Cartridge System

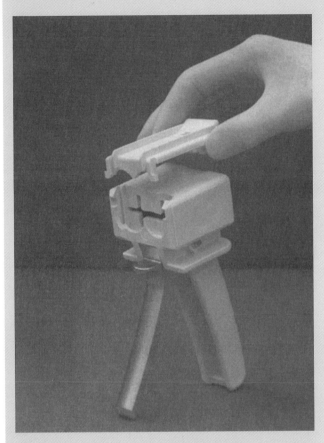

Figure 46-16 Removing retainer plate.

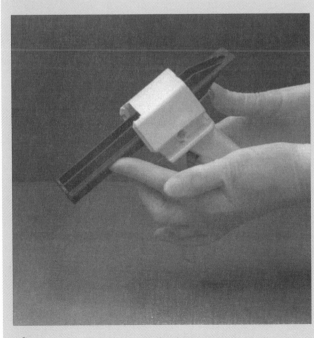

Figure 46-17 Inserting plunger.

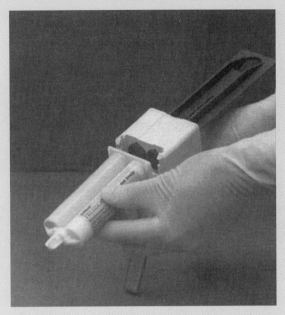

Figure 46-18 Inserting cartridge.

3 Insert dual cartridge into the guide grooves on unit (Figure 46-18).

4 Replace retainer plate (Figure 46-19). Carefully squeeze handle until plunger makes contact with the cartridge.

5 Remove protective cap and seal from the cartridge (Figure 46-20). Check function of unit by expelling a small amount of material onto a paper towel (Figure 46-21).

6 Wipe end of cartridge and insert mixing tip (Figure 46-22). Lock tip into position by giving a one-quarter turn clockwise.

7 Test flow by squeezing handle to expel a small amount of material onto a paper towel (Figure 46-23).

8 With firm and continuous pressure, squeeze handle to expel the desired amount of material needed for the procedure (Figure 46-24). The flow of material is stopped immediately when pressure on the handle is released.

9 Load syringe or putty tray directly from the mixing tip. *Note:* Do not remove mixing tip from cartridge. The impression material left in the mixing tip will harden in a few minutes. The tip helps to seal the cartridge opening, preventing the impression material from hardening.

continued

continued from previous page
Procedure 50 Manipulating an Automix Cartridge System

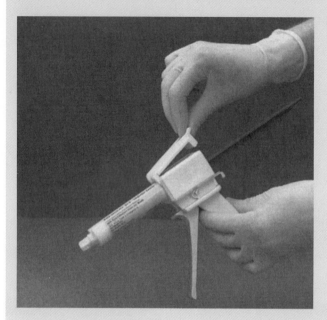

Figure 46-19 Replacing retainer plate.

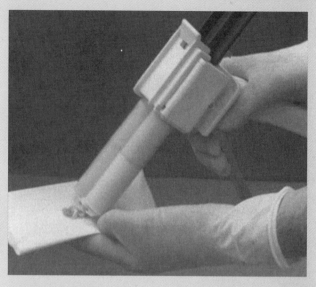

Figure 46-21 Expelling small amount of base or catalyst.

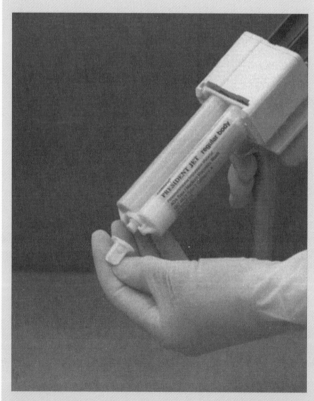

Figure 46-20 Removing protective cap from cartridge.

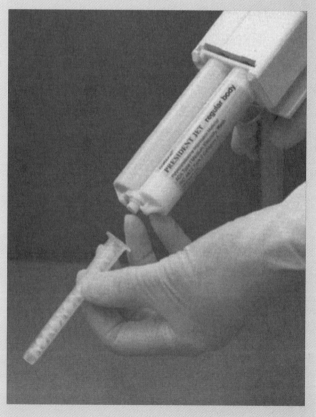

Figure 46-22 Inserting mixing tip.

continued

continued from previous page
Procedure 50 *Manipulating an Automix Cartridge System*

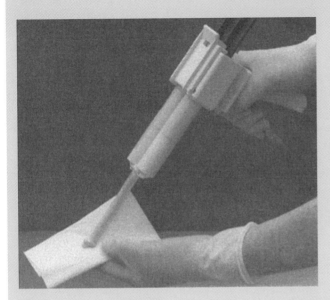

Figure 46-23 Testing flow of material.

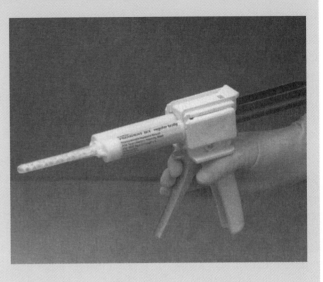

Figure 46-24 Automix system ready for use.

Replacing Used Mixing Tip

1 Remove used mixing tip from cartridge and throw away.

2 Check for hardened material at the cartridge openings.

3 Expel a small amount of material onto a paper towel.

4 Place new mixing tip on cartridge.

Replacing a Cartridge

1 Press release lever up, and hold in position while removing plunger.

2 Remove retainer plate from unit.

3 Remove cartridge.

4 Insert new cartridge, and throw away used cartridge.

Polyether Impression Material

Polyether rubber impression material is a fast-setting and more accurate impression material than either polysulfide or condensation silicone. Examples of this material are Impregum (ESPE), Permadyne (ESPE), and Polyjel NF (Densply/Caulk) (see Table 46-1).

Composition

Polyether impression material is supplied in a two-paste system with light and heavy viscosities. The base material is a polyether polymer, and the catalyst is alky aromatic sulfonate (see Table 46-1).

Uses

Polyether impression material is used for quadrant and full-arch impressions.

Advantages

Polyether is like silicone in that it is easy to manipulate and care for. Polyether also has less dimensional change during polymerization and storing than do polysulfide or condensation silicone. Because polyether is very stable, the finished impression retains its accuracy for extended periods of time; it is unnecessary to pour the impression within the first 30 minutes, as with polysulfide and the condensation silicone materials (see Table 46-1).

Disadvantages

Because polyether is a hydrophilic impression material, it should not be exposed to high humidity or stored in water. Also, the overall stiffness of the set material makes removing the impression from the mouth more difficult. Care should be taken when working with the catalyst to avoid skin contact, as it may cause skin irritation. A custom tray is also required for impression taking (see Table 46-1).

Disinfecting Polyether Impressions

Polyether should be rinsed in the same manner as other elastomeric impressions. However, the ADA recommends that the spray disinfection method be used to disinfect the polyether impression because of its hydrophilic nature. Immersion disinfection could adversely affect the dimensions (shape) and the stability of the material.

Bite Registration

The bite registration is a thin impression of the occlusal relationships of the biting surfaces of the teeth. It is used when the maxillary and mandibular casts are mounted on an **articulator** (a mechanical hinge that acts as the temporomandibular joint). This relationship is needed to construct an appliance.

Materials used for a bite registration are either a thin wax wafer that has a foil laminate sandwiched in the center of the "U-shaped" wax bite or an impression material of very low viscosity such as heavy body polyvinylsiloxane silicone.

Wax Wafer

When using the wax wafer, it must be heated in relatively hot water to make the wax pliable. It is then inserted in the mouth, centered on the mandibular jaw, and the patient bites down in centric occlusion (asking the patient to place the tip of his tongue as far back as possible on the palate may be helpful to register centric occlusion). The wax bite remains in that position until the wax has cooled down. It is removed carefully to avoid distortion and observed for adequate imprints of the teeth in both arches (refer to Figure 44-26A–C). It is rinsed and sprayed with a disinfectant.

Silicone Impression Material

When using heavy-body impression material such as polyvinylsiloxane silicone, it is injected onto the mandibular occlusal/incisal areas of the teeth (Figure 46-25A). The patient bites down in centric occlusion and the material remains in that position until it polymerizes (Figure 46-25B). It is then removed and observed for adequate imprints of the teeth in both arches (Figure 46-25C).

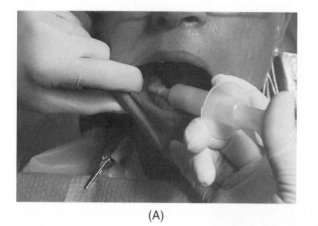

(A)

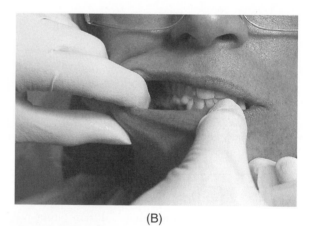

(B)

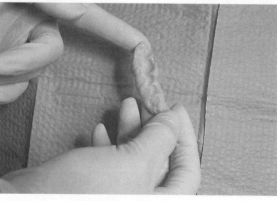

(C)

Figure 46-25 Taking a bite registration using polyvinylsiloxane silicone material.

SUGGESTED ACTIVITIES

- Compare the following materials: polysulfide, condensation silicone, polyvinylsiloxane, and polyether for mixing technique, odor, time frame, and results for each material.

- Practice spatulating the syringe material and loading it into the syringe following outlined instructions.

- Practice spatulating the tray material and lining a custom-made tray.

- Once familiar with spatulation and loading techniques for syringe and tray materials, use the double-mix technique following the step-by-step procedure as outlined.

- Using the automix cartridge system, assemble the unit according to manufacturer's instructions and practice dispensing the mixed material.

- Take an impression using a prepared typodont.

REVIEW

1. What difference(s) may be observed when using polysulfide in contrast to other elastomeric impression materials?
   a. It has an offensive odor.
   b. It is hydrophilic.
   c. It provides excellent tear resistance.
   d. It is one of the newer elastomeric impression materials.
   e. Both a and c

2. The viscosity of an impression material pertains to the:
   a. Capability of taking on moisture
   b. Thickness of a flowable material
   c. Speed of chemical reaction
   d. Tear resistance

3. Condensation silicone impression material has:
   a. Excellent tear strength
   b. A long-term dimensional stability
   c. An objectionable odor
   d. A shorter shelf life than other elastomeric impression materials

4. Polyvinylsiloxane material:
   a. Has a setting time that may be inhibited by the use of certain latex gloves
   b. Has a longer working and spatulation time
   c. Has a catalyst that contains tin octoate
   d. Has poor dimensional stability

5. Polyether impression material:
   a. Is very stable and may be poured in stone after an extended period of time
   b. Is hydrophilic or capable of taking on water
   c. Does not require a custom tray
   d. Both a and b
   e. Both b and c

CHAPTER 47

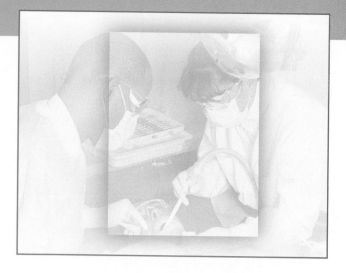

OBJECTIVES

After studying this chapter, the student will be able to:

● Review the construction and placement of accurate temporary acrylic crowns.

● Develop a well-standardized technique for sizing temporary preformed crowns.

● Cement temporary crowns using stated criteria.

● Describe the procedure for placing a Class II temporary restoration using temporary cement.

Introduction

When constructing crowns and bridges, it is necessary to keep the tooth or teeth protected anywhere from a few days up to, in some cases, many months. Placement of accurate temporary crowns and adequate protection and stabilization of the tooth preparation are important in order to:

● Prevent tooth movement and extrusion of the prepared tooth and/or opposing tooth

● Provide for the patient's comfort

● Sedate the pulp of the tooth

● Protect free gingiva from irritation and resulting recession and prevent food impaction into the contact areas, resulting in periodontal problems

● Provide for esthetics

● Prevent unnecessary exposure of the tooth to mouth fluids

● Make up for lost function where possible

● Adjust occlusion in many cases

The placement of well-constructed provisional crowns can also have a great effect on the patient's confidence and attitude. If the restorations are uncomfortable or repeatedly come off between appointments, the patient is apt to become irritable and upset.

Types of Temporary Coverage

Acrylic Temporary Crown

These are made from either acrylic resin or *Bis-acryl composite* and are used as a temporary crown for a tooth until the permanent restoration is placed. They provide a more accurate fit because they are replicas of the patient's original tooth/teeth. One might say they are custom made.

The principle behind constructing a temporary acrylic crown is to approximate the original tooth form with certain modifications. In the majority of cases, the original tooth form will be adequate. However, there are cases where the tooth should not be duplicated such as the pontic tooth or teeth on a bridge. In such cases, the original tooth form is modified on a diagnostic cast. That cast is then used as a model, in constructing the temporary bridge. This is known as the indirect method of constructing a provisional temporary.

When an acrylic resin temporary crown is constructed directly in the patient's mouth, it is known as the direct method. The process requires that an alginate or silicone putty impression be made of the tooth, referred to as the "original tooth" prior to its preparation, for it will be used as a mold also known as a matrix, for the new temporary crown. After the preparation is completed, acrylic resin is mixed and flowed into the impression. When it loses its gloss, it is refitted onto the prepared tooth and left on until the acrylic resin becomes doughy or rubbery. The impression is removed and the new temporary crown begins to take shape while it polymerizes. It must then be gently removed from the prepared tooth without distortion to begin the process of trimming and shaping while taking it "on and off" the prepared tooth until it reaches final **polymerization** [a chemical reaction that occurs between the initiator (peroxide) and the activator (amine) or the use of visible blue light that causes the material to set up or harden] and it resembles the original tooth. This process requires the use of scissors to trim the **flash** (excess material that goes beyond the cavosurface or gingival margins), while doughy. Finishing burs and sandpaper discs ensure that the gingival margins are of adequate fit after polymerization and a polishing agent is used to smooth the temporary crown.

Procedure 51 Fabrication of an Acrylic Temporary Crown

Materials Needed

Safety glasses, gloves, mask
Basic set (mouth mirror, explorer, cotton forceps)
Alginate or silicone putty impression of tooth prior to preparation, quadrant tray
Self-curing acrylic kit (monomer, polymer)
Dappen dish
Cement spatula
Vaseline
Acrylic/finishing burs and sandpaper discs/mandrel
Crown and collar scissors (curved)
Polishing agent such as prophy paste, prophy cup, contra-angle handpiece
Articulating paper with holder
Temporary cement and paper pad or automix temporary cement
Dental engine
Dental floss

Instructions

1 While waiting for the onset of anesthesia, an overimpression is made in alginate or silicone putty. This impression must include, wherever possible, one or more teeth mesially and distally to the tooth to be prepared (Figure 47-1).

2 Store this impression (alginate) in the airtight container. It must be kept moist, as it will not actually be used until after the preparation is completed.

3 The tooth preparation is then accomplished.

4 Lubricate prepared tooth and adjacent teeth with Vaseline when constructing on a typodont.

5 Mix the monomer (liquid) and polymer (powder) in a dappen dish with small spatula, thick enough to trail from spatula 1–2 inches.

6 Flow the mix into the original impression of the tooth. Let it stand until it loses its gloss.

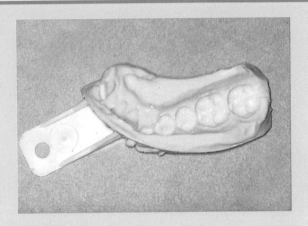

Figure 47-1 Overimpression of unprepared tooth (teeth). (Courtesy of 3M Dental Products Division.)

7 Place the impression with the mix onto the prepared tooth and keep it there until the material becomes rubbery or has reached initial set (about 2 minutes).

8 Remove the impression from the mouth (typodont) and inspect the new temporary crown for possible air voids.

9 Carefully work it off the impression without distorting it.

10 Trim excess flash while in its rubbery stage, with curved scissors (Figure 47-2A)

11 Work it "on and off" while the material undergoes exothermic reaction until it reaches final polymerization. The heat emitted could be significant to cause tissue damage. Continue trimming using an acrylic bur (Figure 47-2B).

12 Accomplish final trimming with finishing burs and sandpaper discs.

13 Use a polishing agent to give the temporary crown a smooth, glossy appearance.

continued

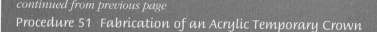

continued from previous page
Procedure 51 Fabrication of an Acrylic Temporary Crown

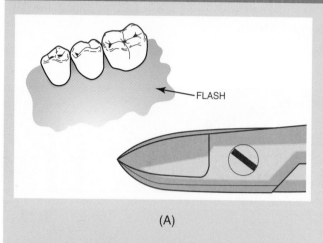

(A)

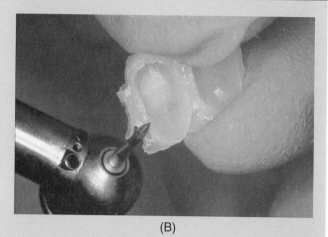

(B)

Figure 47-2 (A) Trimming excess acrylic (flash) with scissors. (B) Trimming excess acrylic with bur.

14 Place acrylic temporary in mouth and adjust occlusion, which will be high in most cases, using articulating paper. Trim the high points (marked areas on the crown) using an acrylic bur.

15 Prior to cementation, lubricate the crown with Vaseline to minimize cement from adhering to outside of crown.

16 Isolate the quadrant with cotton rolls and dry the prepared tooth well.

17 Cement the crown onto prepared tooth with temporary cement mixed to a creamy consistency. Refer to Chapter 42.

18 Remove excess cement from gingival aspect of temporary crown with explorer and use floss to remove any cement particles interproximally.

The process used to fabricate a Bis-acryl composite resin temporary crown, is similar to that used to make an acrylic resin crown in that it also uses either an over-impression of alginate or silicone putty or a thermoplastic matrix. If a thermoplastic bead matrix is used as a mold, the area of placement must be coated with a thin coat of Vaseline and heat must be used to soften the thermoplastic material. Hot water at 150°F or direct flame will soften the material until it becomes pliable or clear. Using pressure, it can then be adapted to the original tooth to make a good imprint of the tooth on the thermoplastic bead matrix (before preparation). When the matrix hardens and returns to a dull appearance, it is ready to be removed. This material will spring open for easy removal and repositioning without distortion. The manufacturer claims that this type of matrix saves time when compared to other techniques.

The Bis-acryl composite is now supplied as a dual cartridge that is automixed and inserted in the matrix or overimpression, filling the desired tooth about three-fourths full within the impression and then repositioning it onto the prepared tooth. It may be self- or light-cured. The procedure for shaping and finishing the temporary crown is the same as for the acrylic resin temporary crown.

Aluminum and Stainless Steel Preformed Crowns

These are manufactured in a series of graduated sizes and in anatomical and nonanatomical forms. They are referred to as preformed crowns (Figure 47-3) and should be used only as an expedient in the rare situation in which, because of time and various other factors, the construction of a plastic temporary is impractical.

A preformed crown is selected that most closely fits the size of the prepared tooth. It should be of adequate dimensions to ensure that it makes contact with proximal teeth. The height of the preformed crown should meet the opposing arch and be able to bear occlusal forces during mastication. The gingival margin should be covered and protected. Trimming of the temporary crown begins by marking the crown to conform to the height (occlusal) of the proximal teeth while seated on the prepared tooth. The amount of material removed from the gingival aspect of the crown should match the same measurement taken earlier on the occlusal surface. When the crown is trimmed, it should be smoothed with sandpaper and rubber discs to avoid injuring the patient's gingiva.

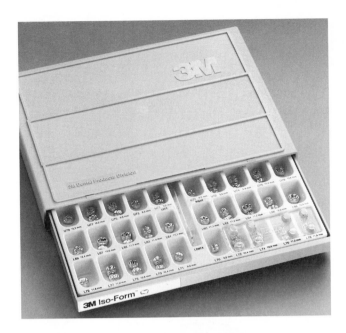

Figure 47-3 Assortment of preformed crowns. (Courtesy of 3M Dental Products Division.)

Preformed Polycarbonate/Acrylic Temporary Crown

This type of crown is generally limited in use to the anterior teeth. They are easily prepared and are selected according to size and shades. They are esthetic in appearance but limited in shade selection. Crown margins are not as well adapted to the tooth and may cause gingival irritation.

Zinc Oxide Eugenol Cements

Zinc oxide eugenol cement can be used alone only in small inlay preparations. The ZOE cements efficiently seal cavities because they undergo minimal overall dimensional change while setting. They are also used routinely in a more workable form to cement all of the previously mentioned types of temporaries.

When used as a temporary restoration, the cement must be mixed to a doughy consistency. If it is used to temporize a tooth with a Class II preparation, a matrix band should be used to create the proximal contact area and be able to preserve adequate space until the inlay is fabricated. The cement is condensed into the prepared tooth until the occlusal cavosurface margin is covered. The matrix band is removed and the temporary restoration is carved down to simulate occlusal anatomy. Refer to Procedure 53.

Procedure 52 Applying Preformed Temporary Crowns

Materials Needed

Safety glasses, gloves, mask
Preformed aluminum or stainless steel crown
Crown and collar scissors
Basic set (mouth mirror, explorer, cotton forceps)
Contouring pliers
Articulating paper and holder
Burlew wheel/mandrel
Dental engine
Dental floss
Cotton rolls
Cement spatula
ZOE cement and paper pad

Instructions

1 Select a preformed crown that most closely fits the size of the tooth being prepared and determine which side of the crown will face the lingual and buccal aspects.

2 Try in a preformed crown to determine the correct width from mesial to distal (Figure 47-4).

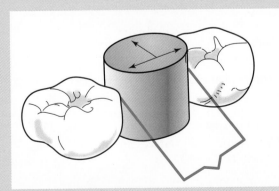

Figure 47-4 Mesial-distal measurement of preformed crown.

continued

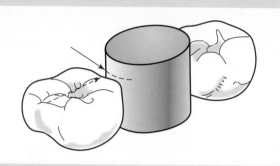

Figure 47-5 Scribing crown to determine height of crown.

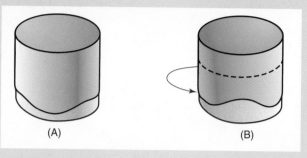

Figure 47-7 (A) Trimming buccal/lingual margin is curved downward. (B) Trimming mesial/distal margin is curved upward.

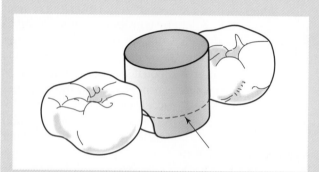

Figure 47-6 Amount to be trimmed from gingival side of crown.

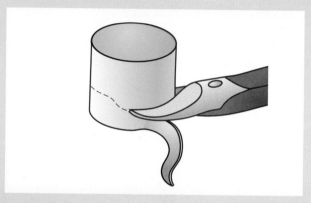

Figure 47-8 Curved scissors are held so beaks are turned upward for buccal/lingual and downward for mesial/distal.

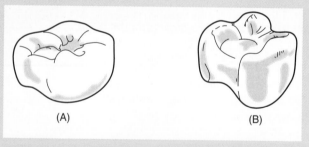

Figure 47-9 (A) Preformed stainless steel crowns used to demonstrate completed trimming for buccal/lingual. (B) Completed trimming for mesial/distal.

3 While the preformed crown is in place, determine the correct height by using an explorer to **scribe** (draw a line on the crown) a line on the mesial and distal surfaces near the occlusal portion of the preformed crown, to match the height of adjacent teeth (this distance will indicate the amount to be trimmed from the gingival portion of the crown) (Figure 47-5).

4 Using the determined distance as outlined above, scribe a line along the buccal and lingual surfaces of the crown near the gingival surface (this is the amount to be trimmed from the gingival portion of crown) (Figure 47-6).

5 Trimming the crown requires the use of a crown and collar scissors. The margins of the buccal and lingual surfaces are trimmed curved downward (Figure 47-7A) while the margins of the mesial and distal surfaces are trimmed curved upward (Figure 47-7B).

6 Trimmed line should correspond with the measured length. Care must be taken to avoid making sharp angles when trimming crown. *Note:*

Scissors are held so beaks are turned inward for buccal/lingual and outward for mesial/distal (Figure 47-8).

7 Gingival margin of the crown must conform to the natural contour of the tooth for buccal/lingual (Figure 47-9A) and for mesial/distal (Figure 47-9B).

continued

continued from previous page
Procedure 52 Applying Preformed Temporary Crowns

8 Margins of trimmed crown are crimped with contouring pliers (Figures 47-10A, B). Correct crimping is depicted in Figure 47-11 and incorrect crimping is depicted in Figure 47-12.

9 The margins of the crown should extend slightly beyond the margin of the preparation but not more than 0.5 mm past the gingival margin of the tooth.

10 The margin of the crown is smoothed with a burlew wheel/mandrel to remove sharp edges.

11 Occlusion is checked using the articulating paper. If there are markings, it may need additional trimming.

12 Prior to cementation, it is a good idea to coat the temporary crown with Vaseline petroleum jelly as this will minimize cement from adhering to the crown.

13 The prepared tooth is isolated with cotton rolls and the quadrant is well dried using air.

14 Cement crown onto prepared tooth with temporary ZOE cement mixed to a creamy consistency. Refer to Chapter 41.

15 Remove excess cement from gingival aspect of preformed crown using an explorer and floss to remove any cement particles.

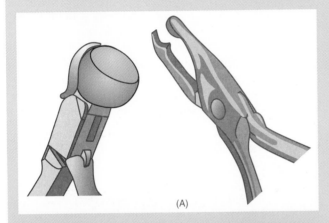

(A)

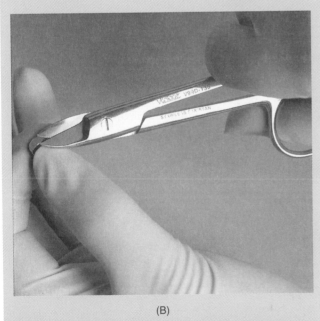

(B)

Figure 47-10 Use of contouring pliers to crimp margin of crown.

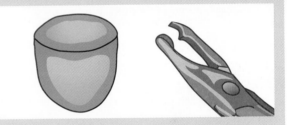

Figure 47-11 Correct way of crimping the crown. Convex or bulbous portion of pliers beak is placed on inside of crown.

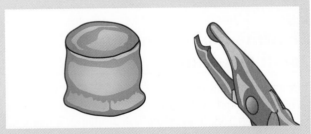

Figure 47-12 Incorrect way of crimping the crown. Convex or bulbous portion of pliers beak is placed on outside of crown.

Procedure 53 Placing a Class II Temporary Restoration

Materials Needed

Safety glasses, gloves, mask
Basic set (mouth mirror, explorer, cotton forceps)
ZOE powder and liquid
Paper pad
Cement spatula
Matrix band, holder, and wedges
Condensers
Carvers
Gold knife, #2
Ball burnisher
Dental floss
Cotton rolls
Articulating paper with holder

Instructions

1 Isolate prepared tooth from moisture with cotton rolls.

2 Place matrix band and holder and desired wedge(s).

3 Adjust matrix band to meet adjacent tooth (teeth) and establish proximal contact with ball burnisher.

4 Place ZOE powder on paper pad and divide into fourths.

5 Place liquid close to powder.

6 Mix powder and liquid in 1 minute or less until it reaches a putty consistency.

7 Coat the small nib of the condenser with powder and start placing small increments into the prepared tooth, starting at the gingival step (box form). If the preparation includes mesial and distal gingival steps, both of these are filled first; then the cement is placed in the rest of the preparation using the larger nib of the condenser.

8 Continue packing the cement until the material reaches the cavosurface margin.

9 Using the explorer, separate the band from the cement at the marginal ridge(s).

10 Remove wedge(s), holder, and band with care.

11 While cement is still in a plastic state, carve the occlusal until it is similar in height to proximal teeth. Check its height with articulating paper. If markings are present, continue to carve until desired height is obtained.

12 Use the gold knife to remove flash from below the gingival step interproximally.

13 Insert floss to remove excess cement and check interproximal contact areas for adequate fit.

Treatment of the Prepared Tooth Structure

It is important that the problem of sensitivity (thermal, in the final restoration) be considered as early as when the tooth is prepared. It has been shown that ZOE cements exhibit less leakage than do zinc phosphate cements, and they also have a sedative effect on the pulp. For these reasons and for ease of removal, the temporaries are cemented with ZOE at preparation time. When the final restoration is cemented, the tooth is treated with varnish. It is very important that the tooth not be dried so vigorously that the dentin is **desiccated** (thoroughly dried up). However, to place varnish or cement, the tooth must be dry. *Note:* The only significant modification required when constructing temporary bridges is that the pontic (artificial tooth) be waxed up in a soft wax on the study cast and the overimpression made on this cast.

SUGGESTED ACTIVITIES

● Use a typodont with tooth preparations and construct a two- or three-unit temporary acrylic restoration.

● Use a typodont to place and finish a Class II temporary restoration using the detailed information in the chapter.

● Use a typodont with a crown preparation to size and shape a preformed aluminum or stainless steel crown.

REVIEW

1. Name the purpose(s) for temporary crowns/
   restorations (1) to prevent tooth movement and
   extrusion of the prepared tooth, (2) to prevent
   unnecessary exposure of the tooth to mouth fluids,
   (3) to provide full chewing function, and/or (4) to
   protect from food impaction and free gingival
   irritation.
   a. 1, 2, 3
   b. 2, 3, 4
   c. 1, 2, 4
   d. 1, 3, 4

2. To construct acrylic temporary crowns, it is necessary to:
   a. Take an impression of the opposing arch
   b. Take an impression of the original tooth prior to
      its preparation
   c. Take an impression of the prepared tooth
   d. Both a and c

3. Preformed temporary crowns:
   a. Are selected by their height size
   b. Are selected by their width size
   c. Must extend at least 2 mm past the gingival mar-
      gin of the tooth
   d. Are cemented with permanent cement

4. A Class II temporary restoration:
   a. Is placed on a tooth that will receive a gold inlay
   b. Provides patient comfort
   c. Is filled with ZOE temporary cement
   d. All of the above

5. Name the purposes for using ZOE cement for temporization: (1) exhibits less leakage than zinc phosphate cement, (2) has a sedative effect on the pulp,
   (3) easily removed, and/or (4) does not fracture
   under great stress.
   a. 1, 2, 3
   b. 2, 3, 4
   c. 1, 2, 4
   d. 1, 3, 4

CHAPTER 48

Gypsum

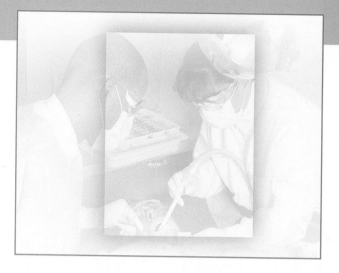

OBJECTIVES

After studying this chapter, the student will be able to:

- Discuss the differences in the structure of dental plaster and dental stone.
- Define the setting time of gypsum (plaster or stone).
- State the difference between wet strength and dry strength of a gypsum product.
- List the factors that influence the strength of plaster or stone.
- Use the chemical balance scale for weighing plaster or stone.
- Use a graduate cylinder to measure water.
- Pour impressions in plaster or stone, according to instructions.
- Mark and prepare a maxillary and mandibular plaster model for trimming.
- Using a model trimmer, trim a set of plaster models to an acceptable standard.
- Evaluate trimmed study models.

Introduction

Gypsum occurs in a massive form as rock gypsum and is mined in many areas of the United States. This dull-colored rock is a commonly found sulfate mineral. Gypsum ($CaSO_4 \bullet 2H_2O$) is the dihydrate of calcium sulfate ($CaSO_4$). The chemical formula indicates that, in its natural state, calcium sulfate is combined with two molecules of water.

When gypsum is heated, some of the water is driven off and forms plaster or stone. This process is termed **calcination**. The resultant powder can be mixed with water, and gypsum is re-formed.

Composition

To understand why plaster sets when mixed with water, it is important to know how plaster is made.

Pieces of ground gypsum undergo a chemical change when heated at atmospheric pressure in open kettles. **Calcining** is simply the process of heating the gypsum particles so that some of the water molecules are driven off in the form of steam. As the water molecules are lost, calcium sulfate hemihydrate is formed. After calcining, the **gypsum powder** (plaster) is dry and contains approximately one-half molecule of water. The water leaving the particles as steam produces pressure that breaks up the particles into finer crystals. They are further dried and ground to provide a variety of particle sizes that provide a plastic (flowable) mass when mixed with water.

Two basic types of calcium hemihydrate are manufactured. The plaster just described is referred to as the beta-hemihydrate form. Gypsum particles heated under steam pressure and in the presence of sodium chloride are designated as alpha-hemihydrate, which is the dental stone. This product is used principally for **stone dies** (a replica of a single tooth or several teeth on which a restoration is fabricated) when constructing metal restorations.

Chemically, plaster and dental stone are identical, but the shapes of the powder particles differ. The powder particles of plaster are generally rough, irregularly shaped, and porous. Similar particles of stone are smooth, regularly shaped, and less porous. The classification of dental gypsum products used in the American Dental Association (ADA) Specification is presented in Table 48-1.

392

Table 48-1 Dental Gypsum Products

ADA *Specification*	Traditional Terminology
Type I plaster, impression	Impression plaster
Type II plaster, model	Model or laboratory plaster, "plaster of Paris"
Type III dental stone	Class I stone or Hydrocal
Type IV dental stone	Class II die stone, Densite
Type V dental stone	High-strength, high-expansion die stone

Type I Impression Plaster

Type 1 plaster may be used for impressions of the edentulous mouth and for selected prosthetic construction work. Great strength is not desired in impression plaster. For this reason, a higher water-to-powder ratio is used for mixing impression plaster than is usually employed with other gypsum products. The chief requirement for the mixture is that it be sufficiently thick so that it will not run out of the impression tray as it is inserted into the mouth.

Type II Model Plaster

Type II plaster is generally used for such laboratory work as construction of study models and for articulating stone **casts** (replica of the teeth or dental arch that is used as a working model) or models.

Type III Dental Stone

Type III stone is originally white and cannot be distinguished by appearance from plaster. For this reason, the manufacturer may color the stone buff or one of the pastel shades. The color does not alter the properties of the stone. Class I dental stone is considerably stronger and more resistant to abrasion than is plaster. It is used extensively for the fabrication of diagnostic casts and opposing arch casts and in constructing removable prosthodontics.

Type IV Die Stone

Class II stone is used for dies. A die is a reproduction of a single tooth preparation on which a wax pattern is fashioned. The wax pattern is invested and then cast in metal. A very hard stone cast is required for a die. Class II stones can be mixed with less water than Class I stones. The surface hardness of a Class II stone is greater than that of a Class I stone.

Type V Die Stone: High-Strength, High-Expansion

Type V stone is utilized in the fabrication of casts and dies for metal-ceramic restorations, particularly when the casting shrinkage of the metal utilized is high and warrants extra expansion in the dies.

Comparison of Water Ratio for Plaster and Stone

Because of the uniform shape and size of the powder particles, dental stone can be mixed with less water than plaster. Probably the best way to mix plaster or stone is under vacuum using a mechanical mixer. To get strong and hard plaster, the powder and water must be carefully proportioned. The powder should be weighed on a chemical balance and the water measured in a graduate cylinder.

Setting Reaction

The setting reaction of plaster and stone is a process of **hydration** (the addition of water to the powder) and of release of heat, an exothermic reaction.

A few scattered crystals of gypsum are always present in any plaster or stone powder. These crystals (nuclei) act as centers of crystalline growth. The more nuclei present, the more rapid the crystallization.

Water-to-Powder Ratio. The water-to-powder ratio determines the physical properties of the final product. Powder particle porosity and size determine the amount of water to use. Because plaster particles are rough, porous, and irregularly shaped, plaster requires more water. This is why set plaster is much weaker than stone. Stone particles are smooth, less porous, and regularly shaped and, therefore, require less water.

The overall strength of plaster and stone really depends on the number of nuclei of crystallization present at the time of spatulation. If more water is used than is required, the final strength of the plaster or stone will be weaker, because the nuclei are widely distributed. Therefore, the plaster or stone and water should be accurately measured. When pouring an impression, the consistency of the plaster or stone mix must be thin enough to pour into the impression. Sufficient water must be added so that the powder particles can be stirred or mixed into the water and poured into the impression. This added water is known as "free" or "excess" water. It is driven off as the exothermic reaction occurs.

Setting Time. The setting times of plaster or stone are known as the initial set and the final set.

The **initial set** is the time between the spatulation and the time the mixture loses its gloss and becomes firm or solid enough to handle but is still moist and slightly pliable.

The **final set** occurs after the plaster or stone has completed its crystallization and all the heat has been driven off. In this stage, the plaster or stone are very hard and fairly dry. As might be expected, the strength of gypsum increases rapidly as the material hardens after the initial setting.

Two strengths of the gypsum product are recognized, the wet strength and the dry strength.

The **wet strength** is the strength present when the water is in excess of that required to bring the gypsum back to its natural water content. When the excess water content has been driven off or the model or cast dried, the strength obtained is called the **dry strength**. The dry strength may be two or more times the wet strength. Factors that influence the setting time of gypsum are:

● Refinement

● Temperature of water and atmosphere

● Time and speed of spatulation

● Water-powder ratio

● Addition of retarders, accelerators, or other ingredients

Spatulation

Within limits, the more the water-plaster or stone mixture is spatulated, the quicker it will set. Nuclei and gypsum crystals that start to form will be broken up by spatulation and will result in a greater number of crystals. The amount of spatulation refers to both the time and speed of spatulation.

Accelerators and Retarders. A few accelerators are:

● Potassium sulfate 2%

● Sodium chloride, very small amounts

● Slurry (a watery mixture of insoluble plaster matter whereby a residue is obtained from the process of trimming models)

Retarders, although seldom used, include:

● Borax

● Hydrocolloid gels

● Sodium citrate

Pouring Plaster Models

When mixing any gypsum product with water, one must be careful to avoid incorporating air into the mix. Not only do the air bubbles cause weakness in the model, they also produce surface inaccuracies.

The actual spatulation is done by rapidly stirring the mixture in a rubber plaster bowl with a stiff-bladed metal spatula.

Air is almost certain to be carried into the water if the powder is dumped in or if the water is poured into the powder. For this reason, the powder should be sifted into the water so that air is not introduced at the same time.

In mixing the powder and water together, begin with a circular motion and incorporate all the powder particles. Next, wipe the blade against the side and bottom of the bowl to ensure that all the powder is being wetted.

Mixing should be done on a mechanical vibrator, with the bowl placed firmly on the vibrator table. When properly spatulated, a plaster or stone mix should be smooth and free from air bubbles.

The amount of time for hand mixing is approximately 1–2 minutes. Any further mixing is likely to break up the crystals of gypsum that begin to form, which tends to weaken the final product. To obtain the maximum strength, the proportions of water and powder must be measured.

When the mixture has been spatulated for approximately 1–2 minutes and appears to be smooth and uniform, the plaster/stone can be poured into the impression.

When the models (casts) are thoroughly dried, they should be removed from the impression(s) and prepared for trimming with a model trimmer.

Pouring the Impressions

Two basic techniques are used for pouring models and establishing a base on them. The inverted technique requires a double pour with the first mix used for filling the teeth, palate, or tongue areas. The second mix forms the base.

The boxed technique employs the use of a wax boxing strip that forms the entire model.

Procedure 54 Using a Gram Chemical Scale and Graduate Cylinder

Materials Needed

Gram chemical scale
Graduate cylinder
Paper cup/paper towel(s)
Plaster powder
Water, room temperature

Instructions

Gram Chemical Scale

1 Remove rubber stoppers and place behind scale.

2 Milligram and gram weights must be at zero (Figure 48-1).

3 Scale must be in balance. If not, add pieces of paper towel to right side of scale until balanced.
   a. Top bar, milligram scale 1/10
   b. Bottom bar, gram scale 10, 20, 30 grams, etc.,

4 Place paper cup or paper towel on left side of the balance.

5 Balance scale again, using milligram scale. Weigh paper cup or towel (Figure 48-2).

6 Set gram scale for given powder ratio (Figure 48-3). Add weight of paper cup or paper towel.

7 Measure powder into paper cup or on paper towel until scale is in balance.

8 Remove cup and set aside.

9 Replace milligram and gram weights on zero.

10 Replace rubber stoppers on scale.

Graduate Cylinder

1 Pour room temperature water into graduate cylinder.

2 Read level of water (meniscus) at prescribed amount (Figure 48-4).

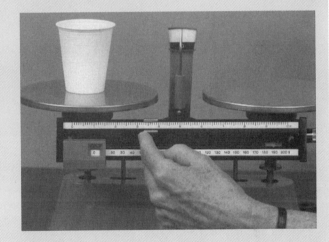

Figure 48-2 Weighing paper cup.

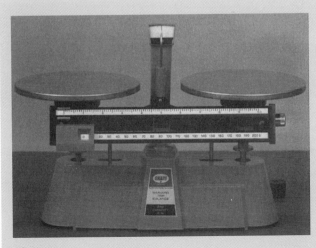

Figure 48-1 Gram scale.

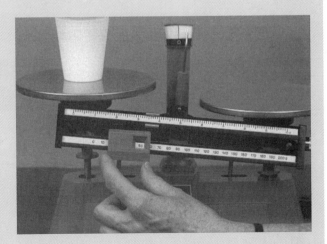

Figure 48-3 Setting gram scale.

continued

continued from previous page
Procedure 54 Using a Gram Chemical Scale and Graduate Cylinder

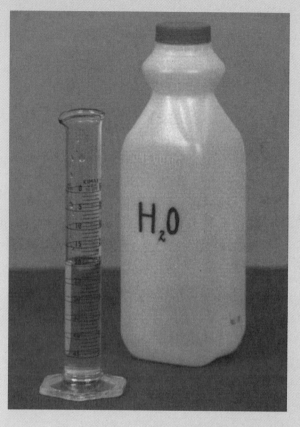

Figure 48-4 Using the graduate cylinder.

Prior to pouring impressions, use a laboratory knife to remove excess impression material from the tuberosity, retromolar pad, and other areas of the impressions. In doing so, care must be taken to avoid losing any portion of the impression(s).

Procedure 55 Inverted Technique

Materials Needed

Alginate impressions
Plaster bowl
Spatula, plaster
Spatula, small (metal)
Vibrator
Glass slab or tile square
Plaster powder

Water (room temperature)
Laboratory knife
Gram scale
Graduate cylinder
Q-tips
Paper cup
Paper towels
Humidor

continued

continued from previous page
Procedure 55 Inverted Technique

Ratio

Maxillary teeth/palate, 75 gr plaster/37 ml water
Mandibular teeth/tongue, 75 gr plaster/37 ml water
Base for maxillary and mandibular, 100 gr plaster/45 ml water for each arch

Instructions

1 Weigh plaster in cup or paper towel.

2 Measure water and pour into bowl.

3 Rinse impression with cool water.

4 Trim excess impression material from tray. Leave a 1/4-in. (6 mm) margin beyond the impression of the tuberosity or retromolar pad and other areas of the impression (Figure 48-5).

5 Remove any visible surface water from alginate impression(s) with Q-tips.

6 Dampen a paper towel and fold in half diagonally.

7 Place maxillary tray or impression in center of folded towel and approximately 1 to 1 1/2 in. from folded edge. This will prevent plaster from flowing onto vibrator.

   Note: When pouring a mandibular impression, it is suggested that the tongue area be blocked out with a damp paper towel.

8 Sift plaster powder into the water.

9 Allow powder to settle in the water for 30 seconds. This will minimize the incorporation of air into the mix during spatulation.

10 Rapidly spatulate plaster for 30 seconds at approximately two revolutions per second.

11 Turn on the vibrator at low speed.

12 Place bowl on vibrator and thoroughly vibrate plaster for another 30 seconds. Remove bowl from vibrator.

13 Hold prepared tray or impression with paper towel in place and rest base of tray or impression on vibrator.

14 Use small cement spatula and begin adding small increments of plaster to the most distal portion of one side of the impression (Figure 48-6).

15 Continue to place small increments of plaster in the same area of the impression, allowing each tooth to be filled in succession. This may necessitate tilting the impression tray until all the teeth are filled. This procedure will prevent the entrapment of air during the process of pouring.

16 With the plaster spatula, continue to add small portions of plaster until the impression is filled to its borders.

17 Remove tray or impression from vibrator and set aside.

18 When initial set takes place, remove paper towel from around the impression tray.

19 Prepare plaster and water for a second mix.

20 Prepare the second mix of plaster according to previous instructions.

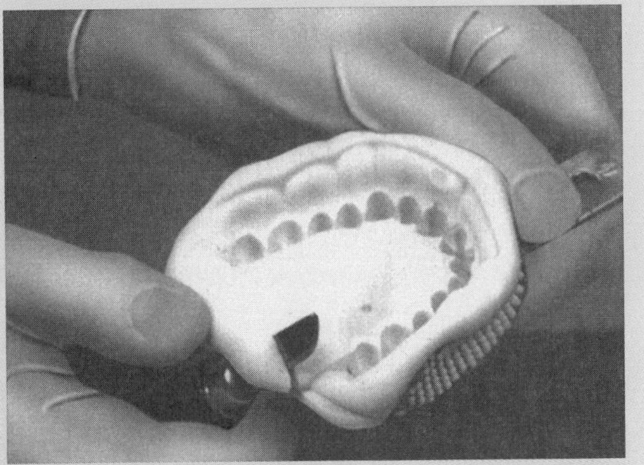

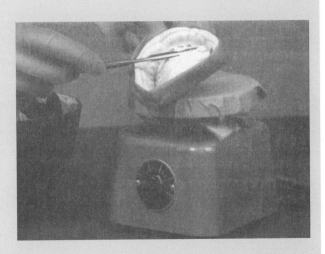

Figure 48-5 Trimming excess impression material.

Figure 48-6 Adding small increments of plaster.

continued

continued from previous page
Procedure 55 Inverted Technique

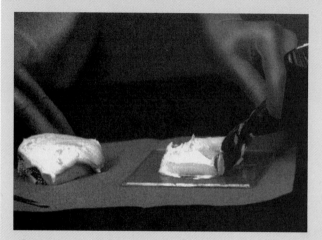

Figure 48-7 Forming plaster patty.

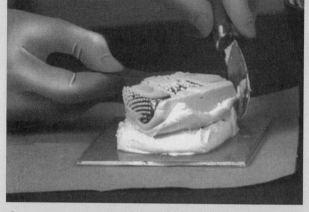

Figure 48-8 Joining patty with impression.

21 Place entire second mix on a glass slab or tile and form a square, thick patty (Figure 48-7).

22 Quickly invert the impression on the patty, which was previously prepared. Seat the patty with sufficient pressure to join the plaster of the patty with the plaster of the impression (Figure 48-8). *Important:* Hold tray handle steady, and hand-vibrate impression, using a fulcrum to support the tray; otherwise, the tray will be buried in plaster, resulting in a shallow base.

23 Soft plaster can be added along the borders of the base at this time. Likewise, excess plaster may be removed. Keep all walls of the plaster base vertical (Figure 48-9). Fill in any voids that may exist. Do not bury tray into plaster. It will be very difficult to separate model or cast from tray.

24 Place poured impression(s) in 100% humidity for 60 minutes.

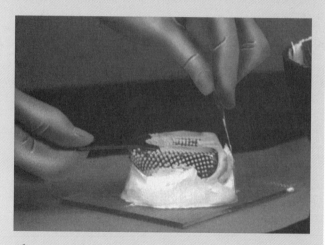

Figure 48-9 Forming the base.

Cleanup

1 Remove excess plaster from bowl and spatulas with paper towel and discard. Never wash plaster or stone products down the sink!

2 Wash and dry bowls and spatulas.

3 Clean plaster from vibrator and return to storage.

4 Clean work station.

Procedure 56 Boxed Technique

Materials Needed

Alginate impressions
Plaster bowl
Spatula, plaster
Spatula, small (metal)
Vibrator
Plaster powder
Water (room temperature)
Laboratory knife
Gram scale
Graduate cylinder
Q-tips
Paper cup(s)
Paper towels
Wax boxing strips
Bowl of hot water
Humidor

Ratio

- Maxillary impression, 100 gr plaster/49 ml water
- Mandibular impression, 100 gr plaster/49 ml water
- Extra plaster, if needed, 50 gr plaster/24 ml water

Instructions

1 Weigh plaster in cup or paper towel.
2 Measure water and pour in bowl.
3 Rinse impression with cool water.

4 Trim excess impression material from tray. Leave a 1/4-in. (6-mm) margin beyond the tuberosity or retromolar pad and other areas of the impression. See Figure 48-5.
5 Remove any visible surface water from alginate impression(s) with Q-tips.
6 Soften boxing strip in bowl of hot water.
7 Place center of boxing strip across posterior part of impression, and bring ends of strip forward, overlapping strip at handle of the tray. Secure overlap by pressing the two ends together (Figure 48-10).
8 The boxing strip must be closely adapted to the impression tray with no visible spaces between tray and boxing strip. The walls of the wax boxing strip must be vertical (Figure 48-11).
9 Dampen a paper towel and fold in half diagonally.
10 Place tray or impression in center of folded towel and approximately 1 to 1 1/2 in. from folded edge (Figure 48-12). Wrap tray or impression with towel, allowing the three points of the towel to come together at the handle of the tray. The paper towel will prevent the plaster from flowing out of the impression and onto the vibrator (Figure 48-13).
11 Sift plaster powder into the water.
12 Allow powder to settle in the water for 30 seconds. This will minimize the incorporation of air into the mix during spatulation.

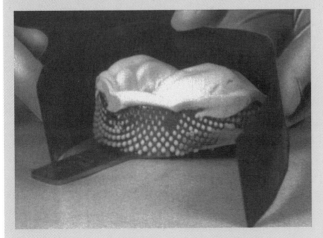

Figure 48-10 Boxing strip and impression.

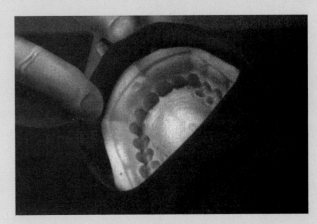

Figure 48-11 Boxing strip in place.

continued

continued from previous page
Procedure 56 Boxed Technique

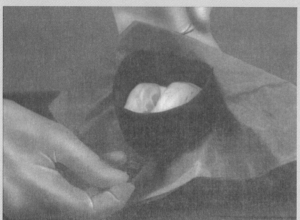

Figure 48-12 Placement of paper towel.

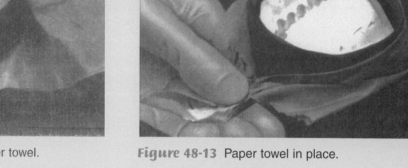

Figure 48-13 Paper towel in place.

13 Next, rapidly spatulate plaster for 30 seconds at approximately two revolutions per second.

14 Turn on vibrator at low speed.

15 Place bowl on vibrator and thoroughly vibrate plaster for another 30 seconds. Remove bowl from vibrator.

16 Hold prepared tray or impression with paper towel in place and rest base of tray or impression on vibrator.

17 Use small cement spatula and begin adding small increments of plaster to the most distal portion of one side of the impression.

18 Continue to place small increments of plaster in the same area of the impression, allowing each tooth to be filled in succession. This may necessitate tilting the impression tray until all the teeth are filled. This procedure will prevent the entrapment of air during the process of pouring.

19 Take the plaster spatula and continue to add small portions of plaster until the impression is filled to top edge of boxing strip.

20 Repeat procedure for mandibular impression, except to fill in tongue area, with a rolled, damp paper towel.

21 Place poured impression(s) in 100% humidity for 60 minutes.

22 Remove from humidor and carefully remove wax boxing strips from impression tray(s). Boxing strips are reusable.

23 Separate models from impression. Where necessary, use laboratory knife to free model from impression. *Caution:* Do not apply force when separating model from impression, as this could cause teeth to be fractured off the model.

Cleanup

1 Remove plaster from boxing strips and straighten strips by placing in water, then on paper towel to flatten.

2 Following previous instructions, clean equipment and work station.

Disinfecting Study Models

To prevent cross-contamination when handling study models, disinfection may be accomplished by soaking the models in solutions of iodophor, glutaraldehyde, or phenol after final set has taken place. None of these solutions should alter the accuracy, surface, or strength of the gypsum material.

Procedure 57 Trimming Study Models

Materials Needed

Safety glasses
Plastic apron
Prepared plaster models
Pencil
Plaster bowl, 2
Laboratory brush
Plastic triangle, 90°

Instructions

Marking Maxillary Model

1 Using pencil, draw a horizontal line about 1/4 in. distal to the tuberosity or molars (Figure 48-14).

2 Mark center tip of maxillary cuspids and extend line to labial fold (Figure 48-15). Mark and draw line division between maxillary central incisors. Extend line on frenum to labial fold (Figure 48-16).

3 Mark and draw a straight line from cuspid to midline of maxillary central incisor along the labial fold, right and left sides (Figure 48-17).

4 Observe occlusal grooves to determine the angle of the buccal cut.

5 Mark and draw a straight line along the buccal fold from the cuspid to the tuberosity or molar line, right and left sides (Figure 48-18).

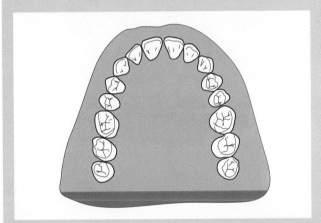

Figure 48-14 Marking peripheral outline of maxillary tuberosity.

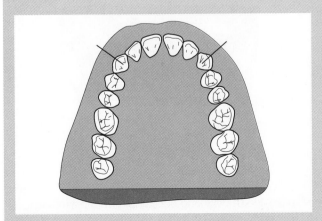

Figure 48-15 Marking maxillary cuspids.

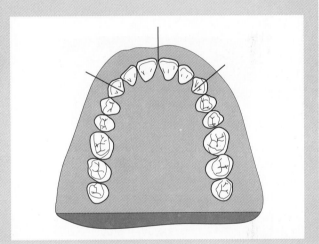

Figure 48-16 Marking division between maxillary central incisors.

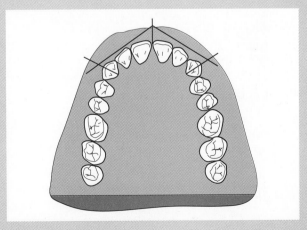

Figure 48-17 Marking cuspid(s) to midline of maxillary central incisors.

continued

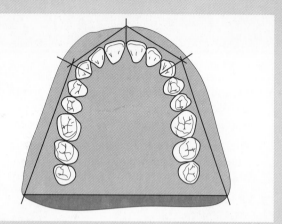

Figure 48-18 Marking buccal fold from cuspid(s) to molar(s).

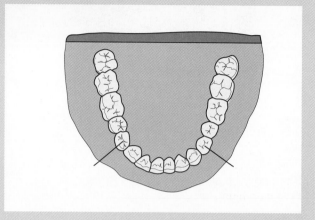

Figure 48-20 Marking mandibular first premolars.

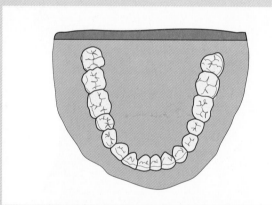

Figure 48-19 Marking peripheral outline of mandibular retromolar area.

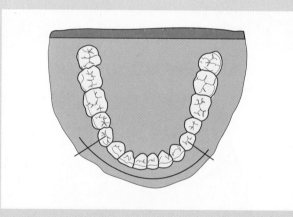

Figure 48-21 Marking anterior curve from first premolar to first premolar.

Marking Mandibular Model

1 Draw a horizontal line 1/4 in. distal to the retromolar pad or molars (Figure 48-19).

2 Mark center tip of first premolar(s), and extend line to buccal fold (Figure 48-20).

3 Draw a curved line from first premolar to the opposite premolar and along the labial fold (Figure 48-21).

4 Observe occlusal grooves to determine the angle of the buccal cut.

5 Mark and draw a straight line along the buccal fold from the first premolar to the retromolar pad or molar, right and left sides (Figure 48-22).

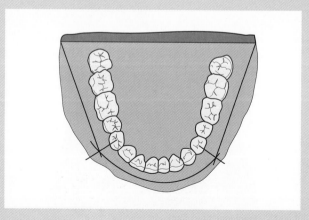

Figure 48-22 Marking buccal fold from premolar(s) to molar(s).

continued

continued from previous page
Procedure 57 *Trimming Study Models*

The Model Trimmer

1 Wear safety glasses and plastic apron.

2 Adjust table to conform to a 90° angle from wheel. Use a plastic triangle (protractor) as a guide.

3 Establish water flow. Turn ON model trimmer switch.

Preparing Models for Trimming

1 Dry models must soak in water for a minimum of 5 minutes.

2 Using a laboratory knife, remove excess extension in posterior area(s) that may prevent occlusion of models.

Trimming Procedures

A grinding wheel cuts faster if the operator does not exert tremendous pressure against the wheel. When trimming models, applying light pressure against the wheel is all that is necessary. Never allow grinding wheel to be used dry without water flow.

1 Invert mandibular model with teeth resting on the countertop. Determine if the base of the model is parallel to the occlusal plane (Figure 48-23).

2 Trim base of mandibular model parallel to the occlusal plane. The base should be at least 1/2 in. thick in tongue area (Figure 48-24).

3 Trim posterior of mandibular model at right angles to the base (Figure 48-25).

4 Occlude maxillary and mandibular models and trim posterior of maxillary model parallel to the base of the mandibular model (Figure 48-26).

5 Occlude models and trim the base of the maxillary model parallel to the base of the mandibular model (Figure 48-27).

6 On the maxillary and mandibular models, trim the buccal line parallel to the occlusal grooves and width of the buccal fold (Figures 48-28 and 48-29).

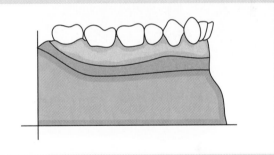

Figure 48-25 Trimming retromolar area at right angle with base.

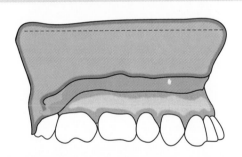

Figure 48-23 Determining plane of base.

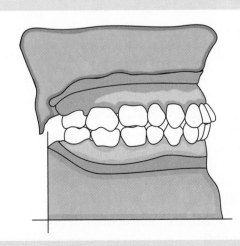

Figure 48-26 Trimming posterior of maxillary model with models in occlusion.

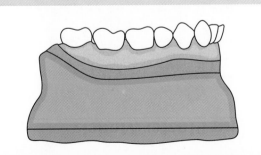

Figure 48-24 Trimming base parallel with occlusal plane.

continued

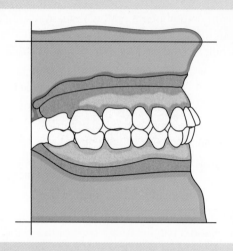

Figure 48-27 Trimming maxillary base with models in occlusion.

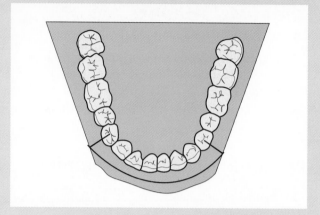

Figure 48-29 Trimming buccal folds of mandibular model.

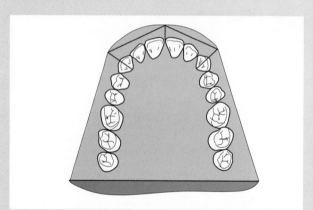

Figure 48-28 Trimming buccal folds of maxillary model.

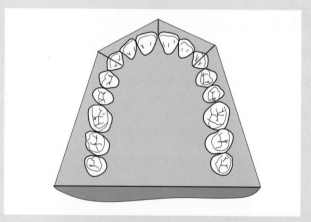

Figure 48-30 Trimming maxillary angles, cuspid(s) to central incisor(s).

7 On the maxillary model, trim from the cuspids to central incisors according to marked lines, left and right side (Figure 48-30).

8 On the mandibular model, trim from the premolar to opposite first premolar along labial fold and according to marked line (Figure 48-31).

9 Occlude both models. With a ruler draw a diagonal line across the maxillary base from the point where the labial and buccal cuts meet (cuspid) to the angle formed where the buccal and tuberosity cuts meet (Figure 48-32).

10 Trim occluded models by aligning point of cuspid area in center slot and forward on grinding table. Adjust posterior angle to fall on the center slot and next to grinding wheel. Trim to form a perpendicular cut to the cuspid line (Figure 48-33).

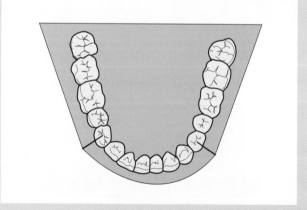

Figure 48-31 Trimming mandibular anterior curve, on first premolar to first premolar.

continued

continued from previous page
Procedure 57 Trimming Study Models

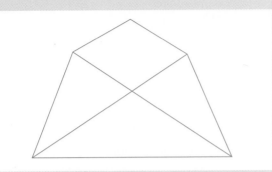

Figure 48-32 Marking maxillary base for buccal angles.

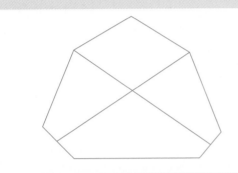

Figure 48-33 Trimming tuberosity or retromolar angle(s) perpendicular to cuspid line.

Evaluating Trimmed Study Models

1 Models must be trimmed in a symmetrical pattern (Figures 48-34A–C).

2 Model must exhibit a 1/2-in. base.

3 Trimmed models will sit on end without losing occlusion.

4 All teeth and supporting structures must be present without loss of any anatomy.

Cleanup

1 Clean model trimmer with laboratory brush. Firmly hold and press brush against grinding wheel while using full flow of water.

2 Turn off water. Switch motor to OFF.

3 Remove guide table. Wash, dry, and set aside. Clean out reservoir beneath the motor where plaster accumulates. *Note:* If the reservoir is not

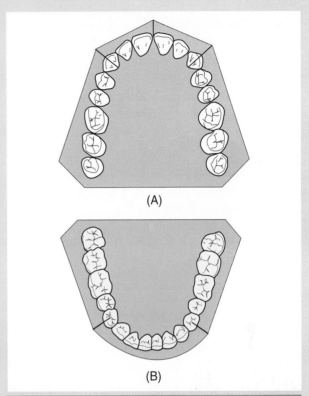

(A)

(B)

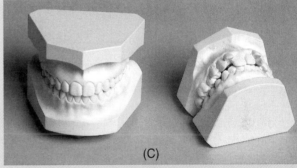

(C)

Figure 48-34 (A) Properly trimmed maxillary model. (B) Properly trimmed mandibular model. (C) Trimmed study models.

kept clean, water backs up, causing the grinding wheel to splash water out.

4 Replace guide table to its correct position on model trimmer.

5 Clean plastic apron with damp towel, fold, and store.

6 Print name on bottom of trimmed models with indelible pen.

7 Trimmed models should be evaluated by both student and instructor.

SUGGESTED ACTIVITIES

● Pour a set of study models from alginate impressions using the inverted technique.

● Pour a set of study models from alginate impressions using the boxed technique.

● Trim each set of study models according to instructions given in this chapter.

● Evaluate both sets of study models according to instructions given in this chapter.

REVIEW

1. Name the process used to change gypsum into dental plaster or stone.
   a. Calcination
   b. Initial set
   c. Hydration
   d. Dihydrate

2. Indicate how stone differs from plaster: (1) stone has irregularly shaped particles, (2) stone has smooth particles, (3) stone has less porous particles, and/or (4) stone particles are generally rough.
   a. 1, 2   c. 3, 4
   b. 2, 3   d. 1, 4

3. How does the water-powder ratio affect the final strength of the gypsum product?
   a. Decreasing the amount of powder in the water-powder ratio
   b. Increasing the speed of spatulation
   c. The number of nuclei present at time of crystallization increasing strength
   d. Driving off water molecules after mixing plaster

4. Name the factors that control the setting time of plaster or stone: (1) temperature of water and atmosphere, (2) time and speed of spatulation, (3) using a mix of plaster and stone, and/or (4) water-powder ratio.
   a. 1, 2, 3   c. 1, 2, 4
   b. 2, 3, 4   d. 1, 3, 4

5. Name one accelerator used to increase setting time.
   a. Borax
   b. Sodium chloride (table salt)
   c. Sodium citrate
   d. Hydrocolloid gels

6. Match the type of plaster with the stated factors.

   ___ a. Type I plaster
   ___ b. Type II plaster
   ___ c. Type III dental stone
   ___ d. Type IV dental stone
   ___ e. Type V dental stone

   1. Class I stone or Hydrocal
   2. Model or laboratory plaster
   3. Impression plaster
   4. High-strength, high-expansion die stone
   5. Class II die stone

7. What is the purpose of using a small spatula to begin adding small increments of plaster when pouring the impression?
   a. To prevent pouring plaster at a fast rate
   b. To increase smoothness of the material
   c. To prevent entrapment of air

8. Prior to trimming models, the dental assistant must (1) remove all undercuts from the models, (2) mark trimming lines on both models with a pencil, (3) soak the models in water for at least 5 minutes, and/or (4) remove excess extensions in posterior area that may prevent occlusion of models.
   a. 1, 2, 3
   b. 2, 3, 4
   c. 1, 2, 4
   d. 1, 3, 4

Pharmacology

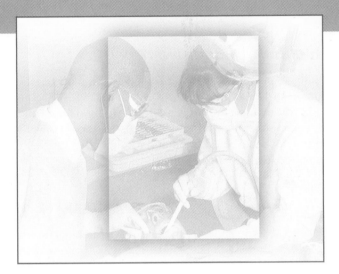

CHAPTER 49

Introduction

Pharmacology is the study of the action of drugs on the tissues and organs of the body. Drugs can be defined as substances used in diagnosis, treatment, and prevention of diseases in the human or animal.

Dental assistants need to be familiar with the administration, actions, and interactions of drugs but may not prescribe or administer them.

Official Regulatory Drug Agencies

Laws have been developed to provide safety to consumers. Therefore, there are agencies that regulate the production, marketing, advertising, labeling, and prescribing of drugs.

Food and Drug Administration (FDA)

The FDA is an agency of the U. S. government that is responsible for evaluation and approval of pharmaceuticals and medical devices. It is involved in the following services:

- Prohibiting false or misleading claims in the labeling of drugs
- Controlling manufacture of drugs for safety, identity, strength, quality, and purity of the product
- Assuring that drugs must be properly tested before being sold to the public
- Ascertaining that manufacturers report any unexpected side effects
- Conducting periodic inspection of manufacturing plants and their laboratories

Federal Trade Commission

The responsibilities of the Federal Trade Commission include:

OBJECTIVES

After studying this chapter, the student will be able to:

- Identify official agencies that deal with drugs and list their responsibilities.
- Explain the five schedules of drugs according to potential for abuse, physical and psychological dependence, and medical usefulness.
- Identify publications that list the action of drugs.
- Describe the sources of drugs.
- Identify drugs by their chemical, generic, and trade names.
- Describe methods of drug administration.
- Describe the conditions that modify the action of drugs.
- Discuss the classification of drugs according to their action.
- Identify cardiovascular, antihistamine, analgesics, CNS stimulants, antimicrobial, and gastrointestinal drugs.
- Describe the essentials and the physical form of a prescription.

- Jurisdiction over advertising, prohibiting false advertising of foods, nonprescription drugs, and cosmetics
- Regulating trade practices of drug companies

Drug Enforcement Administration (DEA)

The DEA oversees the Controlled Substances Act:

- Requires a person distributing any controlled drugs to register annually with the DEA.
- Provides research into problems and prevention of drug abuse.
- Classifies drugs according to potential for abuse, physical and psychological dependence, and medical usefulness, including narcotics, stimulants, and sedatives. Divides drugs into five schedules.

Schedule I. Drugs that have no accepted medical usefulness in the United States and have a high abuse potential. Included in this category are marijuana, heroin, lysergic acid diethylamide (LSD). These may not be prescribed.

Schedule II. Drugs with a high abuse potential with severe psychic or physical dependence liability. The prescription for these drugs cannot be refilled. Included in this category are morphine, codeine, cocaine, phenobarbital (Demerol, Percodan, Seconol), and amphetamines.

Schedule III. Drugs with an abuse potential less than those in Schedules I and II. Included in this category are certain compounds with limited quantities of narcotic such as Tylenol with codeine and nonnarcotics (barbituric acid). A prescription must be written in triplicate (one to the pharmacy, one for the dentist's record-keeping, and one for the federal government), and it may be refilled up to five times within six months.

Schedule IV. Drugs with an abuse potential less than those in Schedule III. Examples in this category are Valium, Miltown, and Darvon. Prescription may be written similar as for Schedule III.

Schedule V. Abuse potential is less than for Schedule IV and consists of limited quantities of certain mild narcotics used for antidiarrheal or cough preparations.

Publications

United States Pharmacopeia (USP)

This publication is issued every five years and is recognized as an official standard by the Federal Food, Drug, and Cosmetic Act. It gives sources, appearances, properties, standards of purity and strength of drugs, setting the manufacturing standards for drugs. When drugs meet these specifications, they bear the label "U.S.P."

National Formulary (NF)

The NF is recognized as an official standard by the Federal Food, Drug, and Cosmetic Act and is issued every five years by the American Pharmaceutical Association. It lists drugs based on extent of use and therapeutic value. It contains drugs of established usefulness that are not described in the USP.

Accepted Dental Therapeutics (ADT)

Published by the Council on Dental Therapeutics of the American Dental Association biannually, the ADT contains information on drugs mainly used by dentists and discusses treatment of oral diseases. It also contains information on hemostatics and astringents not usually included in all pharmacology texts.

Physicians Desk Reference (PDR)

Published annually by pharmaceutical manufacturers, the PDR is a reference guide that gives information about the pharmacology, indications, contraindications, and side effects of prescription drugs. It contains generic, chemical, and brand name indices. It publishes a pictorial identification section and product information section.

Sources of Drugs

Drugs are derived from plants, minerals, and animals and are also produced synthetically (man made).

- *Plants.* From bark, seeds, flowers, leaves, roots. Examples are cocaine, digitalis, morphine, codeine, and antibiotics.
- *Minerals.* From iron, tincture of iodine, silver nitrate, cobalt, magnesium, zinc, and gold.
- *Animals.* Adrenalin, insulin, thyroxine, cortisone, pepsin, and antitoxins.
- *Synthetic Drugs.* Drugs that are produced chemically. Examples are sulfa, antibiotics, and synthetic narcotics. Some may be superior to the natural drugs.

Drug Nomenclature

There are two large groups of drugs, the ones that are dispensed with a doctor's prescription and the ones that are available OTC (over the counter). Each of these types of drugs are further identified by three names: chemical, generic, and trade names.

- *Chemical Name.* This is usually the first name that a drug is known by while it is being investigated for possible clinical use. Example: acetylsalicylic acid.

- *Generic Name.* Before the drug can be marketed, it is given an official name that the pharmacist uses. Example: aspirin.

- *Trade Name.* Also known as the "brand name" and is given when the chemical is determined to be useful and can be marketed commercially. The name is registered as a trademark with the Federal Trade Mark Law and is written in capitalized form. Usually patented under Federal Patent Law giving the company exclusive right to manufacture the drug for 17 years. No competitor may use that name. Example: Bayer.

Drug Administration

Methods of Drug Administration

Drugs may be administered enterally or parenterally. **Enteral** refers to drugs placed directly into the gastrointestinal tract where absorption of the drug takes place in the small intestine:

- Rectal—administered through the rectum
- Oral—administered by mouth

Parenteral refers to drugs that bypass the gastrointestinal tract and are absorbed in a different manner.

- Intravenous (IV)—administered directly into the vein
- Inhalation—administered through the nasal passageways
- Intramuscular (IM)—administered into the muscles
- Intradermal (ID)—administered by injection into the epidermis of the skin
- Subcutaneous (SC, SQ)—administered under the skin

- Sublingual—administered under the tongue
- Topical—placed on the mucosa or skin

Conditions that Modify the Action of Drugs

There are many variations that take place in response to a drug. Some effects will depend on the size and weight of the person, the dose and strength of the drug, and how the person's system will assimilate it.

- Age—A child requires less amount of drug than an adult.
- Weight—Smaller people require less amounts of drug than heavier people.
- **Idiosyncrasy**—An unexpected effect following administration of a drug.
- **Tolerance**—The body builds tolerance to drugs with prolonged use.
- **Allergy**—Reaction to a drug that may be life threatening.
- **Cumulative effect**—The rate of elimination of a drug from the body is slow, leaving excess amounts of the drug present in the body.
- Method of administration—Drugs are absorbed at different rates according to method used.
- Pathologic condition—Type of infective agent determines drug to be used.

Classification of Drugs

See Table 49-1.

Table 49-1	Classification of Drugs	
Types of Drugs	**Use of Drugs**	**Examples (Trade Names)**
Cardiovascular Drugs		
Heart	Strengthen myocardium	Digoxin
	Increase heart rate and force contraction	Epinephrine
	Regulate heart rhythm (arrythmia)	Quinidine
	Dilate coronary arteries	Nitroglycerin
Blood pressure	Dilate blood vessel walls and decrease BP	Hydralazine
	Excrete water and sodium ions	Diuril
	Constrict blood vessels and increase BP	Epinephrine, decongestants
Anticoagulants	Thin the blood and prevent blood clots	Coumadin
Antihistamines	Prevent allergic reaction	Epinephrine, Benadryl

(continued)

Table 49-1 Classification of Drugs (continued)

Types of Drugs	Use of Drugs	Examples (Trade Names)
Analgesics	Prevent or relieve pain	
Nonnarcotic	Relieve mild to moderate pain	Aspirin, Tylenol, Advil
Narcotic	Relieve moderate to severe pain	Morphine, Codeine, Demerol, Darvon
Anxiety Control	Relieve nervousness and apprehension	
Antianxiety agents	Relieve nervousness and apprehension	Valium, Librium
Barbiturate sedative and hypnotics	Depending on dose, may cause sedation, hypnosis, anesthesia, coma, death	Nembutal, Amytal, Seconal
Nonbarbiturate sedative and hypnotics	Promote sleep when suffering from insomnia	Noctec, Dalmane, Halcion
Anticonvulsants	Treat epilepsy	Dilantin, Tegretol
Alcohol	Of no therapeutic value other than as a vasodilator. Interaction with sedatives and narcotics may be fatal.	
Anesthetics		
General anesthetics	Produce loss of sensation in the entire body	Pentothal, Brevital, Fluothane, Penthrane, nitrous oxide–oxygen (used as adjunct for complete anesthesia)
Local anesthetics	Relieve and prevent pain in localized area	Xylocaine, Carbocaine
Topical anesthetics	Produce temporary disensitization of nerve endings in oral mucosa (used in ointment, liquid, or spray form)	Xylocaine, Hurricaine, Cetacaine, Dyclone
CNS Stimulants		
Amphetamines	CNS mood elevator, also to treat narcolepsy	Dexedrine, Ritalin
Other stimulants	CNS stimulants, to encourage breathing	Aromatic spirits of ammonia, cocaine
Antimicrobials	Destroy or inhibit growth of microorganisms	
Antibiotics	Destroy bacteria	Penicillin, Keflex, E-Mycin, Cipro, tetracycline HCl
Antifungal agents	Destroy susceptible fungi that cause "thrush" or candidiasis	Diflucan, Fungizone, Grisactin, Micostatin
Antiviral agents	Treat viral infections (herpes simplex, herpes zoster, HIV, AIDS)	Zovirax, AZT, HIVID
Gastrointestinal Drugs	Treat the stomach and intestinal tract	
Antacids	Neutralize acids in the stomach	Tums, Riopan, Mylanta Tagamet
Emetics	Produce vomiting when poison is swallowed	Syrup of Ipecac
Laxatives	Relieve constipation	Metamucil, Correctol
Antiemetics	Prevent nausea, vomiting, motion sickness	Compazine, Dramamine, Antivert
Antidiarrheals	Treat diarrhea and decrease spasms in bowels	Lomotil, Kaopectate, Imodium

Cardiovascular Drugs

Drugs are given to slow, speed up, or stabilize the heart rate as well as to increase blood flow to the heart muscle and to strengthen the heart beat.

Drugs Affecting the Heart

A. Digitalis glycosides—administered to strengthen the heart muscle (myocardium)

B. Epinephrine—administered to increase heart rate and force contraction

C. Quinidine—administered to regulate the heart rhythm (arrhythmia); reduces heart rate

D. Nitrites—vasodilators that dilate coronary arteries used in the treatment of **angina pectoris** (chest pain resulting from decreased blood supply to the heart muscle):
   1. Nitroglycerin (Nitrostat)—tablet placed under the tongue (sublingually)
   2. Amyl nitrate—inhaler
   3. Transderm-Nitro—transdermal skin patch which has longer action, about 24 hours
   4. Nitrol ointment—ointment applied to the skin every 8 hours as needed

Drugs Affecting Blood Pressure

A. Antihypertensive drugs
   1. **Vasodilators**—act directly on blood vessel walls. Drugs that relax the muscles of the blood vessel walls, increasing their **lumen** (diameter of vessel). For example, hydralazine (Apresoline), is a vasodilator generally used in conjunction with a diuretic.
   2. **Thiazide diuretics**—lower blood volume by promoting renal excretion of water and sodium ions. Example: chlorothiazide (Diuril).

B. **Vasoconstrictors**—drugs that **constrict** (narrow) the lumen of blood vessels. Used to increase blood pressure and stop local bleeding:
   1. Epinephrine
   2. Bronchodilators
   3. Decongestants and OTC cold remedies

Anticoagulants

Patients who are taking anticoagulants will tend to bleed and have poor coagulating properties. These patients should *not* take aspirin. Example: coumarin (Coumadin). They are used:

A. To prevent blood clotting

B. To delay coagulation of blood

C. In stored blood for transfusions

Antihistamines

The body releases **histamines** when a foreign substance (allergen) enters it. The amount of histamines produced may cause itching, hives, asthma, and sometimes anaphylactic shock. **Antihistamines** are histamine **antagonists** (drugs that counteract the action of another drug, decreasing or concealing the effect of the other) that neutralize the symptoms a histamine produces.

● Epinephrine is used to reduce swelling during extreme allergic reactions or **hypersensitivity** (the state of being abnormally sensitive or susceptible to a drug or chemical) such as anaphylactic shock, whereby the airway becomes obstructed due to swelling.

● Benadryl, Dimetane, Pyribenzamine, Dramamine, Marezine, and Vistaril are used to reduce histamine production and its effects.

Analgesics

Analgesics, also known as pain killers, range from the nonnarcotic to the stronger narcotic types.

Nonnarcotic Analgesics. These analgesics relieve mild to moderate pain and do not alter the central nervous system except in an overdose:

A. Purposes and uses:
   1. To relieve mild pain such as headache or arthritis discomfort
   2. **Antipyretic** (an agent that reduces elevated temperatures)—reduces body temperature, only when elevated
   3. **Anti-inflammatory** (counteracting inflammation or its effects) excluding acetylsalicylic acid—relieves joint pain and swelling by stimulating the adrenal cortex to release cortisone

B. Adverse reactions: primarily with acetylsalicylic acid (aspirin):
   1. Causes allergic reactions—edema of the respiratory passage and sometimes the face
   2. Produces painful slough during prolonged contact with the mucosa
   3. Affects the gastrointestinal mucosa, causing bleeding, especially with slow-releasing aspirin
   4. Reduces clotting time even with small doses
   5. Causes poisoning in children when overdose amounts are taken

C. Examples:
   1. Acetylsalicylic acid—Bayer Aspirin, ASA, Ascriptin, Bufferin, Anacin (with caffeine)
   2. Acetaminophen—Tylenol, Datril, Panadol, Vanquish, Sinubid, Anacin-3
   3. Ibuprofen—Ibu-Tab, Motrin, Advil, Nuprin, Ibumed, Pamprin IB

Narcotic Analgesics. These are used for stronger analgesia, sedation, and hypnosis, which will alter the central nervous system:

A. Natural opium alkaloids—must have a prescription for any of these analgesics. They are effective against moderate to severe pain:

1. Example: morphine, methylmorphine (Codeine).
2. Morphine is used as a standard for potency. Codeine is one-tenth as strong as morphine.
3. **Addiction** (physiologic or psychological dependence with a tendency to increase the dosage to achieve original effect) is likely to happen with prolonged use; therefore, it is not used with chronic pain
4. Mental processes are **depressed** (diminished functional activity) causing drowsiness and possibly sleep.
5. Respiration is reduced (depressed) when overdose or toxic amounts are taken.
6. Used only when other analgesics do not work.
7. Tylenol with codeine is widely prescribed following dental surgical procedures. When codeine is added to Tylenol, greater **potentiation** (combination of two drugs are greater than the sum of the independent effects of each drug) is achieved.

B. Synthetic narcotic analgesics—must have a prescription for any of these analgesics:

1. Example: meperidine (Demerol), oxycodone (Percodan), and dolophine (Methadone).
2. Addiction is less than with morphine but greater than with codeine.
3. Dizziness and nausea may occur.

C. Propoxyphene—a synthetic opioid narcotic analgesic that requires a prescription:

1. Example: Darvon, Darvocet (with acetaminophen).
2. Used for mild to moderate pain.
3. May cause drowsiness, dizziness, confusion, headache, and sedation.

Anxiety Control

These are controlled substances and therefore require a prescription.

A. Antianxiety agents—used to control nervousness and apprehension:

1. Suppress mild to moderate anxiety and tension.
2. Less likely to cause excessive loss of alertness than barbiturates.
3. Used as a muscle relaxant.
4. May be used as **premedication** (medication given in advance of the procedure) prior to general anesthesia.

5. Examples: diazepam (Valium), chlordiazepoxide (Librium), meprobamate (Miltown), and hydroxyzine (Vistaril).

B. Barbiturate sedative and hypnotics (sleep producing)—depending on dose, may cause sedation, hypnosis, anesthesia, coma, death:

1. Used as anticonvulsant.
2. May be **cumulative** (drugs not excreted quickly from the body tend to accumulate, causing an increased effect) because of its very slow **excretory** (elimination of waste products from the body) property.
3. May cause skin eruptions (rash) and oral lesions
4. Decrease anticoagulant effect.
5. Decrease contraceptive effect when using oral contraceptives.
6. Examples: pentobarbital (Nembutal), amobarbital (Amytal), and secobarbital (Seconal).

C. Nonbarbiturate sedatives and hypnotics—safer than barbiturates due to less abuse potential:

1. Need larger doses than barbiturates because they are less powerful.
2. Adequate for ordinary **insomnia** (sleeplessness) and daytime sedation; however, may produce confusion and headache.
3. Have a long elimination **half-life** (time required by the body to metabolize or inactivate half the amount of a substance taken in).
4. Should not interact with alcohol, muscle relaxants, antihistamines, analgesics, or any CNS depressants.
5. Contraindications: hypersensitivity, persons with severe liver and renal impairment.
6. Examples: chloral hydrate (Noctec), flurazepam (Dalmane), and triazolam (Halcion).

Anticonvulsants

● Used in controlling **epilepsy** (a central nervous system disorder caused by abnormal electrical discharges within the brain, resulting in abnormal muscular movements and loss of consciousness). Anticonvulsants may cause sedation, dizziness, and confusion.

● Depress the part of the brain that controls motor activity and not the sensory and cognitive (thinking) part.

● Examples: barbiturates and sedatives, including phenytoin (Dilantin), phenobarbital (Luminal), and carbamazepine (Tegretol).

Alcohol

Classified as a CNS depressant and a **psychotropic** drug (any substance that acts on the mind):

● It causes loss of finer grades of attention, judgement, memory, and concentration.

● It is an irritant to the gastric mucosa, leading to possible gastritis, ulceration, and hemorrhage.

● It dilates blood vessels of the skin, producing the flushing and sweating commonly seen with intoxication.

● It causes death in acute alcoholic poisoning or intoxication due to respiratory failure, vomiting, convulsions, **cerebral edema** (fluid in the brain), **delirium tremens** (disorientation with visual and hearing hallucinations due to the habitual and excessive use of alcohol).

● Interactions with other drugs must be avoided.

Anesthetics

See Chapters 50 and 51.

A. General anesthetic—produces loss of sensation through the entire body, producing sleep, unconsciousness, and muscle relaxation:
   1. Inhalation
      • Nitrous oxide–oxygen
      • Halothane (Fluothane)—used with nitrous oxide
      • Methoxyflurane (Penthrane)—contains ether and can be used with nitrous oxide
   2. Intravenous
      • Thiopental sodium (Pentothal)
      • Methohexital sodium (Brevital)

B. Local Anesthetic—injectable solution that relieves and prevents pain in a localized part of the body. Examples: Lidocaine (Xylocaine), Carbocaine, Marcaine, Citanest, Duranest, and Octocaine.

C. Topical anesthetic—an ointment, liquid, or spray that produces temporary disensitization of nerve endings in the oral mucosa. Examples: Xylocaine ointment, liquid, and spray; Hurricaine spray or liquid; Cetacaine spray or liquid; and Dyclone oral rinse.

Central Nervous System Stimulants

These drugs induce stimulation of the CNS, resulting in wakefulness, increased motor activity, and talkativeness. Overdoses can cause hallucinations, which may go into convulsions. They are used to counteract mild states of depression.

A. Amphetamines: Schedule II drugs
   1. CNS mood elevator, causing wakefulness, decreases sense of fatigue, and **euphoria** (a sense of wellbeing) and used to treat **narcolepsy** (sleeping sickness) and attention deficit disorder
   2. Cause loss of appetite and increased alertness and physical activity
   3. Increase blood pressure and heart rate and dilate pupils of the eyes
   4. Slight bronchial relaxant
   5. Examples: amphetamine (Biphetamine, Dexedrine), and methylphenidate (Ritalin)
   6. Abusers: truck drivers, athletes

Other Stimulants

1. Aromatic spirits of ammonia—encourage breathing from reflex stimulation.
2. Cocaine—taken internally, stimulates the CNS temporarily; also gives feeling of pleasure, which later may turn into fear, resulting in violence.

Antimicrobial Agents

Made from organic substances produced by microorganisms, antimicrobial agents have the ability to destroy or inhibit the growth of bacteria and other microorganisms.

Oral infections can spread rapidly and may account for many severe illnesses and fatalities. Individuals with decreased resistance to infection include diabetics, alcoholics, and persons affected with leukemia, Addison's disease (underfunctioning of adrenal gland), and malnutrition. Bacteria can become resistant to antibiotics. Also, antibiotics can kill helpful bacteria. Three types of antimicrobials are identified—antibiotics, antifungals, and antivirals:

A. Antibiotics—used to fight bacterial infections. Hypersensitivity to antibiotics ranges from rash to fatal **anaphylaxis** (life-threatening allergic reaction). Gastrointestinal disfunction and **photosensitivity** (reaction to light or sunlight exposure) may take place.
   1. Penicillins—first antibiotic discovered produced from a fungus. Used to treat many streptococcal, some staphylococcal, and meningococcal infections. The drug of choice when treating such sexually transmitted diseases as gonorrhea and syphilis. Used to premedicate for prevention of recurrences of rheumatic fever or endocarditis. Examples: amino-penicillins (Amoxicillin, Ampicillin, Augmentin) and penicillin V (V-Cillin K, Pen-Vee K).
   2. Cephalosporins—semisynthetic antibiotic produced from a fungus and therefore, related to penicillin. Thus, some patients who are allergic to penicillin may also be allergic to cephalosporins. Examples: cephalexin (Keflex), cefaclor (Ceclor), and ceftriaxone (Rocephin), cefazolin (Kefzol, Ancef).

3. Erythromycins—used on patients who are allergic to penicillin. Considered to be the least toxic antibiotic. Examples: erythromycin (E-Mycin, Ilosone, Eryc) and clarithromycin (Biaxin).

4. Quinolones—a newer drug used primarily on adults. Example: cyprofloxacin (Cipro).

5. Tetracyclines—should be used only when other antibiotics are not effective or contraindicated. They are used in treating rickettsia, chlamydia, and other sexually transmitted diseases, severe acne, and some uncommon bacteria. Example: tetracycline HCI (Achromycin V, Panmycin, Sumycin, Tetram, Tetracap, Robitet).

B. Antifungal Agents—used to destroy specific susceptible fungi.
  1. Good choice against candidiasis ("thrush").
  2. A stronger antifungal agent, fluconazole (Diflucan), may be contraindicated for children under 13 years and pregnant or nursing women.
  3. Examples: amphotericin B (Fungizone), fluconazole, (Diflucan), griseofulvin (Grisactin, Fulvicin), and nystatin (Micostatin).

C. Antiviral Agents
  1. Used to treat virus infections such as herpes simplex, herpes zoster (shingles), varicella zoster (chickenpox), and respiratory infections caused by influenza A virus. Examples: acyclovir (Zovirax), amantadine (Symadine, Symmetrel), and ribavirin (Virasole).
  2. Currently, zidovudine (AZT) is being used for initial management of human immunodeficiency virus (HIV) infections.
  3. Zalcitabine (HIVID) combined with AZT is being used for the management of advanced acquired immunodeficiency syndrome (AIDS).

Gastrointestinal Drugs

These drugs are used to treat the stomach and intestinal tract. They are identified as antacids, emetics, laxatives, antinauseants, antidiarrheals and antispasmodics.

A. Antacid—may contain aluminum, calcium carbonate, magnesium, and sodium. They are sold widely over the counter.
  1. Used to neutralize acids in the stomach, heartburn (esophageal reflux), and indigestion.
  2. They may decrease effectiveness of antibiotics such as tetracyclines and digoxin used to strengthen the heart beat.
  3. Examples: calcium carbonate (Tums), aluminum-magnesium (Riopan, Maalox, Gelusil, Mylanta), and cimetidine (Tagamet).

B. Emetics—used to produce vomiting when poison has been swallowed. Example: Syrup of Ipecac. Vomiting is *not induced* for the following swallowed materials:
  1. Corrosive materials such as drain and oven cleaners, lye, carbolic acid, dishwashing detergent. Additional damage could occur.
  2. Petroleum products such as gasoline, kerosene, lighter fluid, or benzene. Could cause aspiration and asphyxiation.
  3. Convulsant agents such as strychnine or iodine. Could cause seizures.

C. Laxatives—used to relieve constipation. Examples: Metamucil, Milk of Magnesia, phenolphthalein (Ex-Lax), Correctol, and Feenamint.

D. Antiemetics—used to prevent nausea, vomiting, and motion sickness. Examples: prochlorperazine (Compazine), dimenhydrinate (Dramamine), meclizine (Antivert), and scopalomine (Transderm-Scop) 72-hour patch placed behind the ear.

E. Antidiarrheals—used to treat diarrhea and decrease spasms in bowels. Examples: diphenoxylate with atropine (Lomotil), kaolin and pectin (Kaopectate), and ioperamide (Imodium).

Prescription Writing

A prescription is a written order or authorization by a dentist, physician, or veterinarian to the pharmacist to dispense a certain drug or combination of drugs to a patient.

Reasons for Having Prescriptions

A. Assures the patient of proper dose of a drug
B. Designed for the individual patient only
C. For drugs considered habit forming or too dangerous without professional supervision

Essentials of a Prescription

A. It should be legibly written in ink.
B. Date, name, and address of patient should be complete.
C. The name, dosage form, strength, and total number of dosage units should be clearly indicated and number of renewals or no renewals, "NR," should be included.
D. Directions for use that includes the number of times per day and how much should be taken should be included.

(Heading) Name and Address of Dentist

(Superscription) Date ____________
Name & Address of Patient Age ____________
Rx

(Inscription) Name of drug, dosage, form & strength
(Subscription) Directions to the pharmacist – quantities
(Signa) Instructions to patient

(Signature) ______________________
Dentist's signature & degree

(Other)
DEA Number
Refill ________ time(s)

Figure 49-1 Prescription sample.

E. A separate prescription blank for each drug prescribed is used.

F. The prescription should be signed by the dentist.

G. The dentist's federal registry number and address should be included, especially for controlled substances.

H. What was prescribed should be noted on the patient's chart.

Physical Form of the Prescription

See Figure 49-1.

A. Heading—refers to the name, address, and telephone number of the prescriber (dentist)

B. Superscription—refers to the patient's name, address, age, date, and the symbol Rx that means "take thou"

C. Inscription—refers to the body of the prescription that contains the official name and quantity of the drug prescribed

D. Subscription – refers to the directions to the pharmacist regarding dosage form and quantity to be dispensed

E. Transcription or Signa (Sig)—refers to the instructions to the patient for use of the drug (see Table 49-2 for abbreviations used).

F. Signature—refers to the prescriber's signature and professional degree (DDS)

G. Other
  1. Refill information
  2. DEA number of dentist

Table 49-2 Common Latin Abbreviations Used on Prescriptions

a.c. (*ante cibum*)	before meals
p.c. (*post cibum*)	after meals
ad	up to
aq. (*aqua*)	water
h.s. (*hora somni*)	at bedtime
p.r.n. (*pro re nata*)	when needed
q.h. (*quaque hora*)	every hour
q.2h. (*quaque secunda hora*)	every two hours
b.i.d. (*bis in die*)	twice a day
t.i.d. (*ter in die*)	three times a day
q.i.d. (*quater in die*)	four times a day
stat. (*statim*)	immediately

SUGGESTED ACTIVITIES

- In study groups, name one type of drug that would be chosen for the following conditions: severe toothache, infected jaw, fast heart rate, blood clot in the system, headache, to neutralize stomach acid, allergic reaction, high blood pressure, nervousness, and to produce vomiting.
- Go over the following Latin abbreviations used on prescriptions and quiz each other:

  a.c., p.c., p.r.n., q.h., b.i.d., t.i.d., q.i.d., and stat.

REVIEW

1. Which publication contains information on drugs that are used mainly by dentists?
   a. *United States Pharmacopeia*
   b. *National Formulary*
   c. *Accepted Dental Therapeutics*
   d. *Physicians Desk Reference*
2. When drugs are named, they are known by three names. Which name is also known as the brand name?
   a. Trade name
   b. Chemical name
   c. Generic name
3. Describe methods whereby drugs are administered "parenterally" into the body: (1) intramuscularly, (2) intravenously, (3) orally, and/or (4) inhalation.
   a. 1, 2, 3
   b. 2, 3, 4
   c. 1, 2, 4
   d. 1, 3, 4

4. Select the correct answer for column A from column B:

Column A	Column B
___ a. Strengthens the heart muscle	1. Antifungal agent
___ b. Prevents blood from clotting	2. Anticoagulant
___ c. Is able to constrict blood vessels	3. Anticonvulsant
___ d. Type of drug known as pain killer	4. Nitroglycerin
___ e. Type of drug used to control epilepsy	5. Histamine
___ f. Considered to be a psychotrophic drug	6. Epinephrine
___ g. Causes wakefulness and is a mood elevator	7. Amphetamine
___ h. Type of drug that kills bacteria	8. Analgesics
___ i. Type of drug used to destroy fungi	9. Emetic
___ j. Produces vomiting on purpose	10. Alcohol
___ k. Used to prevent nausea, vomiting, and motion sickness	11. Antibiotic
___ l. Drug placed sublingually to dilate coronary arteries	12. Antiemetic
___ m. What the body releases when an allergen enters it	13. Antianxiety agent
___ n. Type of drug that controls nervousness and apprehension	14. Narcotic analgesic
___ o. Codeine is classified under this type of drug	15. Digitalis glycosides

5. Which drug is used to relieve an allergic reaction?
   a. Antihypertensive
   b. Analgesic
   c. Antianxiety
   d. Antihistamine

Anesthesia and Anxiety Control

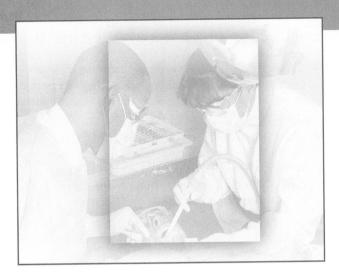

CHAPTER 50

Introduction

Anesthesia is defined as the temporary loss of feeling or sensation by means of depressing the central nervous system or local interruption of nerve impulses to a specific area. Pain control is achieved in various ways: through loss of consciousness as occurs with general anesthesia or by pain and anxiety control using conscious sedation that includes oral, intramuscular, intravenous, and nitrous oxide–oxygen inhalation sedation. Loss of feeling and sensation to a specific area is accomplished by using topical or local anesthesia (discussed in Chapter 51).

Pain Control

Pain

Pain is a feeling of distress, suffering, or agony caused by a stimulus such as bodily injury or disease. It may be described as sharp, burning, aching, cramping, dull, or throbbing. Its purpose is chiefly protective, acting as a warning.

Pain Perception. Pain perception is the conscious mental interpretation of a sensory stimulus or unpleasant experience.

Pain Reaction. Pain reaction is what a person will do about an unpleasant experience. The reactions will differ from person to person and from day to day in the same person. There are two types of reaction—physical and psychological:

- *Physical.* Automatic response to superficial pain by the sympathetic nervous system causing the release of epinephrine (a natural hormone) produced by the adrenal glands. The two adrenals rest on the top of each kidney and play an important role in the chemistry of the body.

- *Psychological.* Dependent on such factors as previous experience with pain, state of health, training to respond to pain, fatigue, tension, and anxiety.

Pain Reaction Threshold. Pain reaction threshold is the degree of reaction a person will show in response to pain.

- *Low Pain Threshold* (**hyperreactive**) is the response from a person who has low tolerance to pain. It is

OBJECTIVES

After studying this chapter, the student will be able to:

- Describe physical and psychological pain reaction.
- Explain the significance of low pain threshold and high pain threshold.
- List methods of controlling pain.
- Explain the difference between sensory and motor nerves.
- Describe the action of general anesthesia.
- List general anesthetic properties.
- Explain what takes place in each stage of general anesthesia.
- Describe advantages and disadvantages for using general anesthesia.
- Give the purposes of conscious sedation.
- Give the rationale for inhalation sedation when using nitrous oxide–oxygen.
- Identify the equipment features in a complete unit of nitrous oxide–oxygen.
- Identify the color of cylinders used for oxygen and nitrous oxide.
- Describe the technique for nitrous oxide–oxygen delivery.
- Describe the symptoms when diffusion hypoxia is evident.
- Explain the purpose for a scavenging system and how it operates.

manifested in persons who feel pain easily and thus, have a quick reaction to pain.

- *High Pain Threshold* (**hyporeactive**) is the response from a person who has a high tolerance to pain. It is manifested in persons who do not feel pain easily and thus have a slow reaction to pain.

Factors Influencing Pain Threshold.
Reaction to pain differs from person to person and in the same person from one day to the next. Therefore, the following considerations exist:

- Situations that may cause lower pain threshold (hyperreactive):
  1. Emotional state could affect a person's attitude toward a procedure, the operator, or the surroundings. Emotionally unstable persons will have a lower pain threshold.
  2. Fatigue.
  3. Generally, Latin and southern Europeans are more emotional and therefore more hyperreactive.
  4. Characteristics of fear and apprehension will tend to mentally magnify the unpleasant experience.
  5. Past experiences may become a factor. Persons either build a tolerance to pain or will expect pain and become hyperreactive.
- Situations that may cause higher pain threshold (hyporeactive):
  1. Age. Older people usually tolerate a greater amount of pain.
  2. Drugs. Analgesics will raise pain threshold while barbiturates will lower it.
  3. Males. Generally have a higher tolerance, possibly due to the "macho" image.

Methods of Pain Control.
To control pain, it is best to remove the cause or block the pathway of the painful impulse through the use of drugs, such as aspirin or narcotics or a local anesthetic injection near the nerve trunk. Having the patient gain confidence in the practitioner helps to put the patient in the proper frame of mind without having to use drugs; moreover, it is wise to keep the patient informed as to what to expect.

Nerves Affected by Pain

- **Sensory** or **afferent nerves**. Carry impulses from one part of the body to the brain.
- **Motor** or **efferent nerves**. Carry impulses from the brain to the muscles in response to pain.

General Anesthesia

General loss of sensation and consciousness (**consciousness** means that protective reflexes are intact,

including ability to maintain airway and capability of rational responses to question or command) caused by an agent or drug that produces a depressing action on the CNS (central nervous system).

Early Developments of Anesthesia

- *1772.* Nitrous oxide-oxygen (laughing gas) was discovered by Joseph Priestley and in 1842 was primarily used in theatres because it caused uncontrollable laughter.
- *1844.* Horace Wells, a dentist, had his student extract his tooth under nitrous oxide. The following year, Wells extracted a patient's tooth in the presence of Harvard medical students. In both cases there was no recollection of pain.
- *1846.* William Morton, a former student of Horace Wells, started using nitrous oxide to quickly build a practice.
- *1847.* In England, James Simpson introduced chloroform as an anesthetic in obstetrics. Queen Victoria used it for childbirth. However, it was not introduced to the United States until the 1890s. Many deaths occurred with increased use of general anesthetics.
- *1896.* Ethyl chloride was used to "freeze" gums, but put patients to sleep if they breathed it. Thus, it was used as a general anesthetic until approximately 1955.
- *1903.* Barbiturates were introduced. Pentothal and hexobarbital were given intravenously.
- *1920.* Ethylene, cyclopropane, and divinyl ether were introduced.

Properties of General Anesthetics

1. Reversible in nature whereby the patient suffers no ill effects following administration of general anesthetic and returns to a normal state
2. Should have a rapid onset and recovery
3. Should be nontoxic
4. Should have minimal side effects
5. Should be stable in preparation and use
6. Should produce minimal nausea
7. Should use an inhalant that is nonirritating to the lungs and respiratory mucosa
8. Should use an intravenous that is readily soluble in physiological solutions and be nonirritating to veins
9. Should meet the surgical requirement

Stages of General Anesthesia (as used with ether):

- Stage I: Analgesia and amnesia
  1. Relieves pain sensation.
  2. Patient starts to lose consciousness, but still responds to instruction.
  3. Patient responds to command and has protective reflexes (able to cough, swallow, and breathe).
  4. Nitrous oxide is used at this stage only.

- Stage II: Delirium or excitement—state of hyperactivity
  1. Begins with loss of consciousness and continues until surgical anesthesia develops.
  2. Excitement with involuntary movements.
  3. Uninhibited reactions may occur.
  4. Vomiting, urination, and defecation may occur.
  5. Blood pressure and pulse rate increase.
  6. It is desirable to pass through this stage as quickly and smoothly as possible to the next stage due to patient's instability.

- Stage III: Surgical anesthesia. The **CNS** (central nervous system) is completely depressed. There is no response to pain. Patient returns to stable breathing, normal blood pressure, and pulse rate. Stage III is divided into four planes indicating increasing depth of anesthesia:

  Plane 1. Surgical procedures requiring minimal anesthesia.

  Plane 2. Most surgical procedures take place at plane 2 or 3.

  Plane 3. Known as the surgical stage.

  Plane 4. **Intercostal paralysis** (paralysis of muscles between the ribs), widely dilated pupils, absence of reflexes, and spontaneous respiration.

- Stage IV: Respiratory paralysis
  1. Cessation of respiration causing circulatory collapse.
  2. Cardiac arrest with imminent death.

Advantages. General anesthesia was instituted to remove temporary pain and memory from the patient who was being subjected to surgical procedures. Advantages include:

- Unconsciousness. The CNS is completely depressed, making it possible for quality dental care to be given in cases where fear or management problems prevented it.
- The patient does not respond to pain.
- The patient experiences amnesia.
- The onset of action of general anesthesia is quite rapid.

- Titration of the anesthetic drug is usually possible (**titration**—small incremental amounts of drug is given until desired dose is achieved).

Disadvantages. Some of the disadvantages may also have been advantages. Disadvantages include:

- Unconsciousness. Due to the many changes in the patient's physiology occurring with the loss of consciousness such as loss of protective reflexes, inability to obey commands, and depression of vital signs.
- Advanced training in anesthesiology is required of the dentist, an additional two years of study.
- Anesthesia team is needed. Ideally, the team should consist of a dentist trained in anesthesiology, an anesthesiologist, a nurse, and an anesthesia assistant.
- Special monitoring equipment is needed, such as a **laryngoscope** (a viewing instrument inserted into the larynx), **endotracheal** tubes (inserted within the trachea), and an **oropharyngeal** tube (inserted into the pharynx through the mouth used to provide ventilation to the patient) or a **nasopharyngeal** tube (inserted through the nose to provide ventilation to the patient's airway).
- A recovery area is needed—a separate room designed as a resting area.
- Patients must not eat or drink 6 hours prior to general anesthesia, as this should prevent the possibility of vomiting during anesthesia, which may cause airway obstruction or severe damage to the lung if vomitus is aspirated.

Conscious Sedation

Sedation is used to allay fearfulness of the patient. One means of sedation used in dentistry is referred to as **iatrosedation** (*iatro* = "doctor," *sedation* = "to calm"). This technique requires no administration of drugs but instead uses psychological reasoning, stress reduction behavior and management, including acupressure, hypnosis, or a manner of communication that promotes trust and confidence in the doctor. Another means of sedation is **pharmacosedation**, which uses sedatives to calm and reduce anxiety by depressing the central nervous system.

With sedation, the patient is conscious and more willing to receive dental treatment, the gag reflex is diminished, and pain is better tolerated. The management of pain and anxiety is controlled by the use of sedatives or nitrous oxide–oxygen. While in the state of conscious sedation, the patient retains the ability to maintain an open airway and respond to verbal commands. There are four methods of pharmacosedation used in dentistry:

- Oral—using the digestive system to introduce a sedative drug into the system
- Intramuscular (IM)—using a needle to inject a sedative drug into the muscle
- Intravenous (IV)—using a needle to inject a sedative drug into the vein
- Inhalation—the act of breathing in an agent (nitrous oxide–oxygen) by way of the nose and trachea through the respiratory system

Oral Sedation

Oral sedation is used preoperatively as well as postoperatively. This method of administering a drug is easy, but controlling its action may be difficult. Patients may react in unexpected ways that create great concern for their well-being. Generally, orally administered drugs are used preoperatively the night before, or just prior to the appointment. In either case the patient should be relaxed and well rested. When this type of sedation is used, a responsible adult should accompany the patient to ensure safe transportation. Once administered, effects of the drug occur in approximately 30 minutes, and the action of the drug may continue 3–4 hours.

Intramuscular Sedation

Intramuscular sedation is administered by injection into a patient's muscle, which bypasses the gastrointestinal tract. It cannot be titrated and therefore is administered by calculated dose. It is used more frequently in the pediatric office than other dental practices. Effects of the drug occur in approximately 15–20 minutes, and the action of the drug may continue 2–4 hours. A responsible adult should accompany the patient to ensure safe transportation.

Intravenous Sedation

Intravenous sedation is administered by injecting the patient's vein. The onset of action is extremely fast, usually about 20–25 seconds and may continue for 1–4 hours. It is possible to titrate it, due to the rapid onset of action, and reach a comfortable level for the patient to experience and for the dentist to manage. Possible management problems may arise that require the expertise of a specifically trained dentist/doctor capable of administering intravenous sedation. A responsible adult should accompany the patient to ensure safe transportation.

When a patient undergoes intravenous sedation, certain health standards should be met; otherwise sedation may be contraindicated. Individuals with serious liver diseases, thyroid dysfunction, or adrenal insufficiency or who are already taking antidepressants may not be suitable candidates.

Advantages

- There is rapid onset of action.
- Titration is possible.
- The patient is able to tolerate the dental procedure.

Disadvantages

- The needle stick may be very uncomfortable and scary for fearful patients.
- It is difficult to maintain the needle in place during the entire dental procedure.
- Continuous patient monitoring by the dentist and/or the dental assistant is required.
- A responsible adult needs to be present to transport the patient when the procedure is completed.

Inhalation Sedation: Nitrous Oxide–Oxygen

Joseph Priestley discovered nitrous oxide in 1772. However, at that time it was viewed as an entertainment tool known as "laughing gas" and not regarded as an anesthetic agent until experimentation with it in 1844 effectively reduced pain during extraction of teeth. Horace Wells, a young dentist, is credited for discovering and successfully applying the uses of vapors or gases whereby operations could be performed without pain. There were others who used it during surgical procedures. However, deaths were also attributed to its use and its popularity diminished.

The use of nitrous oxide–oxygen (N_2O–O_2) returned in 1938 after a long period of time of wavering due to unreliable equipment, failure to produce satisfactory results, and lack of knowledge of the technique. Today it is used simultaneously with general anesthesia, predominantly in oral and maxillofacial surgery offices. It is also used as conscious sedation in general practice, periodontal, pediatric, prosthodontic, and endodontic dental offices.

Nitrous oxide–oxygen is used for various reasons: It is considered to be nearly the most ideal sedative available due to its safe reputation with very few side effects.

Advantages

- More rapid onset than oral and IM; similar to IV
- Easier to control the level of sedation
- Variable duration of action depending on length of time administered
- Rapid recovery time
- Ability to titrate using small increments until desired sedation is achieved

- Rapid complete recovery whereby the patient is usually discharged unescorted
- Needles are not required
- Few side effects with no adverse effects on liver, kidneys, brain, cardiovascular, and respiratory systems
- May not need local anesthesia based on analgesia level experienced by patient and type of procedure performed

Disadvantages

- The equipment is costly, hard to store, and the gases are expensive.
- The desired effect is not always attained for certain patients.
- Chronic exposure to trace amounts of N_2O-O_2 may possibly be harmful to office personnel. Maximum amount permissible in the air is 50 ppm (parts per million). The equipment must have a scavenging system that transports the gases to the outside of the building.
- Training of all staff members is recommended by the American Dental Association (ADA), American Dental Society of Anesthesiology (ADSA), and American Association of Dental Schools (AADS).

Potential Contraindications. When N_2O-O_2 is administered in the intended manner, there is no absolute contraindication. However, there is increased potential for adverse reactions to develop in certain patients:

- Compulsive personality type patients will fight the effects of the drug.
- Claustrophobic patients who cannot tolerate the mask will be uncomfortable.
- Uncooperative children or adults who are crying or screaming will breathe through their mouths, negating the effects of the drug.
- Patients with severe personality disorders who are under psychiatric care should be carefully evaluated to include medical consultation prior to sedative use.
- It is contraindicated in patients who have an upper respiratory tract infection, a contagious disease that may contaminate the equipment, or a respiratory tract obstruction such as emphysema or chronic bronchitis, known as *chronic obstructive pulmonary disease (COPD)*.
- Patients who strongly object to the use of sedation.
- Patients who are in the first trimester of pregnancy, a slight possibility exists that they could abort spontaneously. If they are in their last trimester of pregnancy, there may be a slight possibility of going into labor.

- Patients who are unable to communicate due to a language barrier or mental imbalance.

Physical and Chemical Properties of Nitrous Oxide. Nitrous oxide is colorless, sweet smelling, and nonirritating. It is an inorganic gas that has the capability of depressing the CNS. It is heavier than room air, nonflammable but supports combustion, and relatively insoluble in blood. It is stored in compressed blue gas cylinders. It is an oxidizing gas; therefore substances such as lubricants, grease, or oil should not be used on any nitrous oxide valves. This may cause an increase in temperature to a level that will ignite and cause a chemical reaction resulting in fire or explosion.

Mode of Action. The action of nitrous oxide–oxygen on the body systems, when administered in proper doses and concentration, is usually quite **innocuous** (harmless or benign) to the body since it is excreted almost entirely through the lungs. Some areas of concern include the following:

- High concentration of nitrous oxide for a prolonged period of time has been alleged to cause poor absorption of vitamin B_{12}, which interferes with erythrocyte production.
- Loss of hearing has been observed due to increased pressure causing complications in the middle ear. Patients who have middle ear disturbances or recent infections should avoid using nitrous oxide.
- Caution must be used with patients experiencing altered mental states caused by alcohol intoxication or drugs.
- No allergies have been reported except for latex sensitivity to the nasal hood by patients who experienced contact dermatitis. However, nonlatex nasal hoods are available.
- It is contraindicated during pregnancy, especially during the first and last trimesters. Nitrous oxide crosses the placental barrier; therefore medical consultation is recommended.
- It causes mild depression of the CNS.
- It causes a slight depression of the myocardial contraction.
- It is nonirritating to the respiratory system.
- No significant effect has been noted on the gastrointestinal tract.
- There is no significant effect on the kidneys.

Equipment. Nitrous oxide–oxygen may be delivered using two types of equipment systems: central supply and portable units. Each has its own armamentaria, but they are similar in other respects. The units are either continuous flow or demand flow in how they deliver

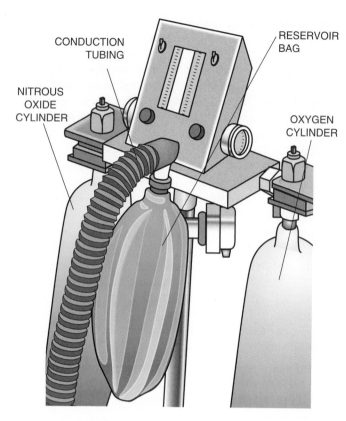

Figure 50-1 Nitrous oxide–oxygen portable equipment.

gases. The armamentaria for a portable unit consists of nitrous oxide and oxygen cylinders, yoke, pin index safety system, regulators, pressure gauges, flowmeters, reservoir bag, conduction tubing, and nasal hood. A face mask or a nasal cannula is also available but is not used in dentistry.

- The nitrous oxide cylinder contains N_2O in liquid form, except for 5% in gaseous form. It vaporizes into gas as it is used. The pressure reading is usually 750 psi (pounds per square inch) at 70°F (25°C). This reading does not change until the tank is fairly empty. The color of the tank in the United States is blue (Figure 50-1).

- The oxygen cylinder contains pure compressed oxygen. It is in the form of gas, with the pressure reading approximately 2000 psi in all cylinder sizes when full. [*Note:* Cylinder sizes vary from Size A (smallest) to HH (largest)]. As the oxygen is used, the pressure gauge indicates the amount of gas remaining. The color of the tank in the United States is green.

- The yoke is the portable stand or framework mounted on wheels that holds the cylinders and equipment in position (Figure 50-2).

- The pin index safety system allows the correct cylinder to be connected to the correct tubing and prevent improper gas flow to the machine (Figure 50-3).

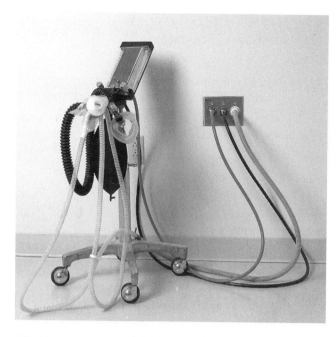

Figure 50-2 Portable stand or yoke (framework) to hold cylinders and equipment.

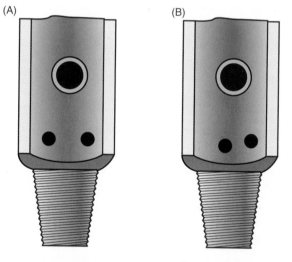

(A)

CGA CONNECTION NO. 870
VALVE YOKE
CONNECTION OXYGEN

(B)

CGA CONNECTION NO. 910
MEDICAL CYLINDER
VALVE CONNECTION
NITROUS OXIDE

Figure 50-3 Close-up of pin index safety system: (A) oxygen on left; (B) nitrous oxide on right.

- The regulators reduce the pressure of gases delivered from the cylinders to the flowmeter.

- Pressure gauges indicate the amount of gas pressure within the cylinders.

- Flowmeters regulate the amount of each gas that passes or flows through the meter to the patient.

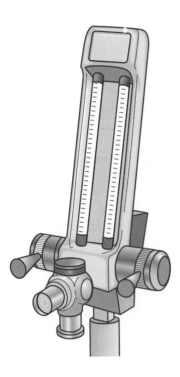

Figure 50-4 Close-up of flowmeters.

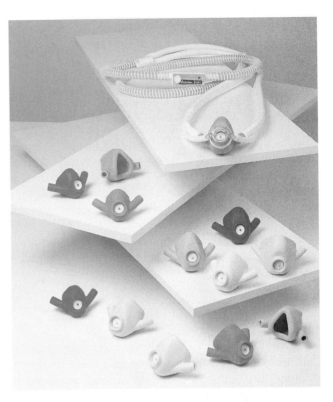

Figure 50-5 Nasal hood assortment and scavenging nasal hood with conduction tubing. (Courtesy of Accutron, Phoenix, AZ.)

Either a rotameter or small balls (floats) located in the flowmeter are used to give a reading for each gas. The gases mix, move into the reservoir bag, and are delivered to the patient in adequate quantities (Figure 50-4).

- The reservoir bag may be used in various ways: as a safety feature that could provide positive-pressure oxygen in an emergency, to monitor the patient's breathing, and to serve as a reservoir for additional gas should the need arise or where the condition of the patient demands its use (Figure 50-1).

- Conduction tubing connects from the unit to the breathing apparatus (nasal hood) (Figure 50-1).

- The nasal hood fits over the patient's nose (Figure 50-5) and allows access to the mouth. The nasal hood should be equipped with a scavenging device (Figure 50-6) that prevents escape of gases into the air. This system uses a second hood or nose piece, placed over the first one, that connects to the vacuum suction whereby exhaled air goes through an outlet and is evacuated into the vacuum system and directed to the outside of the building. The nasal (face) mask fits over the nose and mouth and is not used in dentistry. Likewise, the nasal cannula, due to its inability to seal the nose permitting escape of gases into the environment, is not used in dentistry for nitrous oxide–oxygen delivery.

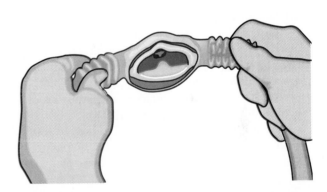

Figure 50-6 Scavenging nasal hood with conduction tubing.

Delivery Technique. There are a number of responsibilities that the dental assistant may assume: preparing the equipment, preparing the patient, assisting in the administration of N_2O–O_2, and cleaning the equipment.

Preparing the Equipment. The dental assistant should prepare the equipment by following a specified routine; this would include checking for:

- Adequate supply of gases in tanks
- Full tank back-ups
- Kinks or leaks in the conduction tubing

- Leaks in the reservoir bag
- Adequate scavenging system
- Correct size of nasal hood

Preparing the Patient. The dental assistant should prepare the patient in the following manner:

- Record the medical history and vital signs.
- Have the patient visit the restroom to avoid interruption and promote comfort.
- Explain the procedure and what may be experienced.
- Explain the importance of breathing through the nose and to not exhale through the mouth.
- Explain that the doctor will maintain communication throughout the procedure.

Assisting with the Procedure. The dental assistant assists the dentist as follows:

- Reclines the patient in a supine position.
- Checks the nasal hood for size and leaks. To fit the hood for comfort, a gauze square may be placed to prevent impingement or to seal the edge of the hood.
- Checks flowmeters and level of oxygen (nitrous oxide tank will always read full).
- Follows the dentist's direction to start the flow of 100% oxygen. The volume of air inhaled and exhaled while the patient is at rest will determine the number of liters administered; this is known as **tidal volume**. Nitrous oxide is then introduced by slowly titrating it according to the patient's response. For each liter of nitrous oxide given, a liter of oxygen is diminished until the desired concentration of nitrous oxide is achieved and the patient's **baseline** (ratio of nitrous oxygen to oxygen that produces the desired level of sedation) is achieved and the patient is comfortably sedated. The dental assistant may leave it at this level until further instruction from the dentist or when the dental procedure is terminated. At no time is the patient left unattended.
- Follows the dentist's direction to shut down nitrous oxide gas administration upon completion of the dental procedure but continues with 100% oxygen flow for a few minutes more in accordance with the length of time the patient was sedated. The more time the patient is sedated, the more oxygen is needed to flush his system. A good rule of thumb to follow is for every 15 minutes of sedation, 5 minutes of oxygen is given. This is to ensure that **diffusion hypoxia** (lack of adequate amount of breathed oxygen causing a person to develop a headache, nausea, and lethargy) is prevented.
- Documents patient's baseline, including the amount of gases used and duration of administration.

- Discharges the patient upon the dentist's approval if vital signs are normal, the patient can respond adequately to questions, and motor coordination is acceptable.

Clean-Up. Equipment requiring clean-up are the nasal hood if it is not disposable, conduction tubing, and reservoir bag. Washing the nasal hood in soap and water only decreases the number of microbes; thus, along with the tubing and reservoir bag, it will need to be steam autoclaved or immersed in glutaraldehyde solution for 10 hours for sterilization to take place. Rinsing in warm tap water for 1 hour should remove the disinfectant solution.

Safety Measures for Equipment

- Oil, hand cream, or other combustible substances should not come in contact with cylinders, regulators, gauges or fittings. Oily materials may act as explosives.
- Flame or sparks should not be in close proximity to cylinders, as the gases will support combustion.
- Regulators specified for nitrous oxide or oxygen should not be used with other gases.
- The gas content should be identified by the label on the cylinder before using.
- Markings on cylinders should not be removed since they are used for identification purposes.
- Cylinders should not be dropped or allowed to strike each other violently.
- Nitrous oxide–oxygen armamentaria should be secured with a lock and not available to unauthorized persons.
- Valves should be opened counterclockwise slowly, never suddenly, and clockwise to close them.
- It is important to remember the color codes for nitrous oxide and oxygen in the United States: blue for nitrous oxide and green for oxygen.

SUGGESTED ACTIVITIES

- Prepare to replace gas cylinders on a portable unit. This procedure may involve two individuals. While one person holds the tank, the other person may place it into the appropriate pin and index guide.
- Check the breathing apparatus for kinks on the conduction tubing and for leaks in the reservoir bag and nasal hood.
- Using the stated procedure, clean and sterilize the breathing apparatus.
- Under a dentist's supervision, establish patient's flow rate for oxygen while observing reservoir bag, indicating patient's tidal volume.

REVIEW

1. Match the terms with their definitions.

___ a. Anesthesia
___ b. Pain perception
___ c. Pain reaction
___ d. Hyperreactive
___ e. Hyporeactive
___ f. Afferent nerves
___ g. Efferent nerves

1. Response from a person who has a high pain tolerance
2. Carry impulses from one part of the body to the brain
3. Temporary loss of feeling or sensation
4. Conscious mental interpretation of an unpleasant experience
5. Carry impulses from the brain to muscles in response to pain
6. Response from a person who has a low pain tolerance
7. Response of what a person will do about unpleasant experience

2. At which stage of general anesthesia does the stage of excitement and delirium occur?
   a. Stage I
   b. Stage II
   c. Stage III
   d. Stage IV

3. Protective reflexes include the ability to (1) cough, (2) swallow, (3) open eyes, and/or (4) breathe.
   a. 1, 2, 3
   b. 2, 3, 4
   c. 1, 2, 4
   d. 1, 3, 4

4. Conscious sedation includes (1) general anesthesia, (2) intramuscular sedation, (3) oral sedation, and/or (4) inhalation sedation.
   a. 1, 2, 3
   b. 2, 3, 4
   c. 1, 2, 4
   d. 1, 3, 4

5. Nitrous oxide–oxygen is used as (1) a general anesthetic, (2) a local anesthetic, (3) a conscious sedative, and/or (4) an inhalant.
   a. 1, 3
   b. 2, 3
   c. 1, 3, 4
   d. 3, 4

6. Match the component parts of the nitrous oxide unit with their respective functions.

___ a. Flowmeters
___ b. Yoke
___ c. Regulators
___ d. Conduction tubing
___ e. Reservoir bag
___ f. Pressure gauges
___ g. Nasal hood
___ h. Nitrous oxide cylinder
___ i. Oxygen cylinder

1. Connects from the unit to the breathing apparatus
2. Indicates the amount of gas pressure within the cylinders
3. Regulates the amount of each gas that flows into patient
4. Green container that contains pure compressed gas
5. Adjusts the amount of gas from cylinders to flowmeter
6. The portable stand that holds cylinders and equipment
7. Blue container that contains liquid form of gas
8. Portion that fits over patient's nose
9. Portion that monitors patient's breathing

7. Symptoms of diffusion hypoxia include:
   a. Headache
   b. Nausea
   c. Abdominal pain
   d. Both a and b

8. The purpose for scavenging nitrous oxide is to:
   a. Prevent escape of gasses into the air
   b. Prevent excessive delivery of gasses
   c. Prevent operator from breathing gasses
   d. Both a and c

Topical and Local Anesthesia

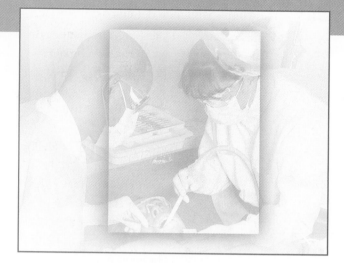

OBJECTIVES

After studying this chapter, the student will be able to:

- Describe the purpose for using topical anesthesia.
- Indicate the types of topical anesthesia used.
- List the ideal local anesthetic properties.
- Describe the purpose for adding vasoconstrictors to local anesthetics.
- List local anesthesia complications.
- Identify parts of the local anesthetic syringe.
- Indicate the importance of using an aspirating syringe.
- Identify parts of the dental needle.
- Describe the procedure for recapping the needle.
- Identify parts of the dental cartridge.
- Recognize a damaged anesthetic cartridge and give the probable cause.
- Explain how to assemble and disassemble an aspirating syringe.

Introduction

In dentistry local anesthesia is the direct application of an anesthetic to oral tissues. It may be applied to the surface of the mucosal tissues to provide topical anesthesia or injected directly into the tissues to provide local anesthesia.

Topical Anesthesia

Topical anesthetics are the agents commonly used in dental offices to provide surface anesthesia to the mucous membranes within the oral cavity. This is one feature that provides relief to patients who are fearful of the anesthetic needle. The numbing sensation only affects terminal nerve endings on the surface of the oral mucosa. It will not be effective in underlying tissues or on the outside surface of the body on intact skin unless the skin is **abraded** (scraped, scratched, or injured).

Indications for Use

The primary purpose of a topical anesthetic is to minimize the traumatic "needle prick" that most patients fear. Other uses include **desensitization** (making it less sensitive) of the gag reflex for easier impression making and film placement, for suture removal, for removal or replacement of a dressing, and for procedures involving the gingiva such as probing and scaling.

Concentration of Topical Anesthetics

Concentrations of the anesthetic agent in topical anesthetics are usually higher than those of local anesthetics. While topical anesthetics vary in concentration from 5 to 20%, local anesthetics contain 2–4% and consequently have a significant overdose potential when used in large amounts. Topical anesthetics are **vasodilators** (agents that expand blood vessels) and do not contain **vasoconstrictors** (agents that constrict blood vessels). Because they **dilate** (expand) the blood vessels, these anesthetics are quickly absorbed into the bloodstream and are capable of reaching toxic levels.

Topical anesthetics are supplied as a liquid, gel, ointment, or spray (Figure 51-1). Some are **insoluble** (incapable of dissolving) in water but are **soluble** (capable of being dissolved) in alcohol; included are benzocaine, lidocaine base, and chlorobutanol. Others are soluble in water with a great potential for toxicity; included is tetracaine hydrochloride.

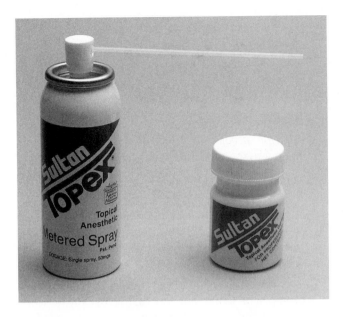

Figure 51-1 Topical anesthetic examples.

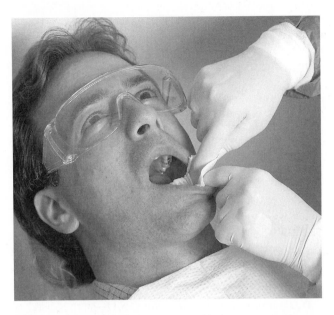

Figure 51-2 Blot drying tissue with gauze square.

Mode of Action

Topical anesthetics that are soluble in water have greater potential of causing overdose reactions because they are quickly absorbed into the cardiovascular system. Whereas those that are insoluble in water are slowly absorbed into the cardiovascular system and are less likely to produce overdose reactions.

Anesthetics are classified as being ester type or amide type. The **ester**-type (alcohol based) anesthetics have a greater potential for causing allergic and toxic reactions due to the fact that they are more soluble in water. The **amide**-type (ammonia-based) anesthetics are insoluble in water and therefore remain in the area of injection for a longer time. This applies to both topical and local anesthetics.

Application of Topical Anesthestics

In some states dental assistants are delegated to perform this procedure. The dental assistant needs to be knowledgeable in the anatomy and nervous system of the oral cavity and to recognize their injection sites:

1. The patient's medical history should be evaluated for overall health status and for any allergies or previous unfavorable experiences with local anesthesia.

2. The procedure should be explained to the patient regarding its anticipated effect and words to avoid using should be "injection," "shot," "hurt," or "pain," but instead, words such as "for your comfort" or "to make you more comfortable" should be used.

3. Using infection control techniques in placing a topical anesthetic, the area should be blot-dried with a 2 x 2 gauze square to ensure full anesthetic strength

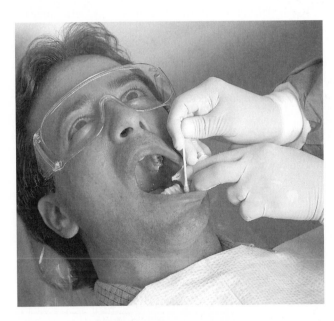

Figure 51-3 Application of topical anesthetic over dry tissue.

without dilution (Figure 51-2). The area should never be rubbed, as this action will bring blood to the surface of the mucosa, promoting rapid absorption of the anesthetic into the bloodstream.

4. Cotton-tipped applicators are used to apply topical antiseptics and topical anesthetics at the injection site. The antiseptic is used to reduce the risk of introducing microorganisms into the tissue.

5. A small amount of the topical anesthetic should be applied (not rubbed) over the dry tissue of a small area (Figure 51-3).

6. The topical anesthetic should be left on for 1–2 minutes, then immediately followed with the local anesthetic.

Placing Topical Anesthetics

Maxillary Arch. Topical anesthetic is placed as follows (see Figure 51-4):

A. *Infiltration (or field block)*—at the apex of any maxillary tooth in the mucobuccal fold

B. *Anterior superior alveolar (ASA)*—at the mesial of the apex of the maxillary cuspid (canine) in the mucobuccal fold

C. *Middle superior alveolar (MSA) and Infraorbital*—at the apex of the second premolar in the mucobuccal fold

D. *Posterior superior alveolar (PSA)*—at the distal of the apex of the maxillary second molar in the mucobuccal fold

E. *Nasopalatine*—at the lateral side of the incisive papilla

F. *Greater/anterior palatine*—above the distal of the second molar at the halfway point from the midline of the palate to the gingival margin using a cotton-tipped applicator to find a natural depression

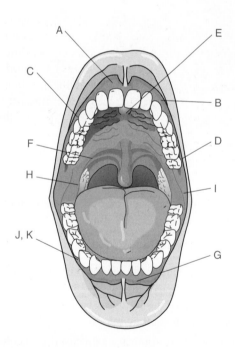

Figure 51-4 Application of topical anesthetic: (A) infiltration, (B) anterior superior alveolar (ASA), (C) middle superior alveolar (MSA) and infraorbital, (D) posterior superior alveolar (PSA), (E) nasopalatine, (F) greater palatine, (G) infiltration, (H) inferior alveolar, (I) buccal, (J) mental, and (K) incisive

Mandibular Arch

G. *Infiltration (or field block)*—at the apex of each incisor in the mucobuccal fold. *Note:* Posterior teeth are unable to be anesthetized using this method due to the **density** (thickness/bulk) of the mandibular bone in that area.

H. *Inferior alveolar and lingual*—distal, superior and lingual to the mandibular retromolar pad

I. *Buccal*—on the buccal side just distal to the third molar or to the most distal tooth in the arch

J. *Mental*—foramen located by palpation, then placed usually between the first and second premolars anterior to the mental foramen in the mucobuccal fold

K. *Incisive*—mental foramen located by palpation, then placed in the mucobuccal fold usually between the first and second premolars in close proximity to the mental foramen

Note: Refer to Chapter 19, Table 19-1 for teeth and tissues affected when each of the preceding nerves is anesthetized.

Local Anesthesia

Local anesthesia is described as loss of sensation confined to a localized area or particular place of the body. Sometimes it is referred to as "regional." It blocks the transmission of pain to the brain and is therefore not interpreted by it.

Local anesthesia was derived from cocaine when it was discovered that when injected into the body, it could numb temporarily but could also cause gangrene, addiction, and death. In the early 1900s, it was mixed with epinephrine to slow down its absorption rate in the system. This lessened the hemorrhage and made it possible to use smaller quantities. By 1905, the first local anesthetic, known as "novocaine," was introduced. Later lidocaine and mepivacaine followed and are still used today.

Ideal Properties of Local Anesthetics

Local anesthetics should possess the following properties:

● Have a rapid onset: One should not have to wait too long to start the dental procedure.

● Possess anesthetic qualities: It should anesthetize tissues for a relatively long duration, from 1 to 4 hours.

● Be reversible without irritating nerves and tissues: The tissues and nerves should be returned to a normal state within a short time.

- Have a low degree of systemic toxicity: Using small quantities of the anesthetic should minimize toxicity.
- Be relatively free of causing an allergic reaction: Choosing amide-type anesthetics and using small quantities can decrease an allergy potential.
- Be sterile.
- Be stable under normal conditions: They should be kept away from heat and sunlight to avoid deterioration.
- Have an average shelf life—approximately 18 months. Expiration date should be checked before using it.
- Be painless when administered and during recovery: They should not sting during delivery or produce discomfort.
- Be economical.
- Be compatible with added vasoconstrictors.

Concentration of Local Anesthetics

The main ingredient in a local anesthetic cartridge is the anesthetic agent itself, which is mixed in a solution of distilled water, preservatives, vasoconstrictor, and sodium chloride. The percentage of the anesthetic varies from 2 to 5%. The label on the canister and cartridge provides information such as, "xylocaine/lidocaine hydrochloride injection 2%" (Figure 51-5).

Dosage

Local anesthetics are supplied in ampules and cartridges, also called carpules, of 1.8 ml. The dosage would depend on the following:

- Type of anesthetic used—ester or amide
- Use of a vasoconstrictor
- Area to be injected
- Size and weight of the patient
- Physical status of the patient

Duration of Local Anesthetics

Duration varies considerably between drugs and between different preparations of the same drug. Anesthetics are categorized as short, intermediate, and long duration:

- Short—approximately 10–30 minutes without vasoconstrictor
- Intermediate—approximately 60 minutes with vasoconstrictor

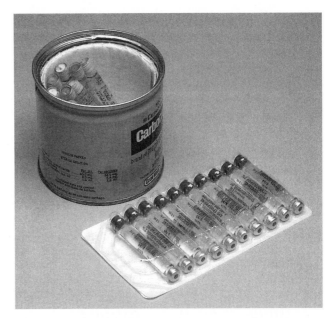

Figure 51-5 Information identified on anesthetic canister and cartridges.

- Long—over 90 minutes for pulpal anesthesia (anesthetizing the tooth) or 60 minutes to 5 hours for soft tissues (anesthetizing the gingiva) with vasoconstrictor.

Vasoconstrictors

All local anesthetics used in dentistry cause vasodilation. As they dilate blood vessels, they cause more blood to flow to the injection site, where more bleeding occurs. This, in turn, causes the anesthetic to be absorbed very quickly into the bloodstream, diminishing its effectiveness and leading to an increase of the amount of anesthetic used. When more anesthetic is used, there is a greater risk of an overdose or toxic reaction.

To counteract the problems with vasodilation, vasoconstrictors are added:

- Vasoconstrictors, such as epinephrine, constrict the blood vessels; therefore there is **hemostasis** (less flow of blood to the injection site causing less bleeding).
- The anesthetic is not absorbed so quickly into the bloodstream; it lasts longer and is more effective.
- Less of the anesthetic is used; there is less risk of an overdose or toxicity potential.

Caution for Epinephrine Use. Three types of individuals who may be at risk if epinephrine is used are those with:

- Hypertension
- Severe cardiovascular disease
- Hyperthyroid (Graves) disease

With each of these diseases, epinephrine may aggravate the health status. It may cause an increase in blood pressure, heart rate, cardiac output, and strength of contraction.

Other vasoconstrictors besides epinephrine are used, though these are not as potent: norepinephrine (Levophed) and levonordefrin (Neo-Cobefrin) are examples.

Concentration of Vasoconstrictors.

There are several ratios of concentration for epinephrine in local anesthetics. It is written in terms of 1 part epinephrine to 50,000 parts anesthetic and observed as 1:50,000 on each cartridge. Other ratios include 1:20,000, 1:100,000, and 1:200,000. The higher the "anesthetic" ratio, the lower the epinephrine content.

Methods of Administration

There are two methods of local anesthetic administration depending on the dental procedure. Starting with the smaller minimal nerve endings and progressing to the main nerve trunks:

1. Local infiltration/Field block
   a. *Local infiltration* is used when only small nerve endings need to be anesthetized, as required for scaling or root planing. Sometimes this method is known as field block.
   b. *Field block*, also referred to as infiltration, is used when only one tooth and surrounding tissues need to be anesthetized. The anesthetic is placed above the apex of a maxillary tooth. This type of injection gives pulpal (within the tooth) anesthesia to the affected tooth. Hereafter, infiltration and field block will be used interchangeably.
2. Nerve block is used when two or more teeth and surrounding tissues need to be anesthetized. The anesthetic is placed near the trunk that feeds those teeth; the anterior superior alveolar nerve block and the mandibular nerve block are examples.

Local Anesthesia Complications

Death, serious illness, or minor reactions may be directly related to dental anesthesia. Such complications can frequently be minimized or avoided by proper pretreatment evaluation.

- *Pain.* To avoid it, a slow injection technique is used. A sharp needle must be employed, not one that is dull from multiple injections on the same person.
- *Paresthesia.* Prolonged anesthesia caused by contaminated solutions, trauma to the nerve, or hemorrhage in the area increasing pressure on the nerve.

- *Muscle trismus.* A condition where muscle soreness develops following local anesthesia, thus causing difficulty in opening the mouth.
- *Hematoma.* Caused by the needle puncturing a blood vessel that leaks into the surrounding tissues turning the skin black and blue, similar to a bruise in appearance. Pressure and ice placed over the affected area should help ease the hematoma. To prevent this condition, the operator uses an aspirating syringe to determine if the needle has penetrated a blood vessel; then the operator redirects the needle.
- *Biting cheek and lip.* Frequently caused by children who inadvertently bite their cheek and lip while tissues are still numb. Children and their parents or guardian should be warned to avoid biting or eating while tissues are still anesthetized. A cotton roll or gauze placed between the teeth may help prevent this condition.
- *Toxic reaction.* Usually due to overdose of anesthetic, too rapid injection, and injection of anesthetic directly into the blood stream. Some signs and symptoms to observe are divided into two levels.

First-Level Symptoms

1. Talkativeness, apprehension, and excitability
2. Slurred speech, stuttering, and muscular twitching
3. Elevated blood pressure, heart rate, and respiratory rate
4. A feeling of light-headedness, dizziness, drowsiness, and disorientation
5. Inability to focus the eyes
6. Hearing disturbances

Management steps to control this condition include reassuring the patient, administering oxygen, monitoring vital signs, administering anticonvulsants if necessary, and allowing patient to recover slowly.

Second-Level Symptoms

1. Generalized seizure activity
2. Generalized central nervous system (CNS) depression
3. Depressed blood pressure, heart rate, and respiratory rate

Management steps to control this more progressive condition include reassuring the patient, administering oxygen, monitoring vital signs, administering anticonvulsants, calling for medical assistance, having a medical doctor evaluate patient, and having someone escort the patient home.

Dental Anesthetic Syringes

Dental syringes used for intraoral injections (local anesthesia) are available in metal and plastic.

Two basic types of metal syringes are the conventional, or *nonaspirating*, syringe and the *aspirating* syringe. The aspirating syringe is the one recommended for use in dentistry as part of the standard of care guidelines.

Luer-Lok Type and Plastic Syringes

Plastic disposable syringes are available in a variety of sizes with assorted needle sizes. The needles that fit are the Luer-Lok screw-on type. These syringes should not be used unless the metal aspirating syringe is unavailable. A cartridge is not used in these syringes; however, the needle is inserted into a vial and the anesthetic is removed by aspiration (Figure 51-6).

A plastic autoclavable aspirating syringe is available and is made like the metal syringe. There is a single-use disposable-reusable syringe. The ring mechanism is reusable, but the rest of the syringe is disposable.

Aspirating Syringe

The aspirating syringe is designed to allow the operator to check the placement of the needle and determine whether or not the needle has entered or penetrated a blood vessel. If the needle has penetrated a blood vessel, a slight amount of blood may appear in the cartridge solution. Should this occur, the needle is withdrawn, redirected, and tested again until there is evidence that the needle is no longer in the blood vessel. The injection is then completed. An aspirating syringe is used for the safety and comfort of the patient.

Parts of the Aspirating Syringe. The parts of an aspirating syringe include the following (Figure 51-7):

- *Thumb ring*—for placement of thumb.
- *Finger grip/bar*—supports the index and middle fingers as the anesthetic solution is introduced into the oral tissues.
- *Syringe barrel*—holds the anesthetic cartridge.
- *Piston rod*—used to push down the silicone rubber plunger of the anesthetic cartridge.
- *Harpoon*—the barbed tip, positioned at the end of the piston rod, engages the silicone rubber plunger in the cartridge. The piston rod and harpoon allow for aspiration to take place during anesthetic delivery.
- *Needle adaptor*—where the needle is attached to the syringe.

The Needle

The needle is used to direct the local anesthetic solution from the anesthetic cartridge into the tissues surrounding the needle tip. Most dental needles used today are made of stainless steel, are presterilized, and disposable.

The selection of a needle for use is based on the type of injection to be given. Two factors that must be considered are the diameter, or gauge, and the length of the needle. The internal opening of the needle, through which the anesthetic solution flows, is called the **lumen**.

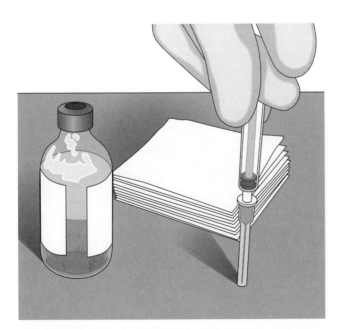

Figure 51-6 Luer-Lok syringe and needle.

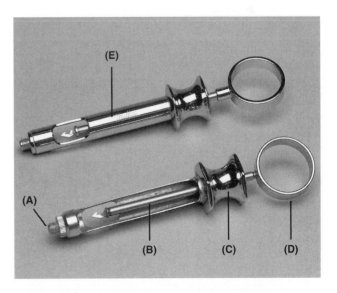

Figure 51-7 Parts of the aspirating syringe: (A) needle adaptor, (B) piston rod, (C) finger grip, (D) thumb ring, and (E) barrel of syringe.

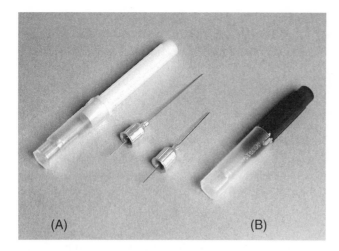

Figure 51-8 Length of dental needles: (A) long, 1 5/8 in.; (B) short, 1 in.

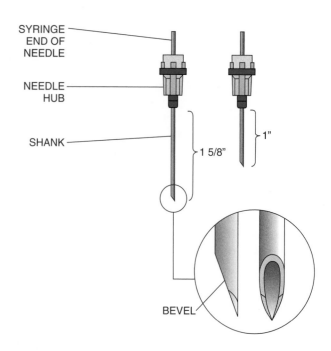

Figure 51-9 Parts of a dental needle.

The needles used in dentistry range from 25 gauge to 30 gauge. The smaller the gauge number, the larger the lumen of the needle; the larger the gauge number, the smaller the lumen. The 25- and 27-gauge needles are recommended for intraoral use.

Dental needles are available in two lengths; long (1 5/8 in.) and short (1 in.) (Figure 51-8). The long needle is indicated when the injection requires the penetration of several thicknesses of soft tissue, such as with a nerve block. Short needles are used for injections that require the penetration of only the surface soft tissue (infiltration).

Parts of a Needle

- *Bevel*—the slanted tip of the needle that will penetrate the soft tissues (Figure 51-9)
- *Shank*—the length of the needle from the hub to the tip of the bevel
- *Syringe adaptor*—the part of the needle that screws onto the syringe and is either metal or plastic
- *Hub*—the part of the needle that attaches to the syringe adaptor
- *Syringe end of the needle*—the end of the needle that punctures the rubber diaphragm of the cartridge

Care of the Dental Needle

1. A needle should never be used for more than one patient.
2. The needle should be changed after three injections for the same patient. Each time the needle penetrates the soft tissue, it becomes a little duller. Failure to change the needle after the third insertion may

result in injury to the patient's tissues and cause postoperative pain.

3. A needle must be covered with its protective cap whenever it is not in use.

Anesthetic Cartridge

The anesthetic cartridge (carpule) is a glass cylinder that contains the anesthetic solution.

Parts of an Anesthetic Cartridge

- *Glass cartridge*—contains the anesthetic solution (Figure 51-10).

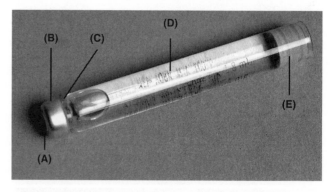

Figure 51-10 Parts of the anesthetic cartridge: (A) rubber diaphragm, (B) aluminum cap, (C) local anesthetic solution, (D) glass cartridge, and (E) silicone rubber plunger.

- *Silicone rubber plunger*—located at the harpoon end of the cartridge. An acceptable silicone rubber plunger in the cartridge is slightly indented.
- *Aluminum cap*—located on the opposite end of the cartridge from the silicone plunger. It fits tightly around the neck of the glass cartridge and holds the thin rubber diaphragm in position.
- *Rubber diaphragm*—located under the aluminum cap at the end of the cartridge where the syringe end of the needle is penetrated.

Color coding of the cartridge plunger is no longer used to identify the drug content of the cartridge. The selection of a cartridge should be based on the information printed on the side of each cartridge.

Recognizing a Damaged Anesthetic Cartridge

Bubbles in the Cartridge. Small bubbles in the solution are bubbles of nitrogen gas and are considered harmless to the patient. A large bubble present may cause the plunger to extend beyond the end of the cartridge. Such cartridges should be discarded.

Extruded Plunger. An *extruded plunger* means that something has happened to the cartridge. The cartridge may have been frozen, causing the solution inside to expand and forcing the plunger past its normal position.

Also, a cartridge with an extruded plunger and with no bubble(s) indicates the cartridge has been stored too long in a chemical disinfectant and that some of the solution has entered the cartridge. Such cartridges should be discarded.

Burning Sensation upon Injection. A burning sensation during the injection may be the result of the cartridge becoming contaminated with disinfecting solution.

Corroded Aluminum Cap. A corroded aluminum cap indicates that the anesthetic cartridge has been immersed too long in a disinfecting solution. Wiping with either 91% isopropyl alcohol or 70% ethyl alcohol should disinfect aluminum-sealed cartridges. A corroded aluminum cap will leave a white deposit on the aluminum cap. Such cartridges must be discarded.

Rust on Aluminum Cap. Rust on the aluminum cap indicates that at least one cartridge has broken in the tin container. This will cause the tin in the container to rust, leaving a red deposit on the cartridge. These cartridges must be discarded.

Common Problems Related to Handling Syringes

Leakage of Anesthetic Solution. Leakage of the solution during injection indicates that the needle did not penetrate the center of the rubber diaphragm. An off-centered needle will prevent the diaphragm from sealing itself around the needle. Therefore, some solution may leak from the cartridge between the needle and diaphragm into the patient's mouth (Figure 51-11).

Broken Cartridges. A cartridge that is cracked, chipped, or damaged in any way should not be used. The pressure exerted on the cartridge during the injection may cause the cartridge to shatter inside the patient's mouth (Figure 51-12).

Bent Harpoon. The harpoon should be sharp and straight. A bent harpoon will puncture the rubber plunger off center, causing it to rotate as it travels down the cartridge. This could cause the cartridge to break (Figure 51-13).

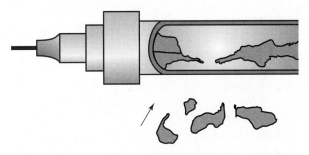

Figure 51-12 Broken cartridge (Courtesy of Astra Pharmaceutical Products, Westborough MA.)

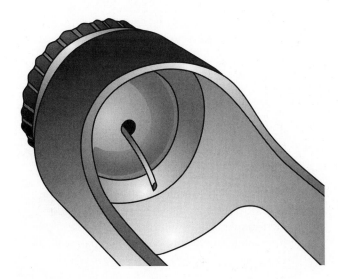

Figure 51-11 Off-centered needle.

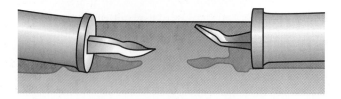

Figure 51-13 Bent harpoon.

Disengagement of Harpoon from Plunger during Aspiration. Aspiration should be completed by gently pulling the plunger in a backward motion. A forceful action is not necessary and may cause the harpoon to become disengaged from the plunger (Figure 51-14).

Taking Care of the Anesthetic Cartridge

1. The anesthetic cartridge must NEVER be used on more than one patient.

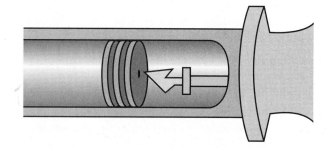

Figure 51-14 Disengagement of harpoon from plunger during aspiration. (Courtesy of Astra Pharmaceutical Products, Westborough MA.)

2. Cartridges should not be used beyond the expiration date indicated by the manufacturer.

3. Cartridges should be stored at room temperature.

4. Cartridges should not be warmed before use.

Procedure 58 Preparing the Aspirating Syringe

Disinfecting the Anesthetic Cartridge

Materials Needed

PPE (personal protective equipment)
Anesthetic cartridges
Aspirating syringe
Disposable needle
Air/water syringe
HVE (high-volume evacuator)
Disinfectant solution (91% isopropyl or 70% ethyl alcohol)
Gauze square, 2 X 2 in.

Introduction

Anesthetic cartridges can be stored in their original containers. When removing the cartridge for use, wipe the rubber diaphragm with a 2 X 2-in. gauze square moistened with 91% isopropyl alcohol or 70% ethyl alcohol.

Prior to loading the syringe, wipe the cap end of the cartridge with alcohol-moistened gauze square.

Loading the Aspirating Syringe

The procedure is for a right-handed individual. (Use opposite hand if left handed.)

1 With washed and gloved hands, select the appropriate needle for the type of injection to be administered.

2 Select correct disinfected anesthetic cartridge to be used for the given dental procedure.

3 Remove the sterile syringe from the autoclave pouch/bag.

4 Hold syringe with left hand, and use the thumb ring to retract the piston rod to its fullest position. Then using the right hand, place the cartridge into the barrel of the syringe, plunger end first (Figure 51-15A).

5 With moderate pressure, gently push the piston rod forward until the harpoon is firmly engaged in the plunger (Figure 51-15B). *Do not* hit the piston rod in an effort to engage the harpoon, as this may cause the glass cartridge to crack or shatter.

continued

continued from previous page
Procedure 58 Preparing the Aspirating Syringe

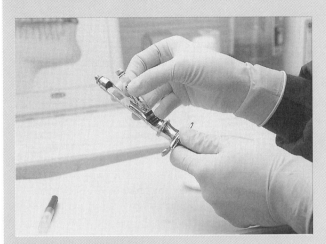

Figure 51-15A Left-handed retraction of piston rod and placement of cartridge.

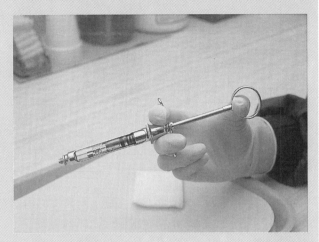

Figure 51-15B Engaging the harpoon prior to needle placement.

6 Place needle on the syringe. Screw the needle onto the syringe (Figure 51-15C). *Note:* A metal-hubbed needle has a threaded hub and can be screwed onto the end of the syringe. If a plastic-hubbed needle is used, the needle is pushed onto the threaded tip of the syringe while constantly turning the needle. Do not screw the needle tightly against the end of the syringe. Leave at least the thickness of a finger-nail between the two. This allows for needle adjustment in positioning the bevel of the needle as needed.

7 Carefully remove the protection cap from the needle and adjust the bevel of the needle for the appropriate procedure. Next, test the syringe by expelling a few drops of solution to test for proper flow of solution (Figure 51-15D). Replace the cap loosely for easy removal.

8 If a second cartridge is required for the dental procedure on the same patient, the first cartridge is removed. See Unloading the Aspirating Syringe, steps 1–3. The capped needle is also removed and a second disinfected cartridge is placed in the barrel. The harpoon is engaged gently and the needle is attached.

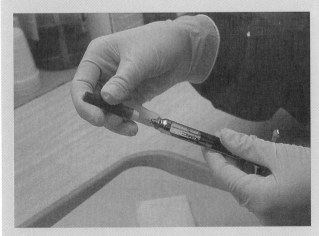

Figure 51-15C Placing the needle on the aspirating syringe.

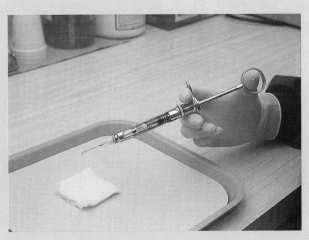

Figure 51-15D Testing the syringe.

continued

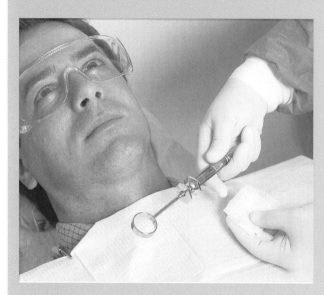

Figure 51-16 Passing to operator below patient's chin.

Passing the Syringe to the Operator

1 Once the topical anesthetic has taken effect, the cotton-tipped applicator is retrieved and the anesthetic syringe is passed to the operator below the patient's chin (Figure 51-16) or behind his head (out of the patient's view).

2 The thumb ring is positioned on the operator's thumb and the finger rest between the index and middle fingers.

3 The needle cap is removed as the operator pulls the syringe away.

4 The operator administers local anesthesia while the dental assistant observes the patient for possible complications.

Recapping the Needle

After the injection, the syringe is removed from the patient's mouth. The needle should be capped immediately. The recapping procedures recommended by most state safety and health agencies are known as the *scoop* technique (Figure 51-17A), or the use of a mechanical recapping device for holding the protective cap.

To prevent a needle stick, the operator (dentist) should not hold the protective cap while recapping the needle. The cap or mechanical recapping device should be placed on a table or counter.

1 Immediately after removal of syringe from the patient's mouth, the operator replaces the protective cap on the needle.

2 Using the scoop technique, the uncapped needle slides into the needle cap that has been placed on the table/counter (Figure 51-17A).

3 The needle must be safely placed within the cap before picking up the capped needle (Figure 51-17B).

4 An uncapped needle should never be placed on a table or countertop. An uncapped needle must never be allowed to touch *anything* before or after the injection.

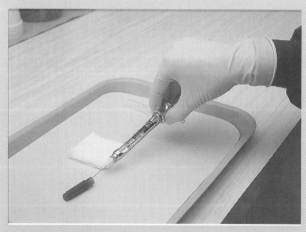

Figure 51-17A Scoop technique for recapping needle after injection.

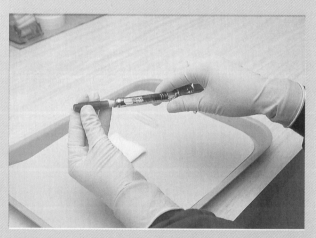

Figure 51-17B Adjusting the needle cap.

continued

continued from previous page
Procedure 58 *Preparing the Aspirating Syringe*

Unloading the Aspirating Syringe

1 Pull the cartridge away from the needle with the thumb and forefinger as the piston is retracted. This will disengage the harpoon from the plunger.

2 Invert syringe, and allow the cartridge to fall freely from the barrel. Discard cartridge in the appropriate container.

3 Carefully remove the capped needle. Should a syringe have its own needle adaptor, care must be taken not to remove the adaptor with the needle.

4 After removing the capped needle from the syringe, the needle and cartridge are placed in a Sharps biohazard container for proper disposal (Figure 51-18).

Taking Care of the Aspirating Syringe

1 After each use, the syringe must be thoroughly washed, rinsed, and dried. The syringe must be free of any anesthetic solution, saliva, or other foreign matter.

2 To help keep the harpoon sharp, prior to autoclaving, a cotton roll can be placed in the cartridge space. The clean syringe should be placed in a labeled autoclavable pouch or bag. The syringe is now ready to be autoclaved. *Note:* It is recommended that after a syringe has been

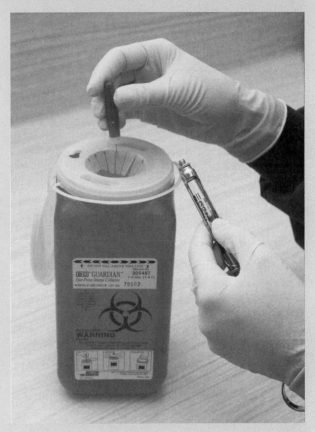

Figure 51-18 Disposal of needle and cartridge in a Sharps biohazard container.

used and autoclaved five times, it should be disassembled and all threaded parts lightly lubricated. Reassemble the syringe, place in a labeled pouch, and autoclave for future use.

Additional Local Anesthesia Techniques

Periodontal Ligament Injection (PDL)

This is an **intraligamentary** (within the periodontal ligament) injection used primarily on the mandibular jaw in place of the inferior alveolar nerve block (injection which anesthetizes half of the mandibular teeth and tissues). When the periodontal ligament injection technique is employed, only one tooth is selected to receive the anesthetic. The anesthetic is deposited through the sulcus and into the periodontal ligament using a pressure syringe better known as the Ligmaject that uses an intraligamentary injection technique. The intraligamentary injection is not generally used on the maxillary arch due to the fact that the alveolar bone is less dense and it is possible to use infiltration in that area. It is employed in anesthetizing one tooth at a time in the mandibular arch where the mandibular bone is very dense, usually the molar area. It provides both pulpal and soft tissue anesthesia in a very localized area such as one tooth (Figure 51-19).

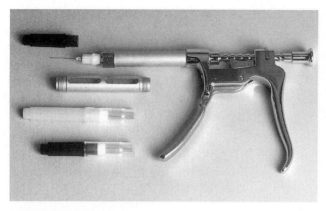

Figure 51-19 Periodontal ligament injection syringe.

Electronic Controlled Local Anesthesia

This method of anesthetic delivery utilizes a microprocessor to automatically pump the anesthetic using constant pressure and volume as it is injected into tissues. A standard anesthetic cartridge is placed in the cartridge holder which is connected to a small microtubing that feeds directly to the handpiece. As it delivers the anesthetic, it compensates for different tissue densities allowing optimal flow of anesthetic solution. The operator uses a foot pedal to control solution delivery. It is named "The Wand" in that it does not employ a syringe but rather a small needle attached to a disposable handpiece (Figure 51-20). The types of injections that can be administered are infiltration, block, periodontal ligament, palatal, and new innovative palatal injections that also affect the maxillary anterior middle superior alveolar (AMSA) block and another one that affects the palatal anterior superior alveolar block (P-ASA). In both cases, the injection is introduced through the palate and affects the two main branches of the maxillary arch.

SUGGESTED ACTIVITIES

● Using cotton-tip applicators, practice finding locations for topical anesthetic placement for all needle insertions.

● Practice loading the aspirating syringe following the step-by-step procedure.

● Practice passing it to another student acting as the operator. Retrieve the syringe and have operator recap the needle using the scoop technique.

● Practice unloading the anesthetic syringe following the step-by-step procedure.

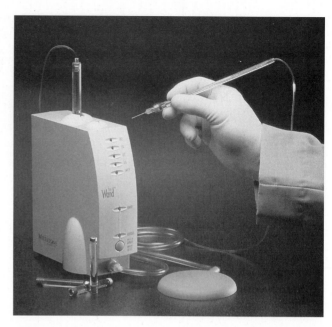

Figure 51-20 Electronic controlled local anesthesia—"The Wand." (Courtesy of Milestone Scientific.)

● Practice disassembling a syringe, lubricate all threaded parts, and reassemble it.

REVIEW

1. The primary purpose for using topical anesthetics in dentistry is to:
   a. Place it on the skin prior to an injection
   b. Minimize the traumatic needle prick on the oral mucosa
   c. Desensitize the apex of the tooth to achieve pulpal anesthesia
   d. Both b and c

2. Name the two factors that should be considered when selecting a needle: (1) the hub, (2) the length, (3) the lumen, and/or (4) the tip.
   a. 1, 2
   b. 2, 3
   c. 3, 4
   d. 1, 4

3. What is the purpose for the operator to use an aspirating syringe?
   a. To prevent injecting directly into a blood vessel
   b. To avoid penetrating a nerve fiber
   c. To provide more comfort to the patient
   d. To prevent penetrating too deeply into the tissues

4. Indicate the sequence for the proper procedure of assembling an aspirating syringe: (1) engage the harpoon into the plunger of the cartridge, (2) remove protective cap from the needle and adjust the bevel of the needle, (3) insert the needle onto the syringe, and/or (4) place the cartridge into the barrel of the syringe.

   a. 1, 3, 2, 4
   b. 3, 2, 4, 1
   c. 3, 4, 2, 1
   d. 4, 1, 3, 2

5. Match the terms on the left with the pertaining complications on the right.

   ___ a. Paresthesia
   ___ b. Hematoma
   ___ c. Toxic reaction
   ___ b. Hematoma
   ___ d. Biting cheek and lip
   ___ e. Muscle trismus

   1. Muscle soreness causing difficulty in opening the mouth
   2. Caused by children who inadvertently injure themselves
   3. Caused by needle puncturing a blood vessel causing leakage
   4. Prolonged anesthesia
   5. Due to anesthetic overdose

Public Health

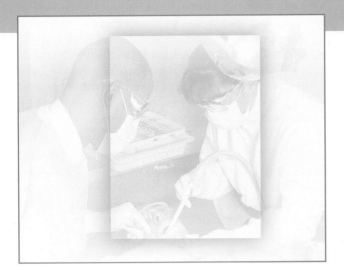

OBJECTIVES

After studying this chapter, the student will be able to:

● Describe the role of dental public health as it relates to the entire practice of dental care.

● Discuss the function of official agencies as a part of local, state, and federal dental health programs.

● Describe the role of voluntary agencies in providing dental health care.

● Discuss the most widely accepted theory of the cause of dental caries.

● Discuss two sets of factors that tend to make an individual susceptible to periodontal disease.

Introduction

Dental public health is involved with the prevention and control of dental diseases, prevention and spread of communicable diseases, and promotion of dental health through organized and shared community efforts.

State and Government Responsibilities

In the United States, the responsibility for the health of the people primarily rests in each state. The federal government has definite responsibilities for health and welfare. One of its functions is to provide guidance and assistance to the several states in developing adequate public health services. The Social Security Acts (SSA) passed by the Seventy-fourth Congress authorized the distribution of funds to improve and enlarge public health services at the national, state, and local levels. The responsibility for the administration of Medicare was transferred from the Social Security Administration to the Health Care Financing Administration (HCFA), and in 1995 it was transferred from Health and Human Services (HHS) to independent agency status in the executive branch of the federal government.

The right of each state to control and safeguard the health of its several communities amounts to police power. It gives to the state government the power to enact laws and to enforce them in order to ensure health, safety, morals, order, comfort, and general welfare.

Health Organizations and Dental Health Education

Dental health education is included in the functions of a number of government agencies. These are called official agencies and operate as a part of the local, state, and federal governments.

At the federal level, the U.S. Public Health Service (USPHS), which is an agency within the Department of Health, Education, and Welfare (HEW), assumes a major role in the dental health programs. The USPHS assists the states in planning and promoting dental health programs. This agency helps to formulate policies for dental health programs in industries and provides special studies and surveys for the evaluation of dental health data. Another function of the USPHS is to provide personnel for demonstration programs.

Demonstration programs provided in a number of states by the USPHS show the techniques, costs, time schedules, and personnel needed for the topical application of stannous fluoride to the teeth of school children. The extensive reports released to the public indicate the value of these caries prevention methods for areas where other means of providing fluoride are impractical.

The Children's Bureau of the USPHS allocates funds to the states for programs of dental health, specifically for mothers and children. The dental consultant of the Children's Bureau advises state agencies concerning dental programs for handicapped children.

The Department of Health and Human Services (DHHS) *Healthy People 2000* lists 297 health objectives to be achieved by the year 2000, 16 of these related to oral health. Among these are concerns that address dental caries reduction, periodontal disease, oral cancer, dental trauma from accidents, dental sealants, and fluorides. Most of the attention is to be focused on the use of fluorides, mouth guards, tobacco use cessation, and periodontal disease. Groups to be targeted are the diabetic, elderly, disabled, and minority populations.

The Department of Education of each state has received from the legislative branch of the state government authority to provide physical examinations of pupils. Where state laws have been enacted in this respect, they frequently employ physicians, dentists, nurses, and other health specialists, including dental hygienists, for the purpose of performing periodic health examinations and inspections. The purpose of these activities is to detect adverse conditions in the school population, to advise concerning the need for care, and to educate parents or guardians and children.

Role of Voluntary Agencies in Dental Health

Voluntary agencies come into existence because of a specific need and are usually organized by groups of people who have financial resources, professional ability, or just plain community spirit and a willingness to contribute to the same cause. The primary purpose of any voluntary agency is to bring to public attention the need for study, treatment, or prevention of a health hazard within the community. Public interest is stimulated, thus demanding government action.

The professional organizations' role deserves notice, for it is through the contributions of the American Dental Association (ADA), the American Dental Hygiene Association (ADHA), the National Education Association (NEA), and a number of others in the field of health and education that authentic dental health information has become available. Through the efforts and controlled research of professional organizations, the aims and purposes for the standards of treatment have been determined.

Four Principles of Establishing a Dental Health Program

Through the ADA Council on Dental Health, four principles were adopted as a basis for dental health programs. Briefly stated, they are:

1. Adequate provisions should be made for research that may lead to the prevention and control of dental diseases.

2. Dental health education should be included in all education and treatment programs for children and adults.

3. Dental care should be available to all, regardless of income or geographic location. Programs should be based on the prevention and control of dental diseases. Dental caries is the responsibility of the individual, the family, and the community in that order. If the responsibility is not assumed by the community, it should be assumed by the state, and then by the federal government. The community, in all cases, shall determine the methods for providing service in its areas.

4. In all conferences that may lead to the formation of a plan for dental research, dental health education, and dental care, there should be participation by authorized representatives of the ADA.

Dental Disease: A Public Health Problem

Public health authorities recognize a situation to be a public health problem if it is widespread and affects the health and life of a wide portion of the population.

Dental disease is known to be **epidemic** (the appearance of a condition or disease that affects many people at the same time) at all times, occurring early in life for most individuals. Studies indicate that less than 2% of the population live the entire life span without some form of dental disease.

According to the ADA, 50% of all two-year-old children have one or more diseased teeth. At five years of age, they have three or more cavities in primary teeth. Fourteen percent of them will have cavities in their first permanent molars. The average youth at age 16 will have seven **carious** (decayed) or restored teeth. Less than 4% of high school students are free of decay.

Dental Caries

Of all dental disorders, tooth caries (decay) is unquestionably the most chronic disease affecting the American people. The cause of dental caries has been attributed to a number of factors.

A summary of research conducted by the ADA Advisory Committee on Research in Dental Caries, states the following: **Caries** is a bacterial disease of the calcified dental tissues (enamel and dentin), producing a typical and abnormal change in the structure of teeth. The active cause of caries is acid produced on tooth areas, often or long enough to enable the acid there to disintegrate the mineral structure. Many secondary factors determine the growth of the bacteria and affect the concentration and confinement of the acids and their resistance to attack. Among these factors are (a) diet as it affects oral environment, products of bacterial growth, and tooth structure and (b) **systemic** (pertaining to the whole body) reaction of the individual, including **metabolic** (pertaining to metabolism whereby the sum of all physical and chemical changes take place within an organism) processes, oral secretions, and tooth construction. Since dental caries is an individual disease, and not communicable, the conditions that allow it to be produced are also individual.

The most widely accepted theory of dental caries, according to the ADA, was expressed as early as 1890 by W. D. Miller. The theory does not completely satisfy the scientists of research as they continue to strive for a more exact explanation. However, the Miller theory of tooth decay remains a reliable one.

As stated by Miller, the process of dental decay follows several steps:

1. Food debris (carbohydrates and sugars) remains on perfect or imperfect tooth surfaces where the cleaning action of saliva, chewing, or toothbrushing cannot reach or dislodge it.

2. The end products of bacteria and enzymes of **fermentation** (the process of decomposition of complex substances through the action of enzymes, produced by bacteria, molds, and yeasts) are in a concentration sufficient to dissolve the mineral content of tooth enamel.

3. **Decalcification** (loss of calcium salts from the enamel in the first step of the decay process), once started, progresses until the enamel surface is broken, and the dentin is subjected to the same action.

4. During the process of decalcification, **decomposition** (process of decay) of the organic structure of the tooth takes place. This process is continuous until the dental pulp is affected.

5. Final putrefaction of the dental pulp occurs. (**Putrefaction** means the chemical breakdown of the tissues, causing the formation of a foul smell and destruction of tooth vitality).

The principal acid-producing bacteria in the mouth is *Lactobacillus acidophilus*, a lactic-acid-forming bacteria. The chemical action of *Lactobacillus* on carbohydrate food debris results in fermentation and the creation of lactic acid. Other bacteria found in the mouth may be contributors as well.

A great contributor to decay in the very young, primarily among disadvantaged children, is the baby-bottle tooth decay (BBTD) syndrome (Figure 52-1), caused by prolonged nursing from a bottle containing milk or other sweet liquids. The only rationale for treatment of this problem is prevention, beginning with education about

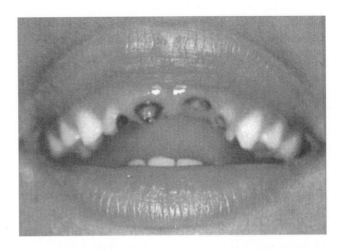

Figure 52-1 Baby bottle tooth decay. (Courtesy of David A. Chin, DDS)

oral care and encouraging the use of a cup in lieu of the bottle at all feedings. Although unsuccessful, there are not many alternative programs.

Conditions such as endocrine dysfunction, emotional instability, improper nutrition, and disease provide a systemic environment for the onset of dental caries.

The diagnosis of dental caries, unlike that of many other diseases, is not a difficult matter. Any layman can observe and detect gross tooth decay. However, the problem of diagnosing interproximal caries calls for radiographic interpretation. Refer to Chapter 71 for more information. Unless small cavities are filled as soon as they are found, extensive amounts of tooth structure must be sacrificed in large cavity preparations.

Factors Involved in Dental Decay. It is a common misunderstanding that food debris remaining on the teeth is the only cause of dental decay. There are other factors involved.

Dental Plaque. Dental **plaque**, a thin filmlike deposit that clings to the teeth, is made up of microorganisms and mucin from the saliva. Mucin is a secretion of the mucous membranes. This deposit covers all or part of the crown of the tooth. It must be constantly removed if dental caries is to be controlled.

Dental plaque accumulates on teeth at varying rates. It can be easily removed by thoroughly brushing and flossing, provided it is not permitted to accumulate and become firmly attached to the teeth.

Although the exact nature of dental plaque is not definitely known, there is evidence that it is a protein substance from the saliva in the form of mucin. This substance traps the microorganisms, specifically *Streptococcus mutans*, and permits them to grow into a matted mass that adheres to the teeth. The same bacteria, acting on the carbohydrates in the food eaten, make the plaque acid. Plaque that has reached a pH of 5.0 is known to cause decalcification of tooth enamel.

Dental plaque accumulates even in a clean mouth during hours of rest. Even after teeth have been thoroughly brushed prior to bedtime, plaque tends to cover the teeth, and a person may arise in the morning with a thick film on his or her teeth. In addition to the role plaque plays in initiating dental caries, it is also one of the factors in producing dental calculus (tartar). A rough, spongy surface of calculus acts as a matrix, thus enabling the inorganic salts of the saliva to adhere to the teeth.

Cleanliness of the teeth greatly depends on the stress used by the teeth in the process of cutting and crushing the food. The more vigorous the chewing, the cleaner are the teeth, and the less chance for dental caries. The value of a diet of natural (unrefined), bulky, fibrous foods that are well chewed cannot be overstressed. Of course, such foods do not eliminate the need for good toothbrushing and flossing.

Fluoride use has made a significant impact in preventing dental caries in the United States. It is used in different ways to prevent dental caries. It may be used by direct application onto the teeth or by ingesting it through the use of vitamins or by community preventive measures of providing fluoridated water. The effectiveness of fluoridation has been well documented. Early studies have demonstrated that 50–70% of caries was prevented in the permanent teeth of children. More recently, about 20–40% effectiveness has been credited to fluoridation due, in part, to the fact that many other fluoride-containing products have been available, such as toothpastes, rinses, dietary fluoride supplements, and treatment applications.

Materia Alba. Materia alba is a thick cream-colored mass that forms on the teeth when toothbrushing is neglected. This condition occurs when the main food of an individual consists of soft carbohydrates. The food debris adheres to the dental plaque and, by bacterial action, becomes highly acid. This accumulation remains undisturbed around those areas of the teeth that are not cleaned by the action of the tongue and cheeks. The retention of materia alba leads to the decalcification of the enamel and the formation of cavities. These cavities are found around the gingival third of the tooth. Routine brushing after each meal will control the deposits of materia alba.

Congenital Malformations

Congenital malformations, or birth defects, that affect the teeth and facial structure of an individual are cerebral palsy, cleft palate, and cleft lip.

Cerebral Palsy. Cerebral palsy is a disturbance of muscular function due to injury of the nervous system during fetal development or during the birth process. The lack of coordination prevents those so affected from receiving dental treatment because of the difficulty in controlling them in the dental chair. Many of these children also have severe orthodontic problems. Because of the unequal tensions exerted by facial muscles, food metabolism may be disturbed, with malformation of teeth as a consequence.

Their problems are definitely within the jurisdiction of those official and voluntary agencies that deal with crippled and handicapped children. Much attention has been focused on this group through efforts of the Association for the Cerebral Palsied. Primarily, this is a fundraising organization for the relief of afflicted children. Efforts have been made to give special training to dentists and dental hygienists in the treatment of the cerebral palsied child.

Education of parents and guardians in the proper care of the mouths of these children is aimed toward helping the child to care for herself or himself, within her or his own limitations. An important phase of the program for rehabilitation of palsied children is continuous care.

Cleft Palate and Cleft Lip. Cleft palate and cleft lip are two recognized malformations, caused by complete or partial failure of the body parts that form the roof of the mouth to unite during fetal development. The deformity results in the lack of a partition between the nasal cavity and the mouth. Correction is started early in life, as the abnormality makes infant feeding difficult. A series of surgical operations may be necessary to close the cleft(s). Through cooperation of the pediatrician, oral surgeon, dentist, orthodontist, and speech therapist, the cleft palate child can be helped to lead a normal life (Figure 52-2A–C).

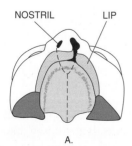
A.

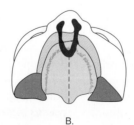
B.

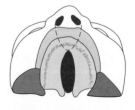
C.

Figure 52-2 (A, B) Cleft lip. (C) Cleft palate.

A.

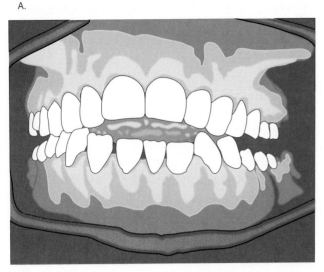

B.

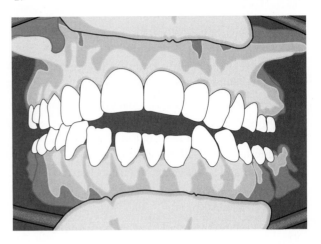

Figure 52-3 (A) Tongue thrust. (B) Open bite.

The role of the dental health advisor is to seek out and recommend to parents and guardians of these children the special services available to them. Poverty need not prevent the correction of these conditions, as there are sources and funds from the crippled children's agencies to provide surgical procedures, prosthetic replacements, and corrective speech, to correct such congenital defects.

Periodontal Diseases

The *Journal of the American Dental Association* (JADA) offered this contribution: The efforts of the dental profession in the field of Public Health Dentistry ought to include a program of preventive periodontia. (**Periodontia** is the science of treating diseases of the supporting tissues of the teeth.) Very often this condition is found to have its inception at an age prior to the teens. If this phase of treatment received emphasis equal to repairing the ravages of dental caries, the interest of our national health economy would be better served.

Because of the involvement of several types of tissues in periodontal disease, no one causative factor can be stated. There appears to be two sets of factors that tend to make an individual susceptible to periodontal disease:

1. Deposits of debris on the teeth, such as calculus and food impactions, are classified as local conditions.

2. Systemic conditions include any irritating force on the tissues, such as dental caries, poor-quality dental restorations, abnormal stress habits (e.g., mouth breathing), **tongue thrusts** [a pattern of swallowing in which the tongue is placed between the incisor teeth or alveolar ridges (Figure 52-3A) that may result in an open bite (Figure 52-3B), deformation of the jaws, and abnormal function], grinding teeth, and chewing on hard objects (pencils and the like).

Acute Necrotizing Ulcerative Gingivitis. **Acute necrotizing ulcerative gingivitis (ANUG)**, otherwise known as Vincent's infection, is a serious, acute infection of the gingiva that tends to become chronic. Caused by disease-bearing bacteria, it is a disease that attacks the individual with lowered resistance, but it is not considered communicable. The disease responds favorably to thorough removal of calculus and other debris by dental prophylaxis, coupled with a strict program of thorough toothbrushing. Individuals who have the infection should complete a physical checkup to determine the cause of low vitality. Corrections of physical illness and the maintenance of optimal good health are the best prevention.

All cases of the simplest types of gingival inflammation should be regarded as conditions that could lead to more serious periodontal disturbances. For instance, children who have heavy deposits of calculus should be treated as potential cases of periodontal disease in later life. However, ANUG is seldom seen in children.

SUGGESTED ACTIVITIES

● Take the opportunity to volunteer and go out to rural areas with a mobile clinic or visit a free clinic that treats economically disadvantaged children The probability of encountering children with baby-bottle tooth decay, gross tooth decay, and severe malocclusion are usually much greater. Learn how to provide instructions to the parents on proper care of the teeth.

● Research what the federal, state, and local agencies provide for disadvantaged persons in your city and make a list for reference purposes.

REVIEW

1. What does USPHS stand for?
   a. United States Public Hygiene Society
   b. United States Persons Health Science
   c. United States Public Health Service

2. What dental health professional organization(s) contribute(s) in providing dental health?
   a. American Dental Association
   b. American Medical Association
   c. American Dental Hygiene Association
   d. a and c
   e. All of the above

3. What is the recommendation for prevention of caries due to the baby bottle?
   a. Removing the bottle entirely
   b. Removing the bottle containing milk or sweet liquid
   c. Replacing the bottle with a cup at all feedings
   d. Both b and c

4. What is the primary active cause of dental caries according to the ADA Advisory Committee on Research?
   a. Bacteria
   b. Acid
   c. Diet
   d. Tooth structure

5. Indicate how the habit of "tongue thrusting" affects the function of dentition: (1) causing an open bite, (2) deformation of jaws, (3) abnormal function of the dentition, and/or (4) causing periodontal disease.
   a. 1, 2, 3
   b. 2, 3, 4
   c. 1, 2, 4
   d. 1, 3, 4

Pediatric Dentistry

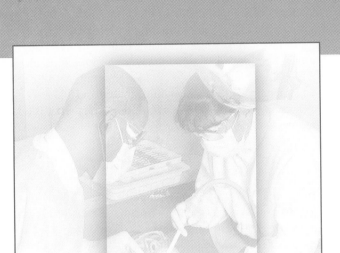

OBJECTIVES

After studying this chapter, the student will be able to:

- Discuss complete pediatric dental care and its importance to a lifelong process.
- Describe methods to gain the confidence of children.
- Describe ways of preparing the child for treatment.
- Explain the purpose of making a radiographic survey on a pediatric patient.
- Explain the difference between a pulpotomy and a pulpectomy.
- Determine how to care for patients who have dental injuries.

Introduction

Pediatric dentistry is the specialty limited to dentistry for children. This branch of dental care includes preventive and therapeutic care while training the child to accept dentistry from birth to the stage of mixed dentition (13–14 years). The pediatric dentist may also care for special patients who are afflicted with mental, physical, or emotional problems. Also included in this dental service are:

- Restoring and maintaining the primary, mixed, and permanent dentition
- Applying preventive measures for dental caries and periodontal disease

- Preventing, intercepting, and correcting various problems of occlusion

The pediatric specialist is concerned with the general health of all young patients. The basic needs and special requirements for treatment, along with a preventive plan as the dentition develops, are all of concern to the specialist.

Pediatric dental practice is maintained by referrals from the general dentist, other dental practitioners, and physicians. The general dentist and the specialist must work cooperatively to ensure ultimate dental care.

The pediatric specialist follows treatment of the child through the eruption of the second permanent molars. As a general rule, the child is referred to the general dentist at this time.

The Pediatric Dental Office

Preparing a child for dental treatment is an approach very different from that for an adult. Children must be made to feel at home by providing a corner of the reception room where furnishings are scaled to a child's size with small tables, chairs, familiar books, coloring books, crayons, pictures, and toys. The reception room may also display an aquarium, have a television/video monitor, or have a special cartoon character theme that would entertain its patients. Becoming acquainted with the dental office gives children a sense of belonging and helps to hold their interest while waiting (Figure 53-1).

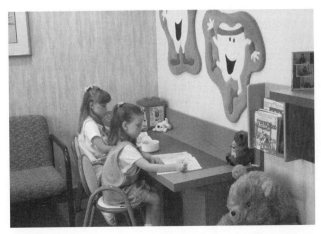

Figure 53-1 Children's corner in the reception room.

447

Many pediatric and orthodontic offices employ the **open bay** philosophy where several dental chairs and units are positioned in one large treatment room. This arrangement affords children to observe other children going through similar treatment. The conventional treatment room, on the other hand, has only one dental chair and unit.

Pediatric offices are outfitted with equipment scaled to children's sizes that may include dental handpieces with smaller heads, burs with shorter shanks, dental dam armamentaria such as smaller dental dam material and smaller clamps, and consumable items such as cotton rolls, matrices, and radiographic film geared for the small mouth.

Informed Consent

When administering treatment to the pediatric patient (less than 18 years of age), the parent or guardian is required to give consent by signing such a form. There are several procedures that would require it:

- Prior to any treatment
- Obtaining radiographs
- Administering sedation/general anesthesia
- Hand-over-mouth (HOM) disciplining technique (A technique whereby the dentist places his or her hand over the child's mouth to get the child's cooperation. When the child cooperates, the hand is removed).
- Surgical procedures

Controlling Fear

When children are placed in an unfamiliar environment, their first urge is self-preservation. In an unknown situation, the first emotion is fear, accompanied by the reaction to resist. Fear of the unknown, fear of pain, or fear of ridicule cause an urge to flee the situation. The confident parent or guardian can do much to reassure the child that he or she is safe in a new experience. Once a child has a feeling of safety, he or she is more likely to become an interested and cooperative patient. Were the child to discover any doubt in the mind of the parent or guardian, a lack of confidence in the dentist might also occur. In this event, dental treatment would literally become impossible.

Sedation. There are also other ways of dealing with children's fears that may require some form of sedation. Children can be premedicated using a mild sedative. They may undergo conscious sedation or inhalation sedation by using nitrous oxide–oxygen. If the fear is extensive, they may need general anesthesia; refer to Chapter 50.

Mutual Respect

Most American children have had some introduction to concepts of dental health in the home and possibly at school. The child hears from others their experiences "at the dentist." A youngster knows that teeth need attention. When placed in an adult situation not experienced before, he or she hopes to act like an adult. A child will respect those who respect him or her and likes to be spoken to as though he or she understands what is taking place.

The Examination

Unless the first visit is an emergency, the child is thoroughly examined. The child's breath, saliva consistency, gingivae, supporting tissues, and oral mucosa are checked. The examination also includes the tongue, tonsils, and pharynx for normal or abnormal conditions.

The surfaces of the teeth are examined with a mouth mirror and explorer. Carious lesions are charted. The eruption pattern of the teeth is recorded.

Following the examination, when only plaque is found to be present, the crowns of the teeth are polished. If any calculus exists, the dentist or dental hygienist performs a prophylaxis.

Medical History. The parent or guardian completes the patient's medical history record. The history of the child's infancy will help to provide information on caries prevention, any previous dental experience, allergies, medications being taken, oral and facial habits, and general development of the child. The family's interest in nutrition and preventive dentistry can be determined at the same time. When all information is gathered, the parent or guardian should sign the medical history form.

Treatment Plan. The parent or guardian meets in consultation with the dentist and is informed of the treatment required and the fee involved for the treatment plan. The parent or guardian must give signed consent for the treatment.

The responsibility of the administrative secretary includes an accurate file of each referral and a letter of acknowledgment should be sent to the referring practitioner.

Preparing the Patient. The dental assistant approaches the child in a friendly manner, calling the child by name. The patient is invited to go meet the doctor. As the patient is seated and draped, and the chair adjusted, the dental assistant will explain what is being done. Conversation between the dental assistant and patient is pleasant, unhurried, and spoken simply and plainly for easy understanding (Figure 53-2). The dental assistant should use comparisons such as "camera"

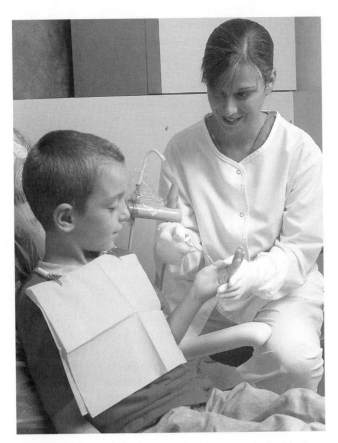

Figure 53-2 Dental assistant communicating with the pediatric patient.

when referring to the x-ray unit, "elevator chair" when referring to the dental chair, and "raincoat" when applying a dental dam. The dental assistant introduces the dentist to the patient, and then the dentist becomes acquainted with the patient. During this conversation, the dentist will explain, in a positive manner, the use of the equipment in the operatory, the procedure to be followed, and why it is necessary.

To maintain a rapport with the child, the dentist and dental assistant must function smoothly, quickly, and comfortably for the patient.

The question of rewards for good behavior has been challenged. Some pediatric dentists feel that the child patient should be given a small gift at the end of each appointment to indicate that the dentist is the child's friend. It is preferable to have the children make their own selection from a chest of small toys. For older children, a word of sincere praise is adequate.

Radiographs. A dental radiographic survey is an important portion of the diagnosis for the pediatric patient. Radiographs will show the condition of the primary teeth and the position and development of the permanent teeth.

Radiographic surveys consist of periapical, occlusal, bitewing, or panoramic radiographs. At times,

it may be difficult to have the child's full cooperation in obtaining radiographs. This situation may require someone to stabilize the film in the child's mouth. The dental assistant should NEVER be put in this position and be subjected to excessive radiation. In this circumstance, the parent or guardian should be summoned to assist. Precautionary measures for radiation hygiene should be used, such as also draping the parent with the lead apron and thyroid collar.

Study Models (Casts). Alginate impressions are made for study models that become a part of the diagnosis. Study models in various stages of development provide growth of the dental arches, supporting structures, and tooth eruption sequence.

Treatment

Children are brought into a pediatric dental office for various reasons. These may include having infectious diseases manifested in the oral cavity, toothaches from badly decayed teeth, accidents involving injury to teeth, or just a "first visit" to the dental office.

Acute Infections of the Mucosa. These infections are generally of brief duration and may recur from time to time. They are due to specific microorganisms. Some are communicable and, therefore, may become epidemic in schools. These infections involve only the soft tissues of the mouth, lips, nose, and throat.

Herpes Simplex. Herpes simplex is commonly seen in children. The onset of the infection may be severe, with fever and general weakness. The entire mouth may be highly inflamed and accompanied by **vesicles** (fluid-filled blisters) on the lips and around the oral cavity. Caused by a virus, herpes simplex may be found in the tissues long after the acute stage is past. It may break out from time to time as the individual's resistance is lowered.

Children suffer considerable discomfort from herpes simplex disease and should be protected from this highly contagious disease by providing a healthful school environment, particularly with reference to drinking fountains and other classroom equipment.

Fluoride Treatment. Depending on the tendency toward dental caries, the dentist may prescribe the topical application of fluoride. After the removal of plaque and/or calculus, fluoride is applied; refer to Chapter 11. These treatments are usually repeated every six months, following the routine prophylaxis. Daily toothbrushing and flossing are a part of ongoing care between prophylaxis appointments.

Pit and Fissure Sealants. If the patient's teeth show a high incidence of caries, the pediatric dentist may prescribe pit and fissure sealants. Sealants are used as preventive treatment to seal hard-to-clean, naturally deep and narrow fissures on the occlusal surfaces of primary and newly erupted permanent teeth; refer to Chapter 42.

When decalcification has already begun, a composite resin restoration may be placed instead of the sealant. Sealants are not used in teeth that have caries, for which a restoration is indicated.

Dental Dam Application. There are many advantages for using the dental dam in pediatric dentistry. The dental dam isolates the teeth away from the tongue and lips to keep a dry environment. It restricts the patient from talking during operative procedures. It prevents aspiration of materials used in the oral cavity and allows for better visibility while maintaining moisture control.

The use of a dental dam in pediatric dentistry is highly recommended for all the stated reasons. When punching the dental dam, only three or four holes are punched within one quadrant at a time. A pediatric dental dam is smaller, usually 5 in. x 5 in. Smaller holes should be selected depending on the sizes of teeth, and the distance between holes should be less when compared to punching for an adult dental dam; refer to Chapter 39.

The sizes of the clamps are much smaller than for adult teeth and should be ligated with waxed floss before placing on the tooth. As the clamp is being placed on the tooth, the operator should explain to the child that a "button" or a "ring" is being placed and that a "raincoat" will be placed next. It is not uncommon for the child to relax sufficiently as to sometimes fall asleep; therefore, a prop or a bite block should be used to keep the mouth open.

Restorative Materials. The materials used in pediatric dentistry are the same materials used in the restoration of permanent teeth. Composite resins are used to provide an esthetic quality to anterior teeth and are sometimes placed in primary molars. However, silver amalgam is most frequently preferred for posterior restorations. When silver amalgam is used on a class II preparation, the choice of a matrix band is important. The Tofflemire retainer may be too bulky and cumbersome for use in a pediatric practice. Instead, the dentist may wish to fabricate one by spot welding it to fit the needed size.

For teeth that need full coronal support due to decay, stainless steel crowns are used (Figure 53-3). The use of stainless steel crowns allows the teeth to function for many more years until they are replaced by permanent teeth; refer to Chapter 47.

Pulpotomy. A **pulpotomy** is performed when decay or injury has invaded the pulpal chamber of a primary tooth. A pulpotomy involves the removal of pulpal tissue from the coronal pulpal chamber excluding the pulpal canals. The dentist anesthetizes the tooth, places a dental dam, removes decay (Figure 53-4A), and cleans out the pulpal chamber (Figure 53-4B). The pulpal chamber is treated with a bactericidal medicament (formocresol; Figure 53-4C) that is left in place for 5 minutes to control hemorrhage in the chamber. Zinc oxide–eugenol (ZOE) cement is mixed to a putty consistency with a drop of formocresol added in the mix and condensed into the pulpal chamber to a thickness of 2–3 mm. (Figure 53-4D), then completed with a more permanent restoration. However, the tooth may be temporarily restored with ZOE until it is determined at a later date that it may be safely restored permanently with an amalgam restoration.

When treating permanent teeth, a pulpotomy is performed using calcium hydroxide instead of formocresol. It is applied at the entrance of the pulpal canals.

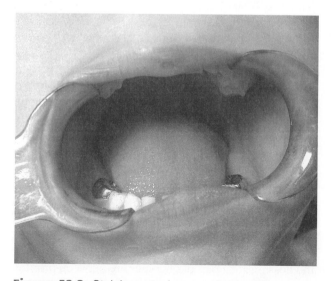

Figure 53-3 Stainless steel crown placement.

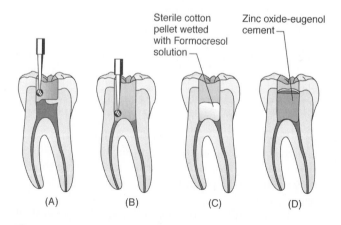

Figure 53-4 Pulpotomy procedure.

The tooth is then restored according to the amount of tooth structure present.

Pulpectomy. A **pulpectomy** is performed on primary and permanent teeth where pulpal tissue of the pulp chamber and canals is removed. There is a difference in how the tooth is restored depending on whether it is a primary or permanent tooth. For permanent teeth, gutta percha is used in the canals and chamber as a restorative material, then the final restoration is completed by using a crown or silver amalgam on the crown portion of the tooth. For primary teeth, gutta percha is not used due to the fact that when the roots begin to resorb, the gutta percha material does not resorb. Therefore, a thin mix of zinc oxide and eugenol is placed in the canals and a thicker mix is condensed into the canals and chamber. The tooth is then restored with a stainless steel crown.

Accidental Injury and Traumatized Teeth. Patients who have experienced a fractured (Figure 53-5) or **avulsed** tooth are treated as emergency cases. An avulsed tooth is one that has been knocked out or torn from its socket.

The person calling in an emergency should be instructed to:

● Try to find the tooth, and any fragments, if it is fractured.

● Rinse it gently and wrap the tooth in a clean wet cloth or place it back into the oral cavity, provided the patient does not swallow it.

● Immediately bring the patient to the dental office.

The lapse of time from the accident to when the tooth can be repositioned (put back into the socket) should be no more than 30 minutes. If the tooth can be saved, it is positioned in the arch and splinted into place.

Splints. A **splint** is a custom appliance whose object is to retain the traumatized tooth (teeth) in approximately the same position in the dental arch as before the injury. The splint may be constructed of cold-cure acrylic and orthodontic wires (Figure 53-6).

Space Maintainers. Following the **premature** (early) loss of a primary tooth, a space maintainer is designed to maintain the space until the normal eruption of the permanent tooth takes place.

A space maintainer may be **fixed** (cemented in place) or **removable** (can be removed and replaced by the patient). A fixed space maintainer consists of an orthodontic arch wire soldered to an orthodontic band that is cemented on a natural tooth, usually a molar. A removable space maintainer is constructed with an acrylic base, an orthodontic stainless steel wire that is shaped into clasps, and a lingual bar to fit a mandibular appliance. The choice of one type over the other depends on:

● The age of the child

● The number of primary teeth present and of permanent teeth not yet erupted

● The patient's oral hygiene

● The need for a **unilateral** (one side) or a **bilateral** (both sides) appliance (Figure 53-7).

Suggestions Concerning Dental Treatment for Children

Most children will accept dental treatment if:

1. Dental appointments do not interfere with their free time. Release time from school has been sanctioned by school administrators for medical and dental appointments.

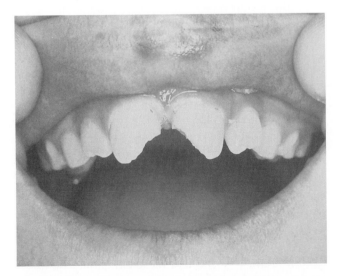

Figure 53-5 Fractured tooth. (Courtesy of Dale Ruemping, DDS, MSD.)

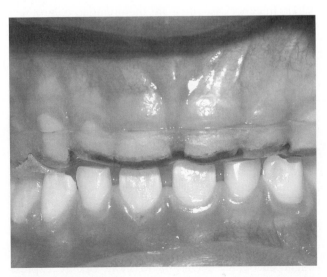

Figure 53-6 Splint holding tooth in place. (Courtesy of Steve Gregg, DDS.)

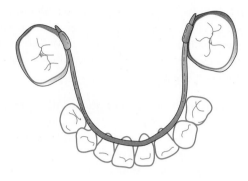

Figure 53-7 Bilateral fixed space maintainer.

2. Appointments for young children are made in the early morning, while they are rested and quiet.

3. Appointments for older children are made for the early afternoon.

4. The apprehensive child is given longer intervals between appointments to aid in relieving nervous tension.

5. The dental visit is shortened if it is noted that the child has a short interest span. The time may be lengthened as the child matures.

6. Discussions about pain are always truthful with the pediatric patient. The pain tolerance of a child should be respected and the dental treatment should never be hurried.

7. Every available means is used to reduce discomfort for the young dental patient.

Special Problems of the Adolescent

Teenagers are often more difficult to treat than younger children. They may be overtalkative or completely silent. In either case, they are attempting to control fear but want no one to suspect they are afraid. Both boys and girls are highly emotional during puberty, and their pain tolerance is low. In treating them, as much of the dental equipment (instruments, syringes, and dental handpieces) as possible should be kept out of sight. Teenagers are highly susceptible to impressions. The amount and appearance of dental equipment are frightening even to a well-adjusted adult patient.

Adolescents are seeking careers and are interested in science. To be allowed to watch what is going on in the dental laboratory holds their interest. For instance, the pouring of plaster models is an excellent opportunity to stimulate their interest in dental careers.

Dental personnel should look for nervous habits that may result in future dental deformities. Subjects that might encourage teenagers to more openly express themselves in a friendly discussion of good dental health include:

1. Personal cleanliness, good appearance, and social advantage of a fine set of teeth in a healthy mouth

2. Adequate diet for clear complexions and good teeth and restriction of sugars, particularly between meals

3. The high incidence of dental decay at this age, stressing the need for regular dental checkups

4. Safety in relation to teeth, encouraging those involved in competitive (contact) sports to wear mouth guards

5. Dentistry and dental research as progressive scientific efforts for the teenagers' particular benefit

Mouth Guards. Mouth guards are designed to fit over the full dentition and to protect the teeth from accidental injury. They are constructed of a pliable material and may be custom molded for a particular patient. Premolded commercial mouth guards (stock guards) can be purchased in assorted mold sizes to approximate the size of the patient's dental arch. These are less accurate in their fit than custom guards but are used by many athletes and are better than no guard at all.

Recognizing Child Abuse

In a practice that deals primarily with children, members of the dental team, as health care professionals, are mandated to recognize incidences of abuse and neglect. Abuse may include physical, emotional, or sexual harm inflicted on another person or child. Neglect may include lack of care by the parent or caregiver for the child's basic needs of food, clothing, safety, or education.

Signs to look for include unexplained injuries such as bruises and cuts, bite or burn marks, wearing clothing with long sleeves and long pants in warm weather that may be used as a cover-up, and overall uncleanliness.

The health professional needs to determine if the bruises match the story told about how the injury occurred. Bruises change color as they heal, which can give the observer an indication about the injury. A bruise looks red or purplish within the first 48 hours. After one week the bruise changes to a greenish color, after two weeks to a yellowish color, and after four weeks to a brown color before it heals. If there are multiple bruises at different stages as already indicated, it could mean that there is chronic abuse.

If bite marks are discovered, the health care professional should inquire if a human or animal inflicted it. To detect a human bite, the skin would not be torn, as characterized by an animal bite, but rather a bite pattern would appear having contusions or a row of small bruises (teeth marks) rather than a puncture wound.

If abuse is suspected, the child should be questioned separately from the parent about the injury. Questions should include when, how, and where it happened, who saw it happen, who did it, and who has been told about it. Then the parent should be questioned to see if the stories are similar. If they are not, abuse should be suspected.

Reporting a suspected abuse case requires a call to be made to the Child Protective Services Unit in the county where the child lives; then a written report is completed by the health care professional within 36 hours after the call (forms are available by calling the Child Protective Services Unit). A social worker will be assigned to the case who will determine if the child is being abused.

SUGGESTED ACTIVITIES

- Using pediatric-size film, practice taking radiographs on a child-size mannequin. Take special care to cover all landmarks for each exposure.

- Practice punching the dental dam for a child. Remember the distance between holes is less and the sizes of teeth are very small.

- Using a typodont, practice demonstrating the procedure used to brush small children's teeth.

REVIEW

1. Indicate for what procedures a parent's or guardian's informed consent should be procured: (1) to obtain radiographs, (2) to administer sedation or general anesthesia, (3) to do an oral exam, and/or (4) prior to any treatment.
   a. 1, 2, 3
   b. 2, 3, 4
   c. 1, 2, 4
   d. 1, 3, 4

2. If a child's fear were extensive, what would be an alternative way of dealing with the fear and provide treatment?
   a. Use general anesthesia
   b. Bring the parent into the treatment room
   c. Use additional local anesthetic
   d. Schedule a lengthier appointment

3. Indicate why it is important to make a radiographic survey on the pediatric patient: (1) to show the positions of permanent teeth, (2) to detect malaligned teeth, (3) to detect rotated teeth, and/or (4) to show the condition of primary teeth.
   a. 1, 2
   b. 2, 3
   c. 3, 4
   d. 1, 4

4. What is a pulpotomy?
   a. A disease process of the pulp
   b. The removal and temporary restoration of the coronal pulp chamber
   c. The removal and restoration of the entire pulp chamber and pulpal canal(s)
   d. Performed on permanent teeth

5. What is the purpose for a splint?
   a. To retain a space until a permanent tooth erupts
   b. To hold the position of teeth that were orthodontically treated
   c. To retain a traumatized tooth/teeth in the same position as before the injury
   d. To protect the teeth from occlusal grinding or attrition

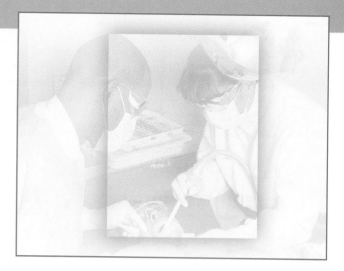

OBJECTIVES

After studying this chapter, the student will be able to:

- Explain the objectives of orthodontics.
- Explain how thumb-sucking, tongue-thrusting, bruxing, and mouth-breathing habits may influence dentition.
- Describe how genetic and hereditary factors may affect dentition.
- Describe normal or ideal occlusion.
- List the classifications of malocclusion and identify each one.
- Describe diagnostic tools used to complete the examination.
- Identify the types of tooth movement that take place during orthodontic treatment.
- Identify the types of separators used in orthodontics.
- Describe the purpose of the arch wire.
- Name parts of a band.
- Explain what a headgear is and the types of force it directs.
- Explain the meaning of tracing lines drawn from a cephalometric radiograph.

Introduction

Orthodontics (*ortho-* "to align or to straighten"; *donto-* "tooth") is the dental specialty concerned with the study and supervision of the growth and development of dentition and related anatomical structures from birth to maturity. Orthodontics is the science dealing with the prevention and correction of dental and oral **anomalies** (any deviation from the normal). An orthodontist is a specialist who, already being a dentist, possesses two additional years of formal education in orthodontics and limits his or her practice to the correction of **malocclusion** (any deviation from normal occlusion).

Orthodontic patients come to the specialist by referral for both preventive and corrective procedures of evaluation and treatment. Orthodontic treatment may be provided for patients of all ages, including adults. The objective of orthodontics includes the maintenance of the functional relationship of the teeth, dental arches, and supporting structures of the face and skull.

Influence of Function

Function is an important factor in the continued growth and development of the human body. In addition to the influence of function, growth is appreciably affected by and dependent on many other factors, namely, heredity, environment, nutrition, and general health.

Dental health and emotional development are interdependent areas. Maladjustment in emotional development is indicated by habits involving the teeth and structures of the mouth.

The orthodontic patient's history is checked for hereditary or physical problems that may affect treatment. The conditions may include heart problems, asthma, diabetes, glandular disturbances, or blood disorders. Therefore, the etiology of **dentofacial** (pertaining to the teeth and face) deformity includes genetic, hereditary, and congenital defects, including local oral problems and systemic influences.

Genetic and Hereditary Origin

Genetic problems present themselves as disharmonies within the jaws and dentition. They include:

- Small jaws and larger than normal teeth
- Large jaws and smaller than normal teeth
- Normal-sized jaws and teeth too small or too large
- Teeth in the maxilla either larger or smaller than teeth in the mandible

Hereditary and congenital problems include:

● Facial and palatal clefts

● Supernumerary teeth or congenitally (present at birth) missing teeth

● Large or small tongue

● Development of muscles and frenum

Systemic Influences

Infectious diseases, endocrine disturbances, and nutritional deficiencies play a significant role in how the teeth develop and function. Many times, when a child suffers from a prolonged high fever, the tooth-forming buds are greatly affected, producing malformed teeth.

Local Oral Problems

These problems include injurious or environmental circumstances that cause malocclusion:

● Early or delayed loss of deciduous teeth

● Early eruption of permanent teeth

● Loss of permanent teeth due to caries or other reasons

● Infections of periodontal structures

● Cysts and growths occurring intraorally

● Injuries

● Bad habits—thumb sucking, tongue thrusting, bruxism, mouth breathing

Habits Influencing Dentition Development

Thumb Sucking. Thumb suckers are of two types. The first type starts at a very early age and stops when the physiological desire is satisfied. The second type starts again, four or five years later, when the child meets with difficulty. Being unable to progress normally with solutions to problems, the child will regress to an early form of gratification.

From infancy to age 5, defects of the teeth and facial structures are not evident. Beyond age 5, defects of the maxillary arch, the palate, and the anterior teeth will become apparent. Should this occur, the orthodontist should recommend corrective treatment.

Tongue Thrusting. Tongue thrusting or reverse swallowing places great forward pressure against the maxillary teeth each time the child swallows. The tongue thrust causes the maxillary arch to move forward, with the teeth pushed into a fan-shaped position. (Refer to Figures 52-3A and B.)

Bruxism. **Bruxism** is the involuntary grinding or clenching of the teeth, other than during normal chew-

ing movements. Bruxism occurs most frequently during sleep, although the grinding sound may also be heard during the waking hours.

Extreme habits of bruxism must be corrected as grinding wears away the enamel and puts pressure on the periodontium. Self-directed suggestions may help patients to overcome their habit. However, a professional psychologist may be called upon, stressing the need to abstain from bruxism. The orthodontist may also suggest wearing a mouth guard at nighttime.

Mouth Breathing. Mouth breathing, referred to as adenoid breathing, may or may not be due to an obstruction of the nasal passages of the respiratory system. A physical examination and consultation with the patient's physician may be indicated before plans for orthodontic treatment are determined.

Mouth breathing can cause a pinched face because of the narrowing of the dental arch. Over a period of years, the entire dentofacial structure of the child may be changed because of prolonged mouth breathing.

Occlusion and Malocclusion

The entire form and function of the face and its structures are directly affected by the manner in which the biting surfaces of the teeth of the maxillary arch meet and close (occlude) with the teeth of the mandibular arch. The exact pattern is called occlusion, further defined as the space relation between teeth in the action of closing and chewing.

The establishment of occlusion of the teeth begins at about the sixth month of life and ends with the eruption of the third molars. It may be said that the development of occlusion in an individual is a long and changing process that begins with inception and continues throughout life.

Normal or Ideal Occlusion

Occlusion is intended by nature where the teeth in the maxillary arch are in maximum contact with the teeth of the mandibular arch. This is associated with a 2-mm maxillary anterior overlap over mandibular anterior teeth, maxillary posterior teeth are positioned one cusp facial over mandibular posterior teeth, and the molar relationship is in neutrocclusion.

Centric Occlusion

Central occlusion refers to the relationship of maxillary and mandibular teeth when the jaws are closed, the teeth are in maximum contact, and the heads of the condyles are in the most retruded, unstrained position in the glenoid fossa.

Table 54-1	Classification of Malocclusion		
Angle Class	**Molar Relationship**	**Profile**	**Occlusion**
Class I	Maxillary first molar mesiobuccal cusp is aligned with buccal groove of mandibular first molar	Mesognathic (straight) (Figure 54-1)	Neutrocclusion (correct occlusion) (Figure 54-2)
	Other teeth are malaligned, tipped, or rotated		
Class II	Maxillary first molar mesiobuccal cusp is aligned between mandibular second bicuspid and first molar	Retrognathic (weak chin) (Figure 54-3)	Distocclusion (jaw too far back)
Division I	Maxillary anterior teeth are overjet		(Figure 54-4)
Division II	Maxillary centrals are depressed and laterals protrude labially and tilt mesially		(Figure 54-5)
Class III	Maxillary first molar mesiobuccal cusp is aligned between mandibular first and second molars	Prognathic (prominent chin) (Figure 54-6)	Mesiocclusion (jaw too far forward) (Figure 54-7)

Malocclusion

Malocclusion is any deviation from the normal pattern of occlusion. Malocclusion tends to:

- Impair mastication
- Increase the susceptibility to dental caries
- Encourage periodontal disease
- Lead to early loss of teeth and cause abnormal respiratory habits
- Provoke abnormal mental attitudes in relation to facial esthetics
- Impair speech

Classification of Malocclusion.

Edward Angle developed the most widely used classification of malocclusion (Table 54-1) based on the position of the maxillary and mandibular first permanent molars.

Angle Class I

- **Mesognathic profile** is a straight profile (Figure 54-1).
- **Neutrocclusion** molar relationship is where the mesiobuccal cusp of the maxillary first molar is aligned with the buccal groove of the mandibular first molar. However, teeth may be malaligned, tipped, or rotated (Figure 54-2).

Angle Class II

- **Retrognathic profile** is a weak chin (Figure 54-3).
- **Distocclusion** molar relationship is where the mesiobuccal cusp of the maxillary first molar is aligned between the mandibular second bicuspid and first molar.

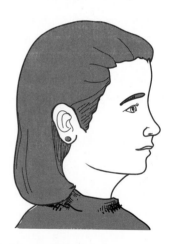

Figure 54-1 Mesognathic profile—straight profile.

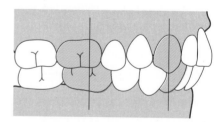

Figure 54-2 Class I: neutrocclusion—mesiobuccal cusp of maxillary first molar is aligned with the buccal groove of the mandibular first molar.

Division I. Anterior teeth are overjet in maxilla (Figure 54-4).

Division II. Maxillary centrals are depressed and laterals protrude labially and tilt mesially (Figure 54-5).

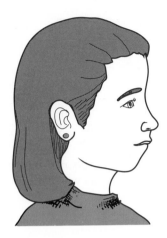

Figure 54-3 Retrognathic profile—weak chin.

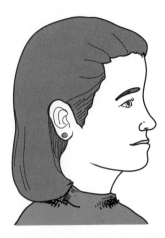

Figure 54-6 Prognathic profile—prominent chin.

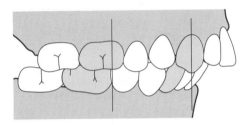

Figure 54-4 Class II, Division I: distocclusion—mesiobuccal cusp of maxillary first molar is aligned between the mandibular second bicuspid and first molar.

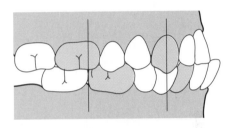

Figure 54-7 Class III: mesiocclusion.

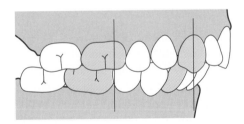

Figure 54-5 Class II, Division I: Distocclusion.

Angle Class III

● **Prognathic profile** is a prominent chin (Figure 54-6).

● **Mesiocclusion** molar relationship is where the mesiobuccal cusp of the maxillary first molar is aligned between the mandibular first and second molars (Figure 54-7)

Malocclusion Conditions

Overjet. An overjet is a horizontal distance that exists due to the protrusion of the most anterior maxillary incisor to the facial aspect of the most anterior mandibular incisors (Figure 54-8). A horizontal measurement is taken while the teeth are in centric occlusion by placing a small sterile ruler at the incisal edge of the most protruded maxillary incisor at a right angle to the facial side of the correspon-

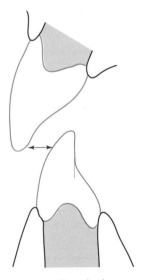

Figure 54-8 Overjet—maxillary incisors protrude over mandibular incisors.

ding mandibular incisor. The distance from the facial surface of the mandibular incisor to the facial surface of the most protruded maxillary incisor is measured in millimeters.

Overbite. An **overbite** is when there is a greater than normal vertical overlap between the incisal edges of the maxillary central incisors and the mandibular central

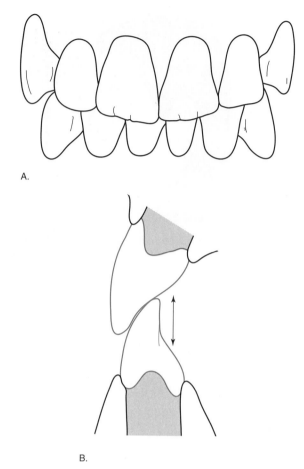

A.

B.

Figure 54-9 Overbite—maxillary incisors in greater than normal overlap over mandibular incisors.

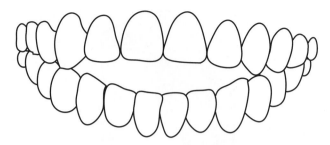

Figure 54-10 Openbite—open space between maxillary and mandibular incisors while posterior teeth are in occlusion.

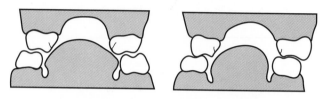

Figure 54-11 Crossbite—maxillary anterior incisals and/or posterior facial cusps in linguaoversion to mandibular teeth.

incisors (Figures 54-9A and B). Normal overbite is when maxillary incisors overlap up to the incisal third of the mandibular incisors. A vertical measurement is taken while the teeth are in centric occlusion by placing a sterile small ruler at the incisal edge of the maxillary incisors at right angle to the facial side of the mandibular incisors. The patient opens the jaws and the measurement is taken vertically on the mandibular incisor between the point of contact with the ruler and the incisal edge.

Openbite. An **openbite** is when there is no overlap but rather an open space between the incisal edges of the maxillary and the mandibular incisors while the posterior teeth are in occlusion (Figure 54-10).

Crossbite. A crossbite is when maxillary anterior incisals and/or posterior buccal cusps are in **linguoversion** (turned toward the lingual side) position and do not overlap mandibular teeth (Figure 54-11).

The Examination

A patient history is completed during the patient's first visit to the orthodontic office. This also includes a back-

ground history of the parents' dental and medical histories that provides growth patterns for the patient.

Photographs

The examination includes two types of photographs, intraoral photographs to document the condition of teeth and soft tissues within the mouth and extraoral to evaluate the patient's appearance, position of jaws, facial symmetry, and proportions. Intraoral photographs require a full anterior view, a lateral view, and a maxillary palate view. Extraoral photographs include a profile and full-face photographs of the patient. Photographs are taken prior to and after orthodontic treatment. They may also be used in patient counseling and education for similar orthodontic cases.

Radiographs

If the referring dentist has provided recent radiographs of the patient, these may be used for comparative diagnosis. Orthodontists usually require periapical, occlusal, cephalometric, and panoramic radiographs.

Radiographs are made to check for positions of teeth, confirm the presence of all teeth, compare the relationship of jaws to each other and to the skull, and verify the presence of dental disease. Periapical and bitewing radiographs confirm the presence of dental disease. Occlusal radiographs verify the presence of supernumerary teeth and the position of unerupted impacted

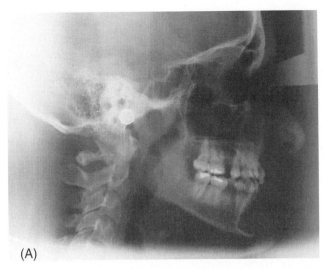 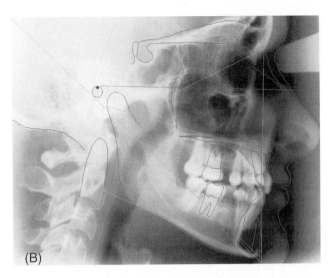

Figure 54-12 (A) Cephalometric radiograph; (B) Cephalometric tracing. (Courtesy of Steven Gregg, DDS.)

anterior teeth. Panoramic radiographs indicate the stages of eruption of permanent teeth as well as the presence of supernumerary teeth and anomalies. The **cephalometric radiograph** (a radiograph of the lateral view of the head and facial structures; Figure 54-12A) is required to reproduce tracings of angular and linear measurements of the anterior cranium base and facial structures (Figure 55-12B). These drawings are very helpful in determining relationships of both dental arches and their supporting bony structures to each other and to the anterior cranial base. The meanings of the landmark designations and linear planes are explained.

Cephalometric Tracing. Landmark designations in a cephalometric tracing are:

- N = nasal bone or nasion
- O = orbit of eye or orbitale
- S = sella turcica, the bone that cradles the pituitary gland within the cranium
- P = external auditory meatus or porion
- ANS = anterior nasal spine
- A = anterior alveolar bone (maxilla)
- B = anterior alveolar bone (mandible)
- Pg = chin or pogonion

Planes drawn in cephalometric tracings are:

- SN plane = from the sella turcica to the nasion
- **Frankfort plane** = from the external auditory meatus to the inferior orbit of the eye
- Mandibular plane = from the lowest point of the angle to the lowest point of the chin
- NA plane = from the nasion to the anterior alveolar bone of the maxilla

- NB plane = from the nasion to the anterior alveolar bone of the mandible
- Facial plane = from the nasion to the pogonion (anterior part of chin)
- A plane from the SN plane through the long axis of the maxillary incisor
- A plane from the mandibular plane through the long axis of the mandibular incisor

Study Models and Working Casts

Alginate impressions to produce study models and working casts are obtained during the initial visit. The dental assistant is usually the responsible person for taking alginate impressions. Every effort should be made to include the crowns of the teeth, supporting structures, and muscle attachments (frenuli). Orthodontic study models are made with extreme care to include a high base and symmetrical cuts when trimmed; see Chapter 48. The study models are further dipped in liquid soap and polished to a high gloss for esthetic appeal and surface protection.

The Case Presentation

The orthodontist will study the diagnostic aids and develop a treatment plan and cost estimate for the patient. These aids will help explain the diagnosis and treatment plan.

The presentation includes the approximate length of treatment and a statement of the responsibility of the patient and/or parent to ensure the successful completion of the procedure.

Financial Arrangements

The fee for the consultation and case presentation is a separate fee usually paid at the time of the visit. When the patient and person legally responsible for the account agree that treatment should proceed, a contract for services is signed.

If the patient requires restorative dentistry before orthodontic treatment, he or she is referred to the general dentist.

When extractions are necessary, they may be performed by the general dentist or an oral and maxillofacial surgeon. After the tissues have healed sufficiently to permit orthodontic treatment, an appointment is scheduled.

Oral Hygiene

Emphasis must be placed on the importance of a clean mouth and teeth during orthodontic treatment.

The teeth and appliances are to be thoroughly brushed after each meal. The orthodontist will recommend a specific type of toothbrush for the patient (Figure 54-13). Particular attention must be given to the ligature ties, the margins of the bands, and the cervical, lingual, facial, and occlusal surfaces of the teeth. If tooth brushing is omitted during treatment, decalcification and decay will occur and the gingival tissue will become inflamed and swollen. Flossing should be an integral part of the daily routine even though it is more difficult.

The patient should be instructed in the technique employed in using a floss threader (Figure 54-14).

Tooth Movement

As orthodontic treatment takes place, tooth movement occurs. The force that is applied to a tooth causes compression of the periodontal ligament on one side of the root, restricting the flow of blood (Figure 54-15A). On the opposite side of the root there is tension on the periodontal ligament (Figure 54-15B). Specialized bone-destroying cells known as **osteoclasts** invade the area of compression where they resorb or cause **resorption** by destroying the alveolar bone, making it possible for the root of the tooth to move in that direction. Other specialized bone-forming cells known as **osteoblasts** begin to deposit or cause **deposition** of new bone cells in the area of tension from where the tooth has moved.

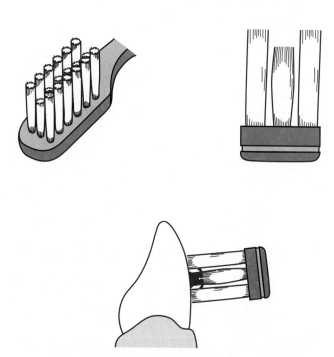

Figure 54-13 Orthodontic-type toothbrush with middle row of bristles recessed.

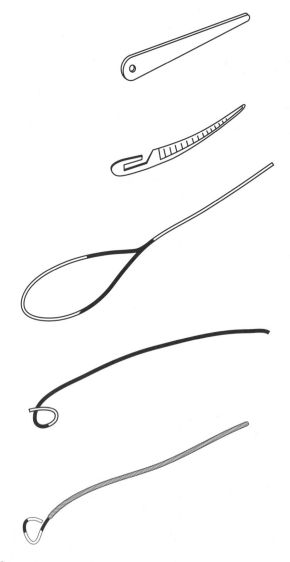

Figure 54-14 Floss threader used to insert floss.

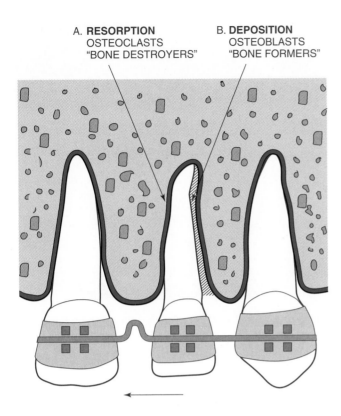

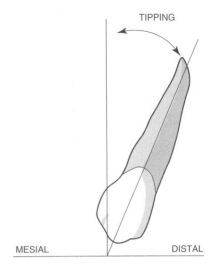

Figure 54-16A Tipping—tooth leans mesially or distally.

Figure 54-15 (A) Resorption takes place where osteo-clasts become activated to destroy bone.
(B) Deposition takes place where osteoblasts become activated to build bone.

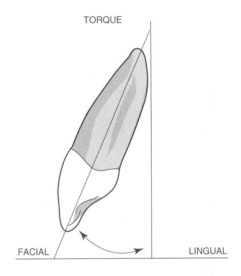

Figure 54-16B Torque—tooth is in linguoversion or labioversion position to arch.

Types of Tooth Movement

Several types of tooth movement occur prior to ortho-dontic treatment:

- *Tipping*—a tooth that leans laterally, mesially or dis-tally and its long axis tips toward a horizontal plane (Figure 54-16A).

- *Torque*—a tooth that is in a linguoversion or labiover-sion position to the arch (Figure 54-16B).

- *Rotation*—a tooth that faces the wrong side but its long axis is positioned correctly (Figure 54-16C).

- *Bodily*—a tooth that is moved in its entirety, both crown and root moved simultaneously mesially or distally, but is otherwise in alignment (Figure 54-16C).

- *Extrusion*—A tooth that is partially displaced out-wardly from its socket due to injury or tooth loss from the opposing arch (Figure 54-17A).

- *Intrusion*—A tooth that is partially driven into its socket and does not meet occlusion with the oppos-ing arch (Figure 54-17B).

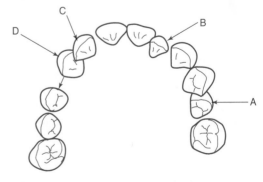

Figure 54-16C A: rotated—tooth is rotated in its long axis, facing the wrong direction; B: torque; C; tipped, D; Bodily—tooth's crown and root move in the same direc-tion from one location to another.

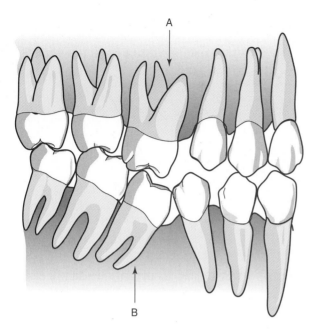

Figure 54-17 (A) Extrusion—tooth partially displaced outwardly from its socket; (B) Intrusion—tooth driven in its socket.

Orthodontic Treatment

Phases related to orthodontic treatment are preventive, interceptive, corrective, and retentive. Appliances used for treatment are categorized as "fixed" or "removable." Fixed appliances include orthodontic bands, brackets, arch wires, ligature ties, and fixed retainers, all of which include appliances that cannot be placed or removed by the patient. Removable retainers include retainers headgear, positioner, and elastics and can be placed and removed by the patient.

Preventive Orthodontic Care

Prior to the interceptive and corrective phases of orthodontic care, the patient may undergo preventive orthodontic treatment that could take place at the pediatric or general practitioner's office. To anticipate some orthodontic problems, the following methods may be suggested: (1) the use of space maintainers on pediatric patients where early loss of primary teeth had taken place, (2) the use of preventive therapy to correct oral habits such as thumb sucking, nail biting, or tongue thrusting (reverse swallowing), and (3) controlling the decay process in primary and permanent teeth to prevent loss of teeth.

Interceptive Orthodontic Care

This phase of orthodontic care occurs prior to full orthodontic treatment or corrective phase. It may include (1)

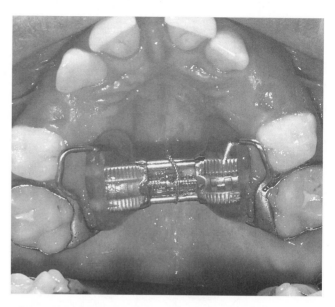

Figure 54-18 Crozat appliance with screw in the center to aid in widening the jaw. (Courtesy of Rita Johnson and Vincent DeAngelis.)

extractions of primary teeth to open up spaces for eruption of permanent teeth, (2) extractions of permanent teeth to allow for tooth movement in cases where overcrowding of teeth exists, (3) using a **Crozat appliance** (palatal spreading appliance consisting of a split plastic palate with a screw in its center that opens or closes the space) to widen the arch in cases of crossbite occlusion or extremely narrow palate with overcrowded teeth (Figure 54-18), and (4) the use of **headgear** (an extraoral device used to control orthopedic growth and tooth movement) to slow down growth of the skeletal bone in a young person on the maxillary jaw, mandibular jaw, or both. Headgear is also used during the corrective phase (Figure 54-19).

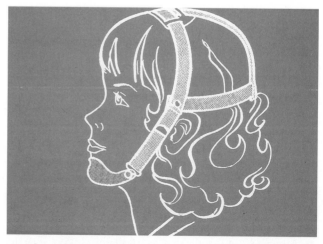

Figure 54-19 Headgear—applies extraoral forces for orthodontic or orthopedic movement. (Courtesy of Rita Johnson and Vincent DeAngelis.)

Headgear Use. The headgear is a device consisting of an outer facebow that connects to an inner bow, which attaches intraorally to the headgear tubes welded on molar bands. Extraorally, the facebow is attached to straps that go over the head or around the neck depending on the type of pull needed.

When the headgear is utilized, it may apply orthodontic forces up to 1 pound per side to move teeth orthodontically or it may apply orthopedic forces up to 5 pounds per side for bony repositioning. Forces are guided according to the direction dictated by the outer straps. Forces applied are:

- High pull—using a strap that pulls in an upward position
- Cervical pull—using a neck strap that pulls in a distal position
- Combination of high pull and cervical—using two straps that pull upward and distally
- Chin cap—to retard growth of the chin

Corrective Orthodontic Care

This phase consists of using fixed and removable appliances to move teeth. To begin treatment, the patient must conform to all preliminary care such as necessary extractions, required restorations, control of destructive habits, prophylaxis, and fluoride treatment.

Prior to the 1970s, banding the teeth was the only method available for fixed orthodontic appliances. Since then, bonding, which is less cumbersome and more esthetically appealing, has largely replaced banding. However, there are still cases that need the strength that banding can provide. Molars are banded to achieve a strong attachment for headgear and arch wires. Banding requires the use of separators to make it possible to fit the band around tight contact areas; band sizing and cementation with permanent type cement follow this.

Separators. **Separators** are used to open up a space interproximally between teeth that will be receiving bands. This process will separate the teeth enough to enable the band to be fitted onto each tooth. There are several types of separators, most of which need to be in place approximately one to two weeks prior to banding. Should a separator be lost or become dislodged, the patient needs to notify the office immediately for replacement. The most widely used separators are elastomeric rings, also referred to as "elastic separators"; others include stainless steel springs, or "TP springs," and brass wire.

Elastomeric Ring Separators. This type of separator is very popular due to ease of placement and removal and comfort for the patient. The shape is similar to a doughnut; thus it encircles the contact area. It is supplied in

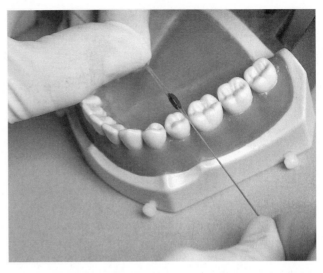

Figure 54-20 Elastomere separating ring placed with floss in lieu of separating pliers.

small or large sizes. The small size is used on anterior teeth and the large size on posterior teeth, distal of the cuspid. The instrument used to place this separator is the elastic separating pliers, and the instrument for removal is the sickle scaler. Prior to inserting this type of separator, each contact area should be tested with dental floss to determine if tight contact areas exist where placement may be difficult.

- *Placement.* An elastomeric ring separator is placed on the beaks of the elastic separating pliers. It is stretched (not overstretched) so that it will fit through the contact area. Only one side of the separator should pass the contact area using a seesawing motion; the opposite side of the separator should remain occlusally or incisally. Another method is to use two strands of floss (Figure 54-20) in lieu of separating pliers the strands are inserted through the separator to aid in stretching it through the contact area. If the separator has been "overstretched," it will not return to its original shape and should be discarded.
- *Removal.* The number and location of documented separators should be compared. The point of the sickle scaler (Figure 54-21) is carefully inserted just under the portion of the separator located above the contact area. Using a proper finger rest and gentle force, the separator is removed occlusally.

Stainless Steel Spring Separator. This type of separator has the advantage of being able to slip into very tight contact areas on posterior teeth. The separator consists of a gingival leg (short leg), occlusal leg (long leg), and the helix (coil) that applies the force (Figure 54-22). The gingival leg is placed below the contact area, the occlusal leg is placed above the contact area, and the helix is placed on the facial side of the contact area. The

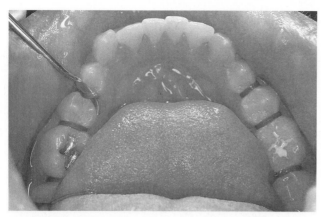

Figure 54-21 Removal of elastomere separator. (Courtesy of Rita Johnson and Vincent DeAngelis.)

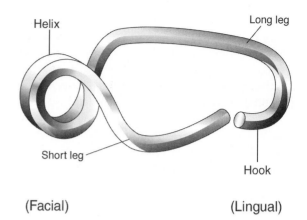

Figure 54-22 Parts of the stainless steel spring, or "TP spring" separator.

instrument used in placement is the bird beak pliers and the instruments used in removal are the sickle scaler and Howe pliers (Figures 54-23A–C).

● *Placement.* The gingival leg is grasped with the bird beak pliers. The hook portion of the occlusal leg is positioned interproximally on the lingual side. While the separator is hooked on the lingual side and the gingival leg is opened enough to place it under the contact area, a finger of the opposite hand should be placed on the occlusal side to stabilize the separator. Once in place, it is released, making certain that both the occlusal and gingival legs surround the contact area. The number and location of separators are documented.

● *Removal.* The number and location of separators are compared with documented separators. The helix of the separator is grasped with Howe pliers while the hook portion is grasped with a sickle scaler, then simultaneously pulled occlusally to disengage it.

Another method of removal is by inserting the sickle scaler in the helix, lifting it occlusally until the hook portion on the lingual side is disengaged. The separator is then removed facially. It is of utmost importance to have a fulcrum, firm grasp and control of the instrument.

Brass Wire Separators. This type of separator provides instant separation upon placement. It is usually more painful to the patient initially. It is supplied in a spool from which the operator cuts off a small length, about 1 1/2 in. in size (Figure 54-24).

● *Placement.* The wire is bent in a loop for ease of placement. One portion is inserted beneath the contact area using the Howe pliers or a needle holder; the other end is brought over the contact occlusally. The two ends are brought together facially and twisted with the pliers or hemostat to form a braid. The excess is trimmed with a ligature cutter (Figure 54-25) leaving a 3–5 mm pigtail. The pigtail is tucked toward the gingiva using a condenser or ligature director/tucker (Figure 54-26). The newly placed separator is checked for roughness that may injure the cheek. The number and location of separators placed are documented.

● *Removal.* The number of visible separators should equal the number documented on the chart. The pigtail is lifted out with a sickle scaler and untwisted slightly with the Howe pliers, enough to insert the beak of the pin and ligature cutter under the wire. The wire on the occlusal closest to the lingual side is cut. The pigtail is grasped using the Howe pliers and gently removed facially.

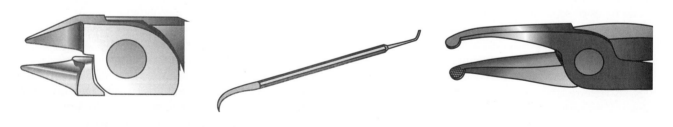

A. BIRD BEAK PLIERS   B. SICKLE-STYLE CEMENT REMOVER AND LIGATURE TUCKER   C. HOWE PLIERS

Figure 54-23 (A) bird beak pliers. (B) sickle scaler, (C) Howe pliers.

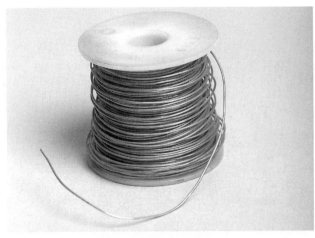

Figure 54-24 Spool of wire for brass wire separators.

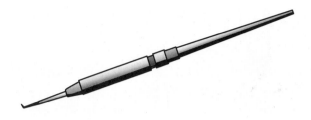

SINGLE-ENDED LIGATURE DIRECTOR

Figure 54-26 Ligature tucker/directed. [Copyright © 3M (IPC) 1999. All rights reserved.]

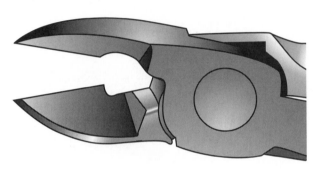

PIN AND LIGATURE CUTTER

Figure 54-25 Pin and ligature cutter. [Copyright © 3M (IPC) 1999. All rights reserved.]

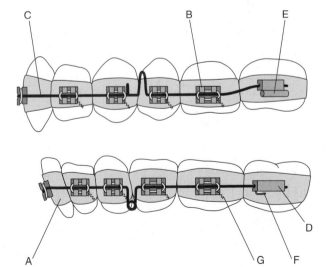

Orthodontic band

Headgear tube

Figure 54-27 Orthodontic band with headgear tube auxiliary attachment. (Courtesy of Rita Johnson and Vincent DeAngelis.)

Banding. The **band** is a fixed appliance consisting of a metallic ring that is cemented on the tooth (Figure 54-27). It has welded attachments including the **bracket** (an attachment on the band or directly on the tooth that provides a means for the arch wire to be secured to the bands or teeth). It holds the **arch wire** (a wire shaped in the form of the dental arch that fits into the buccal tubes and attached to the brackets to provide movement to the teeth). A band may also have welded auxiliary attachments such as a **buccal tube** (where the ends of the arch wire are secured), **headgear tube** (where the inner bow of the headgear is secured), **elastic hook** (a hook that serves to attach elastic bands for additional force) and **seating lug** (an attachment welded to the band used to seat the band to the tooth) (Figure 54-28).

Bands encircle the teeth and are supplied in many sizes for each type of tooth. In some states, a dental assistant with the proper credentials is delegated to perform the duty of band sizing. When choosing the proper size band, it may take a few tries to find the perfect fit.

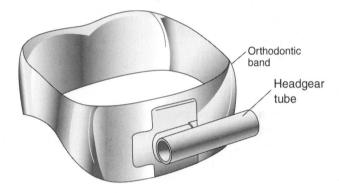

Figure 54-28 Fixed appliances: (A) band (B) bracket (C) arch wire (D) buccal tube (E) headgear tube, (F) elastic hook, (G) ligature tie.

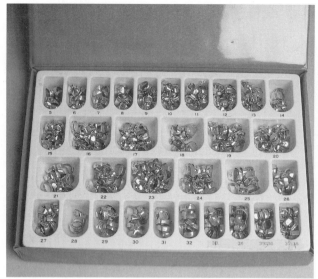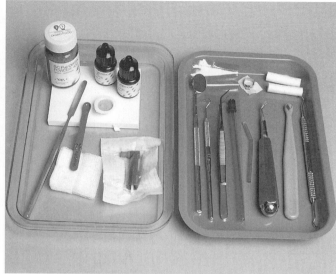

Figure 54-29 Band-sizing armamentaria.

This is one reason why bands may be tried on in advance using the patient's study model to save chair time. Banding takes place after placement and removal of separators (Figure 54-29A).

Selected bands are tried on the patient's teeth using finger pressure initially then seated with a band seater for posterior teeth (Figure 54-30) or a band driver and mallet for anterior teeth. The band must adapt well to the tooth in all areas; there should not be any open spaces between the band and tooth, as this will promote trapping plaque and debris that will contribute to the decay process. If the band adapts well except for a small area, it can be corrected by closing the space with a band pusher (Figure 54-31). The band pusher burnishes the band to conform to the shape of the tooth. Some helpful suggestions to keep in mind while sizing bands are:

- The gingival lumen of the band is larger than the incisal or occlusal lumen.

- The widest circumference of the tooth will determine the band size.

- The band should fit snugly around the occlusal margin.

- The band should not impinge on gingival tissues.

- The bracket should be centered on the facial surface.

- The occlusal margin should be in close proximity to the marginal ridge.

- The band and bracket do not interfere with the opposing arch.

- The gingival margin is well adapted to the tooth.

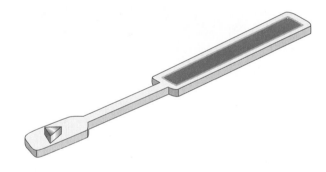

MOLAR BAND SEATER

Figure 54-30 Band seater for posterior teeth.

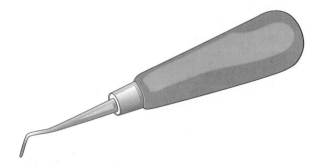

LIGHTWEIGHT BAND SEATER AND PUSHER

Figure 54-31 Band pusher used to burnish the band to the contour of the tooth.

● When force is applied, it should only be applied to welded areas of the band and not the tooth.

● The band should be checked for looseness.

● A bracket-positioning gauge (Figure 54-32) should be used to determine the correct distance between the slot of the bracket to the incisal edge or occlusal plane.

When the bands have been selected and tried in, the orthodontist inspects and makes final adjustments prior to cementation.

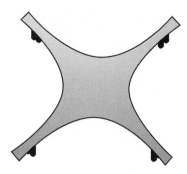

Figure 54-32 Bracket-positioning gauge to determine correct distance from slot of bracket to incisal edge or occlusal plane. [Copyright © 3M (IPC) 1999. All rights reserved.]

Procedure 59 Cementing Orthodontic Bands

Materials Needed

Sized orthodontic bands
Cotton rolls
2 x 2" gauze squares
Chilled glass slab
Orthodontic cement and liquid
Flexible spatula
Squares of masking tape for each band
Band pusher
Band adapter
Band driver and mallet
Anterior band remover
Posterior band remover
Sickle scaler
Bracket wax or Chap Stick
HVE (high-volume evacuator)
Basic set

Instructions (See Figure 54-29B)

1 Document sizes of bands for each tooth receiving one. Thus, if a band becomes loose or fails, it is easier to find a replacement.

2 Arrange all bands in order of cementation according to orthodontist's preference. Place each band on a square of masking tape with the gingival side up.

3 Coat each bracket with wax or Chap Stick to prevent cement contamination in those areas where cement removal may be difficult.

4 Patient's teeth should be coronal polished and ready to receive bands.

5 The teeth should be isolated with cotton rolls and dried using the air syringe.

6 On a chilled glass slab, the dental assistant mixes sufficient cement according to manufacturer's instructions.

7 Using the spatula, the bands are filled with cement from the gingival side, one at a time. It is important that the entire interior of the band is covered with cement.

8 The filled band is passed to the orthodontist, who seats it immediately. The dental assistant passes the seating instruments and continues to keep the isolated teeth dry. The patient is told to bite down on the seating instrument until the band reaches its final position.

9 The next band is filled with cement and passed to the orthodontist and the procedure is repeated until all bands are seated.

continued

continued from previous page
Procedure 59 Cementing Orthodontic Bands

Removal of Excess Cement

1 The sickle scaler is used to remove excess "set-up" cement. Large chunks of cement are removed initially and should be placed onto a 2 in. x 2 in. gauze square rather than into the high-volume evacuator.

2 When removing excess cement in close proximity to the band, care should be taken not to undermine the cement line. The tip of the scaler should be at a 90° angle to the surface where the tooth and band meet (Figure 54-33).

3 The teeth should be flossed and rinsed. The brackets and tubes should be inspected for any excess cement.

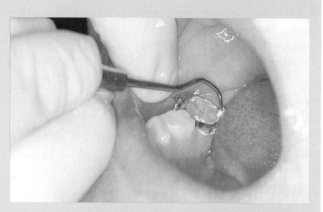

Figure 54-33 To remove excess cement, tip of scaler is placed at 90° angle where the tooth and band meet. (Courtesy of Rita Johnson and Vincent DeAngelis.)

Bonding. Bonding refers to orthodontic brackets that are directly bonded to the tooth. The bracket has a base or pad located behind it. The pad has a mesh screen that aids in retaining the bracket to the tooth. Each pad is conformed to the shape of the tooth for adequate fit. The material used to bond the bracket to the tooth is composite resin, either the self-curing or light-curing type.

Indirect Bonding Method. There are two methods of bonding brackets to the teeth, indirect and direct. The indirect method uses the concept of bonding all the brackets together at one time. To accomplish this, the brackets are positioned on the patient's study model with an adhesive in exactly the same location as when they will be bonded on the teeth. An impression is taken of the model with all brackets in position, which are trapped in the impression and then transferred to the patient's mouth and bonded "en masse" using composite resin material. The teeth receiving the brackets should be prepared by cleaning the facial surfaces with a fluoride-free pumice slurry, rinsed thoroughly, and dried. The facial surfaces of the teeth are acid etched with an etchant gel or liquid, rinsed again, and dried thoroughly just prior to bonding.

Direct Bonding Method. In the direct method each bracket is bonded separately. The teeth to be bonded are usually the anterior teeth and sometimes the premolars (see Procedure 60). Molars are usually banded to provide strength for the arch wire and headgear.

Arch Wires. Arch wires are shaped in the form of the dental arch to fit into the buccal tubes (attachment on the molar band that receives the arch wire; Figure 54-28D) and seated brackets. Arch wires are made of stainless steel, titanium alloy or cobalt-chromium and supplied in a variety of thicknesses, sizes, and shapes. Some very common shapes are the twisted, round, edge-wise rectangular, and square. The arch wire is primarily responsible for tooth movement, and the type of movement will determine which arch wire is used.

The orthodontist bends the arch wire to guide the force that will move teeth. The arch formation card is used to help to determine where the bends are placed. Once prepared, the arch wire is first positioned in one buccal tube, then placed in each bracket of one side of the mouth using the Winegart pliers, and then positioned in the buccal tube of the opposite side of the arch and placed in each bracket on that side. The arch wire is trimmed at its distal ends with a distal end cutter (Figure 54-34). To hold it in each bracket, it must be secured with ligature ties. Some brackets are "self-locking," which require a special tool to open and close the appliance (Figure 54-35).

Ligature Ties. **Ligature ties** are made of thin wire or elastomeric material and utilized to tie the arch wire to the brackets on the bands or teeth. The thin wire ligature ties are made of flexible stainless steel wire that has a loop in the center, which fits around the bracket, and

Procedure 60 Direct Bonding Method

Materials Needed

Selected brackets already prepared and conformed for each tooth

Acid etch gel or solution

Composite resin material

Pumice slurry, prophy cup, and slow handpiece

HVE (high-volume evacuator) and saliva ejector

Sickle scaler

Bracket tweezers

Lip and cheek retractors

Absorbent wedge

Cotton rolls

Basic set

Instructions

1 Selected brackets are placed in order of bonding.

2 Patient's teeth are cleaned with fluoride-free pumice slurry, thoroughly rinsed, and thoroughly dried (the presence of fluoride conflicts with the bonding action).

3 The lip and cheek retractors are positioned, and cotton rolls and absorbent wedges are placed near the Stensen's duct of the parotid gland to control moisture. A saliva ejector is also used.

4 The teeth must not be contaminated by saliva or by any other means.

5 The teeth are etched with phosphoric acid. Caution should be used during this step and the patient should be warned to close the eyes.

6 The etchant is rinsed thoroughly, at least 15–20 seconds per tooth, and evacuated with HVE. The teeth should be thoroughly dried and should appear chalky and dull where etched.

7 The dental assistant prepares the composite resin, spreads it on to the mesh base portion of the bracket, then using the bracket tweezers, immediately transfers it to the orthodontist.

8 The orthodontist seats the bracket on the tooth using a scaler or explorer to push it in place and also begins to remove excess resin with the scaler before it completely hardens.

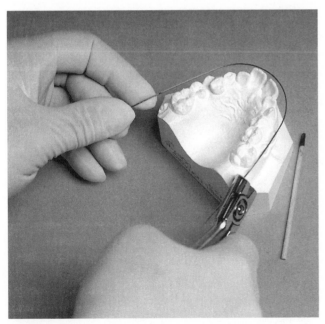

Figure 54-34 Arch wire trimmed with distal end cutter at distal of buccal tubes on molar band (Courtesy of Rita Johnson and Vincent DeAngelis.)

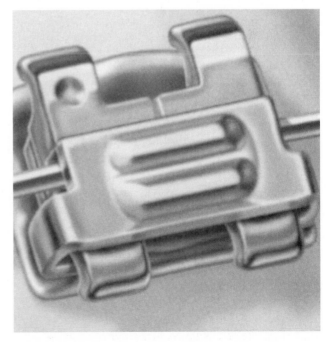

Figure 54-35 Self-locking bracket not requiring ligature ties. (Courtesy of Dwight H. Damon.)

long extensions that are used for tying the pigtail (Figure 54-36). The elastomere ties are doughnut shaped, are made of plastic, and have the ability to stretch when placed around the brackets (Figure 54-37).

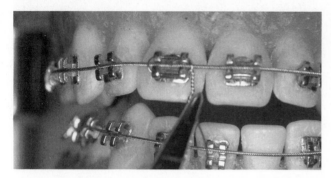

Figure 54-36 Using wire ligature tie to secure arch wire. (Courtesy of Rita Johnson and Vincent DeAngelis.)

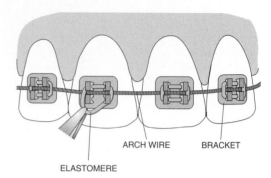

Figure 54-37 Using elastomere tie to secure arch wire with a mosquito hemostat.

Procedure 61 Placing and Removing Wire Ligature Ties

Materials Needed

Wire ligature ties
Ligature-tying pliers or hemostat
Ligature cutter
Ligature tucker or director
Sickle scaler

Instructions

Placement

1 Place a 90° bend on the loop of the wire ligature tie. This will aid in conforming around the bracket when pulled through the bracket wings.

2 Position the bent ligature tie so that it engages both occlusal and gingival bracket wings simultaneously.

3 Once engaged under all four bracket wings, pull both ends away from the tooth.

4 Grasp the two ends and twist them once. Position one wire on each beak of the ligature-tying pliers and lock both wires around the knob of the pliers.

5 Squeeze gently on the handles of the pliers and begin twisting the wires to form a braid, or "pigtail." Rotate the pliers at least six times while gradually diminishing the squeezing pressure on the handles. The pliers are removed and the wire is cut after all tie wires are placed.

6 The wires are cut with a ligature cutter leaving a pigtail of 3–5 mm.

7 Using a ligature tucker, tuck each pigtail under the arch wire. Check with finger tip to see that pigtails are not extended out, causing trauma to tissues.

Removal

1 Using a sickle scaler, pull out the pigtail so it can be grasped.

2 Using the ligature cutter, cut the ligature across from the pigtail (Figure 54-38), grasp the pigtail with the cutter, and gently remove the tie.

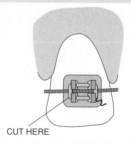

CUT HERE

Figure 54-38 Removing wire ligature tie, cut across from pigtail.

Procedure 62 Placing and Removing Elastomeric Ties

Materials Needed

Elastomere ligature ties
Mosquito hemostat
Sickle scaler

Instructions

Placement

1 Grasp an elastomere ligature tie with the mosquito hemostat, making certain that the beaks of the hemostat go up to the lumen of the tie.

2 Start positioning the tie under one bracket wing and stretch it across to the next bracket wing,

continue until the tie encircles all bracket wings (see Figure 54-37).

3 Release the ligature from the hemostat.

Removal

1 Using a sickle scaler and fulcrum, grasp one portion of the elastomere ligature tie.

2 Start unhooking the gingival bracket wings, and then proceed to the occlusal/incisal bracket wings until the tie is free.

3 Remove tie.

Instructions to the Patient. Once banding and bonding are completed and the arch wire is ligated, the patient needs to be aware of how to care for them. It should be stressed to the patient that if any appliance becomes loose, the office should be notified immediately for a replacement. The patient and parent are given the following instructions:

● How to brush the teeth and appliances using an orthodontic toothbrush and enforce the seriousness of having a daily routine of brushing (see Figure 54-13). Explain that poor oral hygiene will lead to irritated and swollen gums and decalcification with possible caries, especially under the margins of the appliances.

● How to floss the teeth using a floss threader (see Figure 54-14).

● Fluoride rinsing should be used.

● Foods such as hard or sticky candy, nuts, or any hard-to-chew foods, including ice, which would cause appliances to bend or break, should be avoided.

During the corrective orthodontic phase, the patient will be expected to see the orthodontist on a regular basis. Appointments for arch wire adjustments, reinforcing oral hygiene, and progression of tooth movement are evaluated. The amount of time for this phase of treatment differs from case to case. When the corrective phase ends, removal of appliances takes place. This is a lengthy appointment, one that the patient has been waiting for with great anticipation.

Elastics. Small rubber bands are used for exerting forces between maxillary and mandibular arches or within the same arch to close spaces. When ligation takes place from a maxillary bicuspid to a mandibular molar, distal movement will occur for the maxillary bicuspid because molars remain stationary.

Debanding and Debonding. Debanding means that the band is to be removed from the tooth. To accomplish this, it is necessary to first remove the ligature ties, then the arch wire, and lastly the band itself:

● Band-removing pliers are used to remove the band (Figure 54-39).

● The metal beak is placed underneath the bracket and the plastic beak is placed on the occlusal or incisal edge of the tooth; the handles of the pliers are closed,

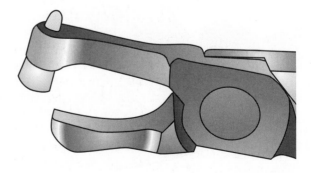

Figure 54-39 Band-removing pliers, used for debanding. [Copyright © 3M (IPC) 1999. All rights reserved.]

placing an occlusal/incisal motion as the band is loosened.

● The remaining cement is removed using a sickle scaler or ultrasonic scaler.

● The mouth is rinsed and an HVE is used to remove loose cement particles.

● The teeth are polished with a prophy cup and paste.

Debonding takes place when the bonded brackets are removed. Sometimes it is preferable to debond brackets while still attached to the arch wire, eliminating the steps of removing ligature ties and the arch wire. Also, by using this method, it is less likely that the patient would swallow or choke on a loose bracket:

● Using the debonding pliers, both beaks are placed underneath the bracket, between the base and the tooth.

● The handles of the pliers are squeezed together to lift off the bracket.

● Once brackets are removed, the composite resin that still remains on the tooth will be removed by the orthodontist. The high-speed handpiece with a carbide finishing bur is used. It is advisable to avoid using the water spray to be able to differentiate the composite resin from the tooth.

After the procedure of debanding and debonding, the orthodontist will take alginate impressions to construct a retainer or positioner that will begin the retentive phase.

Retentive Orthodontic Care

As teeth have moved during the corrective phase, they are now in their newly found positions where they must stay. However, because the newly positioned teeth are not yet completely stabilized, they will tend to return to their former positions. One way to deal with this problem is to use **retainers** (fixed or removable appliances used to hold teeth in place) or **positioners** (an appliance that

will help maintain the teeth in their new positions after orthodontic treatment).

Fixed and removable appliances are used in this phase: fixed retainers, removable retainers, and positioners. If the orthodontist can get the patient's full cooperation, a positioner may be suggested initially.

The Positioner. An alginate impression and a bite registration are taken during the final debanding appointment. The impression is poured in plaster, and construction of the positioner takes place after small changes are made on the models where the teeth are slightly repositioned to simulate final alignment. The positioner is made of soft pliable plastic resembling a mouth guard (Figure 54-40).

The positioner is used only with patients whose cooperation level is high because it covers all surfaces of all teeth, making speech impossible. Its primary function is to allow the alveolar bone to strengthen and to adjust occlusion into its final position.

Instructions to the Patient

● The positioner must be worn for several hours every day, including sleeping hours.

● The patient must exercise by clenching the arches for several seconds and relaxing while wearing it.

● The positioner must be brushed with a toothbrush and toothpaste each time it is removed from the mouth.

● The positioner should be kept in a container when not being worn to ensure that it is kept clean and safe from damages.

Fixed Retainer. A fixed retainer is one that is cemented or bonded to the teeth. It is usually located on the mandibular anterior between the two cuspids or first bicuspids. If cemented, the tooth receiving the band is the anchor for the retainer. If bonded, the retainer is bonded to the lingual surfaces of the anchor teeth. The purpose for using a fixed retainer is to stabilize the anterior teeth and to retain them in their new positions.

Instructions to the Patient

● The appliance is not to be removed.

● Teeth in that area must be brushed very carefully and all food debris should be removed from the wire.

● The office should be notified immediately if the retainer becomes loose.

Removable Retainer. Alginate impressions are made and poured in stone to fabricate the retainer. The new retainer is composed of an acrylic base that fits the palate with clasps that attach to key teeth and a labial wire to hold those teeth in position. Minor adjustments

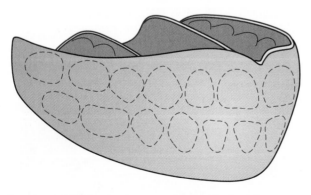

Figure 54-40 Positioner used to retain teeth in new positions.

such as closure of spaces and slight realignment of teeth are made when the retainer is worn. A very commonly known retainer of this type is the Hawley retainer (Figure 54-41).

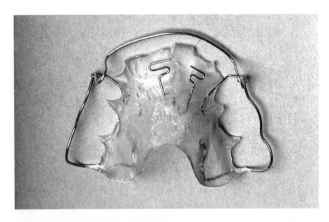

Figure 54-41 Hawley retainer with clasps and labial wire to retain teeth in new positions.

Instructions to the Patient

● The maxillary removable retainer is seated by placing the labial wire facially to maxillary anterior teeth. The thumb is used to place pressure on the palate area and the retainer is pushed up until the clasps are fully seated. Removal is accomplished by pulling down on the clasps, not the labial wire.

● The mandibular removable retainer is seated by placing the labial wire facially to the mandibular anterior teeth. Two index fingers are placed on each side of the appliance and pressed downward to seat. Removal is similar to the maxillary retainer.

● Retainers should be worn most of the time except at mealtime. The orthodontist should prescribe the number of hours per day.

● Retainers should be cleaned daily. The retainers should be held in the palm of the hand and brushed inside and out using a hand brush and soap instead of a toothbrush and toothpaste.

● Care should be taken to not drop the retainers.

● Retainers should be in either the mouth or the retainer case.

● Retainers should never be put in the pocket, as they may be crushed or lost.

● Retainers should never be put in a lunch bag, as they could be thrown away.

● The patient should never adjust retainers; the orthodontist is the only person to do this.

● Retainers should be brought to each appointment to be checked or adjusted.

Posttreatment Diagnostic Records

The orthodontist documents the results of orthodontic treatment by having the patient undergo radiographic and photographic evaluation and impressions for final study models:

● *Radiographs.* Cephalometric and panoramic radiographs are taken to detect the amount of root resorption, position of teeth, and presence of third molars.

● *Photographs.* Intraoral and extraoral photographs are taken to compare the "before and after" graphic results.

● *Study models.* Alginate impressions are taken and poured in plaster of Paris to retain a record and for observation of final position of teeth.

SUGGESTED ACTIVITIES

● On models that already have malocclusions, determine which ones are class I; class II, division I; class II, division II; and class III.

● On a model that was determined to have a class II, division I malocclusion, measure the overjet distance between maxillary and mandibular incisors.

● On a model with an overbite condition, measure the amount of overlapping of maxillary incisors over mandibular incisors.

● Secure a cephalogram and make a tracing on tissue paper using the information provided in this chapter. Find and draw the Frankfort plane, mandibular plane, facial plane SN plane, NA plane, and NB plane.

● Place brass wire separators between mandibular molars, stainless steel spring separators between bicuspids, and elastomeric ring separators between anterior and bicuspid teeth on a typodont.

● Place an arch wire, inserting it in the buccal tubes using the Winegart pliers and ligate it with wire and elastomeric ligature ties using appropriate pliers and instruments.

REVIEW

1. Match the terms on the left with their definitions on the right:

___ a. Neutrocclusion
___ b. Mesiocclusion
___ c. Distocclusion
___ d. Overjet
___ e. Overbite
___ f. Bruxism
___ g. Osteoclasts
___ h. Osteoblasts
___ i. Crossbite
___ j. Openbite
___ k. Prognathic
___ l. Retrognathic

1. Maxillary incisors protrude horizontally over mandibular incisors
2. Specialized bone-forming cells
3. Involuntary grinding or clenching of the teeth
4. When there is no overlap but an open space between incisal edges
5. Specialized bone-destroying cells
6. Mesiobuccal cusp of maxillary first molar is aligned with mandibular first molar buccal groove
7. Greater than normal overlap of incisal edges between maxillary and mandibular central incisors
8. Profile with a prominent chin
9. Mesiobuccal cusp of maxillary first molar is aligned between mandibular second bicuspid and first molar
10. When maxillary anterior incisals or posterior buccal cusps are in linguoversion position and do not overlap mandibular teeth
11. Profile of a weak chin
12. Mesiobuccal cusp of maxillary first molar is aligned between the mandibular first and second molars

2. Match the orthodontic appliances on the left with the appropriate statement on the right:

___ a. Separators
___ b. Band
___ c. Bracket
___ d. Ligature tie
___ e. Buccal tube
___ f. Arch wire
___ g. Elastics
___ h. Headgear
___ i. Removable retainer
___ j. Positioner

1. An extraoral device used to control orthopedic growth
2. A thin wire or elastomeric loop used to tie the arch wire to the bracket
3. A wire shaped in the form of the dental arch that fits into the buccal tubes that is attached to the brackets to provide tooth movement
4. Small rubber bands used to exert forces
5. Made of soft pliable plastic to keep teeth in their new positions
6. An attachment to the band or tooth that provides a means for the arch wire to be secured
7. Where the ends of the arch wire are secured
8. Used to open up a space interproximally to seat bands
9. A metallic ring that is cemented on the tooth
10. Composed of acrylic base with clasps that attach to key teeth with a labial wire to hold teeth in position

Endodontics

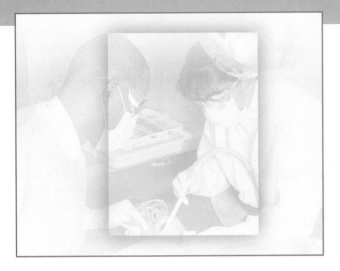

Introduction

Endodontics, also referred to as root canal therapy, is the branch of dentistry that specializes in the diagnosis and treatment of the tooth pulp and periapical tissues. This makes it possible to save a tooth that, otherwise, would be lost by extraction.

Although the general dentist may provide endodontic treatment, the option to refer the patient to an endodontist is often chosen.

When endodontic treatment has been successfully completed, the specialist refers the patient to the general dentist. A permanent restoration is then placed.

Some indications for endodontic treatment are:

● The tooth pulp is grossly inflamed or in a necrotic state. **Necrosis** means the death of cells due to the loss of blood supply, bacterial toxins, or physical and chemical damage.

● The tooth can be restored to function after endodontic treatment.

● Endodontia may be chosen in conjunction with periodontal therapy as a means of saving the tooth.

● The natural tooth (teeth) can be maintained in the dental arch following endodontic treatment.

Endodontic treatment is not recommended for teeth that cannot be restored to function or be maintained because of the weakness of the periodontal support. The tooth may become mobile in the socket, because infection or injury has affected the supporting tissues of the periodontium.

OBJECTIVES

After studying this chapter, the student will be able to:

● Describe the purpose of endodontics.

● Describe various methods of performing clinical examination that aid in providing diagnostic evaluation.

● Explain the contraindications when using an electronic pulp tester.

● Describe the procedure for using an electronic pulp tester.

● Explain the difference between vital pulp capping, pulpotomy, and pulpectomy.

● Explain the difference between apexogenesis and apexification.

● Give the purpose for each item listed for a root canal treatment.

● Explain the reason for using a dental dam when performing endodontic procedures.

● Indicate the rationale for measuring each reamer and file used within the pulpal canal.

● Indicate which medicaments are used for disinfecting the pulpal canal.

● Explain the procedure when performing an apicoectomy.

Planning for Treatment

The potential endodontic patient may call the dental office complaining of severe pain. Others may complain of intermittent discomfort, with a feeling of tenderness and pressure in a particular area of the dental arch.

The general dentist may see the patient and determine the reasons for the complaints. Usually dental radiographs of the periapical area are made to determine the degree of disease. If the tooth appears to have involvement of the apex or apices of a multirooted tooth, the patient will be referred to an endodontic specialist (endodontist) for treatment.

Clinical History and Examination

When the patient is referred to the endodontic office, a complete medical and dental history is recorded. Antibiotics may be prescribed before treatment begins. For this reason, any sensitivity to a particular antibiotic must be determined prior to further treatment.

Radiographs

A periapical radiograph is made of the tooth in question. To ensure that no distortion occurs, it may be wise to expose a second film using a different angulation as a means of comparing the length of the root(s), surrounding alveolus, and periapical tissues. During the process of treatment, radiographs will be made to determine (1) the trial length of the endodontic instrument during the shaping phase of the canals (2) if the master cone is in the desired location and (3) if the final obturation of the canals is satisfactory.

Palpation and Percussion

Palpation of the tooth, surrounding tissues, and soft tissues of the face and neck is performed by the dentist. Palpation means exerting light pressure of the operator's fingers to a body surface. *Percussion* involves tapping of a body part to determine the condition of the body parts beneath. In this case, the incisal edge or occlusal portion of the tooth or teeth in a quadrant are tapped with an object such as the handle of the mouth mirror to establish the amount of sensitivity of the tooth in question. Palpation and percussion are used simultaneously. Not only is the tooth in question tested but adjacent and opposing teeth as well (Figure 55-1).

Thermal Sensitivity

The tooth may be tested for a reaction to hot and cold. A cylinder of ice (made by filling empty anesthetic car-

tridges with water and freezing them) or dry ice [carbon dioxide (CO_2)] held in a gauze square is brought into contact with the tooth. The tooth is then touched with heated gutta percha (Figure 55-2) or a heated ball burnisher instrument or a dry prophy cup is rotated on the tooth to produce frictional heat.

In a clinical examination, cold will stimulate the sensation of pain. The inflamed pulp violently reacts to the application of heat. Relief from this pain may be controlled by a second application of cold. This condition is termed advanced acute **pulpalgia** (severe constant pain in the pulp) associated with **irreversible pulpitis** (inflammation and deterioration of the pulp requiring endodontic treatment).

When the tooth lacks sensation to the cold and hot application, an acute apical abscess may be present and the tooth is said to be necrotic or nonvital (Figure 55-3). If the tooth is vital, it will react with a sharp pain initially that will quickly disappear after removal of the stimulus. If the tooth is nonvital or has a necrotic pulp, the tooth will have no response. If the tooth is diseased, the pain increases in intensity and remains even after removal of the stimulus.

Transillumination

The transillumination test is helpful for teeth in the anterior arch. Because of their position in the arch, a fiberoptic light can be placed on the lingual surface. The light will be reflected through the enamel and dentin.

The dentist can compare the translucency of the tooth with that of other teeth in the arch. Translucency means that the tooth structure allows the light to pass through, making the inner structures visible.

Selective Anesthesia

When a patient complains of pain "somewhere" in the arch but is unable to indicate its source, the dentist may

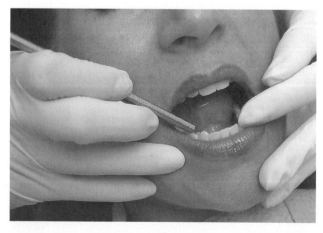

Figure 55-1 Percussion test using instrument handle.

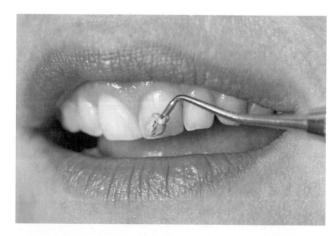

Figure 55-2 Thermal sensitivity test using heated gutta percha.

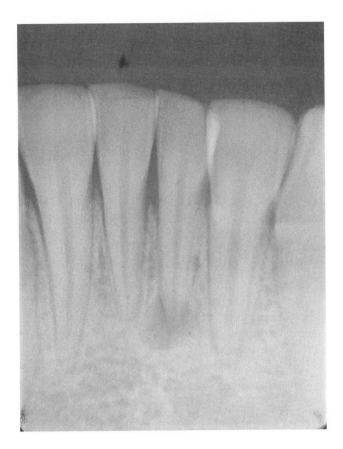

Figure 55-3 Apical abscess viewed on a radiograph. (Courtesy of Clifton A. Caldwell.)

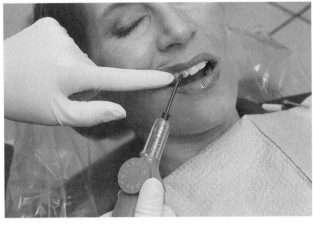

(A)

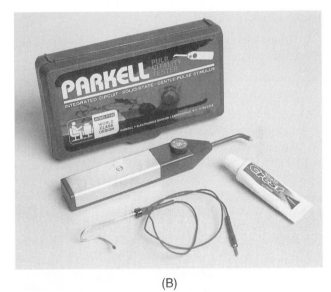

(B)

Figure 55-4 (A) Using a pulp tester. (B) Pulp tester.

suggest selective anesthesia. Local anesthesia is administered and the conclusions drawn by process of elimination. Selective anesthesia is generally limited to the maxillary arch due to the fact that all of the teeth in one quadrant of the mandibular arch become anesthetized when anesthesia is administered there. Thus, selective anesthesia would not be of value in the mandibular arch.

Mobility

The dentist checks the tooth for mobility by using the handle of an instrument and a finger. If the tooth is abnormally mobile, it may be associated with periapical involvement and bone deterioration.

Electronic and Digital Pulp Tester

The pulp tester (vitalometer or digital) is used to measure the vitality of a tooth. It has a control knob to regulate and limit the voltage during the testing period (Figure 55-4A). There are pulp testers that function with electrical current, others that are battery operated, and the latest models have a digital readout. It should be noted that the electric or battery-operated pulp tester uses a control to determine when the patient feels sen-

sation and the digital pulp tester produces a visible readout (Figure 55-4B).

Because of patient apprehension and fear, the use of the test is explained to the patient before the procedure is begun. The patient is told that a slight warm tingling sensation may be felt, and as soon as the sensation is registered, the test on that tooth will cease.

Helpful Factors to Consider When Using the Pulp Tester

1. The current stimulates the nerve fibers in the pulp by way of the dentin layer. The electrode (the point from which a discharge of current takes place) is applied to the cervical third, being the thinnest area of the tooth's enamel.

2. It is used as a diagnostic tool in determining the vitality of a tooth. This procedure involves compar-

ing responses of a suspected tooth with that of a normal tooth.

3. The response of a tooth to an electrical impulse does not mean that the tooth has a healthy pulp, nor does it indicate the degree of pathology of pulpal tissue. It does indicate the degree of vitality or nonvitality of a tooth as compared with other teeth in the same and opposite quadrants.

4. Molars and premolars do require higher intensity than incisors because of their size.

5. The thickness of enamel and dentin combined with recession of the pulp will cause changes in response.

Contraindications. Avoid using the electronic pulp tester on:

1. Patients who wear a pacemaker, as the pulp tester could alter its function

2. Endodontically treated teeth for comparison purposes, as they will be unresponsive

3. Primary teeth, which have large pulp chambers, as they may be subject to intensified electrical current transmission

4. Teeth with extensive metallic restorations that cover three-fourths or more of the crown, as they may be subject to intensified electrical current transmission

5. Persons whose physiological and psychological state is unsuitable, as their confidence must be gained first

6. Teeth not thoroughly dried or electrode placed too close to gingiva, as this will elicit a false reading

Evaluation of Testing Responses

- *Normal pulp*—will react to an impulse, but the pain will disappear as soon as the impulse is removed.

- *Hyperemic pulp*—responds to slightly less current than the normal pulp due to the presence of the first stage of inflammation where excessive blood is present in the pulp. **Hyperemia** means presence of excessive blood. At this stage the pulp should recover without endodontic treatment.

- *Reversible pulpitis*—**reversible pulpitis** responds to much less current than a normal pulp. It is more

---

Procedure 63 Using an Electronic Pulp Tester

Materials Needed

PPE (personal protective equipment)
Pulp tester
Cotton rolls
Toothpaste
Gauze sponge, 2 x 2 in.
Saliva ejector

Instructions

1 Explain the procedure to the patient and instruct him or her to raise a hand when sensation is felt.

2 Isolate the teeth with cotton rolls. Cotton rolls must not touch the teeth.

3 Dry the teeth and surrounding gingiva using air syringe. Presence of moisture will give a false reading. Place a saliva ejector for moisture control within the oral cavity.

4 Place a small amount (pea size) of toothpaste on a 2 x 2 in. gauze sponge. Draw from this toothpaste to place a very small amount on the tip of the electrode probe.

5 Find a finger rest to provide stability and control.

6 With the dial set at zero, place the electrode on the facial side of the tooth at the gingival third. When a tooth has multiple roots, the electrode may also be placed on the lingual side.

7 Begin increasing current flow by turning the knob until the patient responds. Note the reading, return the dial to zero, and remove the electrode.

8 Use the following teeth for comparative purposes: the two teeth adjacent to the suspected tooth and the **contralateral tooth** (a comparable tooth located on the opposite side of the same arch).

9 Record responses on patient's chart for all teeth tested.

hyperreactive. A tooth that is hyperreactive will react more readily to the stimulus than a normal tooth. There is inflammation of the pulp; however, there is still a chance for the pulp to recover without endodontic treatment.

● *Irreversible pulpitis*—response to stimulus is hypoactive. A tooth with a hyporeactive (lower response) pulp will react more weakly to the stimulus. There is inflammation and deterioration of the pulp and the tooth will most likely undergo endodontic treatment.

● *Necrotic pulp*—there is no response to stimulus. A tooth with a necrotic pulp will not register at all. It will need to undergo endodontic treatment.

● *Alveolar abscess* (collection of pus in the alveolar bone surrounding a tooth), **granuloma** (collection of granular tissue at the apex of a tooth due to inflammation), or **cyst** (encapsulated sac containing fluid, semifluid, or solid material)—there will be no response to stimulus and the treatment will include drainage of abscess, antibiotic regimen, and endodontic treatment.

Culture

After the tooth has been opened and prior to final restoration, a culture may be used as a diagnostic tool to determine the presence of bacteria within the canal. A paper point is inserted in the pulpal canal to gather a specimen, which is placed in a test tube with culture medium and incubated for a minimum of 72 hours at 98.6°F temperature. If the specimen becomes cloudy, there is evidence of bacterial growth and the test is termed positive; if it is clear, there is no bacterial growth and the test is termed negative.

Types of Endodontic Treatment

When treating a tooth endodontically, it is essential to use a dental dam. Only one hole is punched for the tooth receiving treatment. Purposes for dental dam use in endodontics are:

● To improve visibility

● To prevent moisture contamination

● To prevent contamination of medicaments with the oral cavity when irrigation is performed

● To prevent contamination of infection with the oral cavity

● To prevent accidental inhalation or swallowing of small instruments

Local anesthesia is used initially in each type of endodontic treatment for patient comfort. However, when treating the same tooth in subsequent appointments, anesthesia may not be required.

Vital Pulp Capping

Pulp capping involves traditional methods of therapy to stimulate pulp regeneration. Indirect pulp capping is used when there is danger of exposing the pulp if all carious tissues (enamel and dentin) are removed. Direct pulp capping is used to treat a pulp that has been mechanically exposed during an operative procedure of preparing a tooth for a restoration. Calcium hydroxide is used when the lesion is in close proximity to the pulp.

Pulpotomy

Pulpotomy refers to partial removal of vital pulp that lies within the crown of a tooth, leaving the root portion intact, therefore keeping the tooth vital. The object of this procedure is to stimulate the tissue in the root canal(s) to form a bridge of secondary dentin over the pulpal root tissue while maintaining vitality of the roots. This procedure, also known as **apexogenesis**, works well for the young patient when the root portion is not fully developed. Thus, the tooth is retained, allowing full development of the root.

If the tooth is necrotic, the pulpal tissues are subject to **debridement** (removal of foreign or dead tissue) and **extirpation** (complete removal or eradication of soft tissue) and treated with calcium hydroxide, extending into the root canals, then sealing the apex with zinc oxide–eugenol (ZOE) followed by zinc phosphate cement. This procedure is called **apexification** (complete removal of pulpal tissues of a necrotic primary tooth with anticipated results of forming a calcified plug to seal the apex). At a later date, the patient is reexamined and a radiograph made of the treated tooth to determine if the apex is sealed and has become calcified. If the treatment was successful, a pulpectomy is performed *without* the use of gutta percha for final pulpal restoration. Refer to Chapter 53.

Pulpectomy

A pulpectomy, also known as root canal treatment, involves the surgical removal of the vital pulp from a tooth. The term pulpectomy is used to describe the method used when removing vital pulp. Trauma-related injuries of the pulp include cysts, periodontal involvement, and other inflammation. The number of treatment appointments depends on the extent of pulpal destruction and the endodontist's discretion.

Procedure 64 Pulpectomy/Root Canal Treatment

Materials Needed

PPE (personal protective equipment)
Topical and local anesthesia set-up
Dental dam set-up
Basic set-up
Friction grip burs for high-speed handpiece
Latch type large round burs for contra-angle handpiece
Luer-Lok or irrigating syringe filled with saline solution (NaOCl)
Luer-Lok or irrigating syringe filled with sodium hypochlorite
Formocresol, Chlorobutanol, Ethylenediaminetraacetic acid (EDTA)
Cotton pellets, 2 x 2 in. gauze sponge
Endodontic explorer
Endodontic spoon excavator
Assortment of endodontic instruments (broaches, files, reamers, lentulos, Peeso reamer, and Gates-Glidden drill)
Endodontic measuring stops
Millimeter ruler
HVE (high-volume evacuator)
ZOE or cavit
Condenser

Instructions

1 Topical and local anesthesia is administered.

2 Dental dam and the clamp are placed only on the tooth to be endodontically treated. The dental dam is disinfected by using cotton pliers and a large cotton pellet dipped in sodium hypochlorite or chlorobutanol to wipe the area.

3 Using the high-speed handpiece and bur, the tooth is opened on the occlusal aspect of posterior teeth or lingual aspect of anterior teeth, as the dental assistant uses the HVE (high-volume evacuator).

4 A large round bur is used in the contra-angle slow-speed handpiece to remove gross decay.

5 A spoon excavator is used to remove debris and pulpal tissue.

6 The endodontic explorer is used to locate the root canal. The pulp chamber is irrigated with saline solution while the dental assistant uses the HVE (Figure 55-5). The dental assistant should be warned not to use the air or water syringe once the pulp chamber is open due to possible contamination.

7 When the root canal is located, a smooth broach is inserted and used as a pathfinder. If the root canal is large enough, a barbed broach is inserted to remove pulpal tissue.

8 A Gates Glidden drill in a contra-angle handpiece is used to further open the canal for easier access and visibility.

9 A small endodontic file is inserted to determine the length of the canal and to start shaping it.

10 While the file is in the canal, a dental film is exposed and immediately processed to determine the length of the canal.

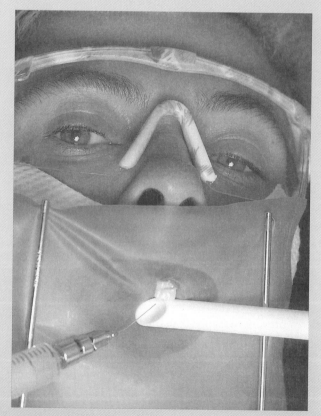

Figure 55-5 Irrigating the pulpal canal using syringe and HVE.

continued

Continued from previous page
Procedure 64 Pulpectomy/Root Canal Treatment

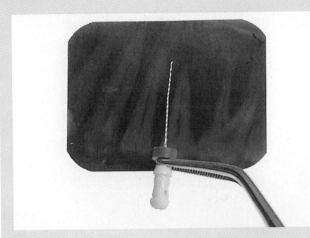

Figure 55-6 Measuring the canal using a radiograph.

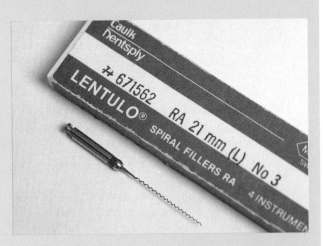

Figure 55-7 A lentulo used for transporting cement sealer to the pulpal canal.

11 If the radiograph indicates the file is of the appropriate length, it is measured with the millimeter ruler and the size recorded in the patient's chart. The dental assistant uses endodontic measuring stops to measure subsequent files and reamers (Figure 55-6).

12 As the canal is being shaped and extirpated while using files, it must be kept moistened with saline solution.

13 The endodontist may opt to use canal enlargement and cleaning materials such as ethylenediaminetetraacetic acid (EDTA), which allows for a chemo-mechanical action to occur. These materials soften the dentin canal walls for easier canal shaping.

14 The endodontic canal is irrigated with sodium hypochlorite solution to cleanse it while the dental assistant uses the HVE.

15 The canal is dried with paper points that have already been trimmed with scissors to avoid penetrating apical tissues. At this point, the canal may be restored temporarily or permanently according to the endodontist's decision.

16 In preparation for obturating (filling) the pulpal canal, a gutta percha point that corresponds to the size of the last file used is measured for length and size. To determine the fit, a radiograph is made. If the gutta percha point fits adequately whereby it fills and seals the canal up to 1 mm from the apex, it is named the **master cone**.

17 The master cone is disinfected and set aside while the root canal sealer is mixed on a sterile glass slab with a sterile spatula. When the cement is ready, a lentulo is used to transfer the sealer to the root canal, where it is deposited (Figure 55-7). The master cone is also coated with the sealer and placed in the canal.

18 A spreader is used to condense the cone laterally and at the same time make room for auxiliary gutta percha points. These are coated with the sealer and added to the canal as space permits (Figure 55-8).

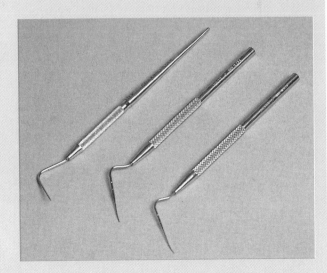

Figure 55-8 Spreaders used for lateral condensation of gutta percha in the pulpal canal.

continued

19 When filled, the protruding gutta percha points are cut off with a heated instrument at the level of the pulpal chamber. Endodontic pluggers are used to condense the material within the chamber (Figure 55-9).

20 The tooth is usually restored with temporary cement such as Cavit or ZOE until a permanent restoration is placed at a later time.

21 A radiograph is made of the restored tooth prior to patient dismissal, the dental dam is removed, and the height of the temporary restoration is checked with articulating paper. The patient is referred back to the general dentist for final restoration.

22 The patient returns to the endodontist at a designated time, usually three months, for a follow-up appointment.

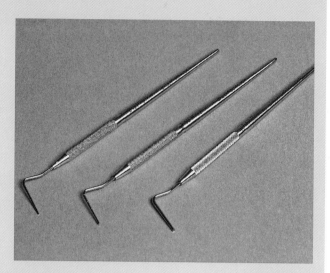

Figure 55-9 Pluggers used for condensing gutta percha in the pulpal canal.

Apicoectomy

An apicoectomy is a surgical procedure where the apical portion of the tooth is excised. Not only is the apex removed but also the diseased infected tissues surrounding it.

A surgical incision on the overlying tissues is made and retracted, and the bone is opened using a high-speed bur and handpiece. While using the bur, the apical portion of the tooth is removed and the apex of the root prepared to receive a restoration (Figure 55-10). Periapical

curettage takes place by scraping and cleaning out the diseased and infected tissues with a dental surgical curette (Figure 55-11). The surgical area is irrigated with saline solution and evacuated using a surgical aspirator.

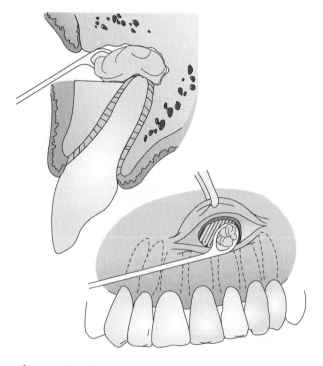

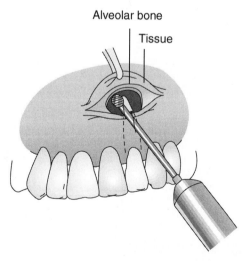

Figure 55-10 Apicoectomy surgical procedure where the apex of the tooth is removed.

Figure 55-11 Periapical curettage whereby infected and diseased tissues are removed with a surgical curette.

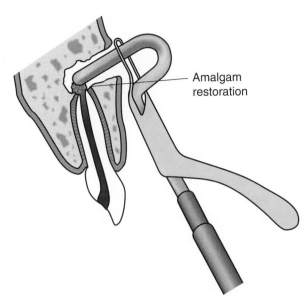

Figure 55-12 Retrograde restoration placed to seal the apex of endodontically treated tooth (Instrument not in proportion with tooth).

The pulpal canal of the tooth is restored with gutta percha. A **retrograde restoration** (tooth is filled at the root end) is placed to seal the apex of the tooth (Figure 55-12). The restorative material may be amalgam, composite resin, or gutta percha. The surgical incision is sutured and the coronal portion of the tooth restored with temporary cement until healing takes place. The patient is given verbal and written instructions to follow in case of bleeding, swelling, pain, antibiotic therapy, foods to avoid, and care of the oral cavity. The patient should be made aware of the importance of informing the office personnel should any problems arise.

Postoperative Follow-up. The patient returns within a few days for postoperative examination and removal of sutures, then is referred back to the general dentist for permanent restoration.

As a general rule, after completion of endodontic treatment and the postoperative appointment, the dentist will request the patient to return at periodic intervals. These intervals may vary from three- to six-month periods up to a period of several years.

A posttreatment radiograph is made to determine the elimination of infections and the extent of regeneration.

Endodontic Instrumentation and Armamentarium

- A *Gates Glidden drill* is a long-shanked bur that only cuts tooth structure laterally. It is used on a slow-

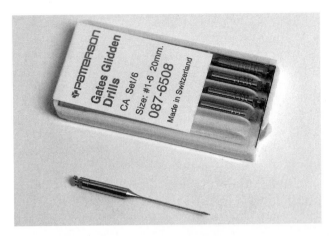

Figure 55-13 Gates Glidden drills/burs.

speed latch-type handpiece to gain access into the canals and further shape and taper the canals (Figure 55-13).

- A *Peeso reamer/drill* is another long-shanked rotary instrument also used on a slow-speed latch-type handpiece to prepare post space for teeth that have lost most of the coronal portion. A post is cemented inside the root canal and a core is built onto it to provide stability for the new crown. The Gates Glidden bur and Peeso reamer/drill are supplied in six sizes, numbered from 1 to 6. To identify which size bur is being used, the manufacturer marks the instruments with notches that correspond to the number of the instrument, i.e., for a number 3 there would be three notches.

- *Broaches* are small instruments that are manufactured as smooth or barbed, are supplied in various sizes from xxx-fine to coarse, and are color coded to match the sizes of files and reamers. The smooth broaches are used initially as pathfinders to explore the root canal and the barbed broaches are used to remove material such as pulpal tissues, paper point particles, or any debris that has become trapped in the canal (Figure 55-14). As a rule, barbed broaches are used

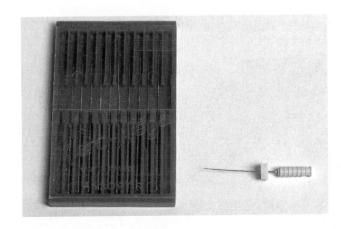

Figure 55-14 Barbed broaches.

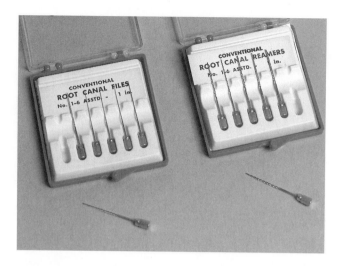

Figure 55-15 Files (left side) and reamers (right side).

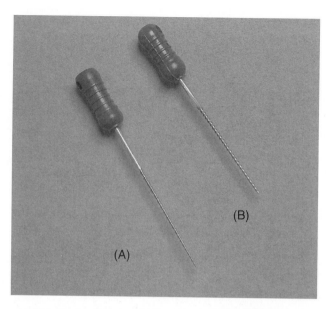

Figure 55-16 (A) K-type file. (B) Hedstrom file.

one time only due to the delicate nature of the instrument as they become brittle after sterilization.

● *Reamers* are supplied in various sizes and are used to clean and enlarge the root canal. There are reamers with longer handles for use in anterior teeth and reamers with smaller handles for use in posterior teeth that may also be used on anterior teeth (Figure 55-15).

● *Files* are also supplied in the same sizes as reamers and are used to enlarge and smooth the root canal. The cutting edges of files are more horizontal and closer together than those of reamers, where the edges spiral down and are further apart. There are two types of files, the standard or K-style (Figure 55-16A) and the Hedstrom (Figure 55-16B). The K-style is rotated within the tooth and pulled out to widen the canal. The Hedstrom file is used without rotating the instrument inside the canal; instead the mode of action is a push-pull in and out of the canal.

Sizing and color coding for reamers, and files. The numbers represent the diameter of the instrument at its tip, i.e., size 15 is 0.15 mm in diameter at the tip (Table 55-1). The length ranges between 21 and 25 mm.

● *Endodontic measuring stops*, also known as rubber stops, are small round discs made of silicone rubber material. They are made with a built-in hole in the center to place on the instrument shaft of files and reamers to mark for proper canal length. The length of the canal is obtained from a radiograph using a millimeter ruler. This information is used to mark the instruments (files and reamers) with measuring stops based on the measurement obtained (Figure 55-17).

● An *endodontic millimeter ruler* is used to determine the length of the root when placing endodontic measuring stops.

● *Lentulos*, also known as paste fillers, are spiral instruments used to carry root canal cement apically in a clockwise rotation. They are used with a contra-angle

Table 55-1	Sizing and Color Coding for Reamers and Files		
Color	Number	Number	Number
Pink	6		
Gray	8		
Purple	10		
White	15	45	90
Yellow	20	50	100
Red	25	55	110
Blue	30	60	120
Green	35	70	130
Black	40	80	140

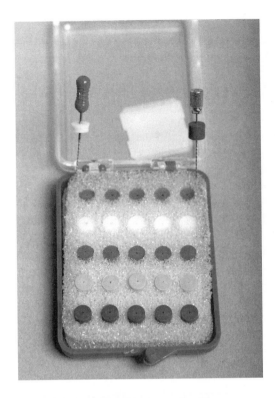

Figure 55-17 Endodontic measuring stops.

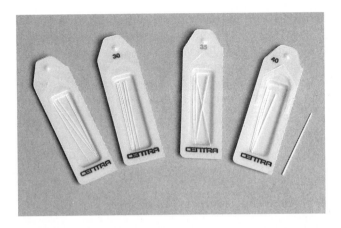

Figure 55-18 Assorted paper points.

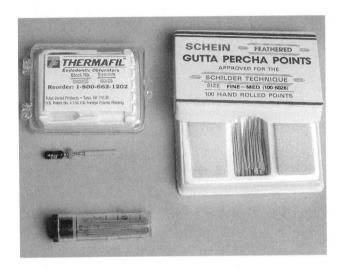

Figure 55-19 Assorted gutta percha points.

handpiece at low speed and are supplied in sizes 25–40, which correspond with root canal instrument numbers.

- *Absorbent paper points* are used to dry endodontic canals, apply medicaments, and take cultures. They are supplied in various sizes that correspond with root canal instrument numbers. They are usually trimmed with scissors to conform to the length of the canal to avoid protruding the apex of the tooth and injuring the periapical tissues (Figure 55-18).

- *Gutta percha points* are used to **obturate** (fill) the canal permanently and are made of a rubbery organic material that changes to a soft consistency when heat is applied. With obturation, root canal epoxy cement is used. Gutta percha points are supplied in sizes that correspond with root canal instrument numbers (Figure 55-19).

- *Silver points* are used to permanently obturate the canal. Although scarcely used currently, they are utilized in combination with gutta percha points to obturate and properly seal the canal.

- An *endodontic spoon excavator*, a double-ended instrument with a long shank capable of reaching deep in the canal, is used to remove deep decay and excess cement material (Figure 55-20A).

- An *Endodontic explorer*, a double-ended instrument with long pointed working ends is capable of reaching into the openings of the root canals (Figure 55-20B).

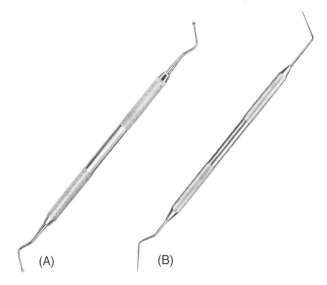

(A)   (B)

Figure 55-20 (A) Endodontic spoon excavator. (B) Endodontic explorer. (Courtesy of Hu-Friedy Mfg. Co., Inc.)

- *Endodontic spreaders* are long pointed instruments used during lateral condensation of gutta percha. When the spreader is inserted between the master gutta percha cone and walls of the canal, it pushes the material laterally while making room for inserting auxiliary gutta percha points. This procedure continues until the canal is filled (see Figure 55-8).

- *Endodontic pluggers* are used after the spreaders. They are long condensors that have a flat surface at the end of the instrument. With all the pieces of gutta percha inserted, the plugger condenses the material vertically into a compact mass (see Figure 55-9).

- *Luer-Lok syringes* with large (size 23 or 25) blunt needles are used for irrigating the pulpal chamber and canals.

- *Endodontic medicaments:*
  1. *Irrigating solutions* are used to irrigate the canals, remove debris and foreign substances, and cleanse the pulp chamber and root canals. For the irrigation process, a Luer-Lok syringe is used to draw the solution from its container. Included are sodium hypochlorite, hydrogen peroxide, saline solution, sterile water, alcohol, and chlorinated soda.
  2. *Preparations used for cleaning and enlarging root canals* are supplied in paste form. The composition of the paste allows for a chemo-mechanical action to occur whereby the material softens the canal walls and smoothes calcium deposits, thus eliminating surface irregularities. Included are Root Canal Prep Paste, EDTA, and citric acid.
  3. *Disinfectants* include formocresol (FC), which contains formaldehyde, cresol, and glycerine. A small amount is applied to the walls and deep in the preparation with a cotton pellet that has been pat dried on a gauze sponge; this preparation will remain in the chamber between appointments. Chlorobutanol and camphorated parachlorophenol (CMPC) are also applied when disinfecting root canals and treating periapical infections.
  4. *Root canal sealer/cement* is utilized for permanent sealing and cementation of gutta percha or silver points. This type of cement usually has a longer working time, sometimes as much as 20 minutes, as opposed to other dental cements. Included are ZOE sealer; Tubliseal, also ZOE type; and Sealapex, a noneugenol calcium hydroxide polymeric resin.

Sterilization and Disinfecting Methods

Several sterilization and disinfection methods are used before, during, and after an endodontic procedure

(Refer to Chapter 8). Autoclave, disinfecting solutions, flame, and glass bead/salt sterilizers, are all used according to the dentist's preference.

- Autoclave is the most desirable method of sterilization. However, there are some instruments that may become brittle after its use.

- Disinfecting solutions are used primarily to ensure that the working field is safer from microorganism contaminants. Wiping down the dental dam with a disinfectant such as iodine solution, sodium hypochlorite, or chlorobutanol will minimize bacterial contamination. Disinfecting the environment within the tooth with medicaments will ensure a more successful treatment.

- Flame is employed chairside to reestablish sterility of instruments during root canal therapy.

- Hot bead/salt sterilizer is the method used at chairside to reestablish sterility of small instruments during the procedure.

SUGGESTED ACTIVITIES

- Using a periapical radiograph, measure the length of the canal in millimeters from the occlusal to the apex of the tooth and practice placing a stop on the instrument.

- Study the small endodontic instruments (reamers and files) and identify them by color and number.

- Identify the long-shanked burs by the number of notches on each bur and determine which type of burs they are (Gates Glidden or Peeso reamer).

- Practice mixing root canal sealer cement and determine how much working time is available.

- Using cotton pliers, practice passing paper points to a fellow classmate, directing the paper point in the appropriate direction (for maxillary or mandibular teeth).

REVIEW

1. Indicate which examination and diagnostic tests are used in endodontics: (1) alginate impressions for diagnostic casts, (2) transillumination, (3) electronic and digital pulp testing, and/or, (4) thermal sensitivity testing.
   a. 1, 2, 3
   b. 2, 3, 4
   c. 1, 2, 4
   d. 1, 3, 4

2. The purpose for using radiographs is to:
   a. Detect incipient caries
   b. Check bone level
   c. Determine if the master cone is in the desired location
   d. Determine the length of paper points

3. Name the contraindications for using a pulp tester: (1) primary teeth, (2) patients who wear a pacemaker, (3) teeth with a class V composite restoration, and/or (4) teeth restored with extensive metallic restorations covering three fourths or more of the crown.
   a. 1, 2, 3
   b. 2, 3, 4
   c. 1, 2, 4
   d. 1, 3, 4

4. Indicate which irrigating solutions are used for cleansing the pulp and root canals: (1) sodium hypochlorite, (2) ethylenediaminetetraacetic acid, (3) hydrogen peroxide, and/or (4) saline solution.
   a. 1, 2, 3
   b. 2, 3, 4
   c. 1, 2, 4
   d. 1, 3, 4

5. Match the endodontic instruments and materials on the left with their purposes on the right:

   ___ a. Gutta percha
   ___ b. Spoon excavator
   ___ c. Pluggers
   ___ d. Spreaders
   ___ e. Measuring stops
   ___ f. Lentulo
   ___ g. Reamer
   ___ h. File
   ___ i. Barbed broach
   ___ j. Peeso reamer
   ___ k. Gates Glidden drill

   1. Used to remove debris trapped in the canal
   2. Used to clean and enlarge the root canal
   3. Long-shanked bur that cuts tooth structure laterally
   4. Spiral instrument used to carry cement apically
   5. Rubbery organic material used to fill the canal permanently
   6. Used to condense gutta percha laterally
   7. Used to enlarge and smooth the root canal
   8. Used to prepare post space in the canal
   9. Small round discs used to mark the length of the canal
   10. Long condensors with a flat surface at the tip of instrument
   11. A double-ended instrument with a long shank used to remove deep decay

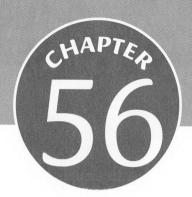

Prosthodontics

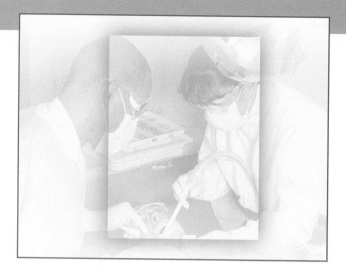

OBJECTIVES

After studying this chapter, the student will be able to:

● Determine the differences between a removable partial prosthesis and a fixed prosthesis.

● Name parts of a removable partial prosthetic appliance.

● Describe the process for delivery of an immediate denture.

● List and describe the types of cast crowns used in fixed prosthodontics.

● Describe the instructions given a patient for prosthetic appliance care.

● Determine the difference between a denture reline and rebase.

● Describe the difference between a three-quarter and a seven-eighths crown.

● Summarize the procedure for preparing a tooth to receive a crown.

● Describe the three types of implants used in dentistry.

Introduction

Prosthodontics is the branch of dentistry that is concerned with the diagnosis, planning, construction, and insertion of artificial devices, or prostheses. A **prosthesis** is the replacement for one or more teeth and associated tissues.

Prosthodontics has three main branches: removable prosthodontics, fixed prosthodontics, and dental implants.

Removable Prosthodontics

The primary objective of removable prosthodontics is to replace missing dentition and restore occlusion with an appliance that the patient removes for cleaning and, with little difficulty, repositions.

Two major groups of removable prostheses are removable partial dentures and removable complete dentures.

A removable partial denture replaces one or more teeth in one arch and is retained and supported by the underlying tissues and some of the remaining teeth.

Removable complete dentures replace all of the teeth in one arch. A full denture is retained and supported by the underlying tissues of the alveolar ridges, hard palate, and oral mucosa.

Removable Partial Dentures.

The basic goals of the partial denture are to restore missing teeth and to preserve the remaining hard and soft tissues of the oral cavity. The partial denture is designed to distribute the forces of mastication between the abutments and alveolar mucosa, enabling them to resist the stress of those forces. An **abutment** is a natural tooth or implant that becomes the support for the replacement tooth or teeth.

Advantages of a Removable Partial. Advantages of a removable partial include:

● Fewer intraoral procedures, chair time, and appointments are necessary.

● Good hygiene of the oral cavity is maintained by the patient, because the prosthesis is removable.

● When several teeth are missing in both quadrants of an arch, a removable partial denture will restore a long span of lost dentition.

● The removable partial denture makes it unnecessary to reduce tooth structure on primary or permanent dentition of children and adolescents. The appliance can also be replaced to compensate for the growth of the child.

- In the case of a cleft palate, the removable appliance may have an added obturator. An **obturator** is that portion of a prosthesis used to close a congenital opening or cleft of the palate.

- The removable prosthesis may be designed to support periodontally involved teeth.

Other Considerations for a Partial Denture

- There must be a number of sufficiently positioned teeth in the arch to support and stabilize a removable prosthesis.

- To retain the appliance, there must be adequate root structure of the remaining teeth.

- The patient must exhibit enthusiasm for maintaining good oral health.

Treatment Planning for a Partial Removable Prosthesis.

The treatment plan may involve operative dentistry, periodontic, endodontic, or surgical procedures before the construction of a partial denture. Such treatment must be completed and healing taken place before prosthodontic preparation can begin.

Diagnosis and Treatment Planning.

A preliminary appointment is scheduled for examination of the patient. Accurate preliminary impressions for producing study models and working casts are taken. Review Chapter 44 for more information on taking alginate impressions.

Radiographic films of the partially **edentulous** (without teeth) mouth are exposed and processed by the dental assistant. Review Chapter 66 for the technique. Instant-type (Polaroid) photographs are made of the patient, including full face, frontal view, and profile, with a close-up of the anterior teeth overbite.

Consultation Visit.

The dentist explains the diagnosis, the proposed treatment plan, and the prognosis and answers any questions and concerns expressed by the patient.

As with other dental procedures, a cost estimate is prepared and presented to the patient during the consultation visit. The dental laboratory fee for constructing the prosthesis is taken into consideration.

When the patient has accepted the treatment plan, a suitable financial plan is approved, and necessary appointments are made for treatment.

Component Parts of a Partial Removable Prosthesis

- The **framework** is the metallic portion of the removable denture that provides strength. It contains the base connector, lingual or palatal bar/major connector, clasps/retainers, and rests (Figure 56-1A).

- The **connector** (palatal strap or lingual bar) is the metal or acrylic bar that connects the right side of the partial denture with the left side (Figure 56-1B). A base connector is the metal portion of the framework that connects to the saddle/base (Figure 56-2C). A

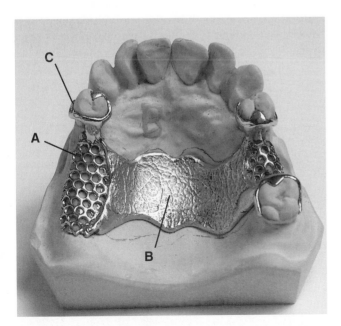

Figure 56-1 Component parts of a maxillary partial denture: (A) framework; (B) Connector (palatal strap); (C) clasp (retainer).

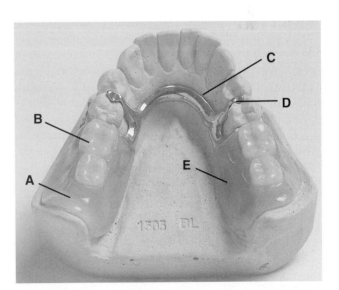

Figure 56-2 Component parts of a mandibular partial denture: (A) saddle (base); (B) Artificial teeth; (C) connector (lingual bar); (D) occlusal rest; (E) flange.

stress breaker is a metal mechanism built in the framework to ease the stresses placed on the abutment tooth during mastication.

- The **clasp/retainer** is the semicircular metallic projection that surrounds the abutment tooth providing retention to the prosthesis (Figure 56-1C).

- The **saddle/base** is the acrylic resin portion attached to the framework that holds the artificial teeth and contacts the tissue (Figure 56-2A).

- **Artificial teeth** are made of acrylic or porcelain. Acrylic teeth are less durable while porcelain teeth tend to fracture and are prone to making clicking noises when the prosthesis is loose. The anterior teeth have a pin on the posterior side and the posterior teeth have a hollow portion underneath, making it possible to connect them permanently to the acrylic base of the prosthesis (Figures 56-2B and 56-4A, B).

- The **rest** is a metallic projection that fits on the occlusal or lingual aspect of a tooth to prevent the prosthesis from seating too far gingivally (Figure 56-2D).

- The **flange** is the acrylic extension of the saddle or base that reaches the border of the prosthesis (Figure 56-2E).

Preparation Appointments. The first appointment, following radiographs and preliminary impressions for study models, is to prepare the abutment teeth located in close proximity to missing teeth where support is needed to anchor and stabilize the prosthesis. Abutment teeth are used to support a clasp and are prepared by grinding a portion of the tooth to receive a rest that will lend support and provide stability for the prosthesis. During this appointment final impressions using rubber-based, silicone elastomeric impression material or polysiloxane are taken to provide an accurate replication of the dental structures. An alginate impression of the opposing arch and a bite registration are made to ensure a good relationship between maxillary and mandibular arches; see Chapter 46 for elastomeric impressions and bite registration. Artificial teeth are selected according to shade and **mould** (shape of artificial teeth). The tooth-shade selection is made according to the age and skin tone of the patient; natural teeth will darken as a person ages. Using a moistened shade guide and in natural light, the shade is selected. The impressions and bite registration are disinfected and readied for the laboratory technician, who pours the impression in stone and begins constructing the framework for the partial denture. A detailed written prescription including the patient's name, age, gender, desired prosthesis design, shade, mould, and due date is made and sent with the impressions. A copy of the prescription is kept in the patient's chart.

The next appointment is made for a try-in of the cast framework with artificial teeth set in wax. During this appointment the patient's occlusion is checked, any needed adjustments are made on the framework, the artificial teeth are repositioned while they are still in wax, and the shade of the teeth is evaluated for esthetic appeal. The framework is disinfected and returned to the laboratory technician, who completes the construction of the partial denture.

Delivery of the Prosthesis. Usually, a 20–30-minute appointment is sufficient time to deliver the removable partial denture.

The new prosthesis is disinfected and rinsed before it is placed in the patient's mouth. The dentist places the appliance in the patient's oral cavity and makes necessary adjustments.

The patient is then given a short 10–20-minute appointment within a few days after the delivery. At this time, the dentist removes the partial denture, checks the mucosa for any discomfort, and makes necessary adjustments.

The patient is given a recall appointment, usually several months later. These recall visits are important and allow the dentist to evaluate the fit and function of the prosthesis. At the same time, the patient's oral hygiene can also be evaluated.

Removable Complete (Full) Dentures

Complete denture prosthesis is the phase of dental prosthodontics dealing with the restoration of all natural teeth and their associated parts in the dental arch with artificial replacements. When one or both dental arches have been rendered edentulous, a full denture is constructed (Figure 56-3).

Other Considerations for Complete Dentures

- Extensive bone loss and lack of support for teeth remaining in the arch

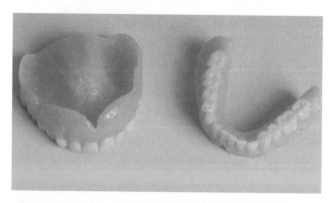

Figure 56-3 Maxillary and mandibular complete dentures.

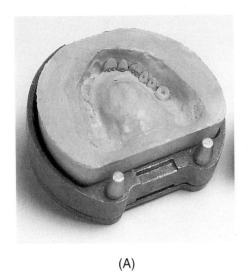

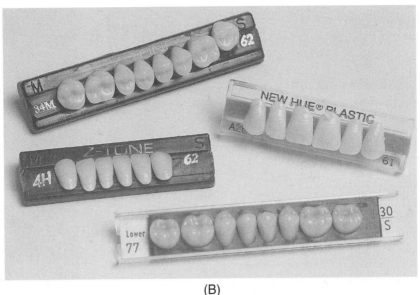

(A)

(B)

Figure 56-4 Artificial teeth (A) showing pins and hollow portions that retain the teeth to the base; (B) sets of artificial teeth.

- Remaining anterior teeth that are involved with gross decay, periodontal disease, or abscesses
- Evidence that oral hygiene has been chronically poor
- Totally edentulous patient

The patient's mental and physical capabilities must be such that he or she is able to accept and wear the prosthesis. Impaired health may contribute to a lack of muscle coordination to retain the denture in place.

Diagnosis and Treatment Planning. A preliminary appointment is scheduled for the dentist and the patient to discuss the need for a complete denture. During this visit, the dentist will examine the patient and review the medical history. The dentist will also prescribe radiographs and alginate impressions for study models (casts). Photographs (instant-type) are made of the full face, frontal view, and profile of the patient.

Preparation of the diagnosis, cost estimate, and treatment plans are much the same as for a partial denture prosthesis.

Component Parts of the Complete (Full) Denture

- The **base** is the portion of the denture made of acrylic resin that seats and makes contact with the tissue underneath. A metallic mesh embedded within the acrylic resin strengthens it.
- Flange refers to the extension of the denture base that reaches from the location of the alveolar ridge to the facial border of the prosthesis.

- Artificial teeth are the same type used on partials and are supplied in groups of six for anterior teeth and in groups of eight for posterior teeth. The moulds of the teeth are designed to be anatomical, simulating the shape of real teeth, or nonanatomical, shaped with little anatomy (Figure 56-4 A, B).

Full Denture Construction. The alginate impressions taken during the preliminary appointment are used to pour stone casts. These may be poured by the dental assistant or referred to the dental laboratory. Custom acrylic denture trays are constructed from the stone casts.

With the custom trays, secondary impressions are taken by using rubber-based, silicone elastomeric impression material or polysiloxane. These impressions are poured in dense dental stone to create the master casts. Secondary impressions provide the basis for the construction of the prosthesis and, therefore, must be accurate.

The maxillary impression must include tuberosities, frenum attachments, and other landmarks of the arch. The mandibular impression must include retromolar pads, oblique ridge, mylohyoid ridge, and the lingual, labial, and buccal frena (frena is plural of frenum).

The dental laboratory will construct a baseplate on the master cast. A **baseplate** is a preformed semirigid acrylic resin material that temporarily represents the base of the denture. Bite rims, made of several layers of baseplate wax, are built on the baseplates. Bite rims register the space provided by the teeth in normal occlusion, or vertical dimension (Figure 56-5).

The baseplate–bite rim is tried in the patient's mouth, and centric occlusion is established by the den-

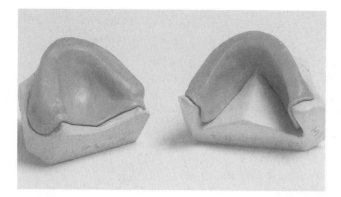

Figure 56-5 Baseplate with bite rims.

tist. Centric occlusion occurs when the jaws are closed in a position that produces maximal contact between the occluding surfaces of the maxillary and mandibular arch.

The final impression involves obtaining the detail of the soft tissues and alveolar ridges. Zinc oxide–eugenol (ZOE) impression paste is flowed into the baseplate.

Artificial teeth are selected according to shade and mould (shape). The tooth-shade selection is made according to the age and skin tone of the patient; natural teeth will darken as a person ages.

The laboratory technician prepares the temporary wax setup of the complete denture(s) on an articulator. This "try-in" consists of the acrylic baseplates, the bite rims, and the artificial teeth set in wax, to resemble gingival tissues. The denture try-in is disinfected before being placed in the patient's mouth (Figure 56-6).

The try-in assembly is disinfected, then returned to the laboratory technician for processing and completion.

The Immediate Denture. The term immediate denture is used to describe a case when the patient's maxillary anterior teeth are the only remaining teeth in the arch. The posterior teeth have been extracted, and the hard and soft tissue areas have completely healed.

The anterior teeth are surgically extracted after the full denture is constructed and ready for delivery. The artificial teeth on the appliance (i.e., the complete denture) replace them. Thus, the patient need not be without teeth, and the denture base will act as a splint during the healing process. Normal resorption during healing of the alveolar ridge will cause changes to occur. The patient returns within 24 hours for the first postoperative follow-up appointment to remove the denture and inspect the surgical site. Sutures are not removed during this appointment but should be within three or four days after surgical extractions.

Because of the changes in the alveolar ridge, the patient must be advised that the immediate denture will need to be relined or rebased within three to six months of the surgery (Figure 56-7A and B).

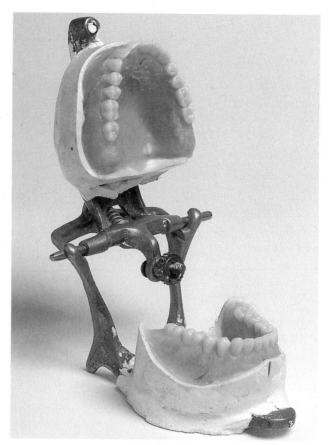

Figure 56-6 Denture temporary wax set-up on an articulator ready for try-in.

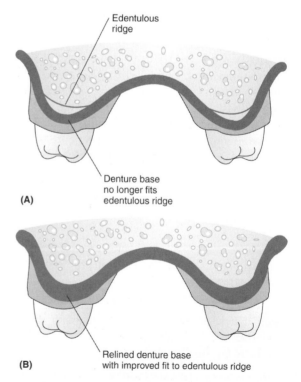

Figure 56-7 (A) Changes in the alveolar ridge. (B) Relined denture base.

Denture Reline. Tissues in the mouth of the patient receiving an immediate denture shrink as healing takes place causing the denture, in time, to have a loose fit. The patient returns within approximately three months for a denture reline. To reline the denture, resin supplied in powder and liquid is mixed according to instructions, spread inside the tissue side of the denture, and repositioned in the patient's mouth where it self-cures in a short time. This resin addition adapts to the tissues and provides a temporary reline.

Denture Rebase. If the denture needs to have a permanent rebase, it means that the entire base of the denture will be replaced, leaving the teeth alone to be reused. The dentist uses the original dentures as trays to take a new impression of the alveolar ridge using elastomeric or ZOE impression paste. The patient needs to understand that the laboratory technician will keep the dentures for a day or two while the procedure is completed. For occasions such as this, it may be prudent for the patient to have a duplicate set of dentures.

Instructions for Prosthetic Appliance Care. Instructions should be given to the patient in verbal and written forms. Prosthetic appliances should:

- Never be allowed to dry out because warping will occur when not surrounded by moisture and so should always be kept in an air-tight, moisture-filled container when not being worn
- Be cleaned and brushed daily with a denture cleaner and water
- Be cleaned over a sink with water, using a towel to cushion the fall if dropped
- Not be soaked in bleach, which may harm it
- Not be worn while asleep, as the tissues of the alveolar ridge need to recover

Fixed Prosthodontics

Fixed prosthodontics is the art and science involved with the complete restoration, or the replacement, of one or more teeth in a dental arch. Fixed prosthodontics is often referred to as crown and bridge work.

Fixed prostheses involve the preparation of abutment teeth to support the replacement of teeth with cast metallic restorations. A **pontic** is the part of the appliance that replaces a missing tooth or teeth. The pontic is fashioned to simulate the incisal edge or occlusal surface of the tooth being replaced. A pontic is the suspended portion of the bridge and has one or more artificial teeth.

The abutment teeth must have stability to support the pontic of the bridge. These restorations are cemented in place to maintain occlusion with the opposing arch.

Diagnosis and Treatment Planning

The dentist reviews the medical and dental history of the patient. Radiographs and impressions for study models (casts) are made. The patient is scheduled for a second visit.

After reviewing the radiographs and study models, the dentist sees the patient to recommend the type of crown and bridge restoration. The fee is explained for the construction of a custom bridge. Often a sample of a crown and bridge is helpful in the patient's decision to accept the treatment plan. The fee for the construction of a bridge is based on the number of units (abutments and pontics) in the bridge.

Types of Crowns

- *Full crowns,* usually made of gold alloy, are precision casts designed to cover the entire anatomic crown of the tooth. Such a crown is often referred to as a full-cast crown or "full gold crown."
- *A Porcelain-fused-to-metal (PFM)* (or veneer) crown is a full metallic crown covered with a veneer. For esthetic reasons, much of the surface of the crown is covered with a thin layer (veneer) of tooth-colored material. Because porcelain is frequently used for the veneer, the crown is so named; however, tooth-colored composite resin materials may be used as well (Figure 56-8A, B).
- *Partial Crowns* are cast restorations that cover three or more, but not all, surfaces of a tooth. A three-quarter crown preparation is made by leaving the facial surface of the tooth intact and by reducing the mesial,

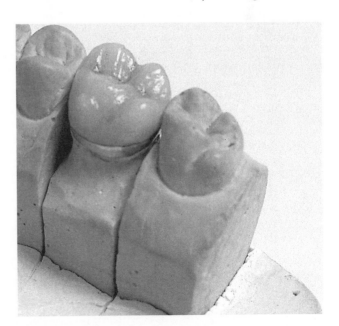

Figure 56-8A Porcelain fused to metal crown.

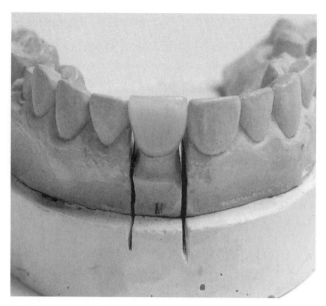

Figure 56-8B Full porcelain crown.

distal, and lingual surfaces, with only a slight reduction of the incisal or occlusal surface of a tooth. A seven-eighths crown preparation is made by reducing the entire crown with the exception of the mesiofacial surface near the occlusal.

Inlays and Onlays

Inlays and onlays are generally made of gold alloy. The tooth is prepared allowing the restoration to be cemented in place as one unit; therefore, the cavity walls are more parallel than the walls prepared for an amalgam restoration. The mechanism that holds the inlay in place is principally the cement. The basic difference between an inlay and onlay is the coverage they provide. Inlays replace the mesial, occlusal, and distal surfaces of posterior teeth, such as MOD, MO, or DO (Figure 56-10A). Onlays replace the same surfaces but also include the cusp tips of the tooth (Figure 56-10B).

Veneers

These are thin layers of tooth-colored material that cover the facial aspect of the tooth (Figure 56-11A, B). They are used in cases of fluorosis or tetracycline-stained teeth and teeth with diastema (large space between two natural teeth) or fractures. The shade for the veneers is selected prior to preparing the teeth. When the tooth is prepared, the preparation includes removing a small amount of tooth structure on the facial aspect extending from the cervical area to the incisal edge. Veneers may be placed on the teeth by either a direct or an indirect method.

Procedure 65 Preparing the Tooth to Receive a Crown (Brief Outline)

1 The anesthetic is administered.

2 The tooth is reduced from all aspects (occlusal/incisal, facial, lingual, mesial and distal) using diamond burs and hand-cutting instruments.

3 Cord retraction is placed in the sulcus of the prepared tooth to isolate it from soft tissues and to control bleeding (hemostasis); (Figure 56-9).

4 Cord retraction is removed, allowing the preparation's margins to be clearly visible.

5 Final impression is made with elastomeric or reversible hydrocolloid materials.

6 The tooth is fitted with a provisional crown.

7 The provisional crown is cemented with temporary cement.

8 The patient is to return for a second appointment within one or two weeks to seat the crown. See Chapter 41 for seating cast restorations.

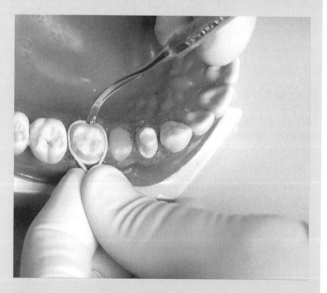

Figure 56-9 Retraction cord placed around preparation for isolation and hemostasis.

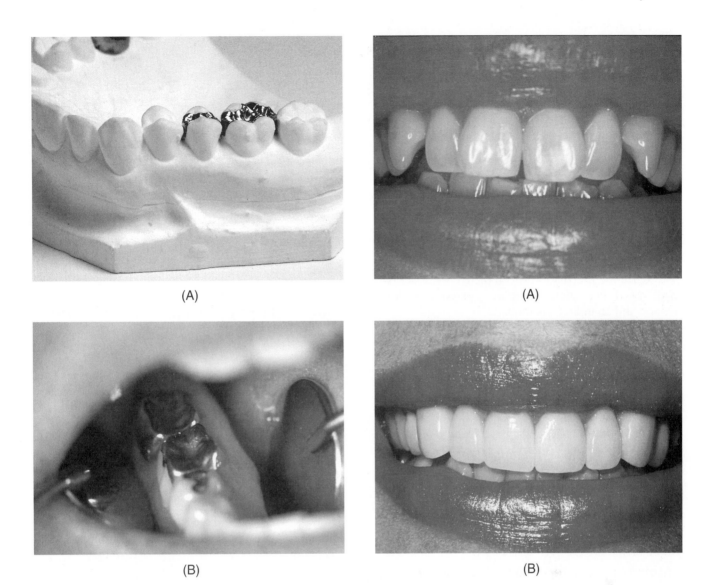

(A)

(B)

Figure 56-10 (A) Gold inlay restorations. (B) Gold onlay restoration.

(A)

(B)

Figure 56-11 (A) Teeth prior to veneer placement. (B) Teeth after veneer placement. (Courtesy of George J. Velis.)

Direct Method. The direct method employs the use of an etchant and bonding agent to prepare the teeth. A composite restorative material is fashioned directly in the patient's mouth. The composite is placed on the facial area and shaped with a plastic form. Excess material is removed before the light cure is applied. After the material is polymerized, the plastic form is removed, and the tooth shape is refined with finishing burs and sandpaper strips. Polishing the tooth completes the procedure.

Indirect Method. The indirect method involves the fabrication of composite or porcelain veneers. After the preparation is completed, a retraction cord is used at the cervical area and impressions similar to that for a crown preparation procedure are taken. The impressions are rinsed and disinfected, then sent to the dental laboratory for construction. If sensitivity is not an issue, the dentist

may opt to not use temporization while the laboratory technician fabricates the porcelain or composite veneers. However, if sensitivity exists, temporary veneers are constructed using bisacryl or other acrylic resins. The procedure for construction and cementation follows the same pattern as for acrylic temporary crowns in Chapter 47.

On the second appointment the veneers are seated. The teeth are prepared by cleaning and drying them thoroughly. To bond the veneers to the tooth, an acid etchant together with a bonding agent and light-cure composite material is used. To finish the procedure, if there is excess composite material around the margins, it is removed with an explorer while the material is pliable before light curing. After the material has cured, diamond burs are used to smooth down and remove excess material. The newly bonded veneers are polished with rubber discs and prophy cups with polishing paste.

Post and Core Restoration for Endodontically Treated Teeth

Endodontically treated teeth are weaker and fracture easier than vital teeth. The purpose for using a post and core is to strengthen the tooth and to provide adequate retention for a cast restoration. The **post** is the metallic pin cemented within the endodontically treated pulpal canal to lend support to a fixed appliance. The **core** is the portion of the endodontic pin that receives the cast restoration. To cement the post, a preparation within the tooth needs to be made. It requires the use of long-shanked burs such as a Peeso reamer/drill. The length of the post is usually one-half to two-thirds the length of the root (Figure 56-12).

Once the preparation is completed, there are two methods of fabricating the post and core, a direct method and an indirect method.

Direct Method. The direct method involves the use of soft wax or acrylic resin to design a pattern for a cast restoration. The wax or acrylic form is fashioned by the dentist directly in the patient's mouth. The completed form will be cast in class III gold alloy by the laboratory technician. A class III gold alloy is a blend of gold with other metals that give it strength. Prefabricated posts are available and may accommodate this method, provided they fit the pulpal canal(s). If compatible, one would be cemented in place, and the dentist could then shape the core to receive a fixed prosthesis that fulfills the needs of the tooth.

Indirect Method. For the indirect method, the dentist will take an elastomeric final impression of the prepared root canal and send it to the laboratory technician, who in turn will fabricate the post and core and cast it in class III gold alloy. The patient returns for final cementation of the post and core. The next step involves preparation of the core to receive a fixed prosthesis, such as a gold crown or PFM. The procedure follows the same pattern as for the crown preparation where final impressions are

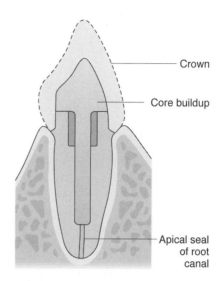

Figure 56-12 Post and core placement in endodontically treated tooth.

taken, a temporary crown is fabricated, and another appointment for seating the permanent crown is made.

Classification of Gold Alloys

To better understand the type of gold used in fixed and removable prosthetics, a summary of available gold alloys is outlined in Table 56-1. There are four types of gold alloys, and they are presented in order of increasing hardness from type I to type IV. The laboratory technician understands the amount of stress that the prosthesis will undergo, and chooses the type accordingly.

Impressions for Fixed Prostheses

Elastomeric impression materials that include polysulfide, silicone, and polivynilsiloxane are used for crown and bridge impressions and are especially suitable for details of impression margins. Review Chapter 45 for construction of custom acrylic trays and Chapter 46 for the use and procedure of elastomeric impression materials.

Table 56-1	Gold Alloys	
Type	**Use**	**Composition**
I	Areas not subject to great stress	Gold, silver, copper, and zinc
II	Primarily for inlays	More copper content than Type I
III	Where stress is greater for crowns and bridge abutments	Additional palladium/platinum, lighter color than gold
IV	Large castings, as for extensive bridges and partial dentures	Considerably more copper

Role of the Laboratory Technician

The dental laboratory technician performs the procedures in crown and bridge construction, including custom trays, pouring the impressions, preparing single tooth dies, articulating stone casts, producing gold alloy castings, and constructing PFMs and porcelain veneers. The technician completes the prosthesis prescribed by the dentist and returns it promptly.

Dental Implants

Dental implants are a stable replacement of natural teeth using a device that is embedded within the tissues. There are three parts to be considered, an anchor, an abutment, and a prosthetic tooth or appliance. The anchor is the metal portion that is surgically implanted within the bone. The preferred metal, titanium, may be coated with a synthetic material that enhances bone formation. The abutment is the connecting part from the anchor to the prosthetic tooth or appliance, and it is inserted surgically after the anchor surgical procedure has completely healed, from three to six months. The prosthetic tooth or appliance (bridge or denture) is constructed by the dentist after healing from both the anchor and abutment surgical placement has taken place.

Authorities in dentistry highly recommend implants when needed. They should be considered only if teeth cannot be saved. An implant should at least have a good prognosis. Determining implant prognosis depends on correct case treatment planning. In other words, the periodontist or oral surgeon must know the medical and dental history and the quantity and quality of remaining bone structure. If these answers are favorable, then an implant can be done. On the other hand, if a tooth has a poor diagnosis and the gingiva is "seeding" bacteria throughout the mouth, the tooth should be removed. According to Thomas J. Kepic, diplomate, American Board of Periodontology, and practicing periodontist, "Keeping your own teeth is inexpensive relative to implants."

Three basic types of implants are used. The endosseous (within the bone) is the most often used dental implant; the subperiosteal (a framework placed under the periodontium and over the bone) and transosteal (transosseous plate that covers a large segment of the mandibular bone), are used in certain conditions.

Metals used most frequently—cobalt alloy, vitallium, ceramic, aluminum, chromium, molybdenum, and titanium—are **biocompatible** (compatible with oral tissues), which makes the implant procedure fairly well received by the tissues.

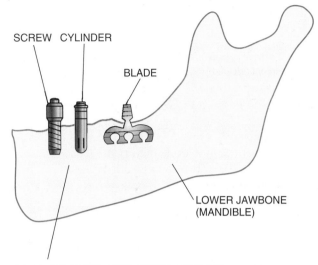

Figure 56-13 Endosseous (endosteal) implant: cylinder, screw, and blade forms. (From *Dental Hygiene Theory and Practice*, by M. Darby and M. Walsh, 1995, Philadelphia: W.B. Saunders. Copyright 1995 by W.B. Saunders. Reprinted with permission.)

The Endosseous (Endosteal) Implant

The endosseous (endosteal) implant is set into the bone and protrudes through the oral mucosa. A fixed or removable partial may be attached to the extension(s) of the implant. Endosseus implants may be designed for a single tooth crown or as an abutment for a fixed bridge. There are two types of endosseous implants, the blade form and the cylinder form (Figure 56-13). The blade form covers a larger span and may include more than one abutment whereas the cylinder form is more widely used and consists of one cylinder with its abutment. This implant involves two surgical appointments. The first appointment is to incise the tissue, then to drill a hole in the bone and fit the implant. Healing time for this procedure and for **osseointegration** (a process whereby the bone grows around the implant and attaches itself) takes three to six months. The second appointment is used to attach the abutment to the implant by surgically opening the tissue above the implant. Once the implant is located through the use of a **template** (a clear plastic device made in the shape of the alveolar ridge with open markings to locate the implant), the abutment is positioned and left on until healing is completed. After final healing, the prosthesis is fabricated and adapted to the abutment (Figure 56-14).

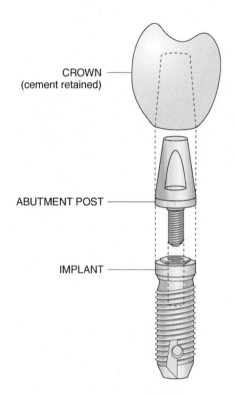

CROWN
(cement retained)

ABUTMENT POST

IMPLANT

Figure 56-14 Parts of an endosseous implant with prosthesis.

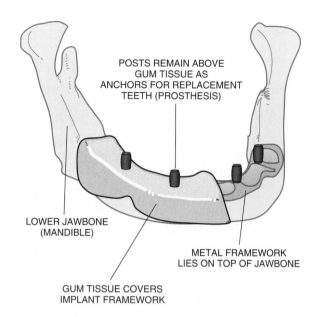

POSTS REMAIN ABOVE
GUM TISSUE AS
ANCHORS FOR REPLACEMENT
TEETH (PROSTHESIS)

LOWER JAWBONE
(MANDIBLE)

METAL FRAMEWORK
LIES ON TOP OF JAWBONE

GUM TISSUE COVERS
IMPLANT FRAMEWORK

Figure 56-15 Subperiosteal implant. (From *Dental Hygiene Theory and Practice*, by M. Darby and M. Walsh, 1995, Philadelphia: W.B. Saunders. Copyright 1995 by W.B. Saunders. Reprinted with permission.)

The Subperiosteal Implant

When a subperiosteal implant is discussed for possible use, the patient must be advised that his or her health must be carefully evaluated. This implant procedure involves at least two occurrences of a surgical nature, and the total health of the patient is something to be considered.

The preparation of an arch for a periosteal implant demands an accurate impression of the alveolar bone of the dental arch. To obtain this impression, the tissue must be surgically incised and retracted to expose the alveolar ridge to the impression material.

After the impression has been taken, the surgical wound is cleansed with a natural saline solution, then sutured. A prepared temporary denture is placed over the wound. The objective is to stimulate the tissue and alveolar bone with a protective covering as healing takes place. Approximately four weeks is allowed for healing.

When the framework implant is ready for insertion, a second surgical procedure is conducted. The original line of incision is reopened and the tissue retracted once again.

After a thorough cleansing with a saline solution, the sterilized framework implant is inserted into place over the alveolar ridge. After the framework implant is seated, the soft tissues are carefully sutured (Figure 56-15). A temporary denture is worn over, and supported by, the protruding projections of the subperiosteal implant.

An alternative way of placing a subperiosteal metal framework implant requires only one surgical procedure. This procedure requires a computerized tomography scan. Using the scan, approximate casts are made. The metal framework implant is constructed on these casts, then surgically inserted in the jawbone.

The Transosteal Implant

The rarely used transosteal implant is limited to the mandible. It consists of a metal plate that is surgically attached to the inferior border of the mandible. It has five to seven pins on the plate located within the bone with two terminal pins that extend into the oral cavity and act as abutments to hold an overdenture. The implant is made of stainless steel, ceramic-coated materials and titanium alloy (Figure 56-16).

The transosteal implant is placed in the patient's mandibular jaw by means of a surgical opening made through the chin. Patients who have an **atrophic** (pertaining to wasting away or reduction in size) edentulous mandible or a deformed mandible are suitable candidates. Implant procedures may be delivered by a dental team, with an oral surgeon or periodontist performing the replacement portion.

Instructions to Patient Following Implant Placement.

● Patient should be encouraged to be meticulous about maintaining good oral hygiene at least once or twice on a daily basis. Using an assortment of brushes of

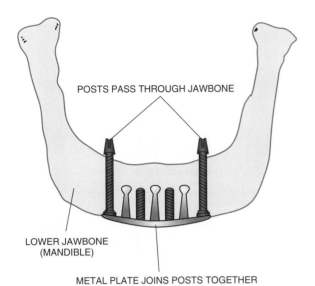

Figure 56-16 Transosteal implant. (From *Dental Hygiene Theory and Practice*, by M. Darby and M. Walsh, 1995, Philadelphia: W.B. Saunders. Copyright 1995 by W.B. Saunders. Reprinted with permission.)

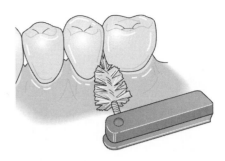

Figure 56-17 Interproximal brush used around implant.

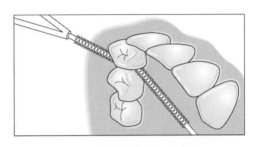

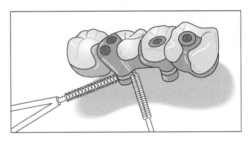

Figure 56-18 Flossing using a shoeshining motion while encircling the implant.

different sizes and shapes with soft bristles that will adapt to the sulcular area of the implant is recommended. These may include small toothbrushes, interdental brushes, electrically powered brushes, and end-tuft interspace brushes (Figure 56-17).

● Toothpastes that are not abrasive should be used. The abrasive type may alter the finish of the implant.

● Flossing must be performed on a daily basis. There are many types of floss that work well. Among these are the regular floss, dental tape, and superfloss; included also are nonfloss items such as shoelaces, yarn, ribbon, and gauze strips. They should be used in a shoeshining motion while encircling the implant (Figure 56-18).

● Weekly appointments should be scheduled following implant placement until healing is completed and the patient is able to control bacterial plaque. Thereafter, three- to four-month recall appointments are made.

● Patients should riinse with an approved antimicrobial (0.12% chlorhexidine gluconate) solution to help minimize bacterial growth during the first month. Thereafter, continued use will stain the teeth.

● Patients should be cautioned about using anything that could scratch or damage the implant, such as safety pins, paper clips, or metal objects, thereby permitting bacteria to become trapped on the implant, causing inflammation or infection.

Awareness of Dental Implant Care within Dental Office. Dental office staff must be knowledge-able in the care of dental implants during the patient's visit. Recently employed staff may not be aware of the special care that must be taken:

● Use of metal instruments should be avoided due to the possibility of marring the titanium surface of the implant, thus encouraging accumulation of bacterial plaque, inflammation, or infection.

● Instruments used for scaling are made of plastic and are Teflon coated, graphite wood tipped, or gold tipped. Gold-tipped instruments cannot be sharpened as this would remove the thin overlay of gold over the stainless steel (Figure 56-19).

● Plastic probe is used.

● Polishing should be done with a rubber cup and a gel dentifrice or tin oxide instead of prophy paste which is abrasive.

● A **porte polisher** (a single-ended handle built with an adjustable loop that holds small wooden points,

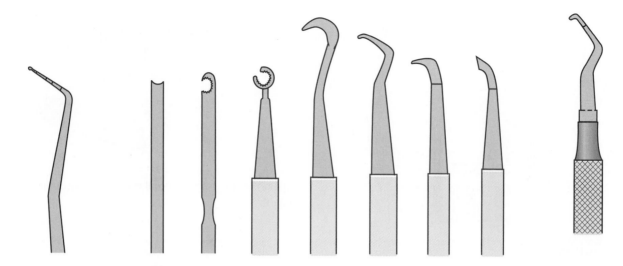

Figure 56-19 Plastic instruments used on implants.

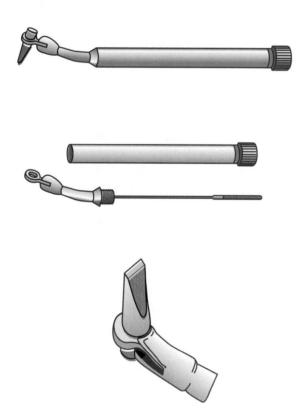

Figure 56-20 Porte polisher assembly with wood points.

used to manually polish teeth) is recommended. However, the wooden points are used only once, then discarded due to the possibility of splintering. The wooden points are available in several standard sizes and shapes (Figure 56-20).

The importance of keeping the implant clean cannot be overly emphasized. This message must be conveyed to the patient for a successful outcome.

SUGGESTED ACTIVITIES

● Find as many different types of prosthetic appliances as possible and describe each.

● Take a set of radiographs on a person who is partially edentulous and process and mount them.

● Holding a removable partial, describe all of its component parts.

● Visit a dental laboratory and inspect the sets of artificial teeth. Identify which ones are anatomically shaped and which ones are nonanatomically shaped.

REVIEW

1. Match the component parts of a removable prosthesis on the left with the description of each part on the right.

   ___ a. Saddle/base
   ___ b. Flange
   ___ c. Connector
   ___ d. Framework
   ___ e. Rest
   ___ f. Clasp

   1. Semicircular metallic projection that surrounds the abutment tooth
   2. Acrylic extension of the saddle that reaches the border of the prosthesis
   3. Acrylic resin portion attached to the framework that holds the artificial teeth
   4. Metallic projection that fits on the occlusal or lingual portion of a tooth to prevent prosthesis from seating too far gingivally
   5. Metallic portion connected to other metallic components that provides strength to the partial denture
   6. Metal or acrylic bar that bridges the right with the left side of the partial

2. During the try-in appointment of a full denture, in what type of material are the artificial teeth placed?
   a. Plaster
   b. Plastic
   c. Impression
   d. Wax

3. What is meant by a denture rebase?
   a. The entire base of the denture is replaced.
   b. The base of the denture is coated with a plastic resin material.
   c. The base of the denture is lined with impression material.
   d. The denture base has self-cured material added while the patient waits.

4. Indicate which of the following appliances are known as fixed prostheses: (1) full gold crown, (2) full denture, (3) porcelain fused to metal crown, and/or (4) veneers.
   a. 1, 2, 3
   b. 2, 3, 4
   c. 1, 2, 4
   d. 1, 3, 4

5. A seven-eighths crown replaces which of the following portions of a tooth:
   a. The entire crown except for the buccal or facial aspect
   b. The mesial, occlusal, and distal portions including the cusps
   c. The entire crown except for the mesiofacial near the occlusal
   d. The entire crown except for the lingual portion

6. The core portion of a restoration for an endodontically treated tooth pertains to:
   a. The portion that was prepared to receive the cast restoration or crown
   b. The portion that is cemented within the pulpal canal
   c. The portion that covers the facial aspect of the natural tooth
   d. The cast restoration that simulates the anatomical crown of a tooth

7. The success of a dental implant is dependent on which of the following: (1) the meticulous care of maintaining good oral hygiene, (2) caution about using anything that could scratch or damage the implant, (3) using any type of toothpaste as long as the teeth and implant are brushed daily, and/or (4) rinsing with an approved antimicrobial solution.
   a. 1, 2, 3
   b. 2, 3, 4
   c. 1, 2, 4
   d. 1, 3, 4

OBJECTIVES

After studying this chapter, the student will be able to:

● Describe factors that contribute to periodontal disease.

● Identify healthy periodontium.

● Identify signs and symptoms of periodontal disease.

● Compare gingivitis with periodontitis.

● Describe the process involved in the formation of a periodontal pocket.

● Identify systemic diseases that contribute to pathological changes in oral tissues.

● Discuss the characteristics of acute necrotizing ulcerative gingivitis (ANUG).

● Identify periodontal instrumentation used for prophylaxis.

● Identify periodontal instrumentation used for surgical procedures.

● Describe an oral prophylaxis procedure.

● Describe the following surgical procedures: gingivectomy, gingivoplasy, gingival grafting, and osteoplasty.

● Explain the procedure for placing and removing a periodontal dressing.

Introduction

Periodontics is the branch of dentistry that deals with the cause, prevention, and treatment of periodontal disease. Periodontia is a generalized term used to describe the many disorders affecting the surrounding and supporting structures of the teeth.

Periodontal diseases are the most common causes of the loss of teeth in adult life. In most cases, they can be prevented before serious damage occurs. The incidence of periodontal disease is not rare in children, although it is commonly believed to be a degenerative disease with aging adults. It should be noted that cases of periodontal disturbances are being reported in ever-increasing numbers. Review Chapter 24 for a clearer understanding of periodontal support.

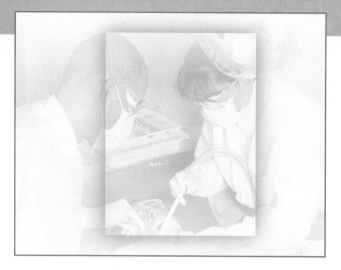

Causes of Periodontal Disease

Disease of the supporting dental structures occurs in childhood, adolescence, and adulthood. However, as one ages, tissues in the oral cavity tend to change and progress to periodontal disease.

Factors that contribute to periodontal disease affecting the periodontium are:

● Plaque harbors microorganisms, producing acids as waste products that inflame the tissues. Calculus promotes roughness, which irritates the periodontium.

● Attrition of the teeth caused by excessive bruxisim and clenching of teeth produces a change in the height of occlusal wear.

● Loss of bone height, due to inflammation, causes a reduction of tooth support.

● Gingival recession, due to poor toothbrushing habits, results in gingival inflammation.

● Malposition of teeth causes bone resorption and mobility of teeth.

● Malposition of teeth and bone loss occur as a result of missing teeth.

● Excessive frenum attachment, due to tight tissue pull, causes gingival recession and exposure of the root portions of teeth.

● Diabetes, a metabolic disorder, inhibits the healing process.

● Aquired immunodeficiency syndrome (AIDS) contributes to quick progression of periodontal disease.

The Healthy Periodontium

Healthy gingiva has a uniform pink color in persons with light skin and darker pigmentation in persons with dark skin. The consistency is firm with smooth free gingiva and stippled attached gingiva. The marginal gingiva is flat with a knife-edge fitting tightly around the tooth and 1 to 2 mm above the cemento-enamel junction (CEJ). The papilla is pointed and fills the interdental space. The sulcus depth is from 0.5 to 3 mm.

The cementum is a very thin, compact, mineralized cellular layer that covers the anatomical root. It provides attachment for the periodontal ligament fibers up to the CEJ.

The periodontal ligament connects the cementum of the tooth to the lamina dura, a compact dense bone located in the tooth socket. Its fibers should not be inflamed or thickened.

The alveolar bone supports the teeth and provides vascular supply to the surrounding tissues. The alveolar crest should be in close proximity to the CEJ.

Signs and Symptoms of Periodontal Disease

When periodontal disease occurs, it may go unrecognized for years because of the insidious (unnoticed) progression in its development. Signs and symptoms to watch for are:

- Bleeding upon brushing, flossing, or probing due to inflammation

- Gingiva becoming red because of irritation, purple as a result of poor circulation, or white, signifying fibrotic (scar) tissue

- Gingiva swelling and exhibiting an abnormal contour, attributable to inflammation

- Sulcus becoming enlarged, trapping food and debris, resulting in pocket formation

- Sensitivity to hot and cold, tenderness of the gingiva while eating, due to gingival recession

- Evidence of foul odor or chronic bad breath associated with infection, entrapment of food debris, and accumulation of plaque

- Teeth becoming loose, malocclusion occuring due to weak periodontal ligament and loss of bone support

Gradual Onset of Periodontal Disease

Gingivitis

Inflammation limited to the gingiva is known as **gingivitis**. Gingivitis in its beginning stages can be reversed and healthy gingiva restored by utilizing preventive measures. Gingivitis does not cause bone loss nor is there evidence that the epithelial attachment migrates beyond the CEJ; however, gingival changes include color from pink to red, contour gingival margin changes from knife-edge to enlarged, and consistency changes from firm to spongy. Gingivitis may be the result of bacterial plaque or in response to other factors such as pregnancy, puberty, and vitamin C deficiency. The three stages of gingivitis are:

- Stage I gingivitis—initial clinical signs of inflammation

- Stage II gingivitis—erythema appearing on the marginal gingiva and bleeding occuring when probed

- Stage III gingivitis—long-standing gingivitis, appearing bluish under the reddened gingival tissues

Periodontitis

Periodontitis begins with inflammation involving the periodontal ligament and supporting structures. A **periodontal pocket** forms when plaque and debris accumulate within the sulcus and are not removed; the depth measures greater than 3 mm. The epithelial attachment progresses apically; some periodontal fibers that attach the tooth to the lamina dura (bone socket) become diseased (Figure 57-1).

Periodontitis is divided into three stages, early, moderate, and advanced:

- Early periodontitis occurs when inflammation from the gingiva progresses into the alveolar bone crest. The epithelial attachment begins to reduce where there is pocket depth formation of 2–4 mm.

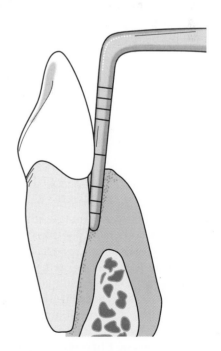

Figure 57-1 Periodontal pocket.

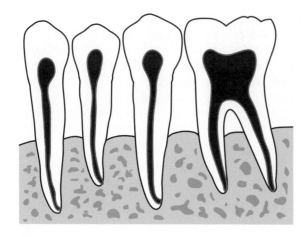

Figure 57-2 Furcation involvement.

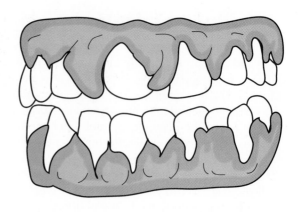

Figure 57-3 Phenytoin-induced gingival overgrowth in a person with epilepsy.

- Moderate periodontitis exhibits continued destruction of the periodontal structures and a pocket formation of 5–7 mm with possible **furcation** (pertaining to the space between two roots in a multirooted tooth) involvement and tooth mobility (Figure 57-2).
- Advanced periodontitis indicates increased pocket depth to 8 mm or more, including furcation involvement and definite tooth mobility.

Systemic Diseases that Cause Gingival Conditions

Diabetes Mellitus

Diabetes mellitus is a disease that results in decreased glucose metabolism. Clinical signs and symptoms in the oral cavity of a diabetic person can include **xerostomia** (dry mouth), enlargement of the parotid gland, **gingival hyperplasia** (overgrowth of the gingiva), alveolar bone loss, periodontal abscesses, and burning or numbness of oral tissues. Lowered resistance and delayed healing are common factors. Periodontal disease is more prevalent in diabetics, even at a young age and likely persisting into adulthood.

Epilepsy

To control epileptic seizures, patients are given phenytoin (Dilantin), an anticonvulsant medication. Overgrowth of the gingiva occurs in 25–50% of persons using the medication. The overgrowth appears bulbous, mostly in the interproximal areas, and tends to wedge the teeth apart. It may also cover a large portion of the enamel and interfere with mastication (Figure 57-3).

Treatment may include a rigorous plaque control program to regress gingival overgrowth while in its early stages. Should it become **fibrous** (containing fibers), it will need to be surgically removed.

Leukemia

Leukemia is a malignancy of blood cells where an overproduction of white blood cells exists. The clinical appearance of the oral cavity includes bleeding of the gingiva and overall gingivitis. Patients who manifest these oral conditions may be mistakenly identified as exhibiting a case of gingivitis. Unless qualified to diagnose a patient with leukemia, it may be difficult to identify one from the other.

Hemophilia

Hemophiliacs must be extremely careful not to abrade or cut themselves because they are missing one of the clotting factors of blood; this can lead to profuse bleeding. However, when caring for their teeth, they must brush sufficiently enough to thoroughly remove plaque yet avoid any abrasion of the soft tissues. Otherwise, the result may be poor oral hygiene coupled with gingival bleeding.

Acquired Immune Deficiency Syndrome

Although similar in appearance to ANUG, gingivitis is manifested by an erythematous (reddish) band of inflammation on the marginal gingiva while in the HIV (human immunodeficiency virus) stage. There is no improvement when preventive measures are employed but rather the condition progresses into ulceration and necrosis.

Acute Necrotizing Ulcerative Gingivitis

Acute necrotizing ulcerative gingivitis (ANUG), also known as Vincent's infection and trench mouth, is a destructive infection of the gingiva. It is characterized by a feeling of illness, bad breath, and appearance of ulcers in the mouth. The thin covering of the ulcer may be easily wiped away, revealing a highly inflamed area that easily bleeds. It can occur in otherwise disease-free mouths, usually among younger people between 15 and 30 years of age who are under a lot of stress, and may involve one tooth, a group of teeth, or the entire mouth.

The patient is advised to get adequate rest and follow a mild but nutritionally sound diet and take an antibiotic such as penicillin. For persons suffering from HIV, which could be fatal due to a compromised immune system, rinsing with chlorhexidine is recommended; in advanced cases where bone is exposed this could cause pain. Smoking and drinking carbonated beverages and alcohol should be eliminated until the condition improves.

When the acute inflammation has subsided, a complete prophylaxis, scaling, and curettage are in order. Thorough preventive home care, good nutrition, rest, and a periodically scheduled recall visit, as prescribed by the periodontist, can keep the condition under control.

Radiographs

Parallel periapical and bite-wing radiographs that include horizontal and vertical exposures are excellent tools to view the height of the alveolar bone because the x-ray is directed closely at a parallel or 90° angle to the object (Figure 57-4). The dentist will evaluate the location, amount, contour of the alveolar crest, and continuity of the lamina dura.

Periodontal Examination and Treatment Planning

A normal sulcus is 3 mm deep or less. When the depth is greater than 3 mm, it is termed a periodontal pocket.

Probing

Six "readings" with a periodontal probe are made for each tooth in the mouth. The periodontal probe is a long, pointed instrument with a scale marked in millimeters. The point of the probe is rounded to avoid patient discomfort or damage to the tissues during probing (Figure 57-5):

- The periodontal probe is inserted into the depth of the sulcus for three measurements on the facial surface of each tooth in the arch: mesiofacial, facial, and distofacial. This procedure is described as walking the probe around the tooth.

- The probing procedure is repeated for three measurements on the lingual of each tooth: mesiolingual, lingual, and distolingual.

- The entire procedure is repeated for the teeth in the opposing arch. All findings are recorded on the patient's clinical record.

Upon conclusion of the examination, the patient may be asked to make another appointment for a diagnosis and prognosis and to discuss the recommended treatment plan.

If periodontal surgery is a part of the proposed treatment, the patient is made aware of the time that will be necessary for the treatment and subsequent healing.

The patient's commitment to the course of treatment, as well as a vigorous home care program, is essential before treatment can be scheduled.

A cost estimate is developed prior to presenting the treatment plan. Questions and concerns expressed by the patient are heard and carefully answered. As soon as the patient and periodontist reach an understanding

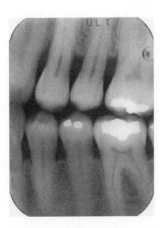

Figure 57-4 Alveolar bone position as viewed on a vertical bite-wing radiograph.

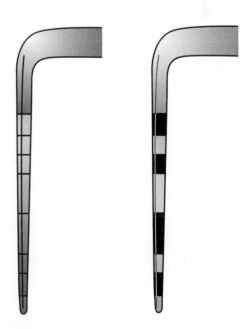

Figure 57-5 Periodontal probes.

of financial obligations for the treatment, an appointment schedule is arranged.

Periodontal Instrumentation

For Prophylaxis

When describing instruments used for calculus removal, one needs to understand there are instruments that remove **supragingival** (located above the gingiva) calculus while others are designed for **subgingival** (located below the gingiva) calculus removal. Instruments used during a prophylaxis appointment may include the following:

● A basic set up consists of a mouth mirror, explorer, and cotton pliers: the mouth mirror for indirect vision, retraction of tissues, and illumination, and the explorer to detect roughness, calculus, decalcification, irregularities in restoration margins, and caries.

● A periodontal probe is an instrument with a blunt or rounded tip with markings to measure pocket depths. The markings on probes may be notched while some are color coded and differ in markings from one manufacturer to another; however, all measure in millimeters. Some mark each millimeter up to 15 mm while others use increments of 3 mm up to 12 mm and still others use a variety of increments (see Figure 57-5). The probing evaluation determines the extent of periodontal disease and includes bleeding upon probing, sulcus depth, and tissue consistency. After a given period of time, the evaluation can be used to determine progress.

● Scalers of many shapes are used to facilitate calculus removal in various locations of tooth surfaces. There are five types of scalers:

1. A sickle is used for supragingival calculus removal. It has two cutting edges on a curved or straight blade and the cross section of the blade is triangular in shape. The straight blade sickle is also known as a jacquette scaler. Both the curved or straight sickles are available with straight or angulated shanks. The straight shank is used primarily on anterior teeth on either mesial or distal surfaces. The angulated shank usually comes as a double-ended instrument and is used on posterior teeth. One end of the scaler gains access interproximally from the facial side, the other end from the lingual or palatal aspect (Figure 57-6).

2. A curet (also spelled "curette") is used for subgingival calculus removal. It has two cutting edges on a curved blade, and the cross section of the blade is similar to a half circle. Curets are available as universal or Gracey (area specific). The universal curets are used on any tooth surface, whereas the Gracey curets are available in pairs and designed for specific surfaces of teeth (Figure 57-7).

3. A hoe is used for heavy supragingival calculus removal. Subgingival use of hoes is contraindicated due to the bulkiness of the instrument and difficulty of adapting a straight cutting edge of an instrument to the curved surface of the tooth. Hoes have a single cutting edge and come in pairs (Figure 57-8).

4. A chisel is used for supragingival calculus removal from proximal surfaces of anterior teeth where the interdental papilla is absent. Chisels have a single cutting edge and are used in only isolated cases (Figure 57-9).

5. A file is used supragingivally or subgingivally to break up heavy subgingival calculus and to smooth the tooth at the CEJ as well as for root planing on the exposed root. Files come in pairs, and the shape of

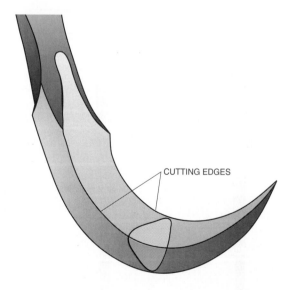

Figure 57-6 Sickle scaler, blade with triangular appearance.

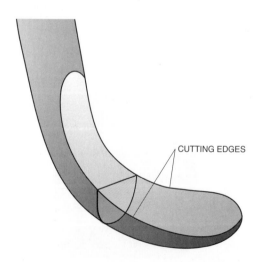

Figure 57-7 Curet scaler; blade with half-circle appearance.

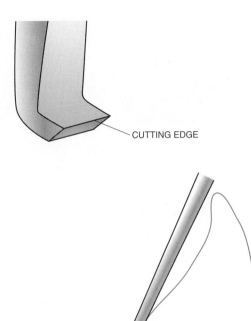

Figure 57-8 Hoe scaler.

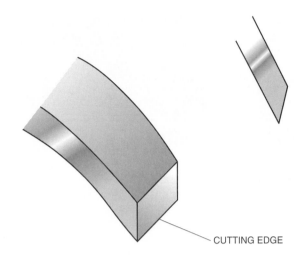

Figure 57-9 Chisel scaler.

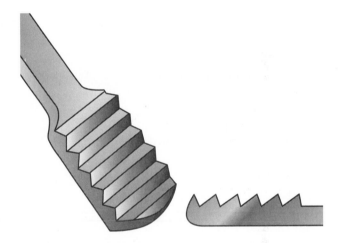

Figure 57-10 File scaler.

the base may be round, oval, or rectangular. Multiple small blades with cutting edges make up the file. It is not generally used during a routine prophylaxis (Figure 57-10).

- Ultrasonic and sonic scalers are electrically powered scaling units producing high-frequency sound waves that create vibrations to break up heavy calculus. Water is used during the scaling procedure to cool the heat-generated vibration. Ultrasonic scalers have made it possible for the operator to remove calculus deposits without the fatigue encountered with manual instrumentation. Currently, smaller tips allow them to be used in the removal of heavy calculus and stain subgingivally as well as supragingivally. Following ultrasonic scaling, manual scaling completes the procedure for residual calculus and stain removal.

There are some precautions to observe when using an ultrasonic scaler (Figure 57-11):

- Aerosol is created when particles of matter become airborne. This promotes the release and transmission of communicable diseases into the atmosphere.

- Microorganisms and pathogenic bacteria from a periodontal pocket may be aspirated by the patient, causing pulmonary infection.

- Although unlikely to occur, operation of a cardiac pacemaker may be disrupted; the patient's cardiologist should be consulted prior to using an ultrasonic scaler.

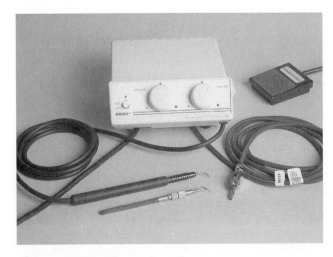

Figure 57-11 Ultrasonic scaler.

Procedure 66 Oral Prophylaxis

Materials Needed

Basic set-up (mouth mirror, explorer, cotton pliers),
   (Figure 57-12)
Periodontal probe
Sickle scalers
Curets: universal and Gracey
Dental floss and tape
Gauze sponges, 2 x 2 in.
Prophy angle with rubber cup and brush (disposable
   prophy angles also available)
Prophy paste and calcium carbonate (chalk)
Saliva ejector, high-volume ejector (HVE) tip, air and
   water syringe tip

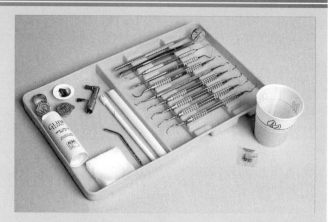

Figure 57-12 Prophylaxis procedure tray set-up.

Instructions

1 The operator examines the patient's mouth for
   overall oral health with the mouth mirror.

2 Each tooth is probed to determine depth of
   sulcus, locate periodontal pockets, identify the
   position of the anatomical root, and detect
   presence of subgingival calculus. The dental
   assistant makes notations of sulcular depths for
   every tooth.

3 Teeth are scaled using a systematic approach.
   The treatment plan may include scaling completion in one or multiple appointments depending
   on the severity of the case. The operator may
   opt to scale one quadrant per week, two
   quadrants or half of the mouth at one time, or
   the entire mouth in one appointment. As large

pieces of calculus and debris are removed, they
are deposited on a 2 x 2 gauze sponge for
disposal.

4 When scaling is completed, the teeth are
   polished with prophy paste utilizing a prophy
   angle, rubber cup, and a prophy brush. Exposed
   roots are polished with a nonabrasive agent and
   a new rubber cup. Dental floss/tape is used to
   polish teeth interproximally while prophy paste
   remains on the teeth.

5 To polish gold restorations, calcium carbonate is
   preferred.

6 With the air and water syringe the teeth are
   rinsed and the mouth evacuated.

Note: During the process of a prophylaxis, the following terms and procedures are likely to occur:

● *Scaling*—takes place during the prophylaxis procedure. The dentist or dental hygienist removes calculus deposits from around the tooth using scalers.

● *Debridement*—involves the removal of plaque and
   calculus deposits from the surfaces of teeth.

● *Root planing*—is performed by using curet scalers to
   remove diseased cementum. The cementum surfaces
   of the root are smoothed until all rough surfaces are
   eliminated, leaving the cementum in a disease-free
   condition. Local anesthesia is used while performing
   this procedure.

● *Gingival curettage*—also referred to as "subgingival
   curettage." After the tooth has been scaled and root
   planing completed, gingival curettage is performed
   using curets to remove diseased necrotic gingival soft
   tissues from within the periodontal pocket lining.
   Local anesthesia is used when this procedure is performed (Figure 57-13).

● *Furcation involvement*—a periodontal condition
   whereby bone loss has extended below the furcation
   of the roots of a multirooted tooth. This condition
   may be visible on radiograph and it signifies marked
   bone loss; refer to Figure 57-2.

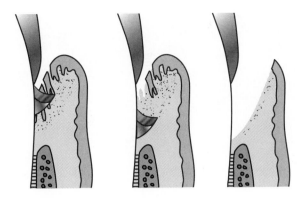

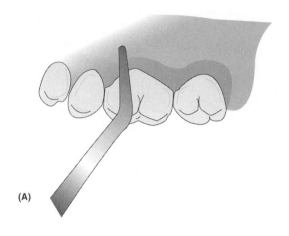

(A)

Figure 57-13 Gingival curettage.

Surgical Instrumentation

Instruments used for surgical procedures include:

- *Pocket markers* resemble cotton pliers; however, one tip has a protruding point built in at a 90° angle from the tip and the other tip is tapered, plain, and not as long. The plain tip is inserted in the pocket to establish its depth while the protruding tip pierces the gingival tissue and marks where the incision will be made for a gingivectomy (Figure 57-14).

- After the pocket marker is used, the operator uses the *scalpel* to make the incision into the soft tissues, as in a gingivectomy procedure (Figure 57-15).

- *Periodontal knives* are of two types. The double-ended, kidney-shaped Kirkland, Goldman-fox, and Buck knives are used to cut and recontour the gingiva

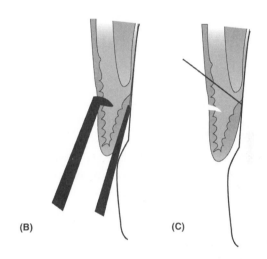

(B) (C)

Figure 57-14 Gingivectomy incision marked with pocket marker.

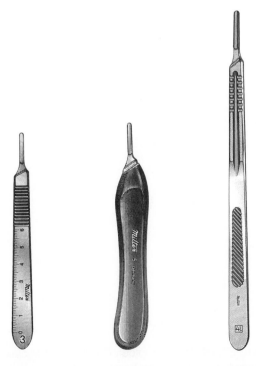

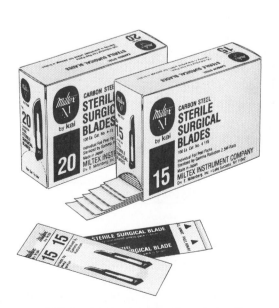

Figure 57-15 Scalpel handles and selection of blades. (Courtesy of Mielex Instrument Co., Inc., Lake Success, NY.)

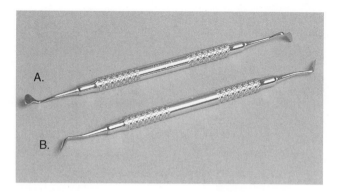

Figure 57-16 Periodontal knives: (A) Kirkland; (B) Orban interdental.

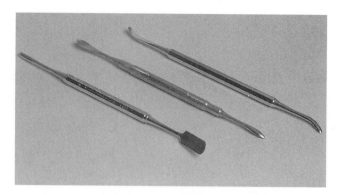

Figure 57-17 Assorted periosteal elevators.

on the facial or lingual surfaces. The Orban interdental knife is also double ended, with long blades and cutting edges on both sides of the blade, and is used to excise interdental tissue (Figures 57-16A and B).

● After the incision is made, and should a flap be raised, the *periosteal elevator*, a double-ended instrument, is used to separate the soft tissue from the underlying bone (Figure 57-17).

● The *surgical curette* is a double-ended instrument shaped similar to a large spoon excavator used to remove loose tissue and debris from the surgical site.

● A special sterile *surgical aspirator* is used during surgical procedures. The lumen is considerably smaller than that of the HVE, and it maintains clear visibility while aspirating blood from the surgical area.

● *Surgical scissors*, available with plain or serrated blades, are primarily used to trim soft tissue and to cut suture material during suture placement (Figure 57-18).

● A *needle holder* is similar in appearance to a hemostat, but unlike the serrated beaks of a hemostat, the inner surfaces of the beaks have a criss-cross pattern, allowing a firmer grasp of the suture needle. It is designed to manipulate a suture needle during suturing procedures (Figure 57-19).

● When surgery is completed, the wound is closed with a *suture needle threaded with suture material*. The periodontist closes the incision, allowing healing to begin.

Surgical Procedures

Gingivectomy

A **gingivectomy** is the surgical removal of the inflamed and diseased gingiva and deep suprabony pockets. **Suprabony** means above the bone. A gingivectomy is performed only after a periodontal pocket has failed to respond to scaling and gingival curettage.

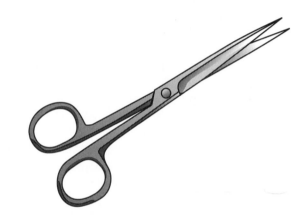

Figure 57-18 Surgical scissors. (Courtesy of Mielex Instrument Co., Inc., Lake Success, NY.)

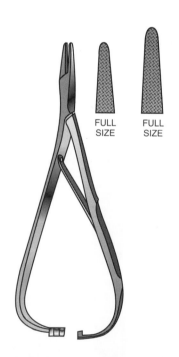

FULL SIZE   FULL SIZE

Figure 57-19 Needle holder. (Courtesy of Mielex Instrument Co., Inc., Lake Success, NY.)

Procedure 67 Gingivectomy

Materials Needed

Basic set-up
Anesthetic set-up
Pocket marker
Gauze sponges, 2 x 2
Scalpel holder and assorted surgical blades
Periodontal knives: Kirkland kidney shaped and
    Orban interproximal
Periosteal elevator
Curet scalers, hoes, files
Sterile water/saline solution
Surgical scissors
Suture needle, suture material, needle holder
Surgical aspirator, HVE tip
Periodontal dressing

Instructions

1 The gingivectomy procedure begins with local anesthesia.

2 A pocket marker is used to mark the depth of each pocket and to guide the periodontist as to where to make the incision; see Figure 57-14.

3 The incision is made using a scalpel or periodontal knives.

4 A periosteal elevator is used to reflect (bend back) the gingival tissue from the bone, also known as a surgical flap.

5 Interproximal periodontal knives or curet scalers are used to remove the interdental gingiva.

6 Calculus deposits are removed with curets and hoes and the root surfaces are smoothed and planed using files.

7 Diseased or **granulation tissue** (tissue that appears granular due to new fleshy projections formed in an area where healing is not taking place) is removed and the area flushed and irrigated with sterile water or saline solution.

8 The flap is repositioned and sutured in place and a periodontal dressing placed on the surgical site; see Procedure 68.

9 Explicit instructions for home care following surgery must be given verbally as well as in written form.

A gingivectomy also includes deep scaling and root planing. The purpose of a gingivectomy is the removal of diseased tissue to prevent the spread of disease not only in the oral cavity but throughout the body as well.

When a gingivectomy is indicated for both dental arches, each quadrant is treated at a separate appointment, usually on a weekly basis.

Gingivoplasty

A **gingivoplasty** is the surgical procedure by which gingival deformities are reduced to create normal and functional form.

Gingivoplasty, unlike gingivectomy, is performed in the absence of pockets with the sole purpose of removing excess tissue and recontouring the gingiva. Gingivoplasty may include (1) tapering the gingival margin; (2) creating a marginal outline; and (3) reshaping the interdental papillae to allow for the passage of food on the free gingiva during mastication.

Gingival Grafting

Gingival grafting is an **autograft** (graft taken from one part of the body and placed in another part) surgical procedure whereby a portion of tissue (the graft) is taken from one area of the mouth (the donor site) and placed in another area such as the gingiva. Preparation of the recipient tissue bed is made by locating connective tissue where the graft will be attached. A template is made of the recipient tissue bed to match the size of the needed graft. The graft is excised, most likely from the palate, and sutured in the new location. Periodontal dressing is used to cover both wounds (Figure 57-20).

Osteoplasty

Osteoplasty is the surgical reshaping of the alveolar bone with maintained basic support of the teeth. **Osseus** (bony) surgery may be either additive or subtractive. *Additive osseus surgery* is directed toward restoring the alveolar bone to its original level. This procedure is

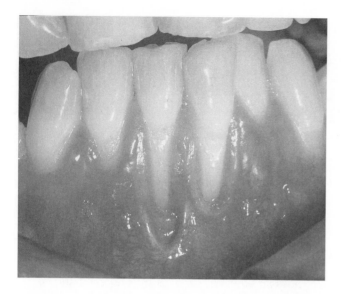

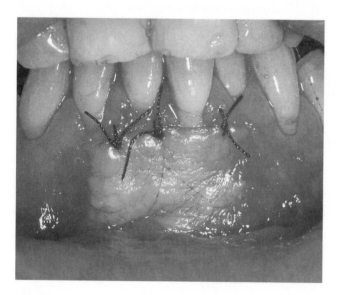

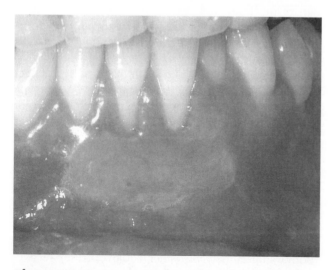

Figure 57-20 Gingival grafting. (Courtesy of Gary Shellerud.)

accomplished by various auto-osseus (auto = "self") implant bone grafts. *Subtractive osseus surgery* procedures are designed to restore the form of the alveolar bone by surgically reducing it, as is the case of tori or exostoses. The bony plate is exposed by reflecting a surgical flap to reveal the bony plate of the alveolar bone and recontouring the area.

Osseus implants are autogeneous (self-producing) bone grafts that are surgically accomplished. For instance, the bony implant material may be obtained from the retromolar area of the patient. A mucoperiosteal flap is prepared at the designated site of the implant. Granulated tissue and periodontal fibers are removed with a surgical curette.

The bony tissue is removed from the donor site and placed in the implant area. After the incision is cleansed with a natural saline solution, surgical suturing closes it. A surgical pack is placed over the closed incision. Healing begins within a period of several days; the pack and sutures are then removed.

Bone allografts (a bone graft obtained from another person) are performed surgically by using the demineralized freeze-dried bone of another human (donor). The donor and recipient are sufficiently unlike genetically to interact **antigenically** (pertaining to antibody production).

Preparation of the donor bone tissue involves medical laboratory engineering to remove the mineral salts from the tissue before it is freeze-dried and retained in a bone bank.

During the surgery, the implant tissue will be precisely positioned, and once implanted in the recipient body, it will act as an enzyme. When introduced into the body, the implant stimulates the production of antibodies. The antibodies will, in turn, neutralize toxins, bacteria, or cells and promote healing.

Recent research indicates that the bone allograft procedure lends itself to periodontal surgery and has proven to be highly successful.

Pericoronitis

Pericoronitis is an inflammation or infection of the gingival tissues surrounding the crown of an erupting tooth. The mandibular third molar is frequently involved, with the tendency of food impactions under the loose margins of the gingivae. Cleansing the area is difficult because of the location of the tooth. The gingival tissue is usually red, swollen, with infection involvement, tenderness, and pain radiating to the ear, throat, and floor of the mouth. In addition, a foul taste and swelling in the general area are common.

Radiographs may determine whether the tooth should be retained or extracted. If the tooth is retained, conservative treatment should be initiated. If the tooth is to be extracted, an antibiotic is normally prescribed prior to surgery.

Placing a Periodontal Dressing

A periodontal dressing is placed on the surgical wound. It acts as a bandage while healing takes place. In some states, the dental assistant places and removes the periodontal dressing. There are three types of periodontal dressings available: zinc oxide–eugenol, noneugenol, and light cured.

When the surgical procedure has been completed and bleeding has ceased, a periodontal dressing is placed. Should the wound continue to bleed or if moisture is present, it will become very difficult to place the periodontal dressing on the surgical wound.

Procedure 68 Placing a Noneugenol Periodontal Dressing

Materials Needed

Basic set-up
Plastic instrument
Gauze sponge, 2 x 2 in.
Tongue depressors for mixing the dressing
Large paper mixing pad
Periodontal dressing base and accelerator
Cotton tip applicators
Lubricant (Vaseline)
Saline solution
Cup with cold water
Gelfoam

Instructions

1 Dispense appropriate amounts of base and accelerator on a large mixing pad, according to manufacturer's instructions. (Figure 57-21A-D).

2 Using a tongue depressor, mix the materials together until homogenous.

3 Gather and place the mixed material on the tip of the tongue depressor and insert it in a cup of cold water.

4 Use the lubricant to coat the patient's lips and operator's gloves.

5 Check the surgical site for bleeding and blot dry any excess moisture and blood using 2 x 2 in. gauze sponges. If sutures were used, locate the knots and cover them with Gelfoam (an absorbable gelatin sponge) to avoid embedding them in the dressing.

6 After the mix loses its tacky consistency, remove it from the tongue depressor and roll it out on the mixing pad. Shape the material into thin ropes by rolling the material between your fingers and the paper pad (if ropes are too thick,

the dressing will need to be trimmed once adapted).

7 Begin adapting the rope on the facial side about the length of the incision of the wound, starting at the distal of the most posterior tooth and working forward. It should cover the incision, the gingival third of the tooth, including part of

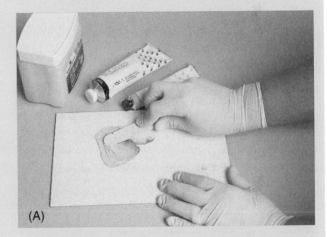

(A)

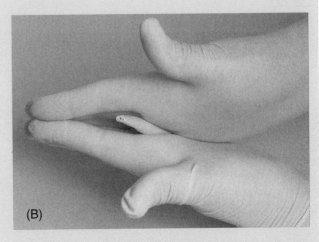

(B)

Figure 57-21 Placement of periodontal dressing.

continued

continued from previous page
Procedure 68 Placing a Noneugenol Periodontal Dressing

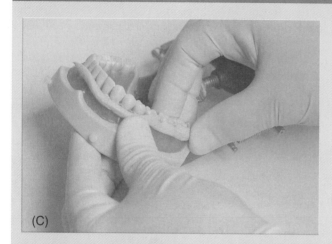

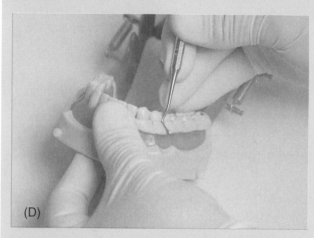

Figure 57-21 Placement of periodontal dressing. (continued)

the gingiva toward the apical side but without interfering with muscle attachments, and provide adequate coverage to include one tooth mesial and one tooth distal of the incision. The dressing should be mechanically locked in each interproximal area using a moist cotton tip applicator. The total width of the dressing should be under 6 mm.

8 The dressing should be thick enough so as to not fracture yet not so bulky to be uncomfortable for the patient.

9 A second rope is adapted to the lingual side of the surgical site starting with the most posterior tooth. The material is adapted as on the facial side. Using a moist cotton tip applicator, the dressing is festooned. It is important that the material be interdentally locked for retentive purposes. When viewing from the occlusal or incisal edges, the mouth mirror is used to detect open spaces in each interproximal area.

10 Using a plastic instrument, the dressing is contoured around the gingival third of each tooth to provide a more esthetic appearance.

11 Have the patient occlude the teeth, making certain the dressing does not interfere with occlusion. Using a small amount of lubricant, smooth the dressing with the index finger.

12 Document the procedure.

Procedure 69 Removing Periodontic Dressing

Materials Needed

Basic set-up
Suture scissors
Plastic instrument
Floss
Saline solution (optional)
HVE tip

Instructions

1 Using a plastic instrument, insert it between the dressing close to the gingival aspect of the tooth and gently pry it loose using lateral forces (Figure 57-22).

2 As the pieces are fractured from the surgical site, check to determine if suture knots are attached

continued

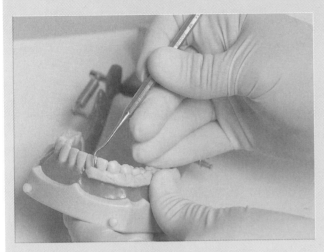

Figure 57-22 Removal of periodontal dressing.

to the dressing. If they are, use suture scissors to cut under the knot and pull the dressing away. Document each suture removed.

3 Remove dressing from interproximal spaces using an explorer and knotted floss.

4 With all dressing pieces removed, irrigate the surgical site with either saline solution or sterile water. Realizing that teeth may be very sensitive once exposed, cautiously use the HVE to remove fluid and fragments.

Postoperative Instructions Following Surgical Procedures

Instructions following surgical procedures should be given to the patient verbally and in written form:

- The patient should be cautioned that slight bleeding may continue for the following 24 hours and to use 2 x 2 in. gauze sponges when needed.

- If sutures were used, the patient should be informed as to the type placed (resorbable or nonresorbable) and when to return for removal of sutures. If a suture is lost, the patient should not be concerned unless bleeding continues.

- The patient should refrain from eating food within the first two hours.

- If a periodontal dressing was used, it will remain in the mouth for approximately one week.

- The patient should avoid smoking (delays healing), drinking alcohol (irritates tissues), and spicy, hard, and hot foods while periodontal dressing is in place.

- Should bleeding occur or large pieces of the dressing become dislodged, the patient should notify the office immediately for dressing replacement.

- The patient should be told to expect some pain; should it become severe, necessary medication will be prescribed.

- Rinsing of the mouth should be avoided for the first 24 hours. Thereafter, a teaspoon of salt in a warm glass of water may be used to cleanse the surgical area.

- Brushing the teeth in the surgical area should be done in a gentle manner, without traumatizing the tissues. All other teeth should be brushed as usual.

- The patient should be scheduled for a postoperative appointment to evaluate healing progress.

SUGGESTED ACTIVITIES

- Place a selection of scalers to include sickles, curets, hoes, chisels, and files in a tray and quiz each other regarding the shape for identification and determine how each scaler is used.

- Set up a tray for an oral prophylaxis procedure.

- Set up a tray for a gingivectomy procedure.

- Using a typodont and periodontal dressing, place dressing to cover the following sites: from tooth numbers 6–11, 2–8, 22–27 and 25–31. Determine the correct thickness and width of the dressing and lock each interproximal site. *Note:* When working on a typodont, a thin coat of Vaseline should be placed preceding the dressing for easier removal; otherwise, the material will adhere to the typodont.

REVIEW

1. Indicate which of the following diseases may cause gingival conditions: (1) leukemia, (2) tuberculosis, (3) diabetes mellitus, and/or (4) AIDS (acquired immunodeficiency syndrome).
   a. 1, 2, 3
   b. 2, 3, 4
   c. 1, 2, 4
   d. 1, 3, 4

2. At what periodontal disease stage does pocket formation of 5–7 mm take place?
   a. Gingivitis
   b. Early periodontitis
   c. Moderate periodontitis
   d. Advanced periodontitis

3. Match the instruments on the left with their uses on the right:
   ___ a. Sickle scaler
   ___ b. Periodontal probe
   ___ c. Curet scaler
   ___ d. Hoe scaler
   ___ e. Chisel scaler
   ___ f. File scaler

   1. Blunt instrument with markings to take pocket measurements
   2. The cross section of the blade is similar to a half circle, has a curved blade with two cutting edges, and may be used on any tooth surface
   3. Bulky instrument with a single cutting edge, used supragingivally for heavy calculus removal
   4. Used to break heavy subgingival calculus, to smooth the tooth, and for root planing exposed roots
   5. The cross section of the blade is triangular and has two cutting edges to remove calculus interproximally
   6. Has a single cutting edge and used only in isolated cases to remove supragingival calculus on proximals of anterior teeth

4. Match the terms on the left with their definitions on the right:
   ___ a. Scaling
   ___ b. Furcation involvement
   ___ c. Root planing
   ___ d. Gingival curettage

   1. Curets are used to removed diseased necrotic gingival soft tissue from within the periodontal pocket lining
   2. Using curet scalers to remove diseased cementum and eliminate rough surfaces on the cementum
   3. A condition where bone loss has extended below the division of roots in a multirooted tooth
   4. Removal of calculus deposits during a prophylaxis procedure

5. Surgical removal of inflamed and diseased gingiva and deep suprabony pockets defines:
   a. Gingivectomy
   b. Gingivoplasty
   c. Osteoplasty
   d. Bone allografts

6. Indicate which of the following are postoperative instructions: (1) if a suture is lost and the surgical site is bleeding, the patient should not be concerned: (2) avoid rinsing the mouth for the first 24 hours, thereafter a teaspoon of salt in a glass of warm water may be used to cleanse surgical area; (3) avoid smoking, drinking alcohol, and eating spicy foods while periodontal dressing is in place; and/or (4) in the surgical area tooth brushing should be done in a gentle manner.
   a. 1, 2, 3
   b. 2, 3, 4
   c. 1, 2, 4
   d. 1, 3, 4

7. What is the main purpose for using a periodontal dressing?
   a. To prevent bleeding in the surgical site
   b. To act as a bandage while healing takes place
   c. To keep food away from the surgical site
   d. To prevent sutures from dislodging

Oral and Maxillofacial Surgery

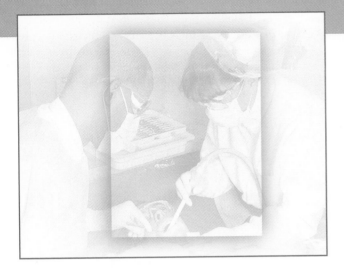

repair, bone and tissue grafts, surgical implants, biopsy, removal of tumors and cysts, and reconstruction of deformities, including the use of general anesthesia.

Examination and Treatment Planning

The oral surgeon will examine the surgical patient and confirm findings of the referring dentist.

Radiographs prescribed by the oral surgeon may include periapical, panoramic, temporomandibular (TMJ), extraoral, and occlusal x-rays. Radiographs obtained from the referring dentist may be used as a comparison of the patient's condition.

Fees for services must be explained by the specialist and accepted by the patient. In the case of a severe toothache, the patient will require immediate attention.

Fees for elective surgery should be presented prior to any service. In cases requiring hospitalization, the patient's medical and dental insurance must be reviewed.

Informed Consent

An informed consent should be signed by the patient or the parent or guardian of a minor at the time it is agreed upon to have the surgical procedure performed. The procedure as well as the outcome should be fully explained by the oral surgeon and understood by the patient or guardian.

Medical History

A detailed medical history should be obtained to avoid an emergency situation. The oral surgeon may need to confer with the patient's physician regarding certain conditions that could compromise the patient's well-being. In particular, the following conditions should be seriously considered:

● A recent heart attack within the last six months may put the patient at risk for further heart damage due to possible secondary infections.

● Heart murmur or joint replacement may potentially cause bacterial endocarditis. When a heart murmur is present or a joint replaced, an antibiotic regimen would be instituted.

OBJECTIVES

After studying this chapter, the student will be able to:

● Describe procedures performed by the oral surgeon.

● Explain why certain medical conditions may compromise a patient's well-being during surgery.

● Identify various surgical forceps.

● Identify the general surgical instruments used in oral surgery.

● Select the surgical instruments needed for a specific oral surgery procedure.

● Select the correct armamentarium for extraction of a specific tooth.

● Indicate the rationale for each postoperative instruction

● Describe the procedures for a frenectomy, osteotomy, and alveolitis.

● Discuss the procedure for cleaning and sterilizing surgical instruments.

Introduction

Oral surgery is the science and specialty practice of removing teeth from the oral cavity. Exodontics is the term used to describe the extraction of teeth. Although the general dentist is trained in dental surgical procedures, he or she may choose to refer the more complicated cases to an oral surgeon. Among other procedures besides extraction of teeth performed by the oral surgeon, the following are included: jaw repositioning due to fracture or overgrowth, temporomandibular bone

- Diabetics who are insulin dependent may have to diminish insulin intake due to partial fasting prior to general anesthesia. The physician must be consulted for approval. The amount of insulin taken depends on food intake.

- Hypertensive patients whose blood pressure may rise when pain is experienced are at risk for stroke or heart attack.

- Patients with kidney and liver diseases may have bleeding problems that could complicate surgical procedures.

- For pregnant patients who are in their first trimester there is a possibility of spontaneous abortion, or in their third trimester they may enter early labor. Elective dental treatment should be postponed until after delivery.

- Monitoring of drugs that the patient takes is imperative. Interaction with drugs used during oral surgery may put the patient at great risk. The patient may have to discontinue taking certain drugs two or three days prior to surgery. Any drugs that thin the blood or contain aspirin should be avoided.

Pain Control

The level of pain tolerance should be determined early in the treatment plan. Premedication in conjunction with local anesthesia may be prescribed for the apprehensive patient.

For more profound anesthesia, the surgeon may use inhalation of nitrous oxide and select a local anesthetic solution of longer duration. Refer to Chapters 50 and 51.

General anesthesia may be indicated for some oral surgery patients. To ensure the patient's safety, a second professional, such as an anesthesiologist, is present to supervise the administration and monitor the patient's vital signs during surgery; refer to Chapter 50.

Surgical Instruments

Forceps

The term *universal*, when associated with forceps, means that the forceps is designed for extracting teeth from either the right or left side of the same arch but not for extracting teeth in the opposing arch. Forceps may also be identified by the angles and the notches on the beaks. A forceps consists of the following parts: the beak, the fraised (indented) portion of the beak, and the handle (Figure 58-1).

Maxillary Forceps

- Maxillary and mandibular incisor forceps (#69). This thin-beaked forceps is used on overlapping centrals

and laterals. It is used, when indicated, to avoid interference with the adjacent teeth or to remove root fragments (Figure 58-1).

- Maxillary universal incisors, cuspid, bicuspids (premolar) and Root Forceps (#150). A forceps used in extracting centrals, laterals, cuspids, bicuspids (premolars), and roots (Figure 58-2).

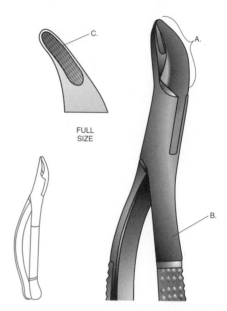

Figure 58-1 Parts of the forceps: (A) beak, (B) handle, and (C) fraised area; maxillary and mandibular incisor forceps #69. (Courtesy of Miltex Instrument Co., Lake Success, NY.)

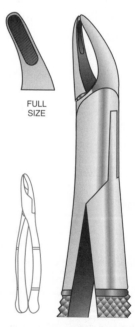

Figure 58-2 Maxillary universal incisor, cuspid, bicuspid, and root forceps #150. (Courtesy of Miltex Instrument Co., Lake Success, NY.)

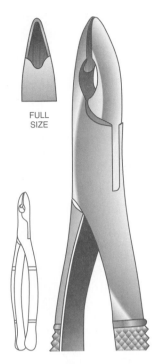

Figure 58-3 Maxillary incisor, cuspid, and bicuspid forceps #99A (Courtesy of Miltex Instrument Co., Lake Success, NY.)

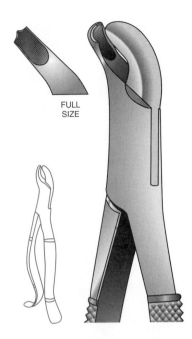

Figure 58-4 Maxillary right first and second molar forceps #18R. (Courtesy of Miltex Instrument Co., Lake Success, NY.)

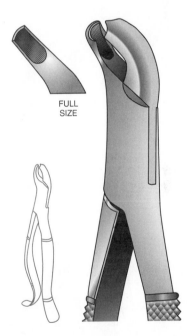

Figure 58-5 Maxillary left first and second molar forceps #18L. (Courtesy of Miltex Instrument Co., Lake Success, NY.)

- Maxillary incisor, cuspid, and bicuspid (premolar) Forceps (#99A). The beaks of the forceps are parallel when placed on the tooth. The design of the forceps allows the beaks to grasp the entire periphery of the tooth at or above the gingival margin (Figure 58-3).

- Maxillary right first and second molar forceps (#18R). The right-side beak is pointed and should be applied to the bifurcation of the two buccal roots; the left-side beak, which is rounded, should be applied to the lingual (palatal) root above the gingival margin (Figure 58-4).

- Maxillary left first and second molar forceps (#18L). The left-side beak is pointed and should be applied to the bifurcation of the two buccal roots; the right-side beak, which is rounded, should be applied to the lingual (palatal) root above the gingival margin (Figure 58-5).

Mandibular Forceps

- Mandibular universal incisors bicuspid (premolar) and root forceps (#103). The forceps has thin, narrow beaks that allow proper application to all the anterior and crowded teeth (Figure 58-6).

- Mandibular universal incisor, cuspid, and bicuspid (premolar) forceps (#151A). The edges of the beaks are sharp to establish good subgingival root contact. This forceps is used for access to large cuspids and bicuspids (premolars) (Figure 58-7).

- Mandibular universal first and second molar forceps (#17). The beaks of the forceps are sharp and pointed and deflect the soft tissue without injury. The beaks engage the bifurcation of the mesial and distal

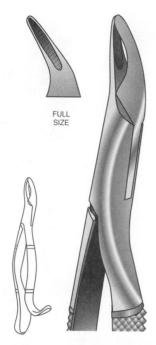

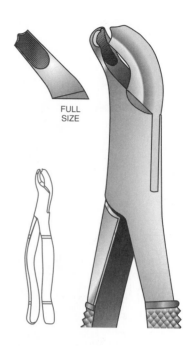

Figure 58-6 Mandibular universal incisor, bicuspid and root forceps #103. (Courtesy of Miltex Instrument Co., Lake Success, NY.)

Figure 58-8 Mandibular universal first and second molar forceps #17. (Courtesy of Miltex Instrument Co., Lake Success, NY.)

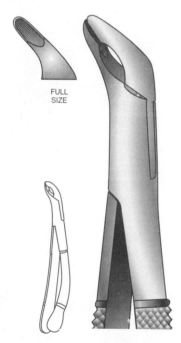

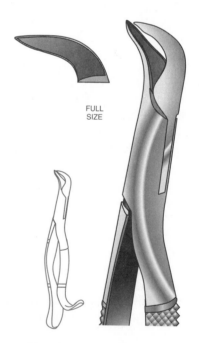

Figure 58-7 Mandibular universal incisor, cuspid and bicuspid forceps #151A. (Courtesy of Miltex Instrument Co., Lake Success, NY.)

Figure 58-9 Mandibular universal first and second molar forceps "cow horn" #16. (Courtesy of Miltex Instrument Co., Lake Success, NY.)

roots and form an extensive coverage of the crown (Figure 58-8).

- Mandibular universal first and second molar "cow horn" forceps (#16). This forceps is known as the "cow horn" and is used on molars when the roots are not fused. The best application of the forceps is with

full crowns or molars with badly broken-down crowns (Figure 58-9).

- Mandibular universal cuspids, bicuspid (premolar), and molar forceps (#85A). The raised portion (raised areas along the horizontal plane forming a curved incline) of the beaks grip almost the entire lingual and buccal surfaces of the tooth. The pressure on the handles pulls the crown into the opening between the forceps beaks and holds the tooth securely (Figure 58-10).

General Surgical Instruments

● *Retractors and mouth props.* There are several types of retractors: lip and cheek retractors for viewing the facial aspect in the oral cavity, tongue retractors to move the tongue away from the operating field, and tissue retractors to move the tissue aside. Mouth props are used to keep the mouth open during sur-

gery, especially when the patient is sedated or under general anesthesia (Figures 58-11, 58-12, and 58-13).

● *Periosteal elevator.* A double-ended instrument with a blade at each end for lifting or reflecting the mucous

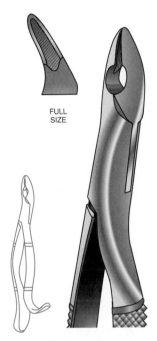

Figure 58-10 Mandibular universal cuspid, bicuspid, and molar forceps #85A. (Courtesy of Miltex Instrument Co., Lake Success, NY.)

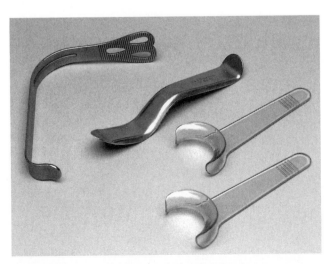

Figure 58-11 Tongue and cheek retractors.

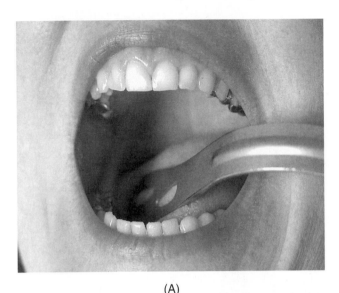

(A)

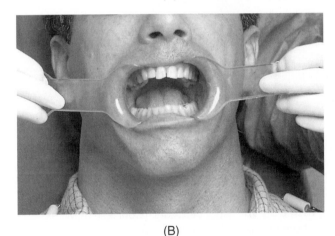

(B)

Figure 58-12 (A) Tongue retractor. (B) Cheek retractor.

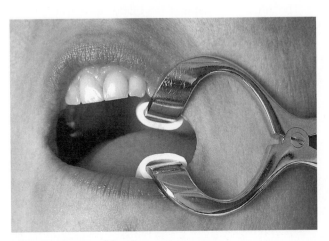

Figure 58-13 Mouth prop.

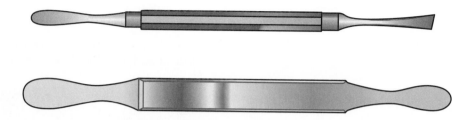

Figure 58-14   Periosteal elevators. (Courtesy of Miltex Instrument Co., Lake Success, NY.)

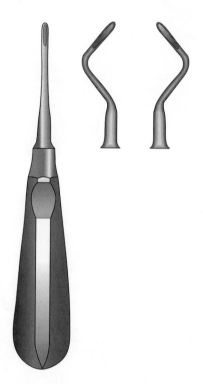

Figure 58-15   Root elevators. (Courtesy of Miltex Instrument Co., Lake Success, NY.)

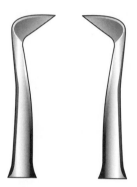

Figure 58-16   Maxillary and mandibular root elevators "Cryers." (Courtesy of Miltex Instrument Co., Lake Success, NY.)

- *Rongeur forceps.* A rongeur is a special type of forceps used to "trim" bone. The beaks may be round nosed or square nosed, with a hard, tough sharp blade extending along one side of the beak and curving around the extreme tip of the beak and along the opposite side. The rongeur may be used on the maxillary or mandibular arch (Figure 58-17).

- *Bone files.* Bone files are used for smoothing the alveolar process after the rongeur forceps, chisel(s), and extractions. The file blade is inserted and the tissue elevated. Pressure on the file causes it to engage the bone, and a pull toward the point of insertion removes rough, sharp fragments of bone (Figure 58-18).

- *Root Tip Picks.* Root tip picks may be straight or contra-angled and are used on the maxillary and mandibular arches. The straight pick is used in the anterior portion of the mouth, and the contra-angled pick is used in the posterior. Their purpose is to remove small root tips and bone fragments (Figure 58-19).

- *Surgical curettes.* Surgical curettes are double-ended instruments used for removing soft diseased tissue and establishing a flow of blood in the tooth socket. They are designed for application in all parts of the mouth. Double-end curettes are used after all extractions (Figure 58-20).

membrane and underlying tissue covering the bone. The angle and shape of the blades give access to all areas of the mouth. This elevator is used before the root elevator (Figure 58-14).

- *Root elevators.* Root elevators are used on the maxillary or mandibular arch, and the concave blade is inserted between the root and the alveolar wall and rotated (Figure 58-15).

- *Maxillary and mandibular root elevators.* A pair of root elevators, right and left, with the blades at a 90° angle to the shank. Maxillary and mandibular molar roots that are not fused can be easily removed with the right or left elevator by applying the point of the blade buccally at the bifurcation of the roots, forcing the point as far into the bifurcation of the roots as possible (Figure 58-16).

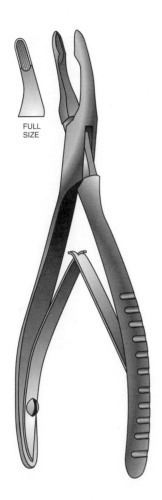

Figure 58-17 Rongeur forceps. (Courtesy of Miltex Instrument Co., Lake Success, NY.)

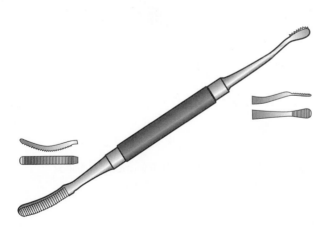

Figure 58-18 Bone file. (Courtesy of Miltex Instrument Co., Lake Success, NY.)

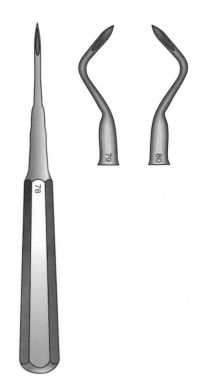

Figure 58-19 Root tip picks. (Courtesy of Miltex Instrument Co., Lake Success, NY.)

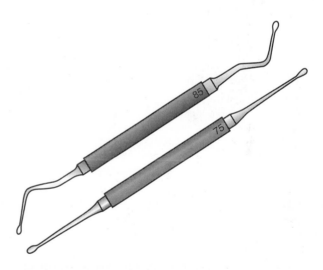

Figure 58-20 Double-end curettes. (Courtesy of Miltex Instrument Co., Lake Success, NY.)

● *Dressing pliers.* Dressing pliers are tweezer-type pliers with a serrated grip and slender pointed beaks for placing needed medication into the tooth socket (Figure 58-21).

● *Scalpels/surgical blades.* The scalpel is a very sharp thin blade placed on a reusable metal handle. Scalpels are used to make the incision. Blades for the scalpel are made of sterile stainless steel or carbon steel and are available in assorted sizes and shapes. Sterile blades are disposed of after one use, but the metal handles are resterilized and reused (Figure 58-22). Some handles are available in plastic and are primarily used in the dental laboratory.

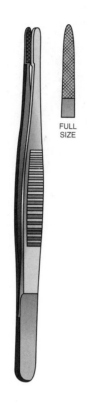

FULL
SIZE

Figure 58-21 Dressing pliers. (Courtesy of Miltex Instrument Co., Lake Success, NY.)

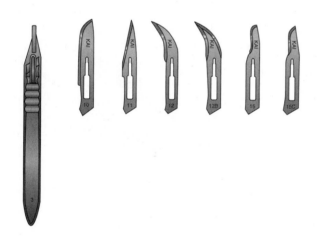

Figure 58-22 Scalpels/surgical blades. (Courtesy of Miltex Instrument Co., Lake Success, NY.)

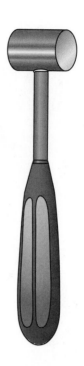

Figure 58-23 Surgical mallet. (Courtesy of Miltex Instrument Co., Lake Success, NY.)

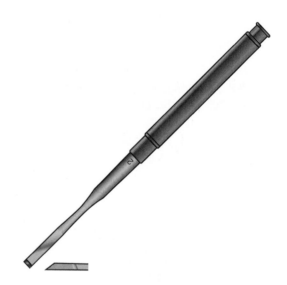

Figure 58-24 Bone chisel. (Courtesy of Miltex Instrument Co., Lake Success, NY.)

● *Surgical mallet.* The surgical mallet is used with bone chisels for reducing bone in selected oral surgery procedures (Figure 58-23).

● *Bone chisels.* Bone chisels are designed for reducing bone structure in the maxillary or mandibular arch. Most bone chisels are used with a surgical mallet (Figure 58-24).

● *Scissors.* Scissors are used to trim soft tissue or for cutting suture material, depending on whether the cut-

ting ends are sharp or blunt. The cutting portion (blades) are available in plain (smooth) or serrated (horizontal, sharp, raised toothlike ridge) patterns. Surgical or tissue scissors with sharp delicate blades are used mainly for trimming soft tissue, and suture scissors with less delicate blades are used for cutting suture material. The shape of the blades may be straight, curved, or angled and of various lengths. Handles may be of varied lengths (Figure 58-25).

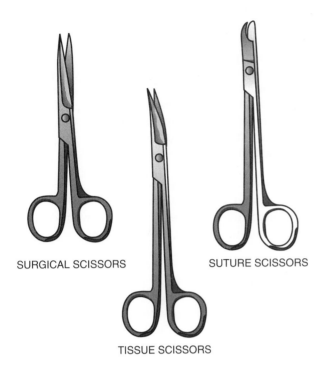

SURGICAL SCISSORS   SUTURE SCISSORS

TISSUE SCISSORS

Figure 58-25 Scissors. (Courtesy of Miltex Instrument Co., Lake Success, NY.)

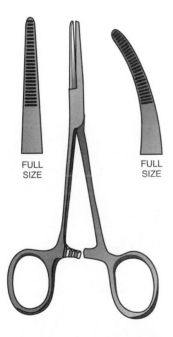

FULL SIZE   FULL SIZE

Figure 58-26 Hemostat. (Courtesy of Miltex Instrument Co., Lake Success, NY.)

● *Hemostat and needle holder.* A hemostat is a scissors-like instrument primarily used to clamp blood vessels. However, it can be used in dentistry to grasp tissue, root, or bone fragments. It is designed with serrated beaks that are either straight or curved. The handles

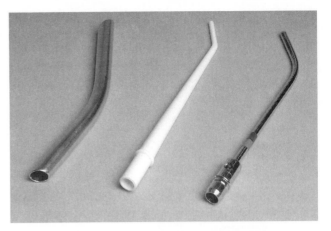

Figure 58-27 HVE and surgical aspirator tips.

are designed to lock in position. The hemostat may be used in oral surgery to direct the suture needle through soft tissue. In endodontic treatment it is often employed to position a radiographic film (Figure 58-26). A needle holder is similar in appearance to a hemostat. Unlike a hemostat's serrated beaks, the inner surfaces of the beaks have a criss-cross pattern, allowing a firmer grasp of the suture needle. It is primarily used to grasp and manipulate a suture needle during suturing procedures (see Figure 57–19).

● *Surgical aspirator.* A surgical aspirator differs from a high-volume evacuator (HVE) tip in that its opening is much smaller. Surgical aspirators are made of metal, autoclavable plastic or disposable plastic and supplied in a variety of sizes (Figure 58-27).

● *Suture needle and material.* Suture needles are supplied with suture material already attached. Suture material is available as nonabsorbable and absorbable. The nonabsorbable type needs to be removed within a few days after placement and the absorbable type remains in the tissues until it disintegrates.

Patient Preparation

Preoperative Instructions

Patients who will be undergoing surgical procedures that involve using general anesthesia or IV sedation should be given preoperative instructions in advance:

1. The patient should have nothing to eat or drink 6 hours prior to surgery.

2. Another person should provide transportation to the patient.

3. The patient should discontinue using aspirin or medications that thin the blood a few days prior to surgery.

4. All prescription drugs that the patient is currently taking should be listed on the medical history form.

5. If the patient has a joint replacement or heart valvular damage, a prophylactic antibiotic medication should be taken prior to and after surgery.

6. The patient should be cautioned that some pain, bleeding, and swelling might take place after surgery.

Preparing the Patient for Surgical Procedures

1. The patient should remove contact lenses and oral prosthetic appliances and give them to the accompanying person.

2. Vital signs are taken before, during, and after surgery and documented in the patient's chart.

3. For patients undergoing general anesthesia, monitors should be positioned ready to be connected to the patient. For patients receiving local anesthesia alone, monitors are not used.

4. Have the patient rinse with an antimicrobial mouthwash to diminish microorganisms in the oral cavity.

Oral Surgical Procedures

Surgical Extractions

Exodontics. (*ex* = "out"; *odont* = "tooth") is the term used to describe the extraction of teeth. The term *oral surgeon* is given to the dentist, who is recognized as having the required skills, knowledge, and training in the specialty of oral surgery. The extraction of teeth is one of many procedures in oral surgery.

The indication for a tooth extraction may vary from the removal of a diseased primary tooth to the removal of a retained tooth (unerupted, embedded, impacted, malpositioned) or the retained roots of a tooth. In some orthodontic cases teeth may be removed to allow space in a dental arch.

Extractions. All extractions are surgical procedures that are rated on a scale from less than difficult to increasingly difficult. Special surgical instruments are used according to the surgical procedure.

Multiple Extractions. When several teeth are extracted, it will be necessary to reshape the remaining alveolar ridge before placing an immediate denture. This procedure is called an **alveolectomy**. A rongeur removes bony projections and a bone file contours the shape of the alveolar bone. The soft tissue is brought together over the bone and sutured.

Impacted Teeth. There are basically two variations of impactions: soft tissue impactions and bony impactions. In a soft tissue impaction the tooth may be partially erupted, with a portion of the tooth visible in the mouth. A bony impaction is blocked from eruption by both alveolar bone and mucosa. These tissues must be surgically displaced before access to and removal of the impaction can be accomplished.

Procedure 70 Surgical Removal of Impacted Teeth

Materials Needed (Figure 58-28)

General anesthetic, IV sedation, patient monitor set-up
Local anesthetic set-up
Basic set-up
Gauze sponges, 3 x 3
Surgical aspirator, HVE tips
Irrigating syringe with sterile saline solution
Scalpel handle with assorted blades
Periosteal elevator
Straight elevator
Root tip elevators
Surgical curette

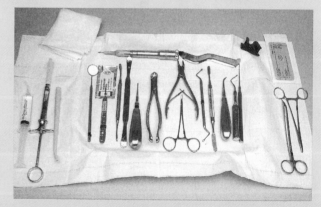

Figure 58-28 Tray set-up for removal of impacted teeth.

continued

continued from previous page
Procedure 70 Surgical Removal of Impacted Teeth

Tongue retractor
Tissue retractor
Maxillary or mandibular forceps
Bone file
Rongeurs
Surgical scissors
Surgical burs, handpiece
Mallet and chisel
Needle holder
Suture needle, suture material
Bite block

Instructions

1 The patient is put under general anesthesia or IV sedation with nitrous oxide–oxygen and is closely monitored throughout the procedure.

2 The oral surgeon administers local anesthesia.

3 Once the area is anesthetized, the oral surgeon is ready to begin the surgical procedure and places a bite block between the patient's posterior teeth on the opposite side of the mouth. In many cases the throat is blocked with gauze to prevent aspiration of debris.

4 The soft tissue is incised with a scalpel and the dental assistant uses the surgical aspirator from this point on and throughout the procedure to maintain a clear vision for the surgeon. The tongue is also retracted with a tongue retractor, especially when removing mandibular impacted third molars.

5 The surgeon uses the periosteal elevator to reflect the tissue from the bone. The flap of tissue is retracted with tissue retractors to gain access to the bone.

6 To expose the tooth positioned under the bone, a bur and handpiece are used together with sterile saline solution. The HVE is used to keep the area clean.

7 When the tooth is exposed, the oral surgeon tries to luxate (displace) it from its socket using a straight elevator. The selected forceps are used subsequently to extract it. If the roots of the tooth are dilacerated (bent or curved), the tooth will need to be sectioned. The bur and handpiece or a mallet and chisel are used to section the tooth into pieces that are removable.

8 Once the tooth is removed, it should be examined for all of its parts. If the tip of a root is still embedded in the bone socket, the surgeon uses root tip picks to remove it.

9 The oral surgeon uses a surgical curette for debridement (clean out debris) of alveolar bone particles and dental sac remnants from the tooth socket.

10 Once the tooth is removed, the bone is contoured using the rongeur forceps to trim bone spicules (sharp bone fragments). The dental assistant should have a 3 x 3 gauze square ready to wipe the rongeur beaks of bone fragments.

11 The surgeon uses the bone file to smooth the edges of the bone, also referred to as alveolectomy, and irrigates the socket while the dental assistant uses the HVE. The socket is cleaned out and evacuated.

12 The surgical site is sutured using a needle holder, suture needle, and material. As the surgeon places the suture, the dental assistant keeps the area clear and may assist in cutting the suture when indicated. The bite block is removed and a folded 3 x 3 gauze square is placed over the surgical site while the patient bites down.

13 If the patient was sedated or given general anesthesia, he or she is transferred to a recovery room until able to respond reasonably and is ambulatory (able to walk). The dental assistant prepares several 3 x 3 gauze sponges, prescription for pain and antibiotic, and postoperative instructions to give the patient or escort.

14 Prior to dismissal, a postoperative appointment is scheduled within a week or less.

Nonextraction Surgical Procedures

Frenectomy. A **frenectomy** is a surgical procedure to remove a poorly attached facial or lingual frenum. Surgery may involve only a small incision to partially loosen the frenum, complete removal of the frenum, or repositioning of the frenum. This surgery is generally performed on children to give added mobility to the lip or tongue.

Maxillofacial Surgery. Maxillofacial surgery is performed to modify or correct facial abnormalities, such as a protrusive or retrusive mandible or maxilla. Protrusive means projected forward to the position of the opposing arch. In the protrusive position, the mandible is projected forward in relation to the maxilla. A retrusive position of the mandible would be far posterior in relation to the maxilla.

Osteotomy. Surgery that involves the cutting of bone is termed an osteotomy. Such dental procedures include the removal of an exostosis. An **exostosis** is an excessive bony outgrowth that may develop bilaterally in the lingual premolar region of the mandible; this is termed torus (on one side) and tori (on both sides) mandibularis. A torus that develops along the palatine suture is referred to as torus palatinus. Surgical removal becomes necessary before a removable partial appliance can be accurately constructed. The tori would interfere with the impression of either arch and subsequent construction of the mandibular lingual bar and saddles and the palatal bar of the maxillary arch. The need for the same surgery would apply for removable full dentures.

Postoperative Instructions Following Surgical Procedures

Instructions following surgical procedures should be given to the patient verbally and in written form:

- Patients should be instructed to keep the gauze on the surgical site for 30 minutes after dismissal.

- Caution the patient that slight bleeding may continue for the following 24 hours, to use a folded 3 x 3 gauze sponge when needed, and to avoid strenuous activity within the first two days.

- Instruct the patient to inform the office staff if excessive bleeding, swelling, or pain occurs. An ice pack should be used for 20 minutes on and 20 minutes off as soon as possible and continued for the first 24 hours to diminish swelling.

- Caution the patient not to rinse forcefully for the following 24 hours. Thereafter, 1 teaspoon of salt in a glass of warm water may be used to rinse gently twice a day.

- Caution the patient to avoid sucking from a straw, which could cause removal of the clot.

- If sutures were used, the patient should be informed as to the type placed (resorbable or nonresorbable) and when to return for removal of sutures. If a suture is lost, the patient should not be too concerned unless bleeding continues.

- The patient should refrain from eating solid food within the first day after surgery but should eat soft nourishing foods and chew on the opposite side of the jaw.

- The patient should avoid smoking (delays healing) and drinking alcohol (irritates tissues) within the first 24 hours.

- Some pain should be expected, which may be controlled with ibuprofen or acetaminophen. Should it become severe, a prescribed medication should be taken. Caution patient not to drive a car or operate machinery while using medication.

- Brushing the teeth in the surgical area should be avoided until the next day when it is done in a gentle manner without traumatizing the tissues. All other teeth should be brushed as usual.

- The patient should be scheduled for a postoperative appointment to evaluate healing progress and suture removal, if applicable.

Postoperative/Suture Removal Appointment. During the postoperative appointment, the patient is evaluated for healing. The surgical site is cleaned with a cotton-tipped applicator soaked in an antiseptic solution such as peroxide or iodophor. Nonresorbable sutures are removed usually within five days. The oral surgeon grasps the knot with cotton pliers and cuts one strand of the suture underneath the knot and removes it. The number of sutures removed is documented in the patient's chart.

Alveolitis (Dry Socket). If the patient is experiencing significant pain following surgical extraction, **alveolitis**, or "dry socket," may be suspected. Alveolitis occurs when the clot that formed after surgical extraction is absent. It may have become dislodged when the patient rinsed vigorously or when drinking with a straw. Treatment for this condition includes irrigation with warm saline solution and insertion of a strip of iodoform gauze in the socket. This will prevent food from entering the socket and provide an **obtundent**, or soothing relief, to the patient. The same treatment is repeated every one to two days until healing takes place. The patient may be placed on an antibiotic and pain control regimen for a few days until the condition subsides.

Biopsy/Exfoliative Cytology (Pap Smear). A biopsy is indicated when there is evidence of excessive tissue growth or change in tissue texture, consistency, or color. For the biopsy procedure, a sample or entire portion of affected tissue is excised and sent to the laboratory to be tested and viewed under a microscope for evidence of malignant cells. The specimen is placed in a bottle of formalin, which is capped and clearly labeled with the date, patient's name, dentist's name, and site of the specimen removal.

When an exfoliative cytology, or Pap smear, is performed, the cells on the surface of the lesion are scraped off and the sample is placed on a glass slide for microscopic evaluation. The slide is clearly labeled with the date, patient's name, and dentist's name and the site from where it was removed.

Hospital Dentistry

Hospital dentistry includes both oral surgery and restorative treatment under general anesthesia. Patients unable to receive treatment in the dental office or clinic under local anesthesia are scheduled in a hospital.

In the practice of hospital dentistry, the dentist must understand and follow operating room procedures and observe all hospital regulations. The dentist, anesthesiologist, and hospital staff should consult on the choice of medication, anesthesia, and course of treatment prior to admitting the patient to the operating room. Certain patients, such as small children, the mentally impaired, the elderly, and medically compromised, should be thoroughly screened for any existing medical problems prior to hospital treatment.

Cleaning, Sterilization, and Maintenance of Surgical Instruments

Instruments

Rinsing. Immediately after surgery instruments should be rinsed under warm (not hot) running water. Rinsing should remove all blood, body fluids, and tissue.

Cleaning. If cleaning is not done immediately after rinsing, instruments should be submerged in a solution of water and neutral (pH7) detergent.

Ultrasonic Cleaning

- For micro and delicate instruments, use manual cleaning.
- Instruments should be processed in the cleaner for the full recommended cycle time, usually 5–10 minutes.
- Hinged instruments should be placed in the open or unlocked position into the ultrasonic cleaner. "Sharps" (scissors, knives, osteotomes, etc.) blades should not touch other instruments.
- All instruments must be fully submerged.
- Dissimilar metals (stainless, copper, chrome plated, etc.) should not be placed in the same cleaning cycle.
- Solution should be changed frequently, at least as often as the manufacturer recommends.
- Instruments should be cleaned with water after ultrasonic cleaning to remove ultrasonic cleaning solution.

Automatic Washer Sterilizers. Manufacturer's recommendations should be followed, making sure instruments are lubricated after the last rinse cycle and before the sterilization cycle.

Manual Cleaning. Most instrument manufacturers recommend ultrasonic cleaning as the best and most effective way to clean surgical instruments, particularly those with hinges, locks, and other moving parts. If ultrasonic cleaning is not available, the following steps should be observed:

- While wearing utility gloves, stiff plastic cleaning brushes with a long handle should be used. Steel wool or wire brushes should not be used except specially recommended stainless steel wire brushes for instruments such as bone files or on stained areas in knurled handles.
- In a basin of water using neutral (pH #7) detergent (prevents breakdown of stainless protective surface), one instrument at a time should be scrubbed under water to diminish aerosolization contamination.
- At this time instruments should be checked for function: scissors blades should glide smoothly all the way (they must not be loose when in closed position). Scissors should be tested by cutting into thin gauze. Forceps (pickups) should have properly aligned tips. Hemostats and needle holders should not show light between the jaws and should lock and unlock easily, and joints should not be too loose. Needle holders should be checked for wear on jaw surfaces.
- Aspirators are cleaned on the inside with adequate long-handled thin brushes.
- Retractors should function properly.
- Cutting instruments have sharp undamaged blades.
- After scrubbing, instruments should be rinsed thoroughly under running water. While rinsing, scissors, hemostats, needle holders, and other hinged instruments should be opened and closed to make sure the hinge areas as well as the outside of the instruments are rinsed thoroughly.

After Cleaning. When instruments are to be prepared for sterilization, they should be allowed to air dry and then stored in a clean and dry environment.

Autoclaving. Prior to autoclaving:

- All instruments should be lubricated that have any "metal-to-metal" or hinged action such as scissors, hemostats, needle holders, self-retaining retractors, etc. Recommended surgical lubricants such as instrument milk are best. Using WD-40 oil or other industrial lubricants is not recommended.
- Instruments should be assembled for autoclaving either individually in pouches or in cassettes, then autoclaved according to manufacturer's instructions.

SUGGESTED ACTIVITIES

● Select and identify the various surgical instruments.

● Explain the use of each selected instrument.

● Practice making a tray set-up for surgical removal of an impacted tooth.

REVIEW

1. The instrument used to reflect tissue from the alveolar bone is the:
   a. Periosteal elevator
   b. Surgical curette
   c. Root elevator
   d. Bone chisel

2. The instrument used to luxate a tooth while in its socket is the:
   a. Root elevator
   b. Straight elevator
   c. Hemostat
   d. Bone file

3. To trim spicules from bone, the instrument used is the:
   a. Bone chisel
   b. Cryer
   c. Surgical scissors
   d. Rongeur forceps

4. To remove debris and dental sac remnants from a tooth socket, the instrument used is the:
   a. Root tip pick
   b. Periosteal elevator
   c. Surgical curette
   d. 2 x 2 gauze square

5. Indicate when a patient who was sedated or put under general anesthesia may be dismissed: (1) if he is escorted home, (2) when he is ambulatory, (3) when he is able to respond reasonably, (4) unescorted, as long as he is coherent.
   a. 1, 2, 3
   b. 2, 3, 4
   c. 1, 2, 4
   d. 1, 3, 4

Oral Pathology

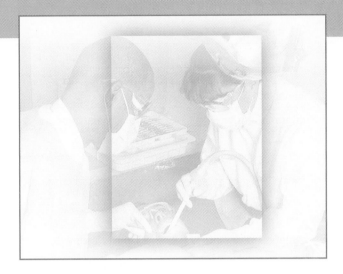

OBJECTIVES

After studying this chapter, the student will be able to:

- Explain which conditions are nonpathologic and which are pathologic.
- Describe and recognize each of the nonpathologic and pathologic conditions found intraorally.
- Define the term oncology.
- Differentiate between benign and malignant tumors based on their characteristics.
- Explain the difference between carcinoma and sarcoma.
- Discuss how the body reacts to chemotherapy.
- Indicate radiation therapy side effects.

Introduction

Oral pathology is concerned with the etiology and nature of diseases that affect oral structures and regions nearby. **Etiology** is the study and cause of disease, which helps in determining how the disease came about.

As a health care professional, the dental assistant should be able to distinguish normal from abnormal conditions (oral lesions). Nonpathologic as well as pathologic conditions may be found in the oral cavity. Nonpathologic are those conditions that may appear unusual but are not disease related. Pathologic conditions arise from viruses, bacteria, and fungi capable of promoting diseased tissues.

Classification of Lesions

Lesions are pathologically altered tissues that appear in several forms. They can be an injury or wound, an infected area, tumors, patches, abscesses, pustules, chancres, ulcers, pigmented skin or mucosa, rash, blisters, crusts, and cysts. Lesions are classified according to location and size (Table 59-1) and color (Table 59-2).

Nonpathologic Conditions

Fordyce's granules are sebaceous glands that are primarily located in the oral mucosa of the buccal vestibule and lips and rarely in other parts of the oral cavity. Fordyce's granules appear as multiple yellowish white papules smaller than 2 mm and are considered to be normal (Figure 59-1).

Hairy tongue is a condition in which the filliform papillae on the dorsum of the tongue become elongated, which results in a hairlike appearance. The papillae may assume a brown, black, yellow, or white coloring. This condition has been associated with poor oral hygiene, smokers, radiation therapy, vitamin deficiency, and gastrointestinal disturbances. Patients may complain of irritation, bad odor, or unusual taste. There is no treatment for it, except that tongue scrapers have been used with some success (Figure 59-2).

Fissured tongue is an **asymptomatic** (without symptoms) condition that for the most part blames heredity as the causative factor. Other factors such as facial paralysis and facial edema are thought to influence this condition. A fissured tongue has deep fissures or grooves on the dorsum and should be brushed to remove trapped debris (Figure 59-3).

Geographic tongue is characterized by loss of filliform papilla within the confines of demarcated areas on the dorsal and lateral aspects of the tongue; however, it could also migrate to the ventral surface of the tongue and other areas on the mucosa. The areas void of filliform papilla appear inflamed and **erythematous** (redness of skin or mucosa). Filliform papilla grows back in a very short time returning the tongue to a normal state.

531

Table 59-1	Classification of Lesions According to Location and Size		
Lesion	**Above the Surface**	**Size**	**Example**
Papule	Solid elevation of skin	< 5 mm	Rash
Nodule	Solid mass elevation of skin	< 1 cm	Enlarged lymph node
Wheal	Elevated area on superficial part of skin that itches	Variable	Hives
Tumor	Solid mass extending deeply	approx. 2 cm	Carcinoma/sarcoma
Vesicle	Elevated lesion filled with fluid	< 1 cm	Herpes blister
Pustule	Elevated lesion filled with pus	approx. 5 mm	Pimple
Bulla	Elevated lesion filled with fluid or blood	> 1 cm	Large blood blister
Lesion	**Below the Surface**	**Size**	**Example**
Ulcer	Open sore on the tissue	3 mm deep or more	Syphilis lesions
Abscess	Deep lesion filled with pus	Variable	Tooth abscess
Cyst	Sac filled with fluid or semifluid	Variable	Gingival cyst
Lesion	**Flat**	**Size**	**Example**
Macule	Flat blemish or discoloration	Variable	Freckle
Petechiae	Small purple or red hemorrhagic spots	Pinpoint or pinhead	Flea bites
Purpura	Hemorrhagic trauma in tissues due to blood disorder	Variable	Purplish lesions
Patch	Of different color and texture	Variable	Leukoplakia

Table 59-2	Classification of Lesions According to Color		
White	**Black**	**Brown, Reddish, Purple, Blue**	**Yellow**
Leukoplakia	Melanoma	Kaposi's sarcoma	Fordyce's granules
Candidiasis		Amalgam tattoo	
Lichen planus		Addison's disease	
Geographic tongue			
Papilloma			

Although the etiology is unknown, it is thought to be related to psoriasis, a skin condition that also has inflamed red patches.

Focal melanosis is an increase of deposition of melanin pigment that may be seen as black, brown, blue, or gray in the mucosal epithelium. It is a benign lesion that has a flat appearance and the size does not usually exceed 1 cm in diameter. The most prevalent areas to observe focal melanosis is on the vermilion border of the lips, middle portion of the lower lip, gingival buccal mucosa, and palate. Affected persons are usually younger to middle-age adults and women more than men.

Median rhomboid glossitis derives its name from the rhomboid or rectangular erythematous area lacking filliform papilla. It is found on the anterior or middle third surface of the dorsum of the tongue. Presently, it is believed to be caused by a fungal infection from *Candida albicans*. There is no specific treatment for this condition, except that an antifungal medication may be applied to the area. Generally, it disappears without treatment.

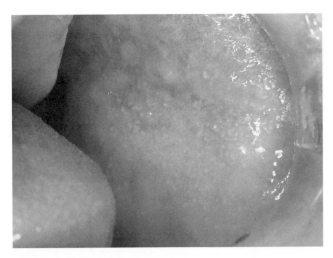

Figure 59-1 Fordyce's granules. (Courtesy of Joseph L. Konzelman, Jr.)

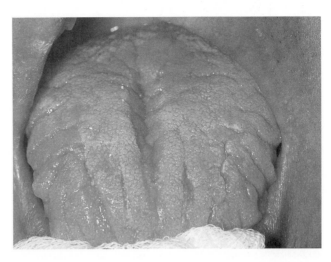

Figure 59-3 Fissured tongue. (Courtesy of Joseph L. Konzelman, Jr.)

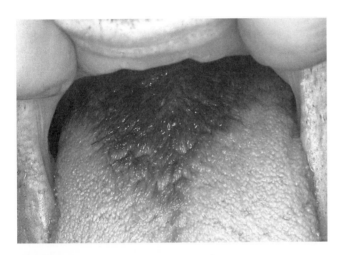

Figure 59-2 Hairy tongue.

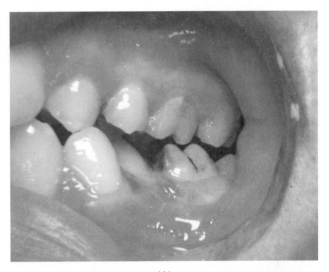

(A)

Lingual tonsils are comprised of glandular tissue located on the lateral posterior of the tongue. They may resemble pathologic lesions due to their nodular texture and erythematous appearance. Examination should include viewing both sides of the tongue to ensure that it is tonsillar tissue.

Ectopic tonsil is tonsillar tissue that is displaced from its normal position. Sometimes it appears on the dorsum of the tongue as a small raised erythematous lesion.

Lingual varicosities are prominent veins located on the ventral and lateral surfaces of the tongue. They are generally found on older individuals over 60 years who may also exhibit varicous veins on the legs.

Amalgam tattoo whose appearance is dark gray or blue, is usually located on the gingiva. The obvious cause is embedded amalgam in the tissues while an amalgam restoration was being placed (Figures 59-4A, B).

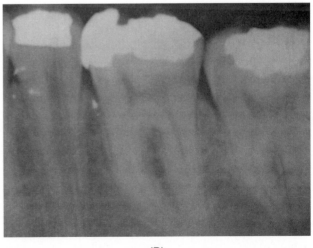

(B)

Figure 59-4 Amalgam tattoo. (Courtesy of Joseph L. Konzelman, Jr.)

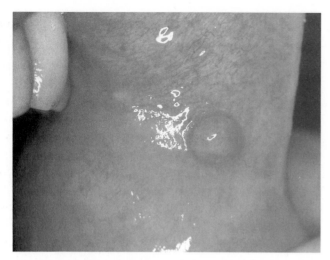

Figure 59-5 Mucocele. (Courtesy of Joseph L. Konzelman, Jr.)

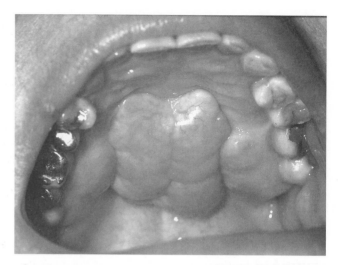

Figure 59-6 Torus palatinus. (Courtesy of Joseph L. Konzelman, Jr.)

Mucocele occurs when the duct of a minor salivary gland is injured. The lesion fills up with fluid and extends itself into the oral cavity, simulating a blister. Its bluish appearance may shrink in size by draining the fluid. The minor salivary gland may be removed to eradicate the problem (Figure 59-5).

Exostoses are classified as "buccal exostoses," "torus palatinus," and "torus mandibularis." They are excess bone enlargements consisting of dense bone with underlying bone marrow affecting the jaws in particular locations. Each of these may be surgically removed for esthetic purposes, for construction of prosthesis, or when constant traumatization occurs. However, they are usually left alone.

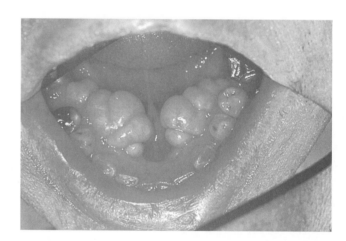

Figure 59-7 Torus mandibularis. (Courtesy of Joseph L. Konzelman, Jr.)

● Buccal exostoses are bony outgrowths of the maxillary or mandibular buccal surfaces. They are usually bilateral, affecting posterior teeth.

● Torus palatinus is another form of exostoses located on the midline of the maxillary palate. It occurs more often in women and appears to be hereditary (Figure 59-6.)

● Torus mandibularis is also a form of exostoses located on the lingual surfaces of the mandibular jaw bicuspid area. It occurs more often in men and also appears to be hereditary, although forces of mastication may be a contributing factor (Figure 59-7).

Ankyloglossia, also known as "tongue tie", is the short lingual frenum attachment between the tongue and the floor of the mouth. This condition limits the tongue movement in an upward or forward direction, thus impeding speech, causing nursing difficulties for babies, and sucking or swallowing problems. To correct this condition, a frenotomy is performed whereby the connective tissue or the frenum itself is surgically cut (Figure 59-8).

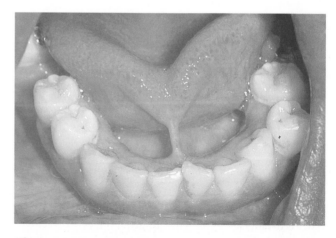

Figure 59-8 Ankyloglossia, "tongue tied." (Courtesy of Joseph L. Konzelman, Jr.)

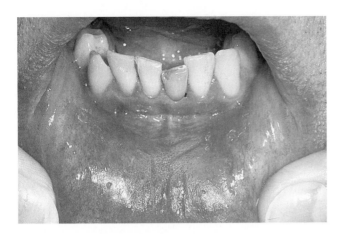

Figure 59-9 Leukoplakia. (Courtesy of Joseph L. Konzelman, Jr.)

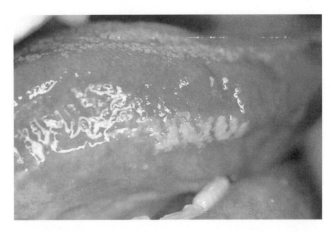

Figure 59-10 Hairy leukoplakia. (Courtesy of Joseph L. Konzelman, Jr.)

Pathologic Conditions

Pathologic oral lesions may develop on various identifiable appearances. Their color, pigmentation, ulcerated state, size, and location may characterize them.

Leukoplakia (*leuko* = "white," *plakia* = "plaque") is a condition that appears as white patches and may be considered to be premalignant. It is usually associated with tobacco smoking and is more commonly seen in males than females. It can be found in all areas of the mouth but primarily occurs in the buccal mucosa, floor of the mouth, lateral borders of the tongue, alveolar ridges, and commissure of the lips. If it continues to progress, the lesion becomes thickened and verrucous (wartlike) and may become cancerous (about 5% may exhibit cancerous changes) (Figure 59-9).

Hairy leukoplakia is one of the lesions found in persons who are infected with HIV (human immunodeficiency virus). Thickened vertical corrugated white lesions on the lateral borders of the tongue occurring bilaterally characterize this condition. This white lesion cannot be removed when rubbed. Temporary treatment can be obtained with systemic use of acyclovir (Figure 59-10).

Candidiasis, or "thrush," is a fungal infection that resembles white patches produced by *Candida albicans*. *Candida albicans* is present in the oral cavity in approximately 45% of healthy adults. This condition usually appears after a person has been through antibiotic or corticosteroid therapy or in persons who suffer from some disease such as diabetes mellitus or acquired immunodeficiency syndrome (AIDS). To distinguish this condition from leukoplakia, the dentist will attempt to remove the white patch with a gauze sponge. Candidiasis will generally rub off, leaving an erythematous patch underneath. It is difficult to remove the lesion by scraping if it has become **keratotic** (hardened). The lesion is commonly found on the tongue,

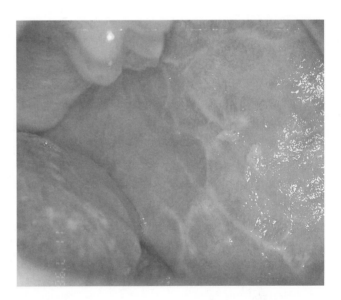

Figure 59-11 Lichen planus. (Courtesy of Joseph L. Konzelman, Jr.)

buccal mucosa, and palate but may also be found in any area of the oral cavity.

Lichen planus is a condition of unknown etiology that affects the skin and the oral cavity. It is more commonly seen in women of middle age. The appearance in the oral cavity resembles white lace or a network of white lines and is commonly found on the buccal mucosa, dorsum of the tongue and gingiva (Figure 59-11). On the skin it may resemble small **papules** (red elevated solid lesions) exhibiting fine scales or white streaks. Sometimes these lesions join together and are found on the inside of the wrists, legs, abdomen, and back. Oral lesions are typically of a chronic nature exhibiting clinical manifestations from time to time and at other times go into **remission** (when signs and symptoms become less severe or are no longer evident).

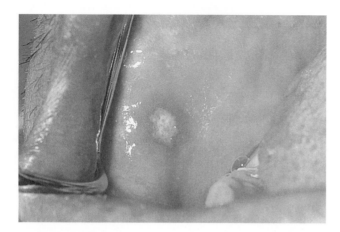

Figure 59-12 Apthous ulcers. (Courtesy of Joseph L. Konzelman, Jr.)

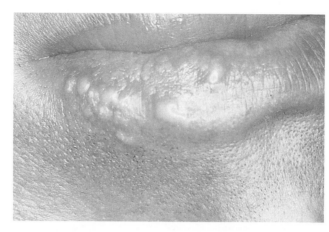

Figure 59-13 Herpes labialis. (Courtesy of Joseph L. Konzelman, Jr.)

Apthous ulcers, also known as "canker sores" or "apthous stomatitis," are lesions found on movable mucosa in the oral cavity and throat. They can be classified as minor, major, and herpetiform. The minor types are most common and are small, usually less than 1 cm in diameter (Figure 59-12). Although the etiology is still unknown, apthous ulcers have been linked to a weakened immune system, heredity, stress, vitamin deficiencies, allergies, and trauma. The length of duration is between 10 and 14 days.

Major apthous ulcers are similar in appearance to the minor ulcers and also occur on movable mucosa. They are larger than 1 cm with several lesions present at one time. It takes about six weeks for healing to take place with a short interval between recurrences. Treatment with systemic steroids and topical elixir (liquid form) has been successful in producing remissions.

Herpetiform apthous ulcers are also similar to minor apthous ulcers except that they are smaller, about 2 mm or less, and occur in greater numbers, up to 100 separate ulcers at one time. They appear as multiple pinhead ulcerations surrounded by reddened tissue on movable mucosa. Treatment for temporary remission has included 2% tetracycline rinse and topical steroid elixirs and gels.

Herpetic ulcers are products of the herpes simplex virus. They are characterized by painful, swollen, red tissue with multiple **vesicles** (small blisters). The lesion begins with a red ulcer, similar to an apthous ulcer except that it is not located on movable mucosa but rather mucosa bound to bone, to the palate, or to alveolus. The ulcer progresses to form a vesicle (blister) within one or two days and later begins to crust until it heals in about 14 days. This disease is communicable and is transmitted by physical contact. Treatment includes acyclovir topical application or taking tablets by mouth, which provides some relief and shortens duration of the lesions.

The virus appears in several areas of the body and is named accordingly:

- Herpetic gingivostomatitis occurs within the oral cavity, on the gingiva, or the palate.
- Herpes labialis, also known as "cold sore" or "fever blister," occurs on the lips and surrounding skin (Figure 59-13).
- Herpetic whitlow occurs on the fingers and thumbs.
- Genital herpes occurs on the genitalia.

Syphilis is a sexually transmitted disease that can also be transmitted through other means, as through blood transfusions, and from an infected mother to her fetus, causing the child to develop permanent incisors with notches or Hutchison's incisors (Figure 59-14) and

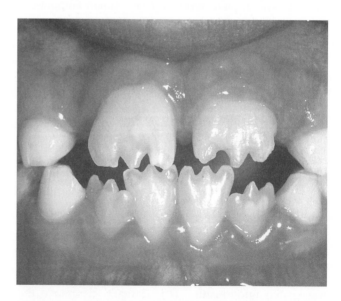

Figure 59-14 Hutchinson's incisors. (Courtesy Dale Ruemping.)

mulberry molars with multiple enamel globules. The disease occurs in three stages:

- In the primary stage, the *Treponema pallidum* bacterial spirochete enters the body through the genitals or by other means. If the point of entry was the oral cavity, a chancre (ulceration) will develop there within 2–3 weeks after **inoculation** (the process by which microorganisms enter the body) and will heal within 3–8 weeks.

- In the secondary stage, about 4–10 weeks after inoculation, the skin develops a rash and an oral lesion called mucous patch occurs that appears as grayish white ulcerated areas on the tongue, buccal mucosa, lips, or gingiva. The lesion will disappear within 3–12 weeks. It should be noted that during the primary and secondary stages, the patient is highly contagious.

- In the tertiary stage the disease progresses to the cardiovascular and central nervous systems and large ulcerations known as "gummas" develop almost anywhere in the body, including the oral cavity. Treatment for this disease consists of antibiotics, particularly penicillin.

Oncology

Oncology is the study of tumors. Tumor means swelling, and the term used for tumor is **neoplasia** (*neo* = "new," *plasia* = "growth"); therefore, it is a new growth of abnormal tissue in which the cells multiply uncontrollably. There are two major types of tumors, benign and malignant.

- **Benign** tumors are contained or encapsulated and do not spread. They carry the suffix *-oma*, which signifies a tumor. For example, a benign tumor of muscle is named "myoma" (*myo* = "muscle," *oma* = "tumor"). Benign tumors are usually surgically removed, which should eliminate them.

- **Malignant** tumors, as is cancer, grow rapidly and can cause death; their cells invade surrounding tissues and are capable of spreading throughout the body. The process of malignant cells spreading to distant parts of the body is termed **metastasis**. Malignant tumors are of two general types. Tumors that originate from **epithelium** (tissue that covers the body, such as the skin, and lines cavities, as in the oral cavity) are called **carcinomas**. An example is **squamous cell** carcinoma (squamous cell is a flat scale-like epithelial cell) because squamous cells are part of the epithelium. Tumors that originate from all other tissues besides epithelium are called **sarcomas** and they take on the name of the tissue they arose from. For example, a malignant tumor of muscle is named "myosarcoma" (*myo* = "muscle," *sarcoma* = "malig-

nant nonepithelial tumor"). Malignant tumors can be removed surgically but must also be treated with chemotherapy and/or radiation therapy due to their ability to spread.

Chemotherapy

Chemotherapy consists of using chemical agents taken internally to destroy or deactivate cancerous cells in all parts of the body. Cancerous cells multiply rapidly because they divide at a fast rate, thus the chemical agents administered in chemotherapy affect all cells that are capable of such proliferation. Cells responsible for hair growth, cells in the intestinal tract, and blood-forming cells in bone marrow fall into this category and, therefore, are affected by chemotherapy.

Chemotherapy Side Effects

- **Alopecia** (hair loss)
- Nausea, vomiting, diarrhea
- Loss of appetite
- Decrease of bone marrow production that leads to anemia
- Decrease of antibody response due to low white blood count

Radiation Therapy

Radiation therapy (radiotherapy) uses ionizing radiation aimed directly at the diseased location to destroy cancerous cells. Not only are the diseased cells destroyed in the oral cavity but also salivary gland cells and bone cells (osteoradionecrosis) together with blood vessels that supply that area.

Radiation Therapy Side Effects

- Decreased salivary production, causing **xerostomia** (dry mouth)
- Change in composition of saliva becoming thicker and more acidic
- Radiation caries, especially on gingival third and any exposed root surfaces
- *Candida* fungal infection due to decreased salivation
- Osteoradionecrosis causing deep periodontal pockets
- Loss of appetite due to diminished saliva, sore mouth, and changes in the sense of taste

Oral Cancer

There are different types of oral cancer. Among them are verrucous, melanoma, squamous cell or epidermoid,

Kaposi's sarcoma, and others. Cancers vary in the way they look and act.

Characteristics of Oral Cancer

- A small granular red lesion or multiple lesions
- A white patch
- Scaly or wartlike appearance
- An ulcer that does not heal within two weeks
- Red and white speckled appearance
- Unusual bleeding or discharge
- Numbness
- Difficulty in swallowing
- Foul odor

Squamous Cell Carcinoma. The most common oral cancer is the squamous cell carcinoma, accounting for 90% of all oral cancers. The primary contributing factors for cancer development within the oral cavity are considered to be tobacco and alcohol. For cancer development on the lip, ultraviolet radiation from the sun's rays is considered the primary culprit. If squamous cell carcinoma is diagnosed early, there is a high probability that recovery will be complete. The five-year survival rate for persons with this intraoral disease is approximately 75%, and for those with lower lip lesions is approximately 90%. Therefore, when inspecting the oral cavity, dental health care professionals should always be on the alert for abnormal changes occurring there.

High-Risk Persons. Persons at high risk affected by squamous cell carcinoma are usually over 45 years of age; however, it may strike persons of any age. Persons using more than half a pack of cigarettes a day, pipes or cigars, smokeless tobacco, or consume 6 oz or more of alcohol per day are also at high risk.

High-Risk Areas. Although oral cancer may appear in any area of the oral cavity, there are some high-risk areas where cancer typically occurs:

- Ventral portions of the tongue
- Lateral portions of the tongue
- Floor of the mouth
- Tonsillar pillars
- Soft palate

Kaposi's Sarcoma. Kaposi's sarcoma is primarily seen in individuals affected with AIDS. The oral lesion is a malignancy of blood vessels usually found on the hard

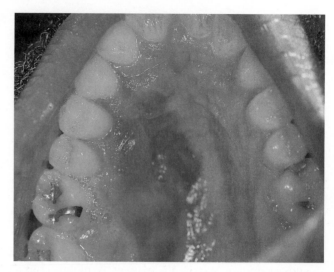

Figure 59-15 Kaposi's sarcoma.

palate and gingiva but may also be found on other intra-oral locations and extraorally on the skin (Figure 59-15). Treatment varies from person to person. Chemotherapeutic drugs as well as low dosages of radiation therapy have been used but have not been proven to be very successful. The best solution at this time is to keep the teeth clean and use chlorhexidine mouthwash. The characteristics of this type of cancer are as follows:

- Purplish to brown in appearance
- May be flat, raised, or appear swollen
- Located close to the teeth on the gingiva and the palate

Benign Neoplasms

Papilloma is a benign tumor of squamous epithelium caused by a virus. It resembles a cluster of cauliflower with many small projections usually located on the soft palate, ventral and dorsal surface of tongue, and the buccal mucosa. It may range in color from white to pink or red and the sizes may be less than 1 cm but in some cases they grow to 3 cm. Treatment consists of surgical removal (Figure 59-16).

Fibroma is a benign tumor of fibrous connective tissue. It is the most common soft tissue tumor of the oral cavity. It forms as a result of irritation and is usually no larger than 2 cm in diameter (Figure 59-17). Treatment consists of surgical removal.

Odontoma is an odontogenic tumor. One type known as a compound odontoma is composed of several small teeth surrounded by a radiolucent "halo" when observed on a radiograph. Another type, named a complex tumor, is composed of enamel, dentin, cementum, and pulp not resembling a normal tooth. Treatment consists of surgical removal.

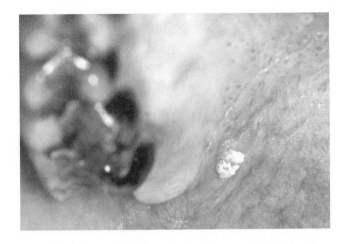

Figure 59-16 Papilloma. (Courtesy of Joseph L. Konzelman, Jr.)

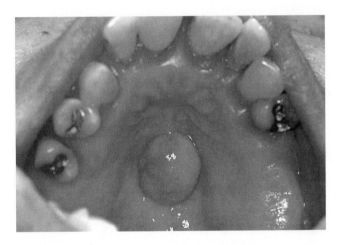

Figure 59-17 Fibroma. (Courtesy of Joseph L. Konzelman, Jr.)

Hemangioma is a vascular benign tumor most commonly occurring on the tongue when located intra-orally. Others occur predominantly in the head and neck area. They are usually present at birth or develop soon thereafter. Treatment may consist of corticosteroids while the patient is young, surgical removal or injecting a sclerosing agent that causes fibrosis and shrinkage.

SUGGESTED ACTIVITIES

● Using flash cards, identify which conditions in the oral cavity are considered to be nonpathologic and which are pathologic.

● Using slides of pathologic lesions, try to identify each condition depicted.

REVIEW

1. Match the nonpathologic conditions on the left with their characteristics on the right:

___ a. Fordyce granules
___ b. Hairy tongue
___ c. Fissured tongue
___ d. Geographic tongue
___ e. Focal melanosis
___ f. Median rhomboid glossitis
___ g. Ectopic tonsil
___ h. Mucocele
___ i. Exostoses
___ j. Ankyloglossia

1. Excess bone enlargements on jaw or palate
2. Displaced tonsillar tissue from its normal position
3. Loss of filliform papilla within demarcated areas on dorsum of tongue
4. Increased deposition of melanin pigment on mucosa not exceeding 1 cm in diameter
5. A lesion filled with fluid due to an injured salivary duct
6. Asymptomatic deep grooves on dorsum of tongue
7. Lack of filliform papilla on the middle dorsal surface of tongue
8. Elongated filliform papilla on the dorsum of the tongue
9. Short lingual frenum attachment of tongue to floor of the mouth
10. Sebaceous glands appearing as small yellowish papules

2. Match the pathologic conditions on the left with their characteristics on the right:

___ a. Leukoplakia
___ b. Candidiasis
___ c. Apthous ulcer
___ d. Herpetic labialis
___ e. Herpetic whitlow
___ f. Lichen planus
___ g. Syphilis

1. Painful ulcer with multiple vesicles on the lip that heals in 14 days
2. Chronic oral condition that resembles white lace generally found on buccal mucosa, dorsum of the tongue, and gingiva
3. Painful ulcer with multiple vesicles occurring on the fingers
4. White patches in any area of the oral cavity that rub off and usually appear after antibiotic or corticosteroid therapy
5. White patch found on buccal mucosa associated with tobacco that may be considered premalignant
6. Sexually transmitted disease causing the offspring to develop Hutchinson's incisors
7. Smaller than 1 cm, known as canker sores, found on movable mucosa and usually linked to a weak immune system

3. Indicate which of the following are side effects of chemotherapy: (1) increased appetite, (2) alopecia, (3) diarrhea, (4) decreased antibody response due to low white blood count, and/or (5) decreased bone marrow production leading to anemia.
   a. 1, 3, 4, 5
   b. 2, 3, 4, 5
   c. 1, 4, 5
   d. 1, 3, 5

4. Indicate which of the following are radiation therapy side effects: (1) xerostomia, (2) thicker and more acidic saliva, (3) leukoplakia, and/or (4) *Candida* fungal infection.
   a. 1, 2, 3
   b. 2, 3, 4
   c. 1, 2, 4
   d. 1, 3, 4

5. Indicate which of the following are high-risk oral cancer areas in the oral cavity: (1) floor of the mouth, (2) ventral portion of the tongue, (3) soft palate, and/or (4) buccal vestibule.
   a. 1, 2, 3
   b. 2, 3, 4
   c. 1, 2, 4
   d. 1, 3, 4

SECTION 14

Principles of Dental Radiography

CHAPTER 60

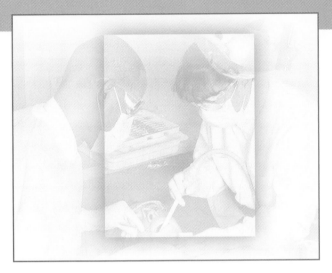

OBJECTIVES

After studying this chapter, the student will be able to:

- Give a brief history of dental radiography.
- State several characteristic properties of x-rays.
- Explain the meaning of ionizing radiation.
- Discuss the three factors that determine the penetrating power of x-rays.
- Explain the principles of x-ray generation.
- Describe the basic components of the x-ray machine.
- State the reasons for filtration of the x-ray beam.
- Explain what is meant by collimation.
- Discuss the different types of radiation as they relate to dental radiography.
- Describe the different ways that radiation interacts with matter.

Introduction

The use of **x-rays** in dentistry has gradually increased as a means of studying underlying structures not visible to the eyes. The **radiograph** consists of shadows or images of a three-dimensional object on film that must be viewed and interpreted by the dental practitioner. The practice of **radiography** requires a basic knowledge of radiation physics and chemistry related to pho-

tography plus a high degree of skill and knowledge of radiation safety techniques.

When the patient seeks the services of a qualified dentist, a full-mouth radiographic survey is often imperative. At times the patient must be convinced that his or her total health may be in jeopardy because of underlying infections that may not have manifested themselves earlier. The profession of dentistry involves causes, diagnosis, and prognosis of disease; therefore, misconceptions and fears of radiation on the part of the dental patient must be overcome if the diagnostic aid, the dental radiograph, is to be used. Times of exposure have been established, and no adverse effect is expected in the person undergoing diagnostic procedures for dentistry if these levels are not exceeded.

Brief History of Origins of X-rays

Wilhelm Conrad Roentgen, a German physicist, discovered x-rays in 1895 during his experimentation with a Crookes-type vacuum tube. As he studied the image formed by the x-rays emanating from the tube, which was covered with black paper, he noticed that when the tube was electrically charged, some unknown rays passing from the tube were affecting a fluorescent tube about 2 meters away. Unaware of the character of these rays, Roentgen named this radiation "x-rays" in order to distinguish them from other types of rays. He presented a paper on the subject to the University of Wurzburg (Germany) Physical Society in 1896. Following the reading of the paper, it was decided by the Society that the rays should be named *Roentgen rays*. Today, the term continues to be used in scientific reference.

Shortly after the discovery of x-rays by Wilhelm Conrad Roentgen, Otto Walkhoff, who used himself in the experiment, made the first dental radiograph in 1896. He used a glass photographic plate wrapped in black paper and rubber and exposed himself to 25 minutes of x-rays. The next pioneer, W. J. Morton, a New York physician, made a dental radiograph using a skull. Later in 1896 a New Orleans dentist, C. Edmund Kells, was the first practitioner to use dental radiographs made on a live patient. He also experimented on himself repeatedly, using x-rays on his hands every day. This amount of exposure eventually caused cancer to develop on his hands, costing him amputation of his fingers, later his hand, and ultimately his arm.

William D. Coolidge invented the first x-ray tube in 1913. This prototype, with some changes, is still in use today. He used the hot filament as opposed to the residual gas that was the source for ionization within the tube. In the same year the first American x-ray machine was made by the Victor X-ray Corporation, later to become the General Electric Corporation and now known as the Gendex Corporation.

Dental radiography is the method of recording images of dental structures on film by the use of *roentgen rays*, or *x-rays*. Shortly after the announcement was made that these rays would penetrate substances known to be **impervious** (not permitting passage) to light, the first dental radiographs were produced. The use of radiographs in dentistry today is considered a necessity to a thorough dental examination. *Note:* For all practical purposes, the terms *x-ray* and *roentgen ray* may be used interchangeably; both terms have the same meaning. Also, when the operator is speaking with patients, it is good technique to use the term *radiograph* (the processed film with an image) since the operator is not really taking x-rays.

Characteristic Properties of X-rays

X-rays are not detected by any of the senses; we cannot see them nor can we taste, feel, hear, or smell them. X-rays, like visible light rays, are electromagnetic rays. This means that they have a definite relationship to electric current and a body of matter that possesses the property of attracting other substances, as a piece of iron or steel is attracted by a magnet. These electromagnetic rays differ from the rays emitted (given off) by radioactive particles. Electromagnetic rays consist of pure energy rather than separate particles of matter.

Wavelengths

The rays are said to radiate, or scatter, in a wheel-shaped path, as waves occur when a pebble is dropped into a pool of water. We refer to the fact that their length varies (from the crest of one wave to that of another) as **wavelength**. This distance between wavelengths is regarded as one frequency. The amplitude is the vertical height from top to bottom of the wave. The trough is the bottom portion of the wave (Figure 60-2A, B).

The electromagnetic spectrum encompasses high-energy waves to low-energy waves that account for the electric and magnetic fields in space. The wavelengths created by each type of energy vary considerably. Wavelengths that are measured in *nanometers* are infi-

nitely smaller, much more powerful, and travel faster than those measured in *meters*. One needs to realize that the speed at which x-rays travel is the same as light, or 186,000 miles per second.

The basic difference in the various types of electromagnetic radiation is wavelength. Beginning with the shortest wavelengths, the range of electromagnetic radiation includes the following (Figure 60-1):

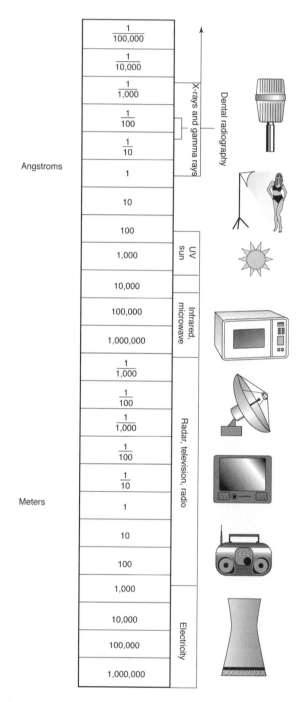

Figure 60-1 Electromagnetic spectrum chart. (From *Delmar's Dental Assisting: A Comprehensive Approach*, by D. Phinney and J. Halstead, 2000, Albany, NY: Delmar)

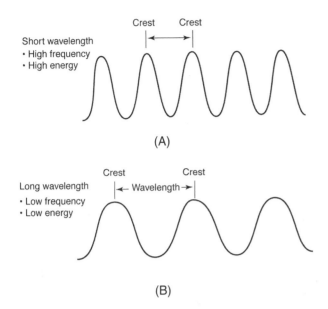

Figure 60-2 (A) Hard radiation waves—short wavelength and high frequency. (B) Soft radiation waves—long wavelength and low frequency.

- X-rays and gamma rays are similar and have the same general properties, i.e., they consist of high-energy photons (elemental units of radiant energy), have short wavelengths, and have no mass or electrical charge.

- Gamma rays, unlike x-rays, are produced by the disintegration of certain radioactive elements (radium, uranium, thorium) and are electromagnetic emissions of that particular radioactive substance. Because of their high penetrating power, gamma rays are sometimes used in the medical treatment of deep-seated malignancies.

- High-energy photons of x-rays and gamma rays have the ability to pass through gases, liquids, and solids and to ionize the substances they penetrate. Because of their very short wavelength and high penetrating power, x-rays and gamma rays are said to produce **hard radiation** (Figure 60-2A). The rays with longer wavelengths that have less energy and do not have the ability to pass through matter, such as electric, radio, television, microwave, radar, infrared, visible light and ultraviolet rays, are said to produce **soft radiation** (Figure 60-2B).

Ionizing Radiation

X-rays and other rays of high penetrating power are capable of producing ions, directly or indirectly, in their passage through matter. An atom (smallest particle of matter of an element) has a nucleus that contains positively charged particles called protons and neutral particles

called neutrons; in the orbits around the nucleus are negatively charged particles called electrons. The orbits, also called shells, are arranged at specific distances from the nucleus. Each shell is identified by a letter, starting with the letter K, which is the closest to the nucleus and the most binding. The shells L, M, N, O, P, and Q follow. The Q shell is the least binding.

Ionization occurs when an x-ray **photon** (a high-velocity mass of radiant energy) strikes an atom and causes the negatively charged particles to be ejected from an orbit. When the balance between the positive and negative particles of the atom is disturbed, the atom becomes unbalanced. This unbalanced atom is called an ion. The ejected electron (negative ion) and the unbalanced atom (positive ion) together are called an ion pair. To again achieve a balanced state, the atom seeks another negatively charged ion (electron) to travel with, thus creating a disturbance or change in the substance. The substance can be *organic* (having lived at one time) or *inorganic* (not living or having been alive) matter. All forms of radiation are capable of causing ionization of matter.

X-rays travel from a common point, as do light waves. They proceed from their source in straight lines and cover an increasingly larger area with lessening intensity. X-rays have a high frequency. The shorter the wavelength, the higher the frequency or the greater the number of oscillations (waves) emitted per second.

The penetrating power of x-rays depends on three factors:

1. The wavelength of the rays—the shorter the wavelength, the higher the frequency, the greater the penetrating power

2. The distance from the source of the x-rays to the object—the shorter the distance, the greater the penetrating power

3. The density of the object penetrated (relative amount of light that the object will allow to pass)—the less the density, the greater the penetrating power of the x-rays

Principles of X-ray Generation

X-rays are produced when any form of matter is struck by electrons traveling at high speed. To accomplish this, it is necessary to have a source of electrons, a high voltage (electromotive force expressed in units called volts) to accelerate the electrons, and a target to stop them.

The X-ray Machine

The x-ray machine is composed of the control panel, the extension arm, and the tubehead. The control panel contains the on and off switch, a peak kilovolt (kVp) selector, a milliampere selector, timing dial, the exposure

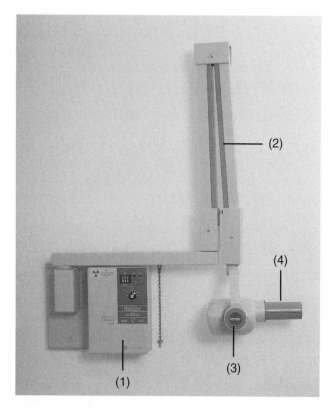

Figure 60-3 X-ray machine: (1) Control panel, (2) Extension arm, (3) Tubehead, and (4) PID.

button on a coiled cord capable of extending 6 feet away, and an indicator red light that lights up when an exposure is made. Newer machines also include an audible sound when exposure is made. The extension arm houses electrical wires that connect the control panel to the tubehead. The tubehead houses the x-ray tube, transformers, oil, tubehead seal, and aluminum filters (Figure 60-3).

The X-ray Tube

Serving as the basis for generating x-rays, the x-ray (vacuum) tube within the x-ray tubehead consists of the following components: a **cathode** (negatively charged electrode), containing a **tungsten filament**, which serves as a source of electrons, controlled by the milliampere dial, and an anode (positively charged electrode, or **tungsten target**), at which the high-speed electrons are directed (Figure 60-4). The filament and target are encased within a lead-lined evacuated vacuum tube. The leaded glass housing for the vacuum tube is treated with lead, which gives it a bluish-gray appearance (Figure 60-5). X-rays are produced when the electrons strike the target. In order to function, an electrical current within the tube creates a charge between cathode and anode, propelling the electrons across at very high speeds (one-third the speed of light).

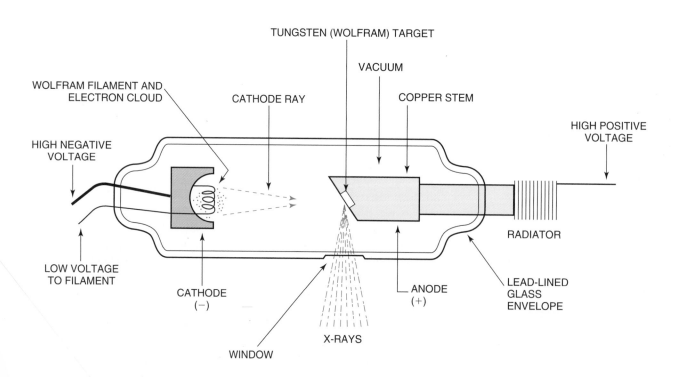

Diagram of the x-ray vacuum tube with components.

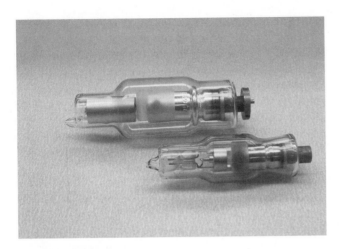

Figure 60-5 Vacuum tubes.

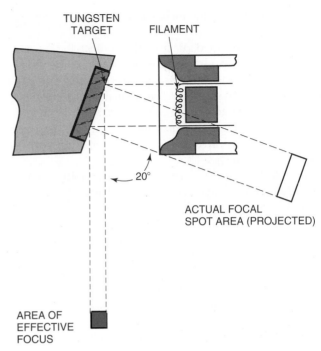

Figure 60-7 Area of effective focus. The relationship between the actual focal spot (target) and the effective focus as projected from a 20° angle.

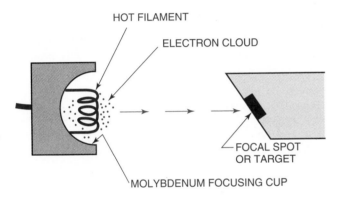

Figure 60-6 Formation of the electron cloud.

Cathode. The cathode of an x-ray tube is composed of two principal parts: the **filament** and the **focusing cup** (Figure 60-6). The filament, the source of electrons within the x-ray tube, is a coil of tungsten (also called wolfram) wire, and is about 0.2 centimeter (cm) in diameter and 1.0 cm in length. It is mounted on two strong, stiff wires that support it and carry the electric current. These two wires lead through the glass tube to serve as connections for the low- and high-voltage source. A **milliampere** (mA, 1/1000 of an ampere) control on a separate side panel provides for fine adjustment of the voltage across the filament, which heats it to a high temperature. Thus, a "cloud" or **thermionic emission** of electrons is produced around the heated coil. The milliampere control regulates the quantity of electrons the filament emits, which in effect regulates the tube current; i.e., the flow of electrons through the tube is measured by the milliammeter.

The tungsten filament is located in the focusing cup, a negatively charged concave reflector cup of molybdenum. The focusing cup electrostatically focuses the electrons emitted by the filament into a narrow beam directed at a small area of the anode called the **focal spot** or target. The electrons are caused to move in this direction because of the strong electrical force imposed between the cathode and the anode by a high negative charge placed on the cathode and a high positive charge on the anode. The high negative charge of the cathode repels the negatively charged electrons while the positive charge of the anode attracts them.

Anode. The anode is composed of a tungsten target and copper stem. The purpose of the target in an x-ray tube is to convert the kinetic (associated with motion) energy of the electrons generated from the filament into x-ray photons. Tungsten is usually selected as target material because of its high atomic number (74)—therefore having many electrons available—high melting point (3370°C), and low vapor pressure, which is important at the high working temperature of an x-ray tube. The tungsten target is embedded in a large mass of copper to help dissipate (scatter in various directions) the large amount of heat created at the target.

About 1% of the energy of the electron beam striking the target is converted into x radiation that exits through the porte or window of the tube; approximately 99% of the energy becomes heat in the anode structure and is dissipated via the copper stem and oil.

The angle of the inclination of the target is important, because it partially determines the *focal spot size*. If the anode is inclined 20° from the vertical and the electrons are projected from the cathode in a rectangular stream, then the projected focal spot can be made square in shape and appreciably smaller than the actual area on the target. Figure 60-7 shows the rectangular stream of electrons bombarding the target, the actual focal spot area projected (area of bombardment), and the area of effective focus.

When x-rays are produced, not all photons possess the same energy and wavelengths. They differ according to the manner in which the high-speed electrons strike the tungsten target. The numbers of atoms of the tungsten target are limitless, and therefore many are affected each time an exposure is made. Two main phenomena take place as x-rays are produced: the **bremsstrahlung**, or "braking," radiation and the characteristic radiation.

Bremsstrahlung Radiation. Bremsstrahlung radiation takes place when high-speed electrons interact with tungsten atoms at the "target" of the anode. One possible way is for a speeding electron to enter the atom hitting its nucleus, which rarely happens, and coming to an abrupt stop, or *braking*. This causes the electron to lose all of its energy, producing a high-energy photon and heat. Another possible way is for a speeding electron to penetrate an atom close to its nucleus without dislodging any of the tungsten atom electrons and being deflected. This reaction can occur repeatedly. The same electron that entered the first tungsten atom exits and enters another atom, causing the same reaction; however, each time it enters a new atom, it loses some of its power and the photons produced each time have less energy or longer wavelengths. About 70% of x-ray photons are produced in this manner (Figure 60-8A).

Characteristic Radiation. Characteristic (pertaining to the interacting material) radiation occurs when another high-speed electron interacts with a tungsten atom at the "target." This time the speeding electron, having more energy than the K-shell electrons that possess 69,000 electron volts, dislodges one, causing ionization to occur and thus forming an ion pair. Cascading and rearrangement of the other orbiting electrons in the outer shells take place to fill in the inner shells of the atom (Figure 60-8B.) Characteristic radiation occurs in machines that operate at 70 kVp and above due to the binding energy of 69,000 electron volts in the K shell. Only a small amount of x-ray photons are produced in this manner.

Power Supply

The primary functions of the power supply are to provide an electrical current to heat the x-ray tube filament

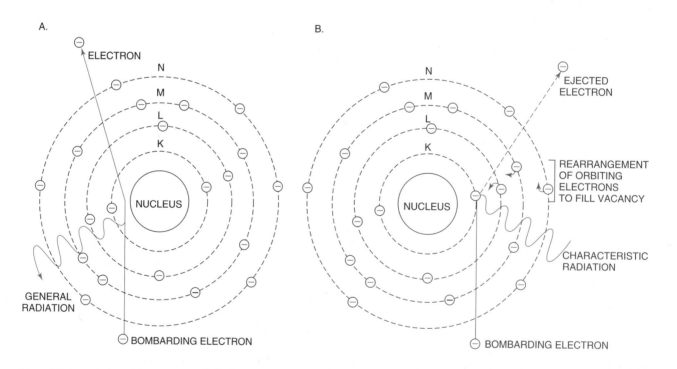

Figure 60-8 (A) Atoms in Bremsstrahlung or general radiation. An electron passes close to the nucleus of a tungsten atom producing an x-ray photon of lower energy or general radiation. (B) Characteristic radiation. An electron ejects an inner shell tungsten atom electron causing a rearrangement of other electrons in the atom, producing a characteristic radiation.

and to provide a potential difference between the anode and the cathode. These functions are accomplished by the use of a **step-down transformer**, a **step-up transformer** or **high-voltage transformer**, and an **autotransformer**.

These transformers and the x-ray tube are contained within an electrically grounded metal housing called the *head* of the x-ray machine. An electrical insulating material, usually oil, surrounds the transformers.

Depending on the make and size of the tubehead, the oil may total as much as 5 quarts.

The step-down transformer that reduces the voltage of the incoming alternating current (AC) to between 3 and 5 volts controls the filament. Its operation is regulated by the filament current control (milliamperage switch), which adjusts the current flow through the filament, its heating, and thus the quantity of electrons emitted by the filament (Figure 60-9).

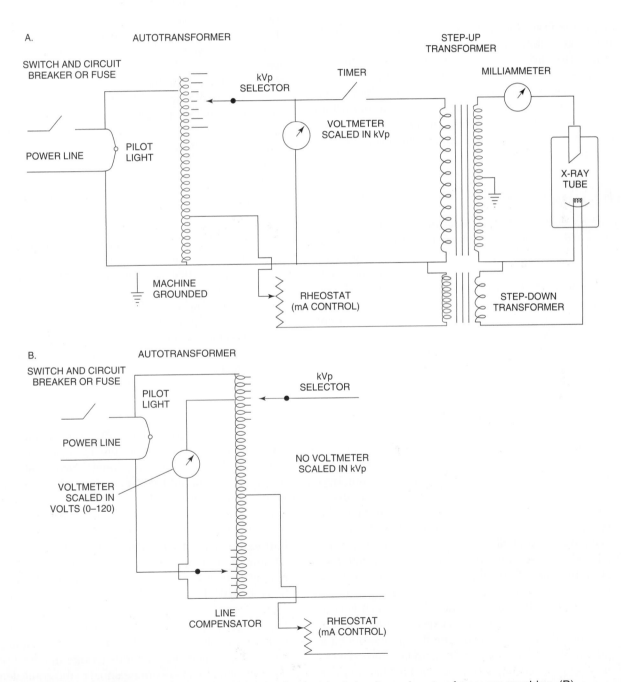

Figure 60-9 (A) A simplified wiring diagram of the basic electrical circuits and parts of an x-ray machine. (B) Alternative voltage regulating the system. (Courtesy of General Electric Company, Medical Systems Division.)

The kilovolt peak selector dial regulates the output of the step-up transformer. It controls the voltage between the anode and cathode of the x-ray tube. The high-voltage transformer provides the high voltage required by the x-ray tube to accelerate the electrons in order to generate x-rays. It accomplishes this by boosting the voltage of the incoming line current to a range of 60–100 kilovolts (kVp), or 60,000–100,000 volts (V). The 60–100 kVp represents the highest, or peak, value of the voltage waves, i.e., the highest voltage that an x-ray machine can produce at a given setting.

The electrons, being negatively charged, will be attracted by a positive charge. The greater the positive charge, the faster the electrons will travel toward it. As the voltage within the tube is increased, the speed of the electrons toward the cathode correspondingly increases.

The autotransformer (Figure 60-9B) makes use of one coil to make small adjustments in voltage. For example, when there is a variation of electrical current within a building, the autotransformer in the x-ray machine takes care of any fluctuations to keep the power supply constant.

The Timer

A timing control device to control the x-ray exposure time is included in the primary circuit of the high-voltage supply. The timer completes the circuit in the high-voltage transformer and controls the time that the high voltage is applied to the tube and thereby the time during which tube current flows and x-rays are produced. To minimize filament use, the timing circuit sends a current through the filament for about half a second to bring it to the proper operating temperature. Once the filament is heated, a time-delay switch applies power to the high-voltage circuit. There is, in many circuit designs, a low-level current passing through the filament that maintains it at a low, safe temperature, so the delay to preheat the filament before each exposure is shortened.

Some x-ray machine timers are calibrated in fractions of seconds and in whole numbers of seconds. On other timers, the time intervals are expressed as numbers of impulses per exposure. The number of impulses divided by 60 (the frequency of the power source) gives the exposure time in fractions of a second. Thus, 30 impulses is equivalent to a half-second exposure. The x-rays are produced only when the operator pushes the button to activate the high electrical input, usually called a dead-man switch. (It should be noted that as long as it takes for the exposure to be made, the dead-man switch is connecting. However, as soon as the exposure is terminated, the connection is broken and even though the operator is still pressing the exposure button, there is no connection.) On more recently developed timers, this is only a fraction of a second of exposure time. To protect the operator, the switch is usually placed outside the operatory or has a long cord, so that it can be activated while the operator is at least 6–8 feet away from the tubehead.

Filtration

Although an x-ray beam is composed of x-ray photons (radiant energy) that are arranged according to their wavelength, only those photons with sufficient energy are useful for diagnostic radiographs. Those that are of low penetrating power (long wavelength) contribute to the patient's exposure but not to the information on the film. In the interest of patient safety, a filter, an aluminum disk, is placed over the aperture or opening of the tubehead, between the tubehead seal and the collimator, to remove the low-energy photons from the beam without affecting those that are able to penetrate the patient and reach the film.

When the amount of filtration for a particular machine is being determined, the operating characteristics of the tube and its housing must be considered. Two types of filtration exist: inherent filtration and added aluminum filtration.

Inherent Filtration. Inherent filtration corresponds to the materials that x-ray photons encounter as they travel from the focal on the target to form the useful beam (primary radiation) outside the tube enclosure. These materials include the glass wall of the x-ray tube, the insulating oil that surrounds many of the dental x-ray tubes, and the barrier material (seal) used to prevent the oil from escaping through the tubehead opening. The tube, surrounded by oil, is encased in a protective metal case called the tubehead, or the tube housing. The window of the tube through which the useful beam passes is chemically treated with lime. Inherent filtration of most x-ray machines ranges from the *equivalent* of 0.5–2 mm of aluminum.

Added Aluminum Filtration. Added aluminum filtration corresponds to the placement of aluminum disks to the tubehead aperture (opening). Increments of 0.5-mm disks may be added. To determine how much aluminum is needed in a given machine, an assessment is made. The aluminum filter would need to reduce the intensity of the x-ray beam by 50%. This is known as the **half-value layer (HVL)**. If a machine has a thickness of 2.0 mm of aluminum, it means that this amount of aluminum is necessary to reduce the energy of the x-ray beam by half (Figure 60-10).

Total Filtration. Total filtration is the sum of the inherent filtration plus any added filtration such as aluminum disks. Governmental regulations require that total filtration in a dental x-ray beam be equal to the equivalent of 1.5 mm of aluminum up to 70 kVp and 2.5 mm of aluminum for all higher peak kilovolt machines.

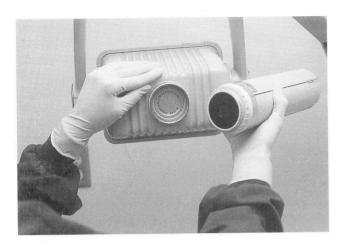

Figure 60-10 Aluminum filter.

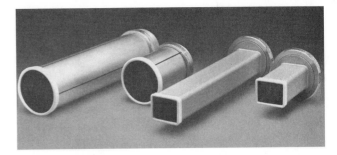

Figure 60-11 Position-indicating devices (PIDs).

Collimation

When the x-ray beam is directed at a patient, tissues absorb some of the x-ray photons, while others pass through to form an image on the film. Many of the absorbed photons generate **scattered radiation**. To minimize the amount of **primary radiation**, **collimation** reduces the size of the x-ray beam and, thus, the volume of scattered radiation within the patient from where the scattered photons originate.

Cylinder and rectangular shaped **collimators** are used in dental radiography (Figure 60-11). These reduce patient exposure and increase film quality.

In many states, radiation protection codes mandate the use of round or rectangular, open-ended, lead-lined cylinders and recommend terminating the use of pointed plastic cones (Figure 60-12).

The diaphragm collimator is a thick washer of radiopaque material (usually lead) (Figure 60-13) that controls the beam size to approximately 2 3/4 in. (7 cm) in diameter at the outer opening of a cylindrical **position-indicating device (PID)** or at the patient's face. This device is usually placed directly over the aluminum filter at the opening of the x-ray head through which the x-ray beam emerges. The size and shape of the aperture of the collimator determine the size and shape of the useful beam (Figure 60-14). The PID also achieves collimation, because it is usually lined with, or constructed of, radiopaque material and can be cylindrical or rectangular in shape. Rectangular collimators limit the beam to a size just larger than the size of an x-ray film. Position-indicating devices may vary in length from 8 to 16 inches.

Types of X-ray Radiation

There are several types of x-ray radiation (Figure 60-15): primary, remnant, secondary, scattered, and stray.

1. Primary radiation is that radiation that emerges from the x-ray tube target (anode), sometimes called

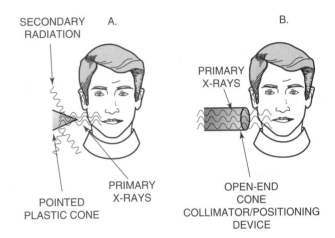

Figure 60-12 (A) Pointed PID causes interaction of the primary beam with the plastic cone causing a major source of secondary radiation. (B) Open-ended lead-lined or metal collimator PID eliminates this source of secondary radiation and patient exposure.

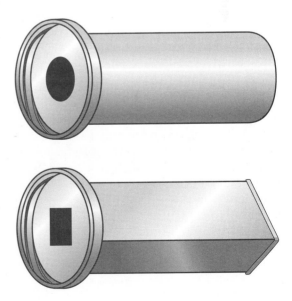

Figure 60-13 Collimator washers: (A) round and (B) rectangular.

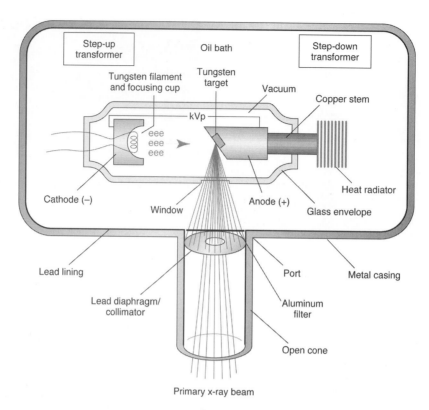

Figure 60-14 Effects of aperture size on divergence of x-ray beams.

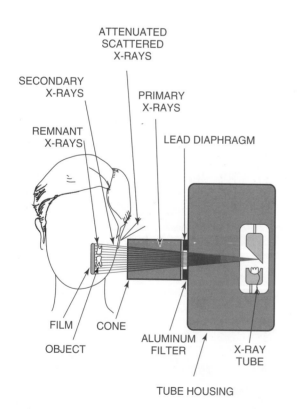

Figure 60-15 Primary, scattered, secondary, and remnant radiation.

direct ray, primary beam, useful beam, or central ray. The quality (penetrating power) of this radiation depends upon the correct settings of milliampere and kilovolt peak controls.

2. **Remnant radiation** is all of the x-ray photons that reach their destination (the film) after passing through the object being radiographed and consist of unabsorbed primary and secondary rays generated in the tissue. Remnant rays produce the radiographic image in the form of the **latent image** (not visible until the radiograph is processed).

3. **Secondary radiation** results from interaction between primary radiation and the atoms of an object it contacts. Some of the primary beam will pass through the object with no contact, and some will irradiate atoms of the object. Secondary radiation, therefore, consists of scattered radiation from primary rays, and the amount produced depends on the quality and quantity of primary radiation and the atomic number of its tissue source. Elements such as water, body tissue, and wood generate large quantities of secondary radiation. The kilovot peak is the primary factor influencing the production of secondary radiation.

4. Scattered radiation, also called secondary rays or secondary scattered rays, consists of rays from the primary beam that have deflected during their pas-

sage through tissues or other substances. These rays may or may not have been **attenuated** (weakened) by absorption or scattering of the photons. Scatter radiation is all of the radiation that arises from the interaction of the x-ray beam with the atoms of an object in the path of the beam, with associated changes in wavelength.

5. **Stray radiation** consists of all radiation other than the primary or useful beam produced *within* the x-ray head and is caused by electrons hitting the glass wall and other parts of the x-ray tube rather than the target. Leakage of a faulty tube or tubehead permits stray radiation to escape.

Exposure to any of these types of radiation contributes to the **absorbed dosage** (this is covered in more detail in Chapter 62).

Radiation Interactions with Matter

There are several interactions with matter that take place when x-ray photons exit the PID. The exiting photons are made up of various penetrating powers that can change in direction as they interact with matter. There are four possible occurrences:

1. *No interaction.* This takes place when the x-ray photon passes through an atom unchanged without disturbing any of the orbiting electrons. It means that the x-ray photon passed through the patient's tissues without any interaction or alteration of atoms. This type of interaction takes place approximately 9% of the time while making bitewing exposures (Figure 60-16A).

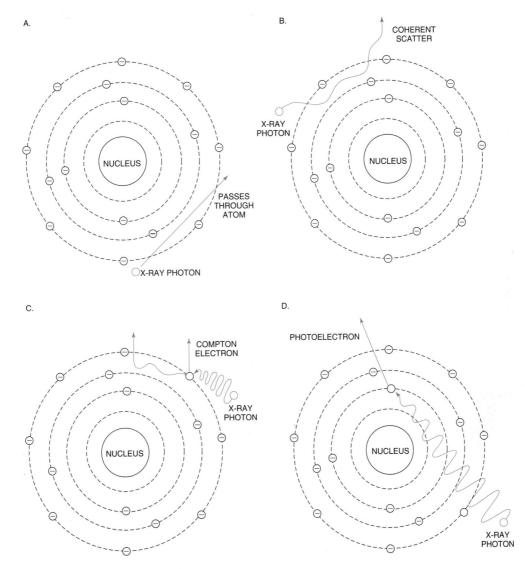

Figure 60-16 (A) No interaction—a photon passes through an atom unchanged. (B) Thompson scatter—a photon is scattered without loss of energy, also known as coherent. (C) Compton scatter—a photon interacts with an outer shell electron and removes it from its orbit. (D) Photoelectric effect—a photon interacts with an inner shell electron, causing the photon to be completely absorbed and producing a negatively charged photoelectron.

2. *Thompson scatter.* Known also as classical, unmodified, or coherent, Thompson scatter occurs when an x-ray photon of low energy interacts with the outer shell of an atom, causing its path to be altered and scattered. There is no change in the atom and no ionization takes place. This type of interaction occurs approximately 8% of the time (Figure 60-16B).

3. *Compton scatter.* When scatter radiation takes place, it is mainly due to this type of interaction. When an x-ray photon of sufficient energy enters an atom, it collides with a loosely bound or outer shell electron, causing it to be ejected from its orbit, thus causing ionization to take place. The ejected electron now has a negative charge and the remaining atom has a positive charge. The same x-ray photon, having lost some of its energy, continues in a different direction to interact with another atom until it loses all of its energy. Compton scatter accounts for approximately 62% of the time while making exposures (Figure 60-16C).

4. *Photoelectric effect.* The **photoelectric effect** takes place when an x-ray photon of sufficient energy enters an atom and ejects a tightly bound electron from one of the inner shells. This causes the photon to lose all of its energy, ceasing to exist, and transfers it to the ejected electron that is now known as a photoelectron. The remaining atom is left with a positive charge since it lost one of its electrons. This is also known as ionization. In this interaction there is no scatter because all of the energy of the x-ray photon was absorbed by the atom and not deflected. This type of interaction accounts for 30% of the time (Figure 60-16D).

SUGGESTED ACTIVITIES

● Compare collimators used on cylinder PIDs with rectangular PIDs and determine the difference.

● Expose one film on a manikin and place another unexposed film nearby within the path of the x-ray beam. Process both films exposed to radiation plus one unexposed film. Compare all three radiographs for density, fogging, and clarity.

REVIEW

1. How does ionization of radiation take place?
   a. When two ions pair up, one with a positive charge and one with a negative charge
   b. When several ions come together
   c. When a balanced atom loses an electron caused by an x-ray photon that displaces it
   d. When a positive ion displaces a negative ion

2. A transformer that reduces the voltage of incoming alternating current to 5 volts to control the required amount of heat needed at the tungsten filament in the cathode is known as:
   a. Autotransformer
   b. Step-down transformer
   c. Step-up transformer
   d. Kilovoltage peak

3. X-rays are produced when the tungsten target is struck by ___ traveling at high speed.
   a. Electrons
   b. Photons
   c. Secondary radiation
   d. Stray radiation

4. Approximately how much of the energy of the electron beam is converted into x-rays?
   a. 99%
   b. 98%
   c. 1%
   d. 5%

5. Match the terms on the left with the statements on the right.

   ___ a. Collimator
   ___ b. Inherent filtration
   ___ c. Added filtration
   ___ d. Anode
   ___ e. Cathode
   ___ f. Focusing cup
   ___ g. Thermionic emission
   ___ h. Focal spot
   ___ i. Tungsten filament

   1. A concave reflector that directs the electron cloud to the target
   2. The target located at the anode where x-ray photons are produced
   3. A coil located in the cathode, which when heated produces electrons
   4. Materials within the tubehead such as the tube window, oil, and seal
   5. A disc made of lead with an aperture that restricts the size of an x-ray beam
   6. A negative electrode that attracts positive ions
   7. A positive electrode that attracts negative ions
   8. A disc made of aluminum located at the aperture of the tubehead to absorb soft or useless waves
   9. The electron cloud produced by the heated filament at the cathode

Measurement of Ionizing Radiation

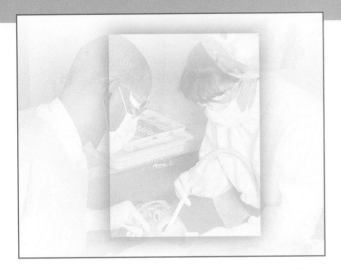

OBJECTIVES

After studying this chapter, the student will be able to:

- Discuss the historical evolution of radiation quantities and units.
- Identify the radiation units of exposure, absorbed dose, and dose equivalent.
- Define *quality factor* as it relates to the different ionizing radiations.
- Explain the differences between rad and rem.
- Explain the ALARA concept.
- State the formula for the cumulative MPD in terms of the traditional unit of measurement, and solve problems using the formula.

Introduction

Natural/terrestrial (backgound) radiaton or ionizing radiation coming from natural sources has always been a part of human environment. Three natural sources include radioactive materials in earth, cosmic radiation from outer space, and **radionuclides** (any atomic nucleus specified by its atomic number, atomic mass, and energy state) existing in the human body. A radionuclide is radioactive and disintegrates with emissions of electromagnetic radiation

The human body contains many radioactive nuclides that exist in small quantities within the tissues. Potassium-40, carbon-14, and strontium-90 are some of the chemical elements. **Cosmic radiation** (from the sun and stars) varies in intensity at different altitudes of the earth's surface. The higher the altitude, the greater the intensity; the lowest intensity occurs at sea level. Thus far, mankind has been unable to control the quantity of natural radiation.

Sources of Radiation

Background Radiation

Existing radiation affecting people can be classified as having a natural background or being man made. The natural background would include *cosmic* coming from the sun and stars and *natural* from radionuclides, atomic breakdown, and isotopes.

Man-Made or Artificial Radiation

Man-made or artificial radiation would include industrial exposure being of occupational nature; industrial waste; nuclear testing; nuclear power plant accidents; and dental and medical radiographic exposures used in diagnosis, therapy, nuclear medicine, and occupational exposure. Other consumer products such as television, smoke detectors, radium in watches and clock dials, cigarettes, and natural gas used in cooking, are included within the artificial radiation (Table 61-1).

The environment we live in produces radiation that occurs naturally and radiation that is man made. The estimated annual dose from naturally occurring radiation exposure is said to be approximately 300 mrems, or 3 mSv, per year. By including medical and dental exposures, the average dose would increase to 360 mrems, or 3.6 mSv, per year. Much of the exposure to radiation is attributed to the environment, when compared to medical or dental exposure. Even though it is estimated that the single largest contributor to artificial radiation is from medical radiation, the potential risk for a person to succumb to terminal cancer related to dental or medical radiation exposure is very low. It has been estimated that about 3 in 1,000,000 may be affected as compared to 3300 in 1,000,000 who develop cancer spontaneously for other reasons.

Standards of measurement for ionizing radiation have been developed throughout the world in an attempt to reduce radiation exposure. It is important that the dental radiographer be familiar with these standardized radiation quantities and units.

Table 61-1 Radiation Sources	
Natural Background Sources	**Man-made or Artificial Radiation**

Cosmic: Sun and stars
Natural: Radionuclides—potassium, carbon, strontium
Atomic breakdown
Isotopes
	Industrial radioactive waste
	Industrial exposure
	Nuclear testing
	Nuclear power plant accidents
	Medical and dental exposure:
	    Diagnostic—Radiography and fluoroscopy
	    Radiation therapy
	    Nuclear medicine
	    Occupational
	Consumer products
	    Television
	    Smoke detectors
	    Radium watch and clock dials
	    Cigarettes
	    Natural gas used in cooking

Standardization of Radiation Measurement

In 1921, the medical and dental community formed the British X-ray and Radium Protection Committee to investigate the alarming number of radiation injuries. The unit of measure at that time was the *skin erythema dose*, defined as a dose of radiation that caused reddening of the skin following radiation. It is unlikely, in modern times, that it would be necessary to expose enough dental films to produce a skin erythema on the patient's face. However, during endodontic treatment, fractures, and other situations when several radiographs are necessary within a short period of time, the limitations of irradiation must be realized.

The International Commission on Radiation (ICRU) was formed in 1925. This commission was charged with the responsibility of defining a unit of exposure in 1928. It was not until 1937 that a report was given to the International Congress of Radiology, defining the roentgen (R) as a unit of measurement of exposure to x- and gamma radiation. In 1962, the roentgen was redefined to increase accuracy and acceptability. Today, there are two systems of radiation measurements: the standard or traditional and the Système Internationale (SI).

Standard or Traditional Measurements

Roentgen

A **roentgen unit (R)** can be defined as the amount of x-radiation that will produce one cubic centimeter of air ions at standard temperature and pressure, carrying one **electrostatic** (the binding force that keeps the negative electrons in their orbits by the positive nucleus) unit of energy either sign (plus or minus). The unit of exposure corresponding to ionization in air of one electrostatic unit is 0.001293 gram of air. Envision a cube of air 1 cm in all dimensions. An x-ray beam passes through it, and the x-ray photons strike electrons orbiting around the nuclei of electrically stable air atoms and separate the electrons from their respective nuclei. This action is **ionization** (ion pair formation); the electron is negatively charged and the remainder of the atom becomes positively charged. When measuring radiation, these charges are collected and counted.

The roentgen has been assigned a quality factor of 1; therefore, 1 R is the traditional unit of x-radiation or gamma radiation (Table 61-2).

Radiation Absorbed Dose

The **radiation absorbed dose (rad)** is the unit of absorbed radiation by the object or patient. One unit of rad is the quantity of energy imparted to a mass of material exposed to any type of ionizing radiation. One rad is equivalent to 1 roentgen. The millirad is 1/1000 of a rad (Table 61-3). X- or gamma radiation does not become a *dose* until it is absorbed. A dose may be defined as the total quantity of radiation in roentgens at a given point measured in air. The dose of ionizing radiation absorbed in human tissue is important in dental radiography, since

Table 61-2 Radiation Quality Factors	
Type of Ionizing Radiation	**Quality Factor**
X-ray photons	1
Beta particles	1
Gamma photons	1
Slow neutrons	3
Fast neutrons	10
Protons	10
Alpha particles	20

From *Radiation Protection for Dental Radiographers* by C. Edwards, M.A. Statkiewics-Sherer, and E.R. Ritenour, 1984, St. Louis, MO: Mosby.

Table 61-3 Traditional Measurement Equivalencies

1 roentgen (R)	=	1 rad	=	1 rem
1 Milliroentgen (mR)	=	1 millirad (mrad)	=	1 millirem (mrem)
1000 mR	=	1 R		
1000 mrad	=	1 rad		
1000 mrem	=	1 rem		

Table 61-4 SI and Traditional Measurement Equivalencies

SI Measurements		Traditional Measurements
1 coulomb/kilogram (C/Kg)	=	3880 roentgens (R)
1 gray (Gy)	=	100 rad
1 sievert (Sv)	=	100 rem

it is responsible for the biological changes that occur in that tissue and specific area.

Because bone contains calcium and phosphorus, it will absorb more ionizing radiation than will soft tissue, which is composed of fat and structures close to that of water. Bone has an effective atomic number (13.8); soft tissue has a lesser atomic number (7.4); the atomic number of water is 7.0. Bone absorbs more ionizing radiation than soft tissue in the diagnostic energy range of 65–90 kVp used in dentistry, because the *photoelectric effect* is the dominant mode of energy absorption within the tissues. Photoelectric pertains to effects produced by increased electrical conduction, as occurs in 65–90 kVp. The higher the atomic number of the materials undergoing a photoelectric effect, the greater the amount of energy absorbed by that material. With a dental x-ray beam, 1 R will produce an estimated 0.903 rad in soft tissue. As the SI measurements are being used today, one needs to know how to convert the traditional units into the newer measurements. For example, the rad is being replaced by the gray (Gy); 1 Gy equals 100 rad (Table 61-4).

Quality Factor

The **quality factor (QF)** relates to radiation in terms of biologic effect in body tissue for equal absorbed doses. X-rays, **beta particles** (high speed electrons), a form of **particulate radiation**, and gamma rays have been assigned a quality factor of 1 and provide the base against which to compare the effectiveness of other types of ionizing radiation in producing biologic damage. For example, the specific ionization of fast neutrons is 10 times greater than x-radiation in producing a given biological effect and is assigned a quality factor of 10. A neutron is an electrically neutral or uncharged particle of matter existing along with protons in the nucleus of atoms of all elements (except the mass 1 of hydrogen). Rays of alpha particles, a type of emission produced by a disintegration of radioactive substance, such as uranium and radium, are used only in radiotherapy (Table 61-2).

Roentgen Equivalent (in) Man

The **roentgen equivalent (in) man (rem)** is the physical and biological effects of the tissues that absorb various degrees of radiation. The rem is the unit of dose equiva-

lent. It is the product of the QF of a particular radiation and the rad dose. In diagnostic radiology, this unit is used to make a comparison between the biologic effects of exposure and the various types of radiation. It is generally accepted that 1 R is equal to 1 rad, which equals 1 rem (Table 61-3). When using the SI units, the rem is replaced by the sievert (Sv); 1 Sv equals 100 rem (Table 61-4).

Système Internationale Measurements

The **Système Internationale** uses the metric units of measurement that are adaptable to international standards. It uses higher values in comparison to the traditional units, i.e., 1 Gray is equivalent to 100 rad or 1 rad is equivalent to 1/100th of 1 Gray.

Coulombs per kilogram is used in place of the roentgen unit. One coulomb per kilogram is equivalent to 3880 roentgens. The **gray (Gy)** is used in place of the rad or one gray is equivalent to 100 rad, and the **sievert (Sv)** is used in place of the rem or one sievert is equivalent to 100 rem (Table 61-4).

Relative Biologic Effectiveness

Relative biologic effectiveness (RBE) is similar to QF and is used only in reference to laboratory investigations.

The effects of radiation on living tissue may vary because of the many different physical and biologic circumstances. Two generalizations can be made: (1) Ionization is the underlying phenomenon by which changes occur and (2) all ionizing radiation is hazardous but the degree of hazard varies.

Dose-Limiting Recommendations

Report No. 39 (1971) of the National Committee on Radiation Protection and Measurements (NCRP) establishes certain criteria for the use of radiation on human subjects:

- Methods providing maximum information with minimum dose should be utilized.

- Determination should be made as to whether radiation is the preferable agent for performing the survey or study.

- The possible need for repetition of radiation should be considered in the original plan. In other words, dental x-radiation should not be used when other media can make the determination.

ALARA

Included in the 1954 report by the NCRP is the stated principle that radiation exposures should be kept "as low as reasonably achievable" **(ALARA)**. The concept of ALARA is accepted by all regulatory agencies. The employment of all proper radiation control procedures is the shared responsibility of all persons working in radiology.

Consumer-Patient Radiation Health and Safety Act of 1981

The Consumer-Patient Radiation Health and Safety Act of 1981 provides federal legislation requiring the establishment of minimum standards for accreditation of educational programs for persons who administer radiological procedures and for the certification of such persons. This legislative act was signed in August 1981 by then President of the United States Ronald Reagan. The purpose of the act is also to ensure that dental and medical procedures are consistent with strict safety precautions and standards. Legislation governing the practices of radiological technology (radiography, radiation therapy, and nuclear medicine) includes dentists, dental assistants, and dental hygienists.

The Secretary of Health and Human Services has the responsibility for establishing minimum standards for certification and accreditation. Individual states are urged to enact similar statutes and to administer appropriate programs for such certification and accreditation.

Maximum Permissible Dose to Operator

The first recommended limits of radiation exposure were developed in 1928 by the NCRP. These limits or guidelines have been revised downward, and the cumulative maximum permissible dose is not set below levels where any damaging effects have been observed. The NCRP Report No. 17 (1954) defined the **maximum permissible dose (MPD)** as "that radiation dose which should not be exceeded without careful consideration of the reasons for doing so." Persons engaged in the operation of x-ray equipment are classified as "occupationally exposed"; however, it is not expected that the absorbed dose that has accumulated over the course of an individual's career (cumulative MPD) will cause any detectable bodily injury to the radiation worker in his or her lifetime.

The NCRP recommends further that the MPD be held to close limitations. For educational and training purposes it is necessary and desirable that students exposed during educational activities not receive in excess of 0.1 rem per year in the context of their educational activity. This is considered to be a part of the annual dose limit of 0.5 rem for persons under the age of 45, not supplemental to it. Furthermore, operators or x-ray units should be limited to 0.1 R per week.

The NCRP Report No. 35 (1970) recommends that the operators in daily contact with roentgen rays receive no more than 0.3 R in any one week, or more than 3 R in a 13-week period (calendar quarter), or in excess of 5 R per year:

$$MPD = 5(N - 18) \text{ rem}$$

This formula was developed by the NCRP and has been used since 1957. The number 5 represents the maximum number of whole-body rem that a radiation worker is permitted to receive in any one year. The letter N represents the actual age (in years) of the individual concerned, and the number 18 specifies the legal age at which a person may be employed as a radiation worker.

Problem. Determine the maximum whole-body dose of x-radiation that a 25-year old radiographer may receive.

Solution.

MPD	=	$5(N - 18)$ rem
	=	$5(25 - 18)$ rem
	=	$5(7)$ rem
	=	35 rem

Although the NCRP and similar organizations have no legal status, their suggestions and recommendations are highly regarded. Regulatory bodies have used them to formulate legislation controlling the use of radiation in the dental office.

SUGGESTED ACTIVITIES

- Using your own age and the formula for determining cumulative MPD, determine whole-body rem.

- Using the conversion chart, determine how many R (roentgens) would equal 5 C/kg. Also, how many rad would equal 5 Gy. Also, how many rem would equal 15 Sv.

REVIEW

1. What is the traditional unit of measurement for x-ray exposure in air?
   a. Coulomb/kilogram
   b. Gray
   c. Sievert
   d. Roentgen

2. The unit of absorbed radiation is termed:
   a. Rem
   b. Rad
   c. Roentgen
   d. Sievert

3. What does the term ALARA represent?
   a. As long as reasonably allowed
   b. As long as radiographically acceptable
   c. As low as reasonably achievable
   d. As low as roentgens (are) acceptable

4. What is the maximum permissible dose of whole-body rem to a radiation worker in one year?
   a. No more than 5 R
   b. No more than 3 R
   c. No more than 0.5 R
   d. No more than 0.3 R

5. Name the three SI standards of measurement: (1) coulomb/kilogram, (2) rem, (3) gray, and/or (4) sievert.
   a. 1, 2, 3
   b. 2, 3, 4
   c. 1, 2, 4
   d. 1, 3, 4

CHAPTER 62

Radiation Protection and Radiobiology

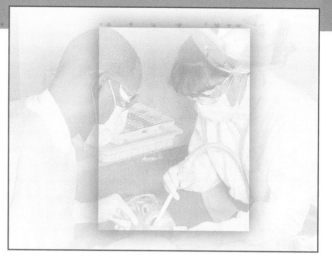

OBJECTIVES

After studying this chapter, the student will be able to:

- State the benefits and hazards of radiation
- Explain the direct and indirect effects of damage to cells during ionization.
- Explain the dose-response curve.
- Explain genetic effects of ionizing radiation.
- Explain the symptoms experienced with whole-body irradiation.
- Describe the symptoms experienced at each therapy stage in oral cancer irradiation
- Describe various protective measures for the patient.
- Discuss protection for the operator of radiographic equipment.

Introduction

The public today is fairly well informed about the hazards of radiation; on the other hand, they are often misinformed. The responsibility for radiation protection of the dental patient lies with the dentist and dental auxiliary personnel. The dental practitioner should base the need for a radiographic examination by obtaining necessary information to enable patient diagnosis.

Every exposure of a dental patient to radiation carries with it the dual features of diagnostic benefit and risk of biologic harm. Therefore, all exposure to radiation should be kept to the minimum that is necessary to meet specific diagnostic requirements. It should be emphasized that failure to obtain radiographs that are clinically indicated is more likely to harm patients than the slight possibility of suffering radiation injury as a result of exposure. Modern equipment and current safety techniques make the actual hazard from a dental radiograph an improbability.

It should be noted, however, that radiation of any type should be used sparingly and that a record of previous exposures be entered on the patient's chart.

Benefits of Radiation

For a complete dental oral diagnosis, a series of radiographs is extremely important. Many systemic and oral diseases can be detected on radiographs before they are clinically apparent. For example, decay between the teeth can be detected much earlier and more accurately with the aid of radiographs. In addition, abscesses (infection at the root tip), bone diseases, periodontal disease, and the eruption of permanent teeth can be detected with the use of radiographs.

Hazards of Radiation

All radiation is ionizing radiation and therefore hazardous. However, the degree of hazard varies; it depends a great deal on the operator's safety techniques. Ionizing radiation affects living tissue through a process that causes atoms and molecules to become electrically unbalanced. Keep in mind that (1) all living substances are composed of atoms and (2) they are arranged in a particular fashion and known as molecules (the smallest particle of a substance that retains the properties of the substance). There are two theories regarding cell damage: the direct effect and the indirect effect.

Direct Effect Theory

Although most cells do not sustain much damage as photons interact with them, there are others, as in the photoelectric interaction, where ionization takes place or where x-ray photons strike the DNA of a cell, causing direct injury to the organism. The result of this type of injury causes the cell to die immediately or at the time of cell division (mitosis).

Indirect Effect Theory

Atoms prefer to be in balance; in an effort to regain balance after ionization with water, the **free radicals** (hydrogen and hydroxyl) may combine with other atoms, creating a new and different substance. This new substance may be harmful to the organ or cell. An example of this is the subtle change from H_2O (water) to H_2O_2 (hydrogen peroxide). The former is essential for a cell; the latter is poisonous or toxic. This process is also known as **radiolysis**. This type of injury can occur frequently due to the high content of water in cells, and the effect takes place when a hormone balance is altered or the functions of the cell are changed in a destructive manner. The more cells affected or killed in a body organ, the more rippled that organ becomes. If few alterations occur, the effect may be so slight that the organ functions properly and is unaffected by the radiation. Cells can recover by repair if an x-ray dose is not high enough to kill the cell before it divides or if many cells in the area are only damaged, not killed.

Dose-Response Curve

A **dose-response curve** refers to the direct correlation between the dose of radiation given and the response (damage) to tissues.

The premise by which the dose-response curve works is to create awareness of how much radiation it would take that would result in tissue damage. There are two concepts that demonstrate when damage is perceived to take place.

One concept is called a **threshold dose-response** curve. It is based on the premise that there has to be enough radiation dosage (a threshold) to cause damage to tissues and that prior to that dose, no response (injury) was noted.

The other concept is called a **nonthreshold dose-response** curve, based on the premise that no matter what amount of radiation dosage is absorbed, damage to tissue cells does take place. Therefore, there is no safe amount of radiation.

Radiobiology

Radiobiology is the study of the effects of ionizing radiation on living tissues. Tissues are separated in two groups to see how radiation affects them. Those that are sensitive are called radiosensitive and those that are more resistant to ionized radiation are called radioresistant.

Radiosensitive and Radioresistant Tissues

Some cells are more **radiosensitive** than others. Radiosensitivity is directly proportional to the reproductive cycle of the cell or due to its high metabolism. In other words, the more rapid the mitotic and metabolic activity, the more radiosensitive the cell. Those cells that are constantly dividing, undergoing differentiation, or have high metabolic activity are considered to be more radiosensitive. Following is a list of cell types ranked from the most radiosensitive to the least radiosensitive. The second list ranks cell types from the least **radioresistant** to the most radioresistant:

Radiosensitive (from most to least)

- Germinal cells of the ovary
- Seminiferous epithelium of the testes
- Blood-forming cells, lymphocytes, and other blood-forming tissues (bone marrow)
- Intestinal epithelium
- Skin

Radioresistant (from least to most)

- Glandular tissue (other than genetic)
- Muscle
- Nerve
- Bone
- Enamel

Radiosensitivity varies among species. Also, there is individual variability depending on the age of the species, the intensity of the x-ray, the length of exposure, and the area of exposure. Areas that may be affected by dental radiography include the thyroid gland, lens of the eye, bone marrow, and skin.

Cumulative Effects

Repeated exposure to radiation is additive, increasing the risk of absorption and accumulation in tissues. Tissue injury may depend on cellular alteration, repeated dose rate, and total dose given. If cumulative effects from repeated exposure were of great magnitude, they could lead to development of thyroid, blood and skin cancer, cataracts, and birth defects.

Latent Period

The elapsed time from the time of exposure and when observable clinical signs are manifested is known as the **latent period**. The amount of time elapsed would depend on the dose amount and rate of exposure to radiation. In other words, the more radiation, the less will be the latent period. In dental radiography, there are no observable signs immediately following radiation exposure. Injured cells tend to repair themselves and are not considered to have permanent damage. However, the possibility of injury still exists.

Acute and Chronic Radiation Exposure

A differentiation between acute and chronic radiation exposure is necessary to understand how this applies to dental radiography. **Acute** exposure does not apply to dental radiography but rather to large doses of radiation exposure such as in radiation therapy or nuclear power plant accidents. This can produce **short-term effects** where the person affected develops classic symptoms of radiation sickness in a short period of time.

Exposures to small amounts of radiation over a long period of time are considered to be **chronic**. Effects of such exposures that are manifested after many years are known as **long-term effects**. These cumulative effects could include birth defects, cancer, and cataracts.

Somatic Effects

Somatic refers to all body tissue except genetic or reproductive tissue. Residual effects of radiation that remain in the body are termed **cumulative**. The first signs of radiation illness are blood changes. However, it takes a great deal of **whole-body exposure** to radiation to have this occur. Radiation used in dentistry is termed **localized** or specific-area radiation, as only a small area of the body is exposed. It would take hundreds of times more radiation than a dental x-ray machine is capable of producing to cause even erythema or reddening of the skin.

The lens of the eye is one area of somatic tissue that deserves special consideration. Tissues of the eye are nonrepairable. Even though it would take much more radiation than is used in dentistry to harm the eye, the safest approach is to avoid subjecting the eye to any radiation by asking patients to close their eyes during exposure of the film.

Genetic Effects

All types of radiation, including radiation in the atmosphere, can affect the body. The cumulative effects of radiation on the chromosomes, or genes, is an important consideration, as the possibility of mutations is involved. Mutations may be beneficial or harmful to the species and may not appear for several generations. Because we cannot detect **genetic effects** (effects passed on to future generations) and because genetic damage is nonrepairable, it is important that the patient and operator be exposed as little as possible to radiation from medical and dental sources. Proper use of all radiation equipment is imperative.

Localized and Whole-Body Exposure

Localized Exposure

Localized exposure pertains to a small area of the skin exposed to an x-ray beam diameter such as 2 3/4 inches in dental exposures made of the oral cavity. Only 1% of the body is affected, and the amount of radiation absorption in that area is estimated to be 1 rad for each gram of tissue. Remember that this is a very small area in comparison to the entire body. Some pertinent areas of concern when a person is subjected to localized dental exposures are the thyroid, bone marrow (representing only 5% of total bone marrow in the body), skin, and eyes. However, as depicted in Table 62-1, it would be very unlikely for a person to develop injuries due to dental radiographs.

Whole-Body Exposure

Whole-body exposure may take place in an accidental nuclear power plant disaster where 100% of the body is affected and the radiation absorption is estimated to be 1 rad for each gram of tissue. Depending on the amount of radiation incurred by such an exposure, it may be lethal or cause "radiation sickness."

There are several stages of sickness that take place after a person has been subjected to whole-body exposure of great magnitude. The following will demonstrate stages of illness according to radiation absorption doses (Table 62-2).

Oral Cancer Irradiation

It is wise for the radiographic operator to understand the implications presented when a patient has undergone

Table 62-1 Localized Radiation Risks

Rads	Gy	Area of Exposure	Number of Radiographs Required	Injury
6	0.06	Thyroid	20,000	Cancer
5	0.05	Bone marrow	2000–5000	Leukemia
250	2 1/2	Skin	500+ in 14 days	Erythema
200+	2+	Eyes	3000+	Cataracts

Table 62-2 Whole-Body Irradiation

Rad	Gy	Acute Radiation Syndrome	Symptoms	Latent Period
200 and less	2 and less	Prodromal syndrome (symptoms indicating the onset of disease)	Nausea, vomiting Diarrhea Headache Malaise Anorexia	4–5 days Erythema Hair loss Internal bleeding
200–1000	2–10	Hemopoietic syndrome (formation/development of blood cells in bone marrow)	Nausea, vomiting Diarrhea Anemia [red blood cells (↓RBC)] Leukopenia [white blood cells (↓WBC)] Hemorrhage	10–30 days death
1000–10,000	10–100	Gastrointestinal syndrome	Electrolyte imbalance Septicemia, infection	3–5 days death
10,000+	100+	Neuromuscular/central nervous system (CNS)	Fluid in brain, seizures	1–2 days death

irradiation (radiation therapy) for oral cancer. This type of exposure is considered to be of acute nature on a localized area. The treatment requires daily doses of 200 rad (2 Gy) within a six-week period. There are several stages that the patient undergoes within a five-year period. At postexposure, when tissues have had a chance to heal, a number of long-term effects are observable. Patients may exhibit **radiation caries** (rampant caries that usually affect the cervical portion of the teeth); **osteoradionecrosis** where underlying bone dies causing teeth to loosen; **xerostomia**, drying of the mouth; **dysphagia**, causing difficulty in swallowing; and *mucositis* where there is inflammation and sloughing of the mucous membrane (Table 62-3). When some of these clinical signs are apparent, one needs to be aware that the patient may have undergone significant radiation exposure. It may be wise to explore this possibility and to refrain from further exposure to radiation.

Table 62-3 Oral Cancer Irradiation Therapy Stages

Stage I: Acute Clinical Period (within the first 6 months)

Painful mouth	Dysphagia (difficulty swallowing)
Susceptible to trauma and infection	Swollen tongue
Loss of appetite and sense of taste	Throat feels congested
Thick (ropey) saliva	Mucositis (inflammation and sloughing of mucous membrane)
Xerostomia (dry mouth)	

Stage II: Subacute Clinical Period (within the next 6 months)

Xerostomia	Oral ulcers
Oral mucosa blanched (pale in appearance)	Radiation caries

Stage III: Chronic Clinical Period (second year through 5th year)

Salivary glands and taste recovery	Inflammation of gingiva
Oral ulcers continue	Osteoradionecrosis (bone cells die, loosening teeth)

Long-Term Effects (postexposure healed tissues)

Radiation caries	Dysphagia
Osteoradionecrosis	Mucositis
Xerostomia	

Radiation Protection for the Patient

Radiation subjected to the patient in the usual dental radiographic examination is but a small fraction of the amount that would produce bodily harm. However, the dental auxiliary should make it a habit to ask every patient if he or she has been exposed to radiation for **therapeutic** (pertaining to the treatment or curing of disease) or diagnostic purposes. A history of all radiographic exposures (medical and dental) should be made. Thus, the supervising dentist must determine if radiographs would be required to achieve maximum diagnostic results.

A policy regarding pregnant patients should be established and strictly observed. Many experts recommend that elective radiographic procedures be postponed until the patient is no longer pregnant.

On a patient's initial visit to the dentist, a thorough clinical examination should be followed by a radiographic survey. The decision to complete a full-mouth survey should depend on the dentist's professional judgment. A complete survey is taken for two reasons: first, to determine the condition of the teeth and underlying bone; second, to establish a basis for future comparison. As a rule, the dentist need not repeat a full-mouth (complete) series for several years unless the patient has a history of trauma, extensive oral surgery, or orthodontic treatment. Individual radiographs should be made whenever necessary for preventive reasons or in cases of a toothache, a loose tooth, or pain in the jaw or to evaluate the progress of dental treatment. Such intraoral radiographs are obtained by use of modern dental x-ray equipment (refer to Figure 60-3).

Guidelines for prescribing dental radiographs have been published by the American Dental Association and the Food and Drug Administration. These guidelines are made available through the Eastman Kodak Company (Table 62-4).

Using Protective Lead Shields

Lead aprons and thyroid protective shields are constructed of various light and flexible materials with the thickness of lead varying from 0.25 to 1.25 mm depending on the kilovoltage peak used; the higher the kilovoltage peak, the thicker the lead shielding. The apron should protect the patient's reproductive organs and be draped over the pubis in males and over the lower pelvis in females. Lead aprons should be used to protect *all* patients. The lead collar, also called thyroid protection collar, provides more complete patient protection (Figure 62-1). It may be attached as part of the lead apron or used as a separate shield to protect the radiosensitive thyroid gland. A thyroid collar cannot be used effectively with a panoramic x-ray machine because it blocks out parts of the jaws. It should be common practice to extend the life of lead aprons by hanging them on specially made hangers and avoid folding them when not in use. This practice would prevent development of cracks and defects.

Using Appropriate PIDs

Three position-indicating devices (PIDs) were identified in Chapter 60: the pointed, cylindrical, and rectangular. It was mentioned that the pointed PID, made of plastic, caused x-ray photons to interact with the plastic, producing scatter or secondary radiation that contributed to excessive radiation to the patient and is no longer appropriate for use; see Figure 60–12A. The cylindrical PID is open ended, does not produce scatter radiation, but does allow excess radiation to interact with the patient's skin at the face, due to its large diameter of 2.75 inches. The rectangular PID is also open ended and is very close to the size of the film and therefore does not produce scatter radiation or allow excess radiation to interact with the patient's skin. Both the cylindrical and rectangular PIDs are lead lined and come in 8-, 12-, and 16-inch lengths (see Figure 60-11). It is for the benefit of the patient that lead-lined open-ended PIDs be used.

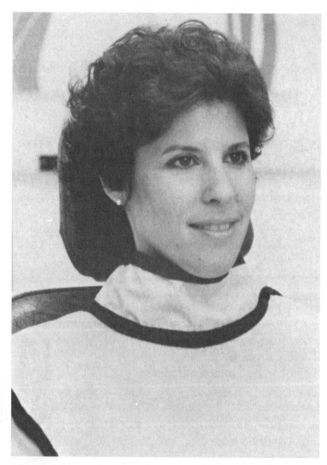

Figure 62-1 Use of lead apron and thyroid protective shields.

Table 62-4 Eastman Kodak Table for Prescribing Radiographs

[The recommendations in this chart are subject to clinical judgment and may not apply to every patient. *They are to be used by dentists only after reviewing the patient's health history and completing a clinical examination. The recommendations do not need to be altered because of pregnancy.*]

Patient Category	Child		Adolescent	Adult	
	Primary Dentition (prior to eruption of first permanent tooth)	Transitional Dentition (following eruption of first permanent tooth)	Permanent Dentition (prior to eruption of third molars)	Dentulous	Edentulous
New Patient* All new patients to assess dental diseases and growth and development	Posterior bite-wing examination if proximal surfaces of primary teeth cannot be visualized or probed	Individualized radiographic examination consisting of periapical/occlusal views and posterior bite-wings or panoramic examination and posterior bitewings	Individualized radiographic examination consisting of posterior bite-wings and selected periapicals. A full mouth intraoral radiographic examination is appropriate when the patient presents with cliniical evidence of generalized dental disease or a history of extensive dental treatment		Full mouth intraoral radiographic examination or panoramic examination
Recall Patient* Clinical caries or high-risk factors for caries**	Posterior bite-wing examination at 6-month intervals or until no carious lesions are evident		Posterior bite-wing examination at 6- to 12-month intervals or until no carious lesions are evident	Posterior bite-wing examination at 12- to 18-month intervals	Not applicable
No clinical caries and no high-risk factors for caries**	Posterior bite-wing examination at 12- to 24-month intervals if proximal surfaces of primary teeth cannot be visualized or probed	Posterior bite-wing examination at 12- to 24-month intervals	Posterior bite-wing examination at 18- to 36-month intervals	Posterior bite-wing examination at 24- to 36-month intervals	Not applicable

*Clinical situations for which radiographs may be indicated include:

A. Positive Historical Findings
1. Previous periodontal or endodontic therapy
2. History of pain or trauma
3. Familial history of dental anomalies
4. Postoperative evaluation of healing
5. Presence of implants

B. Positive Clinical Signs/Symptoms
1. Clinical evidence of periodontal disease
2. Large or deep restorations
3. Deep carious lesions
4. Malposed or clinically impacted teeth
5. Swelling
6. Evidence of facial trauma
7. Mobility of teeth
8. Fistula or sinus tract infection
9. Clinically suspected sinus pathology
10. Growth abnormalities
11. Oral involvement in known or suspected systemic disease

(continued)

Table 62-4 Eastman Kodak Table for Prescribing Radiographs (Continued)

Patient Category	Child — Primary Dentition (prior to eruption of first permanent tooth)	Transitional Dentition (following eruption of first permanent tooth)	Adolescent — Permanent Dentition (prior to eruption of third molars)	Adult — Dentulous	Adult — Edentulous
Periodontal disease or a history of periodontal treatment	Individualized radiographic examination consisting of selected periapical and/or bite-wing radiographs for areas where periodontal disease (other than nonspecific gingivitis) can be demonstrated clinically	Individualized radiographic examination consisting of selected periapical and/or bite-wing radiographs for areas where periodontal disease (other than nonspecific gingivitis) can be demonstrated clinically	Individualized radiographic examination consisting of selected periapical and/or bite-wing radiographs for areas where periodontal disease (other than nonspecific gingivits) can be demonstrated clinically	Individualized radiographic examination consisting of selected periapical and/or bite-wing radiographs for areas where periodontal disease (other than nonspecific gingivits) can be demonstrated clinically	Not applicable
Growth and development assessment	Usually not indicated	Individualized radiographic examination consisting of a periapical/occlusal or panoramic examination	Periapical or panoramic examination to assess developing third molars	Usually not indicated	Usually not indicated

12. Positive neurologic findings in the head and neck
13. Evidence of foreign objects
14. Pain and/or dysfunction of the temporomandibular joint
15. Facial asymmetry
16. Abutment teeth for fixed or removable partial prosthesis
17. Unexplained bleeding
18. Unexplained sensitivity of teeth
19. Unusual eruption, spacing or migration of teeth
20. Unusual tooth morphology; calcification or color
21. Missing teeth with unknown reason.

**Patients at high risk for caries may demonstrate any of the following:

1. High level of caries experience
2. History of recurrent caries
3. Existing restoration of poor quality
4. Poor oral hygiene
5. Inadequate flouride exposure
6. Prolonged nursing (bottle or breast)
7. Diet with high sucrose frequency
8. Poor family dental health
9. Developmental enamel defects
10. Developmental disability
11. Xerostomia
12. Genetic abnormality of teeth
13. Many multisurface restorations
14. Chemo/radiation therapy

The recommendations contained in this table have been developed by an expert panel composed of representatives from the Academy of General Dentistry, American Academy of Dental Radiology, American Academy of Oral Medicine, American Academy of Pediatric Dentistry, American Academy of Periodontology and the American Dental Association under the sponsorship of the Food and Drug Administration (FDA). This chart has been reproduced and distributed to the dental community by Eastman Kodak Company in cooperation with the FDA (Reprinted with permission of Eastman Kodak Company. KODAK is a trademark)

Using Film Holders

The use of film holders greatly reduces the need for excessive exposures, thus reducing the amount of radiation to the patient. They provide stability by holding the film in position, eliminating the need for the patient to hold the film, thereby eliminating radiation to the patient's hand (Figure 62-2).

Using Fast Film

Another way to reduce radiation exposure to the patient is to use the fastest film possible. With the introduction of the E-Speed (Ektaspeed) film, it is possible to reduce exposure by half. It requires half of the exposure time as did the D-Speed (Ultra-Speed). However, the quality of the radiograph is compromised due to the larger silver halide crystals used on the film, producing a grainy appearance on the image.

Avoiding Retakes

The importance for the operator to have a thorough knowledge of radiographic techniques cannot be overemphasized. There have been too many errors made that required retakes. One should be mindful that when a retake is made, the area is being subjected to two exposures within a very short time. There are many variables that may warrant retakes, some of them are listed here:

- Using improper radiographic techniques
- Allowing the patient to hold the film by digital retention with possible movement
- Improper machine settings for exposure time, kilovoltage peak, or milliamperes
- Improper film processing

Suggestions for the Dental Radiographer

Dental radiography is a skill that must be learned and practiced. There are no short cuts to developing a high degree of competence. Effort and self-application are the keys to success. Bear in mind that mistakes will be made. Making these mistakes is part of the learning process. The concept of the ALARA (as low as reasonably achievable) should be practiced at all times.

Suggestions for improvement in radiographic skills would include the use of mannequins or skulls for exposure during the learning process prior to patient exposures. This practice will help in correcting mistakes in film placement, angulation of the PID, and processing procedures. An exposure time chart is usually posted near the control panel of the x-ray unit.

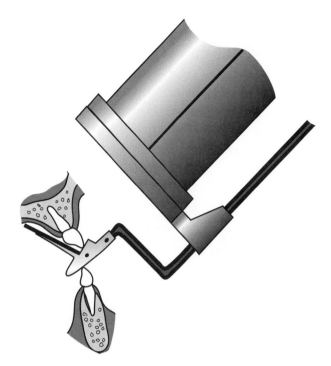

Figure 62-2 Use of film holders vs. patient's finger. (Courtesy of Rinn Corporation, Elgin, IL.)

Radiation Protection for the Operator

It is essential to reemphasize that under usual circumstances any patient radiation reduction will have a direct effect on the amount of radiation received by the operator. The term operator includes the dentist and the auxiliaries who expose film. The operator may receive radiation in the form of secondary radiation when the primary beam strikes the patient or objects in the operatory. If the operator foolishly stands in the path of the primary beam, he or she receives radiation exposure. Direct exposure to ionizing radiation is cumulative. In other words, the effects of yesterday's are added to today's and tomorrow's exposures. The resulting accumulation, when great enough, can cause harmful effects. Overexposure may be avoided by observing a few basic safety guidelines.

By having adequate equipment, good education in radiographic techniques, and a well-defined monitoring system, it should be improbable for the operator to be exposed to radiation. However, the possibility of exposure may exist if the operator does not adhere to safety guidelines used in the prevention of occupational exposure.

At present, the maximum permissible dose (MPD) set by the National Committee on Radiation Protection and Measurements in 1971 allotted the operator is 5 rem or 0.05 Sv radiation of whole body per year. Recently, the International Commission on Radiation Protection (ICRP) has recommended that operators be limited to 2 rem or

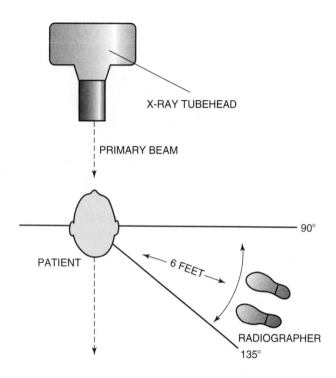

Figure 62-3 Operator protection from primary beam.

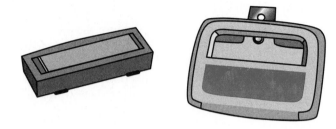

Figure 62–4 Use of film badge or dosimeter to monitor amount of radiation affecting the operator.

0.02 Sv per year instead of 5 rem per year. Nevertheless, it is good practice to strive for "zero" exposure.

Operator Safety Guidelines

The operator must always avoid being in the path of the primary beam while exposure is being made, by following the stated guidelines:

- Using a full-length protective lead shield.

- Stepping behind a thick wall.

- Standing at a distance of at least 6–8 feet from the source of radiation, at a perpendicular angle of 90°–135° degrees from the primary beam, toward the back of the patient (Figure 62-3).

- Never holding the film in the patient's mouth or on any radiographic training mannequin.

- Never holding a drifting tubehead.

- Making certain that the x-ray machine meets all standards for operation and safety as regards filtration, shielding, and collimation. Having a periodic check of x-ray equipment made by a competent radiation expert.

- Using a personnel-monitoring badge at all times to detect unwanted exposure. There is minimal cost to acquire the services of a radiation monitoring company. The service provided includes a film badge for personnel who may come in contact with radiation and a monthly report of any detected radiation exposure (Figure 62-4). The film is maintained by the monitoring company and constitutes a permanent legal record of personnel exposure. Manufacturers recommend one month as the maximum period of time that a film badge should be worn as an effective monitoring device.

Safety of Shockproof Units

All dental x-ray equipment and tubes are shockproof for the operator and the patient. In self-contained units, the high-voltage elements (x-ray tube and transformer) are immersed in oil in a single, grounded metal container. This oil immersion serves to both insulate the high-voltage circuits and help cool the tube. Insulation of this type eliminates the danger of electric shock if the tubehead is touched during exposure.

SUGGESTED ACTIVITY

- Compare E-Speed film with D-Speed film: Expose each type on a mannikin using the average exposure time for D-Speed film, and process. Then expose each type again, this time using half the exposure time that was used for D-Speed film, and process. Look for density and clarity on each film and determine which type of film provided the most adequate radiograph.

REVIEW

1. Identify the type of body cells that are more radiosensitive: (1) cells that are constantly dividing, (2) cells that have a high metabolic activity, (3) reproductive cells, and/or (4) bone cells.
   a. 1, 2, 3
   b. 2, 3, 4
   c. 1, 2, 4
   d. 1, 3, 4

2. Identify radioresistant tissues: (1) muscle, (2) intestinal epithelium, (3) enamel, and/or (4) nerve.
   a. 1, 2, 3
   b. 2, 3, 4
   c. 1, 2, 4
   d. 1, 3, 4

3. The elapsed time from the time of exposure and when observable signs are seen is known as:
   a. Cumulative effect
   b. Acute exposure
   c. Chronic exposure
   d. Latent period

4. How may a person be exposed to whole-body radiation?
   a. When exposing the patient to chest x-rays
   b. When a person is present in an accidental nuclear power plant disaster
   c. When the operator stands at less than 6 feet from the source of radiation
   d. When a patient's lower extremities are subjected to radiation exposure

5. Indicate the methods that may be used to minimize dental radiation exposure to the patient: (1) using D-speed over E-speed film, (2) using a rectangular PID, (3) using film holders as opposed to having the patient hold the film, and/or (4) avoiding retakes by possessing thorough knowledge of radiographic techniques.
   a. 1, 2, 3
   b. 2, 3, 4
   c. 1, 2, 4
   d. 1, 3, 4

6. Match the terms associated with irradiation therapy on the left with their meaning on the right:
   ___ a. Erythema
   ___ b. Dysphagia
   ___ c. Osteoradionecrosis
   ___ d. Prodromal syndrome
   ___ e. Mucositis
   ___ f. Xerostomia

   1. Difficulty in swallowing
   2. Drying of the mouth
   3. Redness of skin
   4. Inflammation and sloughing of the mucous membrane
   5. Destruction of bone
   6. Early symptoms of radiation sickness after whole-body exposure to radiation

CHAPTER 63

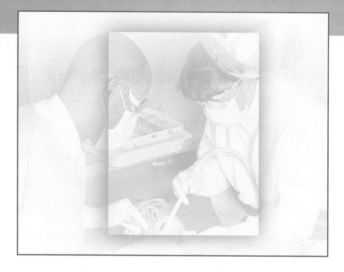

OBJECTIVES

After studying this chapter, the student will be able to:

- Describe film emulsion and state its purpose.
- Analyze the components of an x-ray film.
- Describe the various film packets.
- Distinguish between different film sizes.
- Discuss the speed of film.

Introduction

When handling film, it is wise to know about its component parts and the effect that light, radiation, chemicals, and heat would have on it. This should alert the radiographer about proper storage, how to care for film, and how to use protective measures. Failure to adhere to safe practices could cause repeated radiation exposure to the patient.

X-Ray Film

Film Composition

Dental x-ray film has two principal components: the base and the emulsion. The base, made of transparent polyester, is the supporting material onto which the emulsion is coated. The emulsion records the radiographic image and is sensitive to x-rays and visible light rays.

The Base. The base of the x-ray film consists of transparent polyester. This transparent base serves to support and retain the emulsion on the film and lends some degree of stiffness throughout the handling of it. Its thickness is approximately 0.2 mm (0.007 inch). A blue tint is added to the polyester during the manufacturing process, which increases the contrast of the exposed and processed film. (This subject will be discussed in Chapter 65). Added to the film base, on both sides, is a thin adhesive material; this enables the emulsion to adhere to the base material.

The Emulsion. The emulsion of the x-ray film consists of **silver halide crystals** suspended in a gelatin matrix (framework). A halide is a compound of a halogen (bromine, iodine) with a chemical element of silver or potassium. All halogens are of a closely related chemical family and combine easily with chemical elements. Silver halide is the product of virgin silver dissolved in nitric acid. This silver solution is mixed with potassium bromide to produce silver bromide. To a lesser extent, silver iodide serves as the remainder of the chemical components of the emulsion. Silver iodide adds greatly to the sensitivity of the emulsion, thus reducing the dose of radiation to produce a diagnostic image. The size of the crystals determines the speed with which the emulsion reaction occurs during radiation.

Silver halide crystals (grains) are suspended on both sides of the base, with the gelatin serving to keep the silver grains dispersed. During processing (Chapter 65), the gelatin absorbs the processing solution and thereby allows the chemicals to act on the silver halide grains.

A supercoating on the surface of the film is added to provide a protective barrier during the frequent handling of the film (Chapter 65). This coating is, typically, an additional coating of gelatin. This added coating also helps to protect the film from damage by the rollers of an automatic processor (Chapter 65). The emulsion retains much of its rigidity during normal processing; it has strength when wet but is sensitive to high temperatures.

Various manufacturers in the United States supply intraoral film. Each film is double coated, i.e., the emulsion is coated on each side of the film base. Double-emulsion "ultraspeed" and "ektaspeed" film is used in modern radiography, because the added thickness of the emulsion allows less radiation to be used when exposing an object (Figure 63-1).

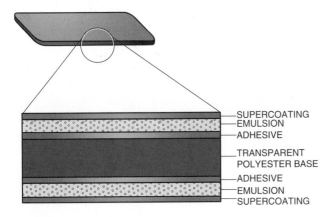

Figure 63-1 Cross section of a film.

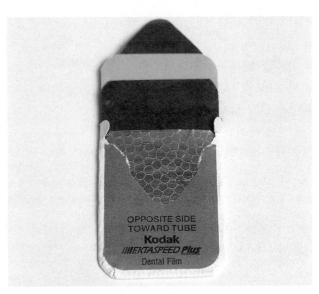

Figure 63-2 Inside the film packet.

Film Packaging

The x-ray film is sensitive to such things as light, x-rays and gamma rays, various gases and their fumes, and heat and moisture. Films that are placed within the mouth are termed *intraoral* and, for protection against light and moisture, are individually wrapped in the **outer wrapping**, a packet of fairly waterproof material, either white plastic or stippled-surface paper. These materials aid in the retention of the film as it is positioned against the mucosa of the patient. The film is further protected by a **black paper envelope** or sheath and backed by a thin sheet of **lead foil**. The lead foil backing prevents much of the secondary radiation, which originates in the tissues of the patient, from *fogging* the film through "backscattering." It also helps to reduce radiation fog during exposure. The metal foil absorbs x-rays that have passed through the object and film and helps to reduce exposure to the tissues behind the film. The lead foil is embossed with a pattern that will appear on the film, resulting in a light image of the object if the film is placed with this surface toward the x-ray beam during exposure. To identify the tube side of the film, the plain, white, unmarked surface is to be placed toward the x-ray source. The manufacturer places an **identification dot** (a circle or indentation) at one corner of the film packet, and the side with the depression is placed toward the patient's tongue. After the film is processed, the depression, or *identification dot*, is used to identify the patient's right or left side (Figure 63-2).

Films are packaged as either single or double packets, with either a single sheet of film or two sheets of film in each packet. When double packets are used, the second film becomes a duplicate record.

Double Film Packets. A double film packet makes it possible to produce an exact duplicate of a film, thus eliminating the need for additional radiation exposure to the patient or duplication procedures.

Original radiographs should always be kept in the office with the patient's record. Should the doctor need to refer the patient to another doctor for treatment or verify an insurance claim, dual film packets should be used.

Intraoral films vary only in size and clinical use; the composition of the film is identical.

Film Types

Intraoral Film

Current intraoral film sizes are the result of a demonstrated need by the practicing members of the dental profession. They are manufactured in the following sizes (Figure 63-3):

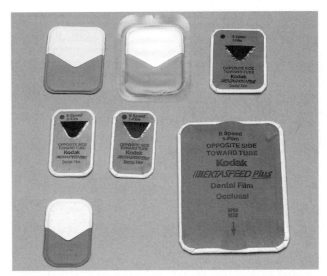

Figure 63-3 Various sizes of x-ray film: top size, #2; middle size, #1; lower left size, #0; lower right size, #4.

- Size 0 (7/8 x 1 3/8 in.)
- Size 1 (15/16 x 1 9/16 in.)
- Size 2 (11/4 x 1 5/8 in.)
- Size 3 (11/16 x 2 1/8 in.)
- Size 4 Occlusal (2 1/4 x 3 in.)

The #0 film packet is half the size of the adult packet and is used for children. This so-called pedo film resulted from the practice of early pediatric dentists who specialized in the care of children's teeth of folding a standard #2 size packet in half lengthwise to produce a small packet for small children.

The #1, or narrow, film was created as the result of requests from the profession for a film narrow enough to be accepted in the anterior portion of the mouth with less distortion than could be obtained with the use of the standard #2 packet.

The #2 (standard size) packet is a **periapical film** that has been traditionally used for adult full-mouth surveys and bite wings. It is used to record the crowns, roots, and periapical areas of the teeth.

The #3 is longer and narrower than the #2. It comes with a tab already attached to it; therefore, it is only used for posterior bite wings on adults.

Bite-Wing Film

With a wing or tab attached, a #2 size periapical film becomes a bite wing. The patient bites on the wing that is placed on the tube surface of the film. This film is used to record interproximal caries and conditions of the alveolar crest. It may be purchased with the wing fixed in position, or a paper loop may be placed over a periapical film. Film-holding instruments for bite-wing projections are available. A child's bite wing consists of a #0 or #1 size film with a tab attached (Figure 63-4).

Occlusal Film

Size #4 occlusal film is more than twice the size of a #2 film. It is generally used to observe larger areas of the maxilla and mandible than may be seen on a periapical film. The film is held in position by having the patient bite lightly on the film to retain it between the occlusal surfaces of the teeth (Chapter 66).

Other Film Characteristics

Film Speed

The American National Standards Institute developed a film speed classification that groups x-ray film by speeds ranging from A through F. "A" represents the slowest speed film (requiring the most exposure); "F" represents the fastest speed group. Currently, the fastest available

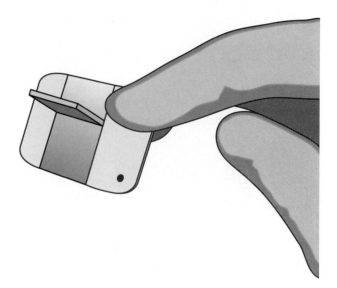

Figure 63-4 Bite-wing tab attached to periapical film.

film on the market is E speed, as type F has not been released. Of the various types of film, D and E are commercially available. It should be noted that the use of "Ecktaspeed" E film requires less radiation exposure, almost 50% less, being more sensitive to radiation and light, and requires precise exposure techniques and darkroom handling due to the incorporation of larger silver halide crystals in the emulsion.

Film Storage

Unexposed x-ray film should be stored in a lead-lined container in a location where the atmosphere is cool. X-ray film is inherently sensitive to high temperature, moisture, chemical fumes, and all forms of x-radiation. Since unexposed sensitive materials deteriorate with age, films should be stocked only to the level that they would be used. When the number of unbroken boxes of film is in such excess that they will need storage, they should be placed in the refrigerator and removed at least 12 hours before exposing them. In either case, the time limit indicated by the expiration date printed on the box should be observed and noted.

SUGGESTED ACTIVITY

- Select a film to determine its physical characteristics and contents:
  1. Determine the tube side of the film.
  2. Open the film packet to reveal its component parts and identify each part.
  3. Observe the black envelope and its location.

4. Observe the film itself. Is there more than one film present?
5. Determine the position of the lead foil backing. Look for the pattern embossed on it.

REVIEW

1. What is the purpose of the lead foil in the x-ray film packet?
   a. To alert the operator that the film is reversed during exposure
   b. To absorb secondary radiation
   c. To minimize secondary fog on the film during exposure
   d. Both a and b
   e. Both b and c

2. What is the purpose of having a dot on the film?
   a. To identify the top from the bottom of the film
   b. To identify the upper right side of the film
   c. To identify the patient's right from left side
   d. To identify the front from the back of the film

3. What is the composition of emulsion?
   a. Silver halide crystals suspended in gelatin
   b. Supercoating gelatin
   c. Adhesive material
   d. Polyester

4. In what sizes is intraoral film supplied?
   a. 00, 0, 1, 2, 3
   b. 0, 1, 2, occlusal
   c. 0, 1, 2, 3, occlusal
   d. 00, 0, 1, 2, 3, occlusal

5. In what way does D speed differ from E speed film?
   a. In the processing technique
   b. In the size of the silver halide crystals
   c. In the size of films
   d. In the number of films per packet

CHAPTER 64

Quality Assurance and Infection Control for Dental Radiography

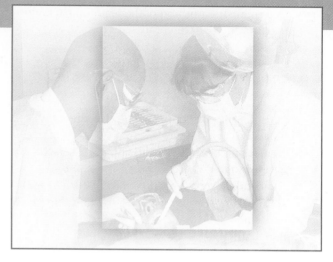

OBJECTIVES

After studying this chapter, the student will be able to:

- Define quality assurance as it relates to dental radiography.
- Identify the components of a quality assurance program.
- Explain the function of a reference radiograph.
- Describe the method for testing x-ray machine effectiveness.
- Explain how to determine if processing solutions are of adequate strength.
- Describe the method used for replenishing solutions.
- State infection control measures used for personal protection.
- Describe the meaning of plastic barrier envelopes.
- Describe types of barriers used in dental radiography.
- Explain the step-by-step procedure when processing contaminated film in the automatic processor with daylight loader.
- Discuss the means by which contaminated film packets are processed in the darkroom using infection control measures.

Introduction

The term **quality assurance (QA)** in dental radiography describes a systematic approach to control and ensure that all components in a radiographic system are functioning at an acceptable level of proficiency.

An established *quality assurance program* should maintain a standard of operation that will produce quality dental radiographs while reducing the level of ionizing radiation to both patient and operator.

The first step in a quality assurance program is to establish a reference or baseline value by which the x-ray equipment and film processing system can be monitored before a problem occurs that could adversely affect the diagnostic quality of radiographs. A program of this type has been shown to lower the level of radiation exposure to patients through the decrease in the number of retakes.

Many changes have evolved regarding infection control in the practice of dentistry. The awareness of incurable infectious diseases has had a major impact on personal and patient protection from cross-contamination.

Infection control procedures in radiography should follow the same basic guidelines imposed by the Centers for Disease Control and Prevention (CDCP), Occupational Safety Administration (OSHA), and the American Dental Association (ADA). Using universal precautions means that each patient must be treated in the same manner as though infected by a deadly communicable disease.

Quality Assurance

X-Ray Unit

Monitoring of generators (transformers) and other electronic components (kilovoltage peak, milliamperes, and exposure timer) of the unit should be done by a qualified physicist or x-ray engineer at least once a year. Additional methods for testing may be found through the Eastman Kodak Company, who publishes a free pamphlet entitled "Quality Control Tests for Dental Radiography." It contains step-by-step procedures to test x-ray machines that may be performed by any member on the dental team.

One way to evaluate the x-ray machine's performance and exposure factors is to coordinate it with the time solutions are changed. Having fresh solutions allows films to be processed in solutions that have appropriate strength. It is important to follow the steps outlined below.

Reference Radiograph

The use of a **reference radiograph** (a radiograph made previously under ideal conditions of exposure and processing, kept as a measuring device for subsequent radiograph assessment) is one method to monitor the quality of film, x-ray unit, and processing solutions. It is placed on a **viewbox** (a source of light that uses fluorescent tubes under a frosted window to examine radiographs) and used for comparison purposes.

Using a Step Wedge

1. A film is exposed using a step wedge at a similar anode-to-film distance as projected on a patient and the same exposure settings as were used on the reference radiograph. If there is more than one x-ray machine, film is exposed for each one. (Figure 64-1).

2. Film(s) should be processed using fresh chemicals and ideal techniques. It is important to use fresh chemicals for the first test because subsequent tests will be based on this initial test film.

3. The processed radiograph should reveal 10 distinct steps of the wedge (normal contrast and density) (Figure 64-2). The processed radiograph should be compared with a reference radiograph to see that all 10 steps are revealed and to see that the densities match. If the steps are lost on the lighter end of the scale, radiographs may be underexposed, requiring an increase in either exposure time or milliamperes. Should some of the steps be lost on the darker end of the scale, the radiograph is overexposed and will require a decrease in exposure time or milliamperes.

Assessment Program for Darkroom

Test Safelight or Other Light Leakage

Radiographs may become fogged in the darkroom due to factors that can be controlled. It is essential that the safelight be of excellent quality. A **safelight** consists of a low-intensity 71/2–10 W red-orange light with a filter that sufficiently illuminates a darkroom without exposing or otherwise causing a foggy appearance on the processed radiograph.

Reasons for film fog include using a faulty safe-

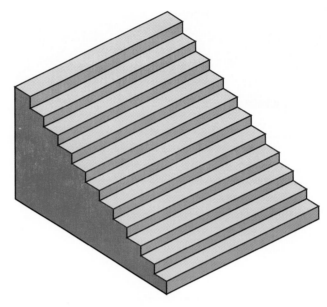

Figure 64-1 Step wedge.

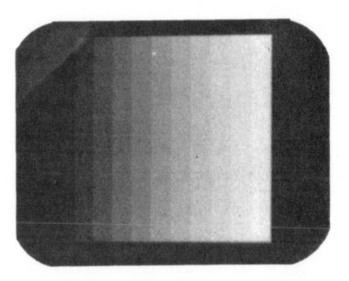

Figure 64-2 Radiograph depicting shades of gray on step wedge.

light, one that is too bright, or one whose filters are defective or scratched. Also, the darkroom door must be **light tight**, with no light leakage around the door. To check a light-tight door, it should be closed and the knob allowed to latch, while all lights are turned off. If, while inspecting from the inside of the darkroom there are openings around the door or a keyhole allows white light to enter the room, it is determined that the room is not light tight. To test for light leakage, the following techniques should be used.

Procedure 71 Testing for Safelight Leakage

Materials Needed

Unexposed film
Coin
Processing rack
Processing solutions
Safelight
Timer

Instructions

1 Use an unexposed film.

2 Close darkroom door and turn on safelight.

3 Remove film from packet, and place on clean, dry countertop.

4 Place a coin in the center of unwrapped film.

5 Allow the coin to remain on film for 5 minutes.

6 After 5 minutes, remove coin and process film.

Note: If processed film shows an outline of the coin, faulty safelight or other light leakage is fogging the film (Figure 64–3).

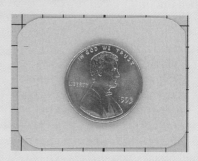

Figure 64-3 Coin placed on x-ray film and radiograph of same.

Procedure 72 Testing for White Light Leakage

Materials Needed

Unexposed film
Coin
Processing rack
Processing solutions
Timer

Instructions

1 Use an unexposed film.

2 *Do not* use a safelight.

3 Unwrap the film; place a coin over it and leave on for 5 minutes.

4 Proceed with processing.

Note: Should the coin's image occur in either case, replace safelight, use weather stripping to close gaps around the doorway and key hole if applicable, and take steps to eliminate the cause.

Daily Evaluation of Processing Solutions and Darkroom Equipment

Processing solutions need to be in optimum condition at all times. Information on the radiograph is largely dependent on the processing technique; therefore, one must be certain that processing solutions are in good working order. To maintain adequate levels and strength of solutions, the following guidelines should be followed.

Procedure 73   Evaluating Processing Solutions

Materials Needed

Two cups (one for develop, one for fixer)
Processing solutions
Replenishing solutions
Stirring rods
Film exposed with step wedge
Step wedge
Processing rack
Timer

Instructions

1 Replenishing solutions on a daily basis is recommended. Take away one cup-full (approximately 6 oz) of existing solution from each tank and discard properly.

2 Fresh developer and fixer replenisher solutions should be stirred and added to maintain proper levels in processing tanks (Figure 64-4).

3 Solutions should be changed at regularly, prescribed intervals.

4 Solutions should always be stirred prior to each processing procedure to achieve a homogenous mixture.

5 To determine the strength of solutions, expose a film using a step wedge that will test the densities on the radiograph and process it. If the densities appear light, the strength of the solutions may be exhausted. The "test radiograph" should reveal 10 distinct steps and match the densities to the

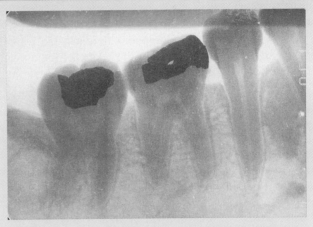

Figure 64-4 Radiograph processed in low-level solutions.

reference radiograph. The reference radiograph should be taped to a viewbox for daily comparison.

6 If the fixer solution is suspected of being weak, an unexposed film can be placed directly in it, *bypassing* the developer. The *time* it takes for the silver halide crystals to be removed is essential in determining how effective the solution is.

Note: If it takes 2 minutes to clear the film, the solution has adequate strength. If it takes 3–4 minutes to clear the film, the solution is weak and should be changed.

Test the Quality of Film

Film should be stored in a cool, dry place, away from radiation, heat, and chemicals. It should be used prior to the stated expiration date found on the side of the package. To test the quality of the film, the operator should process an unexposed film each time a new package is open:

● If the processed film appears clear with a blue tinge, it is considered to be of good quality.

● If the processed film appears dark or fogged, it should be discarded as its optimum use has expired or it has been contaminated by radiation, heat, or chemicals.

Other Factors to Consider

To achieve optimum results in producing high-quality radiographs, besides using established guidelines already mentioned, there are other factors that need to be considered:

● *Have adequate working equipment.* As already mentioned, the x-ray machine should be monitored on a yearly basis or more frequently if needed. This should include not only the quality of the beam but also the unit as a whole. If the arm that suspends the tubehead begins to drift, it could cause the beam to affect other areas other than the intended one.

- *Maintain clean working areas.* When films are unwrapped in the darkroom, it is imperative that working areas are free of solutions; otherwise the incidence of having artifacts increases. If unwrapped, unprocessed films come in contact with fixer droplets, the image in that area will be permanently removed.

- *Control temperature of processing solutions.* The darkroom should be equipped with adjustable water valves to be able to change the water temperature. Thus, on a cold morning, the temperature of the water could be increased to a warmer level by adjusting the valve. Otherwise, the quality of the radiograph may be compromised, causing it to appear light. The optimum temperature is 68°F.

- *Use adequate safelight.* The operator should be keenly aware that when processing panoramic films that are so sensitive to light, only Kodak GBX-2 safelight or others of similar illumination are recommended for use; otherwise the film will be light fogged and not exhibit any images.

- *Maintain processing racks in good working condition.* Many films have been "lost" while processing them. One certain way for this to happen is by assuming that the clips on the processing racks will securely hold the film. The operator needs to test *each* clip by tapping on the film as it is loaded to avoid this problem (Figure 64-5).

- *Use reliable timers.* Film processing requires exact timing based on the temperature of solutions. If the timer is not reliable, it will greatly affect the quality of the radiograph. Not only does it affect the developing time where film can become chemically fogged if allowed to remain in the tank for an extended time, but it can also affect the fixing time where the film can lose density if left in for too long.

- *The viewbox.* The viewbox should be checked periodically. Fluorescent tubes that show blackening at the ends should be replaced.

Radiation Safety Assurance: Patient and Operator

Patient

1. X-ray exposure to the patient must be based on diagnostic need.

2. A lead apron and thyroid shield or collar should be used.

3. The D or E speed film should be used.

4. High-kVp exposure technique should be used.

5. Open-ended, lead-lined cylinders or PIDs should be used. The rectangular PID is considered more ideal.

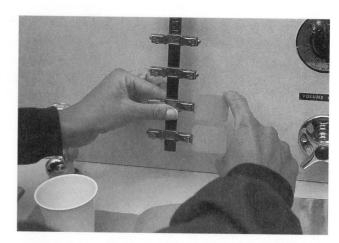

Figure 64-5 Testing film for film security on a processing rack.

6. Appropriate techniques should be used in exposing and processing radiographs.

Operator

1. Monitoring devices such as film badges (known as dosimeters) are recommended to provide a useful record of occupational exposure.

2. An accepted radiographic technique should be used to observe all safety practices.

Monitoring Records

A monitoring log should be kept for each quality assurance procedure. Records of yearly x-ray equipment evaluation should be on file. Log sheets should be posted in nearby areas for processing and step wedge exposures. Thus, each time a step wedge is exposed and processed, the log should state what was being tested, the findings, and the management used for rectifying the problem.

Infection Control

Although radiographic procedures are not considered to be **invasive** (allowing infective microorganisms to gain entry into the body), nevertheless, the risk of infection transmission is present. During the radiographic examination, it will be necessary to work inside the patient's mouth. Infection control procedures are in order for every patient to avoid exposure to the operator and cross-contaminating other patients. Refer to Chapters 7 and 8.

While using universal precautions, properly prepared equipment and infection control procedures, marked by common sense and good judgment, should be strictly followed. There are some major areas that need to be dealt with when following infection control techniques:

1. Protective attire and immunizations for the operator
2. Protective attire for the patient
3. Areas that need barriers
4. Type of barriers available
5. Disinfecting and sterilizing equipment
6. Film processing

Protective Attire and Immunization for the Operator

It has been established by the CDCP that dental health care professionals need to follow specific guidelines to aid in effective infection control. The presence of infectious diseases in the dental office is inevitable. The dental professional must guard against the possibility of becoming infected by these microorganisms; thus immunization for specific diseases such as hepatitis B is a must. In following the CDCP's guidelines, it is stated that protective attire consisting of gown, mask, eyewear/face shield, and examination gloves be worn when spatter is anticipated. It behooves the dental professional to determine if these protective measures are applicable in radiographic procedures. However, in the best interest of the operator and patient, above items should be used at all times (refer to Chapters 7 and 8).

Protective Attire for the Patient

Two primary concerns for patients are protection from excessive radiation exposure and protection from disease transmission. Providing them with necessary attire would include the lead apron and thyroid collar, minimizing radiation exposure (see Figure 62–1). It should also be remembered that these items might become contaminated with patient's saliva. Therefore, they must always be disinfected after each patient use. It is good practice to use a patient's bib with a paper towel or tissue attached to blot saliva from the film packet as it is removed from the patient's mouth.

Areas That Need Barriers

Areas where possible contact made by the operator who is wearing contaminated gloves should be noted. Barriers need to be placed in all possible contact areas as follows (Figure 64-6):

- Foil or plastic adhesive film for light handles and switches.
- Plastic adhesive film or plastic wrap for tubehead/position-indicating device (PID)/yoke handles and extension arm.
- Large plastic bag for dental chair and headrest.
- Plastic wrap for control panel.

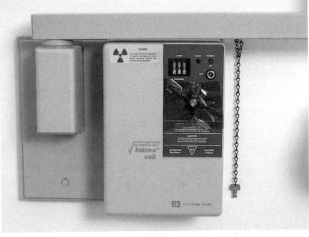

(A)

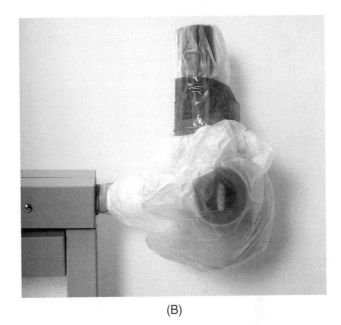

(B)

Figure 64-6 Barriers placed on (A) control panel and (B) tubehead.

- Plastic wrap or bracket tray covering for countertop.
- Plastic adhesive film for film dispenser and receptacle lid.
- A baggie for exposure timer switch.
- Plastic adhesive film for doorway handle.

Types of Barriers Available

When choosing a barrier, it must be impervious and be able to adapt to the area being placed. There are several disposable barriers from which to choose:

- Plastic bags—small, medium, and large
- Plastic baggies

- Plastic wrap, the type used in most kitchens
- Plastic adhesive film
- Aluminum foil

Disinfecting and Sterilizing Equipment

After the patient is dismissed, the treatment room needs to be prepared for the next patient to enter. It is cleaned and disinfected.

- To remove barriers and disinfect areas that may have been contaminated, the operator wears protective **utility gloves** (protective, puncture-resistant gloves). The contaminated barriers are placed in the same larger bag that covered the chair confining them to one specific location, then placed in a biohazard bag marked for contaminated materials. The protective utility gloves are washed thoroughly with a bacteriostatic soap, dried, sterilized, and stored for future use.

- A disinfectant registered by the EPA (Environment Protection Agency) is applied to areas where barriers cannot be used. The types of disinfectant selected for this procedure should be iodophors, sodium hypochlorite (chlorine dioxide) solutions, or synthetic phenolics. One needs to determine the shelf life of these compounds and use them accordingly. For example, if using a chlorine-based solution, it should be mixed daily at 1 : 100 dilution and replaced daily; if using an iodophor, it should be mixed at 1 : 213 dilution and also be replaced daily; some phenolics already come mixed and will last longer.

  All instruments used on the patient are sterilized in an autoclave. Only autoclaveable film holders should be exposed to high heat.

Film Processing

As exposed films are removed from the patient's mouth, the retained saliva on the packet is blotted with a paper towel or tissue and placed in a receptacle containing a plastic cup or baggie that is protected from radiation until completion. The operator removes examination gloves and washes hands thoroughly. Film packets are transported in the cup or baggie to the darkroom or automatic processor.

Keeping in mind that the film packets are contaminated, the operator must use caution not to further contaminate anything by proceeding as follows:

In the Darkroom

1. Operator puts on new "powder-free" examination gloves to unwrap contaminated film packets.

2. Uncontaminated films are dropped into another cup or container.
3. The wrappings are placed in a paper towel and discarded with contaminated gloves.
4. At this time, the uncontaminated films are handled with ungloved hands and placed on a processing rack.
5. Processing continues.

Using Automatic Processor with Daylight Loader

1. Operator feeds contaminated film packets in cup or baggie, extra cup for uncontaminated films, paper towel or small bag, and powder-free gloves through the daylight loader lid.
2. Operator closes lid and places hands through daylight loader cuffs (assuming there has not been any contamination to cuffs; otherwise, double gloves should be worn—one set to unwrap film and one set to handle uncontaminated film).
3. Operator puts on gloves and unwraps contaminated film packets.
4. Uncontaminated films are dropped into a clean cup or clean surface.
5. Contaminated wrappings and gloves are placed in paper towel or small plastic biohazard bag or in the same cup that transported films.
6. Uncontaminated film is placed in the processor and processing is continued.

   Note: The above recommendations are intended for film packets *without* plastic barrier envelopes.

Film "Barrier" Packets

Film barrier packets are film packets equipped with a plastic wrapping (envelope) for infection control purposes and are sold in sizes #0, #1, and #2 in either "D" or "E" speed periapical film. It is also possible to purchase only the plastic barrier envelopes to cover and seal individual film packets. When film packets *with* plastic barrier envelopes are used, the procedure is as follows:

Plastic Barrier Envelopes

1. Barrier envelopes may be removed prior to transporting films for processing. The envelope is torn open and the film packet is allowed to fall out into a cup or paper towel without touching anything, especially operator's contaminated gloves.
2. Operator's contaminated gloves and barrier envelopes are discarded.
3. Operator's hands are washed and dried.

4. Uncontaminated film packets are transported and are ready to process in the darkroom or automatic processor.

Daily Infection Control Protocol

- *Disinfection.* Using utility gloves, the operatory is cleaned and prepared for the next patient. All areas are disinfected that may have been touched by the operator, to include lead apron/thyroid collar, light switches, door handle, counter top, film dispenser, head rest, cabinet drawers/doors, control panel, tubehead, and extension arm.

- *Hand washing.* Hand washing using bacteriostatic soap must be done at the following times: prior to preparing the patient, prior to donning gloves, after gloves are removed upon completion of film exposure, after removing barriers from film packets, after processing films, and after disinfecting the treatment room.

- *Gloves.* Latex, vinyl, or nitrile examination gloves are used when possible contamination with patient's saliva or blood exists. The operator should don gloves *after* the patient has been seated and draped, *during* the x-ray exposure procedure, and *while* unwrapping contaminated films. Contaminated gloves should *never* be worn while removing lead apron/thyroid collar, upon leaving the operatory (contaminated gloves need to be removed if operator has to step out of the operatory, i.e., to get more film, answer the telephone, or get instruments from the sterilizer), or when leaving to process films. Utility gloves are used during clean-up/disinfection and preparation of instruments for sterilization.

- *Sterilization.* Film-holding devices and instruments such as mouth mirror, cotton pliers, and hemostat must be sterilized by heat. Cold sterilizing solution may be used for devices that are not autoclaveable.

- *Barriers.* Barriers should be used primarily in areas where continuous "touching" by the operator occurs, such as tubehead/yoke handles, control panel, counter top, dental light handles and switch, dental chair/head rest, door handle, and exposure switch.

SUGGESTED ACTIVITIES

- Test the darkroom for safelight or other light leakage.
- Using the step wedge, expose a film to test each x-ray machine and process in the darkroom and/or automatic processor to test the effectiveness of fresh chemicals.

- Practice positioning barriers in the treatment room and using infection control techniques on a fellow student as if exposure of film were to take place.
- Practice infection control techniques in film processing when using the darkroom and automatic processor.

REVIEW

1. Describe what a reference radiograph is.
   a. A radiograph made to check the effectiveness of the x-ray machine
   b. An exposed film processed in fresh solutions that tests their effectiveness
   c. A radiograph that appears to have ideal densities
   d. A radiograph made previously under ideal conditions of exposure and processing for subsequent radiographic comparisons

2. When performing a coin test in the darkroom, the coin is placed on:
   a. A film packet for 5 minutes, then processed
   b. An unwrapped exposed film for 1 minute, then processed
   c. An unwrapped unexposed film for 5 minutes, then processed
   d. An unwrapped unexposed film for 1 minute, then processed

3. A step wedge: (1) is used to evaluate the x-ray machine for effectiveness, (2) has 10 steps of densities, (3) is used to expose a film that compares to a reference radiograph for density on all steps, and/or (4) is exposed only after the x-ray machine is tested by a qualified physicist once a year.
   a. 1, 2, 3   c. 1, 2, 4
   b. 2, 3, 4   d. 1, 3, 4

4. Daily infection control protocol while making radiographs should include (1) using impervious barriers such as plastic material, (2) using disinfectants on all contaminated surfaces, (3) using disinfected film holders, and/or (4) practicing universal precautions.
   a. 1, 2, 3   c. 1, 2, 4
   b. 2, 3, 4   d. 1, 3, 4

5. Areas that need barriers while exposing film on patients include (1) exposure timer switch, (2) control panel, (3) tubehead, and/or (4) film holders.
   a. 1, 2, 3   c. 1, 2, 4
   b. 2, 3, 4   d. 1, 3, 4

Film Processing

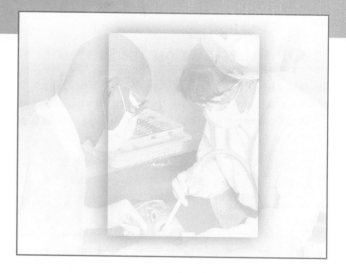

OBJECTIVES

After studying this chapter, the student will be able to:

- State the function and composition of the developer.
- List components of the fixing solution and the action of each.
- Discuss the importance of the water bath.
- List the three basic principles for effective darkroom procedure.
- List and explain the 12 steps in proper darkroom preparation procedure.
- State the importance of using care when processing film.
- Describe the procedure for developing film using an automatic processor.
- Compare darkroom processing with automatic processing of radiographic film.
- Describe the procedure for duplicating radiographs.
- Explain possible ways that film fogging may occur.
- Explain how a processed film appears clear without an image.
- Explain how processing spots appear on a radiograph and give the rationale for each type.

Introduction

Film processing that will produce the highest quality radiographs depends on several factors: The primary principles for effective darkroom procedure are (1) absolute cleanliness, (2) absolute light-tight security, and (3) proper use of time and temperature techniques. There is also a need for the operator to have a clear understanding of the function, chemistry of solutions, and manner in which they react on the film. Knowledge of their sensitivity to temperature changes and oxidation is of value. The darkroom should be well equipped and the procedure for film processing should be followed with accuracy. Processing errors take place when improper equipment is used or inadequate procedures are implemented.

Chemistry of Development

Developer is the solution that removes the bromide from the metallic silver, chemically known as **reduction**. The black metallic silver remaining behind forms the image of the exposed object (teeth). The function of the developer is to bring out the **latent image** (the invisible radiographic representation of dental structures on an exposed but not processed film). It reduces the exposed area of the emulsion so that it will be visible to the human eye. It is generally composed of hydroquinone, elon, sodium sulfate, and other chemicals in solution. Two chemicals used in the developing solution that are *reducing* agents and have a definite action on the photographic emulsion are hydroquinone and elon. The composition of the developer is given in Table 65-1.

Chemistry of Fixation

After development of the film, the undeveloped silver halide salts are removed by immersion of the film in what is called the **fixer**. The composition of the fixer is sodium thiosulfate/ammonium thiosulfate, also known as hyposulfite of soda or **hypo**. Fixing is accomplished by means of the hypo only. This chemical is the *fixing agent* and removes the unexposed silver halide crystals that were not affected by the developer. Only the dark images that were produced by the developer are now visible. Sodium sulfite acts as a preservative. Acetic acid is used to compensate for the alkaline chemicals. Potassium alum is the hardening agent that also shrinks the gelatin that was softened and swollen in the developer (Table 65-2).

Table 65-1 Composition of Developer

Chemical	Action	Purpose
Hydroquinone	Reducer	Works slowly to gain density by converting exposed silver halide (bromide) crystals to black metallic silver. Very sensitive to temperature changes.
Elon	Reducer	Works quickly to bring the image gaining density slowly. Not readily sensitive to temperature changes.
Sodium carbonate	Accelerator	An alkali that softens the gelatin of the emulsion. Promotes developing to take place. Too little slows developing action. Too much may cause chemical fog.
Sodium sulfite	Preservative	Prevents oxidation and prolongs life of developer.
Potassium bromide	Restrainer	Prevents too rapid development and fogging of transparent areas of the film (unexposed silver halide crystals).

Table 65-2 Composition of Fixer

Chemical	Action	Purpose
Sodium thiosulfate/hypo	Fixing agent/clearing agent	Removes unexposed silver halide (bromide) crystals not affected by developer
Sodium sulfite	Preservative	Prevents deterioration of sodium thiosulfate
Acetic acid	Acidifier	Maintains acidity and neutralizes alkaline developer by stopping development action
Potassium Alum	Hardener	Hardens and shrinks gelatin

Distilled Water

Distilled water should be the vehicle for all developing and fixing solutions. Water containing chemicals may combine with the chemicals of the developing and fixing solutions and have a damaging effect on the silver halide (bromide) salts of the emulsion.

Processing Solutions

Processing solutions are supplied in two forms: concentrate and "ready to use." The concentrated form must be diluted with water. To prevent contamination with chemical agents, distilled water should always be used. Ready-to-use solutions are available in both quart and gallon sizes. This form is used in automatic processors. Solutions should be stored in a cool, dark place, away from direct light or heat.

In normal processing situations, it is recommended that solutions be changed every three to four weeks with daily replenishing to maintain solutions at appropriate strengths and levels.

Procedure of Washing

The actual time of washing may best be understood by remembering that, as the washing proceeds, the amount of hypo remaining in the gelatin emulsion is continually halved in the same period of time. An average film will give up one-half of its hypo in 2 minutes, so that at the end of 2 minutes one-half the hypo will be remaining in it; after 4 minutes, one-quarter; after 6 minutes, one-eighth; and so on. In a short time, the amount of hypo remaining on the emulsion will be minimal. However, this assumes that the film is continually exposed to circulating water. During processing, films should always be washed between solutions. After fixing, they should remain in running water for at least 20 minutes before drying.

The temperature of the water in which the films are washed is of great importance. If the temperature is too high, the films will become pitted or **reticulated** (a condition in which the emulsion softens and tends to slide off the film base), caused by the softening or swelling of the emulsion. Reticulation can also be caused by sudden temperature changes between the solution and the water bath. Keeping the water bath under 70°F (21°C) is recommended.

Darkroom Procedures

Darkroom Equipment

A well-equipped darkroom should have the capability to process periapical and panoramic x-ray films in a clean environment (Figure 65-1). It should possess some basic components to carry out effective darkroom procedures. The component parts should include the following:

Light-Tight Security. It is imperative that the darkroom is light tight. This means that when the door is closed and lights are turned off inside the darkroom, white light from the outside should not enter. If light is visibly coming in under or around the door, installation of weather stripping should remedy the problem.

Safelight. The safelight is used to give the operator visibility while unwrapping film without affecting it. For increased security, the safelight may be connected to an outside warning light that lights up when it is turned on.

White Overhead Light. Darkrooms need to have a white overhead light to be able to see while cleaning and changing processing solutions, reading the thermometer, and reading the time/temperature chart. One item of importance is to place the switch at a much higher level than the usual place to guard against accidental bumping or activation.

Processing Tank. The processing tank consists of a main tank with two one-gallon insert tanks, one for the developer and one for the fixer; a circulating water bath; hot and cold water intake valves with a thermostat control valve; an overflow pipe; and a light-tight tank lid. A stainless steel tank with plastic inserts will prevent any chemical reaction with the solutions and provide easy

upkeep. The circulating water that surrounds the developer and fixer containers controls the temperature of the solutions. The thermostat control valve controls the temperature of the water, allowing one to select the temperature setting. The overflow pipe allows the circulating water to move across the tank and spill excess water into it. The light-tight lid protects the solutions from **oxidation** (when solutions combine with oxygen, causing them to deteriorate), prevents evaporation, and protects the films from white-light exposure while processing (Figure 65-2).

Water Thermometer. The water thermometer is a necessary item because it establishes the time that films should remain in the developer and is placed in the *developer*. It is very critical to have this information since the *time/temperature chart* in Table 65-3 is consulted to determine appropriate developing time. Without it, film will be either chemically fogged when left in too long at

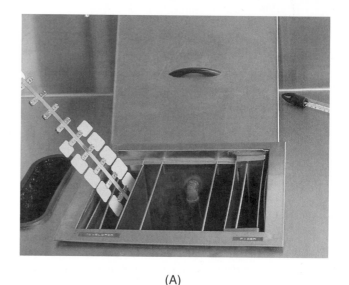

(A)

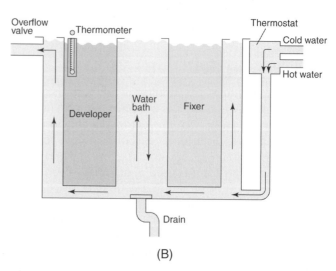

(B)

Figure 65-2 Manual processing tanks.

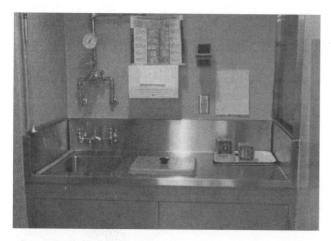

Figure 65-1 Darkroom.

Table 65-3	Time-Temperature Chart
Temperature of Developer (°F)	**Time**
60–62	9 (min)
64–66	7 (min)
68–70 (optimum temperature)	5 (min)
66–76	4 (min)
78–80	3 (min)

Note: Fixing time: 10 min (generally twice the time for developing). Washing: 20 min.

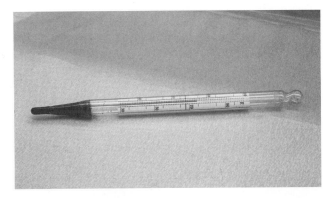

Figure 65-3 Floating thermometer.

higher temperatures or underdeveloped as evidenced by lack in contrast if left in for too short a time at lower temperatures in the developer. The ideal processing temperature is 68°F at 5 minutes time (Figure 65-3).

Interval Time Clock. The interval time clock works hand in hand with the water thermometer. The time clock is set depending on the temperature reading of the developer. The clock should be set, activated, and placed in a location that can be heard by the operator. The operator should know how to set the clock prior to processing. Mistakes have occurred due to being unfamiliar with a clock (Figure 65-4).

Film Hangers and Drying Racks. Film hangers are used to carry the films through the processing procedure. They are made of stainless steel and come with clips that hold the film in place. Hangers are available for intraoral film with a single clip or from 2 to 20 clips. For processing panoramic or extraoral film, hangers are designed for the film to slide-in and are named "slide-in" type. They will hold either 5 x 12 or 6 x 12-in. film. Racks are labeled with a tab, tape, or label. It is recommended that felt tip pens *not* be used to label racks as they will smear when wet. If a tape is used, it is best to use a ballpoint pen as opposed to a pencil, which may be rubbed off (Figure 65-5).

The darkroom should be equipped with drying racks. Film hangers can be placed there, away from splatter and the possibility of being knocked off. If the drying rack has two levels, one above the other, it may be best to place wet hangers on the lower level below others that may already have dried; this confines water droplets to the lower level and eliminates any interference with dry films (Figure 65-6).

Storage Compartments. Every darkroom should be equipped with storage compartments. Items such as extra film hangers, processing solutions, powder-free gloves, and cleaning agents should have a place in the darkroom.

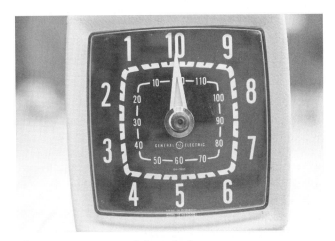

Figure 65-4 Interval time clock.

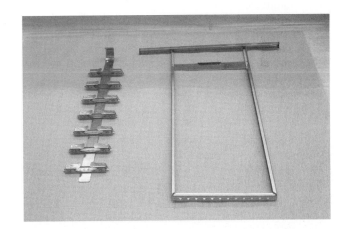

Figure 65-5 Intraoral and panoramic film hangers.

Stirring Rods. Stirring rods should be kept nearby processing solutions. They are made of plastic, wood, or glass and are used to stir the solutions each time processing takes place to equalize the temperature of the solution and to ensure a homogenous mix. They are rinsed, dried, and stored until the next time processing

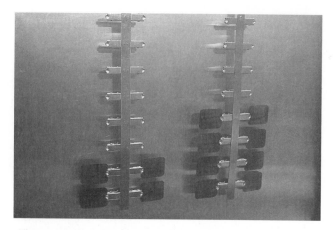

Figure 65-6 Drying rack.

takes place. If solutions are not stirred, there is a possibility that processed radiographs will exhibit varying degrees of density.

Viewbox. The purpose for having a viewbox in the darkroom is for convenience. When radiographs are removed from the processing tank, they are wet, and thus when carried to another part of the office, a trail of water spots will most likely appear. This is not only unsightly but also dangerous. Water on polished floors may cause someone to slip and fall.

Manual Processing

Basic principles for effective darkroom procedure are:

- Absolute cleanliness
- Absolute light-tight security
- Proper use of time and temperature techniques

Rationale for Preventing Problems

Wiping Working Surfaces. The first step to undertake when entering the darkroom is to wipe and dry all work surfaces. Frequently, someone may have inadvertently sprinkled some developer or fixer on the work surfaces; these droplets subsequently evaporate and leave a highly concentrated crystalline residue of processing chemicals. If film is dropped or placed in contact with this chemical combination, it will become spotted, often in such a manner as to indicate possible pathology on the processed film.

Stirring Solutions. Both developer and fixer should be stirred with separate stirring rods. These rods should be washed in water between each stirring operation. The reason is relatively simple; the chemicals of both developer and fixer are heavier than water and tend to settle to the bottom of the tank inserts. Processing without stirring produces a developing "tree" whose films are quite dark at the bottom of the rack, possibly reasonably accurate in the middle, and very frequently quite light at the top. Therefore, for overall consistency of radiographic result, thorough stirring is essential.

Determining Temperature. As mentioned, an effective temperature range is generally between 68 and 70°F (20–21°C). When developers are used at temperatures below 65°F, they may not be effective. Chemicals used at temperatures above 75°F present two problems: (1) reticulation and (2) demands on accuracy in terms of processing time that are unjustified. This situation implies the availability of both hot and cold water inflow to the tank.

Referring to the Time-Temperature Chart. Table 65–3 contains recommended time for a given temperature to achieve complete development of the film.

Setting the Timer. The time should correspond to the recommended time for the temperature available in accordance with the charts published by each manufacturer for each solution.

Opening the Film. The white overhead light should be turned off and the safelight turned on before the film packet is opened. Care must be taken when opening dental film and extracting the film from the covering in order to avoid injury of the emulsion through crimping, scratching, or finger marking. Fingernail markings appear as crescent-shaped images on the developed film. This damage usually occurs at the time the film is softened before it is placed in the mouth or at the time that the bite-wing tab or strip is placed on the film. Crimping (bruising) of the emulsion may occur as the film is placed in the film holder prior to exposure or as the film packet is opened. If the fingers grasp the film, marks may occur on the emulsion as the packet is opened and placed on the hanger. These fingerprints will remain on the film. Caution of harming or contaminating the film should be exercised at all times.

Securing the Film. All too frequently, films are lost from the processing hanger in the tank because of improper fastening of the film. Introducing the film to a clip hanger in the following manner can eliminate this problem:

1. Hanger is grasped with clips in an "up" position.
2. Selected clip key is depressed.
3. Film is placed on the edge nearest the embossed dot and the upper edge of the clip introduced at a 45° angle. While holding the film at this angle, clip key is released. This will permit the film to be grasped by the three securing prongs rather than the one central prong frequently employed.

4. The security of each film on the hanger is tested by gently tapping each with the index fingertip; if the film is not secure, it will fall off before it is immersed in the developer solution.

Immersing the Film and Starting the Timer.
In as simple an action as the immersion of the hanger, specific procedural steps must be followed. The hanger and its films should be immersed in the stirred developer, then lifted out completely from the developer, and then reimmersed and agitated in the developer. The timer is set according to the manufacturer's direction. The reason for this is relatively simple to explain once the problem is understood. There are small globules of air suspended in the solutions. Because the film surface is dry as it enters the solution, these air bubbles are frequently attracted to the surface of the film where "surface tension" will cause them to cling to the emulsion. This, in turn, prevents the developer from reaching the emulsion, causing one or more white spots to appear on the radiograph.

Removing and Washing the Film.
When the timer rings indicating completion of the development process, the hanger and films are removed from the developer. Upon removal, the hanger is tilted over the developer to drop excess developing solution to avoid depletion of the solution. Films are inserted into the water bath and washed thoroughly in the clean, running water for at least 30 seconds.

Large quantities of valuable chemicals are lost in hanger movement from one compartment to another, because the clips of the hanger tend to retain a substantial amount of fluid. The hanger should be given a quick vertical shake over the appropriate compartment, then turned diagonally and again shaken over the same compartment. This action will reduce the loss of fluids.

Fixing the Film.
A simple formula for proper fixation is 3 + 7 = 10. At the end of 3 minutes, the films may be removed from the fixing solution and quickly washed by dipping the hanger in the water bath for study or "*wet reading*" only. After the films have been studied, they are returned to the fixer for 7 minutes more for complete fixation or a total of 10 minutes. In the event the films were out of the fixer sufficiently long enough to dry, they should be washed in the circulating water bath before placing them in the fixer and allowing a full 10 minutes of fixation.

Note: If proper processing is observed and the temperature of the solution does not exceed 70°F (21°C), it is reasonably impossible to "overdevelop" or "overfix."

Washing and Preparing to Dry Films.
Following fixation of films, a second wash period removes all chemical residue from the hanger and films. This wash period should be approximately 20 minutes in the flowing water bath. Again, within the limitations of cleanliness and temperature, one cannot reasonably "overwash."

Films are removed from the water bath and held under running *cold tap water*. The water is allowed to run over the hanger, clips, and film. The surface of the films is tested for any residual chemicals while water is contacting them. The films may have a slick surface if they are not completely washed; this residue will gather at the lower surface of films as they dry. To remove the slick surface, films are gently rubbed using the ball of the thumb and fingers until they feel clean to the touch. The excess water from the hanger and films is shaken off and dipped in a solution of *Photo Flo* (solution used in photography to eliminate spots) for a few seconds until all films are immersed, then shaken off again.

Drying the Films.
Films on the hanger are placed on a drying rack until they are completely dry. Any residual moisture in the emulsion offers the serious risk of a scarred film surface. Films should not be mounted until absolutely dry.

Note: Working area surfaces in the darkroom and film hangers should be cleaned thoroughly. Such a simple safeguard can eliminate many future problems.

Procedure 74 Manual Operating Procedures and Processing

Materials Needed

Exposed films
Processing solutions
Stirring rods
Thermometer

Labeled hanger/rack
Interval timer
Powder-free gloves
Paper towel/cup
Photo-Flo solution
Fan

continued

Instructions

Preparation

1 Enter darkroom and turn on overhead white light.

2 Check level of solutions and replenish (should be done on a daily basis).

3 Wipe all work surfaces thoroughly.

4 Check temperature of developer solution. Thoroughly stir solutions using marked stirring rods: one for the developer and one for the fixer. (Avoid contamination between solutions.) Rinse stirring rods, dry, and put away.

5 Set interval timer according to temperature of developer and time temperature chart. (Do not activate it).

6 Label hanger with patient's name, date of exposure, and number of films.

7 Close door tightly, turn on safelight, and turn off overhead white light.

8 Don gloves.

9 Unwrap contaminated film packets, allowing them to drop into a cup or onto a paper towel (Figure 65-7). (If plastic envelopes were used and if not already opened in the operatory, open them, allowing film packet to drop onto a paper towel, remove contaminated gloves, and proceed to remove film.)

10 Remove contaminated gloves and dispose with film wrappings.

11 Clip uncontaminated films onto film hanger, handling film by the edges and being mindful of finger marks and scratches that damage the film (Figure 65-8).

12 Check stability by tapping on top edge of each film. If any films are unstable, reattach and check again or do not use a loose clip.

Developing

1 The hanger with films is ready to be immersed in the developer. Place films in the solution and lift out completely from developer, then reimmerse and agitate the rack up and down for at least eight times. (This action will remove surface tension air bubbles.)

2 Place hanger on side of tank, making certain that all the films are below the level of the solution and not touching the wall of the tank or other films.

3 Activate the interval timer already set according to developer temperature.

4 Close the tank lid.

Rinsing

1 When timer rings, lift and drain excess developer from hanger into developer solution.

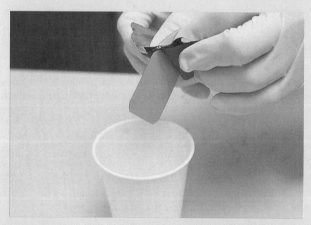

Figure 65-7 Unwrapping a contaminated film packet.

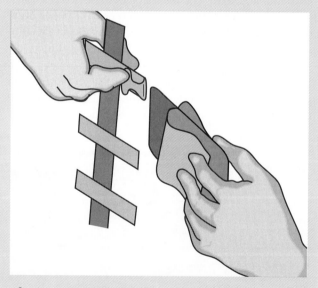

Figure 65-8 Clipping film to hanger.

continued

continued from previous page
Procedure 74 *Manual Operating Procedures and Processing*

2 Place hanger into water bath and agitate up and down gently for at least 30 seconds.

3 Drain excess water from hanger into water bath.

Fixing

1 Place hanger with films into fixing solution; agitate gently up and down a few times.

2 Place hanger on the side of the tank, making certain that the films are below the level of the solution and not touching the wall of the tank or other films.

3 Close the lid and set the interval timer for 10 minutes or double the time of developer processing.

Washing

1 When timer rings, lift hanger and drain excess fixer from hanger into fixer solution.

2 Place hanger into water bath and allow circulating water to rinse films for a *minimum* of 20 minutes (more time is preferred).

Drying

1 Remove hanger from water bath and hold under cold tap water. Allow the water to run over films and clips.

2 Test the surface of the films by gently rubbing them while water runs between the thumb and forefinger. They should be free of any residual solution and feel clean to the touch. (At this time they may be dipped in Photo-Flo, ensuring that all films are immersed and shaken off to aid in more uniform drying, preventing possible water spots.)

3 Hang films up to dry, making certain the air is circulating and the fan is on.

4 Do not attempt to remove films from the hanger until they are *completely dry*.

5 When films are dry, remove them carefully from hanger and place them on a labeled mount.

6 Clean working surfaces and film hangers to remove solutions.

Automatic Processing

Automatic film processing is a technique that depends on the interrelation of mechanics, chemicals, and film. Automatic processors use a roller transport system to move the film through the developer, fixer, and wash and dry cycles. Special chemicals have been developed to meet the needs of this processing device (Figure 65-9).

In addition to very quickly developing and fixing the image on the film, the processing chemicals must prevent excessive swelling or a slippery or gummy emulsion and must allow the film to be rapidly washed and dried. Equally important is the use of a replenisher solution for chemicals.

Automatic processors may be loaded in a conventional darkroom using a safelight or can be loaded in the presence of white or daylight when a daylight loader is attached to the processor. Some makes require plumbing. An automatic processor *does* require an electrical source for the rollers and heater bar to function.

Manufacturers will recommend chemical solutions that are compatible with a particular model and brand

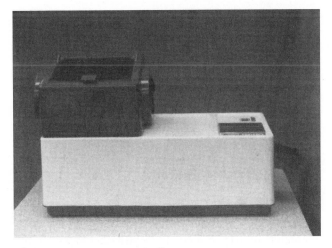

Figure 65-9 Automatic film processor.

name. The developer and fixer tanks have a capacity of 1 quart each, and the slightly larger wash tank contains 11/2 quarts.

Procedure 75 Preparing the Automatic Processor

Depending on the brand name and model, instructions for use may vary slightly; however, there are basic principles that apply to automatic processors (Figure 65–10):

1 Set the base of the unit on a level surface. Be sure the surface is stable, so chemicals do not splash or spill.

2 Remove the cover and note the three tanks.

3 Fill water tank to the recess level with room temperature distilled water.

4 Fill the developer tank with 1 quart of solution. Pour carefully to avoid splashing and contamination with the other tanks.

5 Fill the fixer tank with 1 quart of solution. Pour carefully to avoid splashing and contamination with other tanks.

6 Insert the transport (roller) system. Carefully lower into place. Be sure the transport sits squarely on the unit.

7 Place the cover and film receptacle.

8 Follow the instruction manual for processing films to obtain best-quality radiographs.

9 Use infection control measures when unwrapping contaminated film (see Chapter 64).

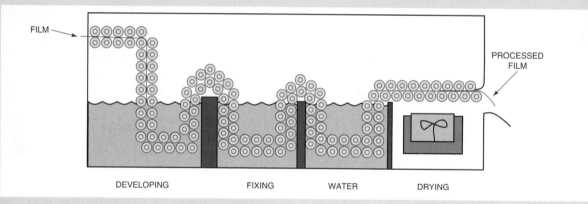

FILM

PROCESSED FILM

DEVELOPING   FIXING   WATER   DRYING

Figure 65–10 Schematic drawing of an automatic film processor.

Helpful Hints

● To minimize the possibility of deposits of chemical particles that may float in the wash tank, *water should be changed every day.*

● The chemical levels in the developer and fixer tanks should be checked daily and processing solutions replenished.

● A log of the number of films processed should be maintained as an accurate record. Chemicals should b e changed every 300–350 films or every two weeks, whichever is sooner. The calendar date of the most recent change should be placed in a conspicuous location and the entry updated when chemicals are changed.

● Manufacturer's instructions should be strictly followed for care and maintenance of an automatic processing unit.

Duplicating Radiographs

It is often necessary to duplicate radiographs to make them available to other practitioners or insurance companies. When a request is made to forward radiographs to another office, the original radiographs must never leave, but instead, a duplicate should be made and sent.

Duplicating film is available in a variety of sizes including periapical size (similar to a size 2 film), 5 x 12 inches (similar to panoramic film), and 8 x 10 inches (similar to a head plate film). To differentiate them from regular film, they have a notch on one side of the film. They are coated with emulsion only on one side, which appears dull, while the opposite side appears shiny.

A duplicator has a light source that affects the duplicating film when exposed to it. It has a diffuse glass top where the radiograph and duplicating film are placed, a timer that shuts off automatically when film has been exposed to the desired time, and a locking device that secures the radiograph and duplicating film in place.

Procedure 76 Duplicating Radiographs

Materials Needed

Duplicating film
Duplicator
Radiograph being duplicated
Rack to process the new film
GBX-2 safelight in darkroom

Instructions

1 The radiograph to be duplicated is placed directly above the light source, on the glass top or light screen. One must make certain that the right and left sides of the radiograph are adequately positioned or marked, as duplicating film does not have a dot to determine right from left. Be sure the duplicator light is turned off before placing the duplicating film.

2 The duplicating film is placed over the radiograph to be duplicated, with the "dull" side contacting the radiograph and the "shiny" side facing the operator. Placing the notched side of the duplicating film at the upper right side may be helpful in determining the correct side (Figure 65-11).

3 The lid is closed tightly to ensure that there is contact between radiograph and duplicating film;

otherwise, the duplicate will not have sharp detail—it will appear fuzzy.

4 The timer is set. If the timer is set for a shorter time, the duplicate will appear *darker* (more dense); however, if the timer is set for a longer time, the duplicate will appear *lighter*. Generally, the timing will depend on the duplicator machine used.

5 The new "duplicate" film will be processed using the same guidelines as for processing panoramic films.

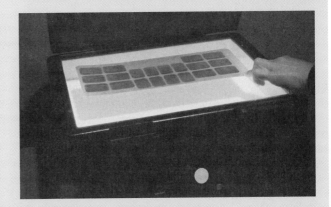

Figure 65-11 Loading duplicator.

Processing Errors

It has been stated that 90% of all errors taking place in radiography occur in the darkroom while processing films. Therefore, one must take every precaution to avoid making errors and use quality assurance techniques to produce diagnostic radiographs. Some of the most common processing errors are fogged radiographs, clear film, underdeveloped radiographs, low-level solutions, reticulation, spots on radiographs, artifact, and scratched raidographs.

Fogged Radiographs

The appearance of a fogged film is darker (dense) overall, without much contrast or detail. There are several reasons for fogged film. It may be due to excess chemical contact, warm solutions, white light/faulty safelight, or exposure to radiation.

1. If caused by chemicals, it was chemically fogged or "overdeveloped" and left in the developer for an extended period of time.

2. If caused by warm solutions, the developing time should have been shortened or temperature of solutions reduced.

3. If caused by white light or faulty safelight, it was exposed to light while processing in a darkroom with light leaks.

Correction

1. If films were chemically fogged, the timing in the developer was excessive, which may be due to a faulty interval timer. The timing for the developer is very critical and must be adhered to unconditionally according to the temperature of the solution.

2. If the solution was too warm, using the control valve to attain cooler water input should reduce water temperature.

3. If fogging was due to white-light exposure due to light leaks or a faulty safelight in the darkroom, the room needs to be inspected to see that it is light tight from white light and check that its safelight is not too bright.

Clear Film

The appearance of a clear film is a transparent film without an image.

1. It may be due to placing the film in the fixer initially, which removed all the silver halide crystals.

2. The films were left in the fixer or water for 24 hours or more, which caused the emulsion to fade or slide off the film base.

3. The film was processed never being exposed to radiation.

Correction

1. Solutions are tested by doing a quality assurance (QA) test to see that the fixer and developer were not switched. The operator should always be aware of their positions. However, this problem could happen to a novice who was not familiar with the darkroom.

2. Films should never be left in the fixer solution or water beyond the stated processing times.

3. One should not confuse exposed with unexposed film.

Underdeveloped Radiographs

The appearance of an underdeveloped radiograph is light with little density. It is apparent that not all the silver halide crystals were affected by the developer. It can be caused by weak or cold developer solution or diminished developing time.

Correction. A test should be done each day to ensure that solutions are not weak. The test should consist of using a step wedge film that is processed and compared to a reference radiograph for density. Moreover, solutions should be changed regularly. If the solutions are cold, adjusting the water temperature valves should warm them. Each time processing takes place, adequate time should be used based on the temperature of the developer solution and a time-temperature chart should be followed.

Low Level Solutions

The appearance on a radiograph processed in low-level solutions will be evidenced by a horizontal straight line at the superior border of the radiograph. It will affect the top radiographs on the film hanger (see Figure 64-4).

Correction. To avoid losing information on a radiograph that was not immersed fully in the solutions, a QA should be done on a daily basis. Solutions need to be replenished every day.

Reticulation

Reticulation on a radiograph appears as if it were cracked. This error takes place when there is a wide temperature difference between solutions and water. If the film was processed in an elevated temperature developer and then immersed suddenly in the cold water bath, the swollen emulsion shrinks and gives a wrinkled appearance.

Correction. Temperature differences between solutions and water should be avoided. If temperatures were elevated, it is wise to allow them to cool down prior to processing.

Spots on Radiographs

There are many types of spots that occur on radiographs:

1. Developer spots appear as dark spots that contaminated the film prior to processing.

2. Fixer spots appear as white spots that contaminated the film prior to processing.

3. White round spots are due to air bubbles that remained on the film while processing in the developer; the developer never reached the film.

4. Yellow stains appear on a radiograph due to improper rinsing or fixing. If due to improper rinsing, films were rushed through the water bath and were not fully rinsed. If due to improper fixing, the fixer may have been exhausted or films were not fixed for an adequate time.

Correction

1. To avoid developer spots, the counter top in the darkroom should be wiped clean of wet solutions or dry solution crystals. Cleanliness is of utmost importance.

2. To avoid fixer spots, the counter top in the darkroom should be wiped clean. Fixer has the ability to remove silver halide crystals, eliminating the image in that area. *Note:* If spots are detected immediately

upon removal from the fixer compartment due to contact with the wall or another film, they may be returned to the fixer and agitated for better fixer contact with film.

3. When round white spots appear on a radiograph, it is suspected that films were not agitated to break surface tension when first inserted into the developer. Therefore, films must be agitated when inserted into any compartment.

4. As films are being processed, one cannot impose "shortcuts." If fixing time is set for 10 minutes, it must be for 10 minutes, or if final washing is set for 20 minutes, it must be for 20 minutes; otherwise, radiographs will discolor and turn brown in time. One must realize that radiographs are used as legal documents and should be handled with extreme care.

Artifacts

Any image that appears on a radiograph that was not intended to be there is known as an **artifact**. There are many types of artifacts:

1. Static electricity appears as thin black lines in the shape of a tree branch, caused by a spark of light while opening a film packet rapidly.

2. Fingernail marking appears as a dark crescent-shaped marking caused by bruising the emulsion during improper handling of film.

3. Fingerprint marking appear as a dark fingerprint caused by handling film on the flat portion as opposed to only handling the edges.

4. Fluoride, if it is stannous, produces black marks on the radiograph where contacted. If the operator's hands are contaminated by stannous fluoride, it may be transferred to the film while processing.

5. Light leak in the film packet will cause a dark artifact to appear. If there is a pin hole or a tear in a film packet, light leakage will occur that will affect the film.

Correction

1. Static electricity usually takes place when the air is dry, while walking on a nylon carpet, or by rapid movement. When unwrapping film, especially panoramic, it is best to do it slowly to avoid possible static electricity.

2. Fingernail markings should be avoided by handling film by the edges with extreme care and by keeping fingernails short.

3. Fingerprints can be avoided by handling film by the edges only, taking extreme care not to touch the center of the film with fingerprints.

4. Fluoride, particularly stannous, contamination should be avoided by using a new pair of gloves or washing hands with soap and acid such as vinegar or lemon juice prior to handling film and not exposing someone who has just undergone a fluoride treatment.

5. Light leak on film should be eliminated by checking every film prior to exposure. If a film looks defective or if damaged by a film holder, it should not be used.

Scratched Radiographs

When radiographs are scratched, white lines appear and part of the image is missing due to removal of emulsion. This condition is due to overcrowded conditions in the processing tanks where other racks, when moved, affected films in this manner.

Correction. To prevent scratched films, it is necessary to take extreme care not to make contact with other racks that are already in the solutions. It is also advisable to remove racks that have been fixed and washed sufficiently and not expose them to secondary problems.

SUGGESTED ACTIVITIES

- Using two outdated films, expose one to white light and bend one corner of both films and practice processing them manually in the darkroom. Determine the results. Which one was black, and did it have an artifact on the corner? Which one was clear except for an artifact on the corner?

- Practice filling the three tanks before the electrical source is plugged in. Then, in the automatic processor, practice processing a double-film packet that has been exposed on a mannequin or skull:

  1. Mount one of these radiographs in the corner of a view box and retain it as a standard reference radiograph.

  2. Periodically, place another radiograph next to the standard reference radiograph.

  3. Compare the density and contrast of the two radiographs. Is there a difference? *Note:* Be sure both radiographs used for comparison were exposed using the identical technique factors.

- Using a full-mouth mounted set of radiographs, duplicating film, a labeled rack, and adequate safelight (GBX-2), make a duplicate set of radiographs.

REVIEW

1. What is the main function of the developer?
   a. To soften the gelatin of the emulsion
   b. To bring out the latent image
   c. To harden the emulsion
   d. To act as a preservative

2. What is the main function of the fixer?
   a. To remove the undeveloped silver halide crystals
   b. To increase action of silver halide crystals
   c. To soften the emulsion
   d. To produce density and contrast

3. Match the developer chemicals on the left with their purpose on the right:
   ___ a. Hydroquinone
   ___ b. Elon
   ___ c. Sodium carbonate
   ___ d. Sodium sulfite
   ___ e. Potassium bromide

   1. A preservative that prevents oxidation and prolongs solution life
   2. Converts exposed silver halide crystals to black metallic silver
   3. Prevents too rapid development and fogging of unexposed crystals
   4. Works quickly to bring the image gaining density slowly
   5. Softens the gelatin to promote developing to take place

4. Match the fixer chemicals on the left with their purpose on the right:
   ___ a. Sodium thiosulfate
   ___ b. Sodium sulfite
   ___ c. Acetic acid
   ___ d. Potassium alum

   1. Prevents deterioration of sodium thiosulfate
   2. Hardens and shrinks gelatin
   3. Removes unexposed silver halide crystals not affected by developer
   4. Maintains acidity and neutralizes alkaline developer

5. What is the optimum temperature and time for manual processing in the developer?
   a. 65°F and 4 minutes
   b. 68°F and 5 minutes
   c. 75°F and 7 minutes
   d. 78°F and 8 minutes

6. When duplicating films, the radiograph is placed:
   a. Over the duplicating film
   b. Under the duplicating film
   c. So that dull side of duplicating film is contacting the radiograph
   d. So that shiny side of duplicating film is contacting the radiograph
   e. Both b and c

7. Match the processing errors on the left with possible cause(s) on the right:
   ___ a. Fogged
   ___ b. Clear
   ___ c. Underdeveloped
   ___ d. Reticulation
   ___ e. Artifacts
   ___ f. Scratched
   ___ g. Spots

   1. Sudden temperature change between solutions
   2. Film placed in fixer before developer
   3. Air bubbles preventing developer to reach film while processing
   4. Faulty safelight or light leakage
   5. Weak or cold developer solution
   6. Spark of light caused by static electricity while opening film packet
   7. Overcrowding of racks in processing tank

Intraoral Radiography

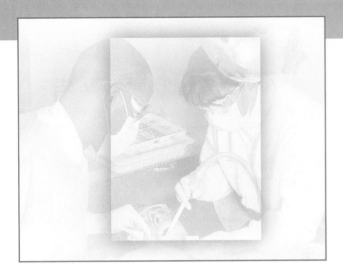

- Determine the proper position of the film, PID, and paralleling instruments for the anterior film exposures.
- Determine the proper position of the film, PID, and paralleling instruments for each posterior quadrant of the oral cavity.
- Determine the angle of projection of the central ray for occlusal radiographs.

Introduction

Generally, a complete dental radiographic examination, in addition to the periapical radiographs, includes **bite wings** (interproximal radiographs of the bicuspids and molars). It is not always necessary to include bite-wing interproximal radiographs of the incisor and cuspid regions.

Certain areas of the teeth cannot be examined except by radiographs. Cavities may invade the tooth pulp before being discovered by visual examination or periapical radiographs. However, when interproximal radiographs are used, the carious area becomes clearly visible and can be restored before the pulp becomes involved.

Bisected angle and paralleling are two techniques used to make intraoral periapical radiographs. Each technique employs corresponding bite blocks that give adequate results.

The occlusal technique bears its name because the film is placed on the occlusal plane for exposure and is used to show a topographic large area of each arch.

Interproximal Bite Wings

Purpose

The interproximal or bite-wing examination serves to reveal the presence of interproximal caries, pulp changes (abnormal or otherwise), overhanging restorations, improperly fitted restorative crowns, recurrent caries beneath restorations, and resorption of alveolar bone. It is superior to the periapical examination in certain respects for two reasons:

1. The film surface is placed parallel to the long axes of the crowns of the teeth. The x-rays pass through the teeth at nearly a 90° angle, which results in more accurate images of structures (Figures 66-1 and 66-2).

OBJECTIVES

After studying this chapter, the student will be able to:

- Prepare a set of four film packets for a bite-wing survey.
- Explain how to position the x-ray tubehead and PID for premolar and molar interproximal bite-wing exposures.
- Demonstrate the complete procedure for completing a bite-wing survey, using a manikin, then a patient.
- Describe the basic principle used in the bisected-angle technique.
- Demonstrate correct collimator or positioning device and film placement for the maxillary and mandibular arch using the Rinn Eezee-Grip holder.
- Assemble the Rinn bisecting-angle components for anterior and posterior film placement.
- Demonstrate correct film and position-indicating device (PID) placement for each region of the oral cavity.
- Compare the bisecting-angle technique with the paralleling technique.
- Determine the proper film placement and angulation of the central ray for various areas of the oral cavity, using the paralleling technique.
- State the principles used as a basis for the Rinn extension cone paralleling (XCP) technique, using a 12- or 16-in. PID.
- Discuss four advantages of the XCP technique.
- Assemble the components of the Rinn XCP instruments.

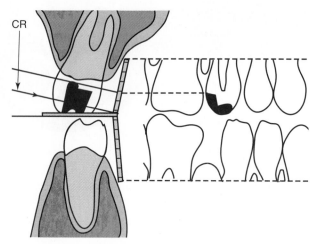

Figure 66-1 Angle of projection of central ray in a premolar bite-wing radiograph.

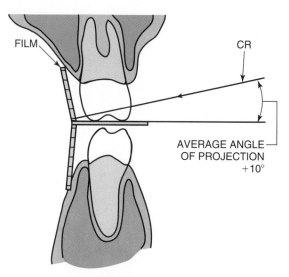

Figure 66-2 Angle of projection of central ray for a molar bite-wing radiograph.

2. Images of the coronal and cervical portions of both the maxillary and mandibular teeth and the alveolar borders of the region are recorded on the same film.

The bite-wing film should provide the most accurate representation of the anatomical structure present. Consideration of the vertical and horizontal angulations is of extreme importance. There should be no overlapping of the interproximal areas of the teeth. When this occurs, the film should be retaken as it is not useful for diagnosis.

Interproximal film for posterior bite-wing exposures is supplied with a tab that extends across the middle of the long aspect or horizontal portion of the exposure side of the film packet. Anterior interproximal film (vertical bite wing) has a tab that extends across the short aspect or vertical portion of the exposure side of the film packet.

Periapical film may be used for making interproximal radiographs. When preferred, special tab loops or adhesive tabs are placed on the film. In the mouth, the tab extends from the film packet between the teeth of the maxillary and mandibular occlusal or incisive surfaces. The film is held in place by having the patient close his or her teeth firmly on the tab.

Vertical angulation is the alignment of the central ray using an up-and-down motion to position the PID (tubehead cone) at a positive (+) directing the ray downward or negative (-) angulation directing the ray upward. This controls elongation or foreshortening.

Horizontal angulation is the alignment of the central ray using a horizontal movement to position the PID at a mesial or distal angulation. This controls open or closed interproximals.

Procedure 77 Bite-Wing Technique

Materials Needed

Patient's chart
Basic setup
Tab film loops or adhesive tabs
Required number of film
Position-indicating device (PID)
Paper cup (with patient's identification)
Facial tissues
Gauze squares, 2 x 2 in.
Cotton rolls

Petroleum jelly
Exam gloves

Preliminary Considerations

Whenever exposing film on patients, it is assumed that the operator has completed disinfection, placed infection control barriers on the x-ray equipment, and will be using disposable or sterile film placement accessories.

continued

continued from previous page
Procedure 77 Bite-Wing Technique

The operator is attired in a disposable or washable gown, wearing protective eyewear, face mask, and exam gloves.

The patient chart should be available for recording the date, prescription, number of films exposed, total kilovolt peak (kVp), milliamperes (mA), and total x-ray exposures. A prescription for radiographs should always be kept with the patient's records.

Instructions

Preparing the Film

1 Wash and dry your hands.
2 Prepare the film.
   a. Select four #2 films.
   b. If you are affixing the tab or loop, assemble all films, making certain the tab is located on the tube side of the film. In placing the loop, allow your index finger to direct the film through the loop. By exerting slight pressure on the film edges, with your thumb and forefinger, the film now has a slight convex shape and will slide easily into the loop (Figure 66-3).
   c. Soften the four corners of each film by gently rolling them from the tube side toward the lingual side between the ball of your thumb and forefinger (Figure 66-4). Do not crease the corners or you will damage the emulsion as well as the seal of the packet, resulting in

artifacts on the processed film. Place prepared films into a lead-lined storage receptacle.
   d. Prepare for placement. Always position the dot on the film toward the sagittal plane (midline) of the patient. It will appear on the lower corner for the right (Figure 66-5) and the upper for the left (Figure 66-6).
   c. Before positioning film, slide the tab back (distally) for the premolar exposure. For the molar exposure, slide the tab forward (mesially). This will position the tab on the mandibular first molar for either exposure. Figure 66-7 shows four bite-wing films with loops and tabs in position.

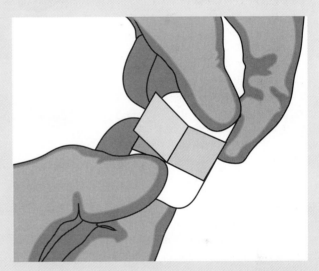

Figure 66-4 Softening the corners of the film.

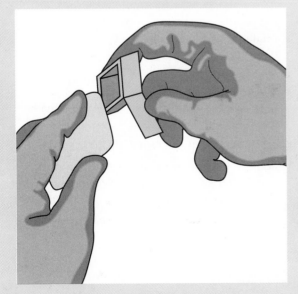

Figure 66-3 Placing the film loop.

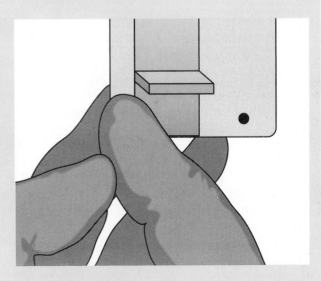

Figure 66-5 Position of dot, right side.

continued

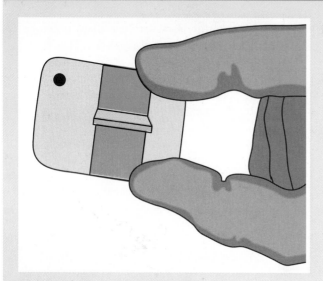

Figure 66-6 Position of dot, left side.

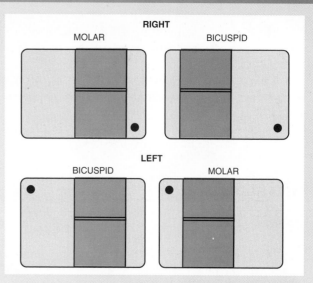

Figure 66-7 Films with tab / dot in position. (A) For bicuspid (premolar) film, place so that more of the film is *forward of tab*. (B) For molar film, place so that more of the film is *back of tab*. (C) Tab will be placed over *mandibular first molar* for both bicuspid (premolar) and molar films.

Preparing and Positioning the Patient

1 Check the x-ray control panel: master switch on, kVp, mA, and electronic timer.

2 Assemble all necessary equipment: film, paper cup with patient information, and basic setup before the patient is seated.

3 Seat the patient upright in the chair with the head firmly positioned in the headrest.

4 Place the lead apron and protective thyroid collar; refer to Figure 62-1.

5 Place the dental napkin, with an additional facial tissue folded and secured under one clip of the neck chain.

6 Thoroughly wash your hands with germicidal soap and water. Rinse and dry. Don disposable exam gloves.

7 Ask the patient to remove removable appliances and eyeglasses, if any. Place these items in a safe place, preferably within the patient's view. Direct patient to remove lipstick; offer a tissue. Ask the patient to remove drop earrings if they interfere with the procedure.

8 Lubricate the corners of the mouth using a small amount of petroleum jelly on the tip of a cotton roll.

9 Using the mouth mirror and a gauze square, examine the mouth. The gauze square will aid in moving and lifting the tongue.

10 Move the x-ray tubehead to the side (area) of the patient being surveyed.

11 To open the contact areas and interproximals, observe the occlusal surfaces of the teeth. Retract the cheek while standing at the side of the patient, positioning yourself with your eyes on the same plane as the x-ray beam will be directed to. Often, teeth may be rotated or positioned out of normal occlusal alignment.

12 Move the PID into position near the patient's face; adjust the vertical and horizontal angulations. Make the exposure.

13 Move the PID away from the patient's face.

14 Remove the film from the patient's mouth and wipe it free of moisture (saliva) using the folded and secured facial tissue or dental napkin.

15 Drop exposed film into the prepared paper cup; store behind the leaded protective shield until films are processed.

16 Repeat steps 10–15 until all prescribed films have been exposed.

continued

Positioning the Bite-wing Film

1 Select a prepared film from the lead-lined storage box. It is good practice to begin with a premolar exposure, then proceed to the molar area. *Note:* For patient comfort, a moistened 2 X 2 in. gauze square or cushions already fabricated for this purpose may be placed on the portion of the film touching the floor of the mouth to cushion the soft tissues. Grasp the film with the middle and index fingers of one hand (Figure 66-8).

2 With the opposite hand, retract the patient's cheek using the index finger (Figure 66-9).

3 Carry the film into the mouth in a horizontal position, over the tongue, and gently bring the film into a vertical position as it is placed in the sulcus between the tongue and teeth. With the cheek retracted, bring the tab to rest on the mandibular first molar (Figure 66-10 for bicuspid and Figure 66-11 for molar).

4 As soon as the packet is in proper position that includes the distal of the mandibular cuspid, the operator positions the index (retraction) finger to stabilize the film by pressing against the tab on the occlusal surface of the mandibular first molar.

5 To avoid impingement into the soft tissues in the floor of the mouth, and while continuing to retain the positioned film, gently shift the anterior corner of the packet toward the tongue. By positioning the film toward the tongue, it provides more vertical space, preventing the film to

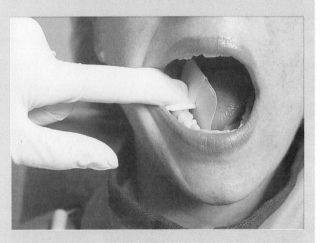

Figure 66-10 Premolar (bicuspid) placement. Anterior portion of film should include distal portion of cuspid (canine).

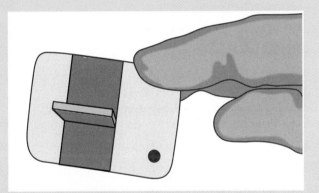

Figure 66-8 Finger grasp of film.

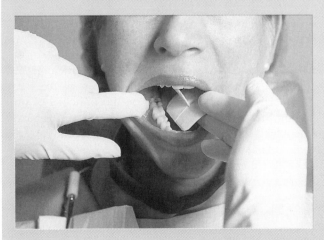

Figure 66-9 Film in horizontal position as it is introduced in the mouth.

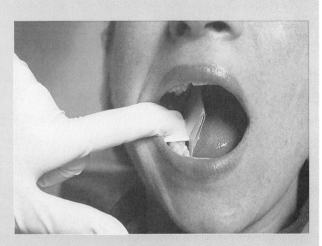

Figure 66-11 Molar placement. Anterior portion of film should cover the distal portion of second premolar.

continued

continued from previous page
Procedure 77 Bite-Wing Technique

be driven into the floor of the mouth, resulting in unnecessary pain for the patient and an inferior quality radiograph.

6 Ask the patient to *slowly* close on the tab. As the maxillary teeth begin to contact the operator's index finger, the finger is rolled toward the patient's cheek, thus permitting the patient to close on the tab. This places the film half lingually covering the maxillary teeth and half lingually covering the mandibular teeth. The tab should be seen facially when the cheek is retracted.

7 Position the PID, and adjust vertical and horizontal angulations.

8 Make any final adjustments of the patient's head.

9 As a general rule, direct patients to close their eyes during each film exposure to diminish exposure of these sensitive tissues to x-radiation.

10 Direct the patient to temporarily not move during the film exposure to avoid a blurred image on the radiograph.

11 Step behind the leaded shield. Make the exposure.

12 Remove the film from the patient's mouth and wipe it free of moisture (saliva).

13 Drop exposed film in the prepared paper cup and store behind the leaded shield.

Premolar Bite Wings

● Follow procedural steps for positioning the film, 1–13.

● Position the PID using +5° vertical angulation. Direct the horizontal angulation on the bite-wing tab toward the center of the film, *between* the premolars, and toward the occlusal plane. This angulation will prevent a **cone cut** (improper positioning of the PID rendering a radiograph with an unexposed area) on the processed film (see Figure 66-10). This projection provides an interproximal image starting with the distal area of the cuspid, the contacts of the premolars, and the first and second molars on the processed film.

Molar Bite Wings

● Follow procedural Steps 1–13.

● Position the PID using a +10° vertical angulation. Direct the horizontal angulation on the bite-wing tab toward the center of the film, between the contacts of the first and second molars, or at right angles to the linguals of molars and toward the occlusal plane; see Fig. 66-11. This projection provides an interproximal image of the distal area of the second premolar, the contacts of all dental molars, plus some of the tuberosity and retromolar area.

Finishing Up

When all interproximal prescribed film exposures have been completed:

● Process the films prior to dismissing the patient.

● If all radiographs are acceptable, return the patient's belongings and dismiss the patient.

● Remove all barriers, clean and disinfect the x-ray equipment, and sterilize accessories.

Bisected-Angle Technique

Principles of the Bisected-Angle Technique

The term **bisected-angle** technique describes a method followed for determining the angulation of the x-ray beam. The technique is based on the principle of projecting the x-ray beam at right angles to an imaginary line which **bisects** (cuts in half) the angle formed by the longitudinal axis of the tooth and the plane of the film packet. This commonly used technique is based on a geometric principle, **Ciezynski's rule of isometry** (the normal ray is directed perpendicularly to a plane which lies midway between the plane or long axis of the teeth desired and the plane of the film). Vertical angulation of the central ray is based on this principle (Figure 66-12).

The correct angle of projection for the maxillary central area is shown in Figure 66-13. If the ray is direct-

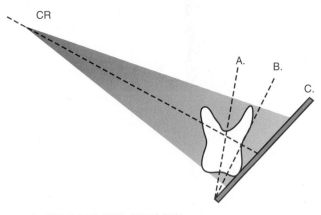

A. LONGITUDINAL AXIS OF TOOTH
B. IMAGINARY BISECTING LINE
C. PLANE OF FILM
CR CENTRAL RAY

Figure 66-12 Angulation of the central ray.

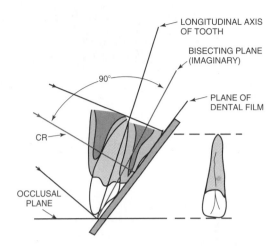

Figure 66-13 Correct vertical angle (90°) for projection of central ray (CR).

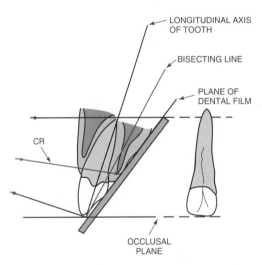

Figure 66-14 Incorrect vertical angle that produces an elongated image.

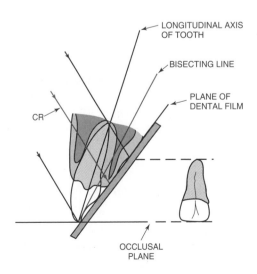

Figure 66-15 Incorrect vertical angle that produces a foreshortened image.

ed at right angles to the long axis of the teeth, the image in the resultant radiograph will appear **elongated** (images of teeth appear longer than the actual teeth due to insufficient vertical angulation), as shown in Figure 66-14. If the ray is directed at right angles to the plane of the dental film, the resultant image will appear **foreshortened** (images of teeth appear shorter than the actual teeth due to excessive vertical angulation), as in Figure 66-15. Because it is difficult to determine accurately the position of the bisecting plane, the technique relies heavily on the experience of the operator. To say the least, it is difficult to master the technique. Even the most proficient operator must use approximate angles based on head position. At best, the bisected-angle angulation technique lacks some accuracy and consistency.

When a high vault of the maxilla causes the packet to assume a more vertical position, the vertical angle should be decreased about 5°. When a low vault causes the packet to be less vertical in position, the vertical angle should be increased about 5°. In the mandibular region, the vertical angle is increased 5° when the teeth are inclined or the floor of the mouth is shallow; it is decreased 5° when the teeth are more vertical or the floor of the mouth is deep.

For the edentulous (without teeth) patient, the film must be placed more nearly horizontal than for the average dentulous mouth. Angulation is increased 5–10° more. When surveying the maxillary teeth on children, the angle must be increased 5–10° because the arch is not fully developed and the film packet is difficult to adapt properly.

Projection of the Central Ray at a Horizontal Angle. The horizontal angulation is determined by directing the central ray through the interproximal

INCORRECT   CORRECT

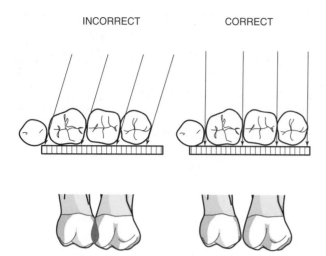

Figure 66-16 Horizontal angle.

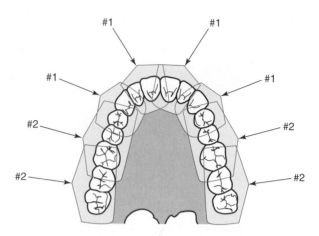

Figure 66-17 Maxillary arch showing correct film position and projection of the x-ray beam for each periapical radiograph of the teeth. Size #1 film used on anterior teeth and size #2 film on posterior teeth.

spaces (between the teeth) without overlapping adjacent teeth. Examples of correct and incorrect horizontal projections are illustrated in Figure 66-16.

Both the vertical and horizontal angulations are dependent on specific head positioning of the patient and correct film placement for success with the bisected-angle technique. Dimensional distortion is an inherent characteristic of this technique.

Size and Number of Films. As the form of the dental arch is studied, it becomes obvious that variation of width and depth can be noted. Using a 19- or 20-film full-mouth survey is now becoming a more common practice. This particular arrangement produces better end results, although it uses a greater number of films. The film placement shown in Figure 66-17 will be used as a guide, producing eight maxillary periapical films and either seven or eight mandibular periapical films plus four bite-wing radiographs to complete the survey. Depending on the width of the mandibular central to cuspid region, two central-lateral and two cuspid films may be taken. This type of survey uses two sizes of film; the #2 (standard) size is used in the posterior regions and for bite-wings and the #1 (narrow) for the anterior survey.

The #I (narrow) size film used for the anterior exposures permits a greater degree of patient comfort and lesser tendency for the film to bend and produce distortion. Since each #1 film will cover two or three teeth and their related interproximals, the placement of the PID for the anterior radiograph becomes less complicated than with the use of three #2 films for anterior projections.

Rinn Bisected-Angle Instruments

The Rinn bisecting-angle instruments (BAIs) are designed to reduce to a minimum some of the variables of angulation, specific head positioning, and dimension-

al distortion. These inherent characteristics of the bisected-angle technique may be reduced by:

1. Automatically indicating the correct horizontal and vertical angulation, thus eliminating the need for numerically setting the angulation and for placing the patient's head in a predetermined position.

2. Simplifying the technique, making it easy to master and teach

3. Standardizing the technique, making accurate duplication of postoperative radiographs the same as the preoperative

4. Minimizing curved film plane distortion (Chapter 69)

5. Eliminating cone cutting (Chapter 69).

Rinn BAI Instrument Components

Bite Blocks. designed to hold all sizes and brands of periapical x-ray film. The BAI bite blocks differ for anterior and posterior (Figure 66-18).

Aiming Rings. Plastic rings used to bring the film "on target." Aiming rings for anterior and posterior films differ (Figure 66-19).

Indicator Rods (Arms). Two-pronged rod used by inserting into openings (holes) on the bite block. Anterior and posterior aiming rods differ (Figure 66-20).

Assembly Instructions. The same procedure for assembly of the BAI components is followed for all instrumentation (Figure 66-21). However, prongs of the posterior rod should be positioned in the openings on the left side of the bite block for left maxillary and right mandibular placement. This is accomplished by inverting

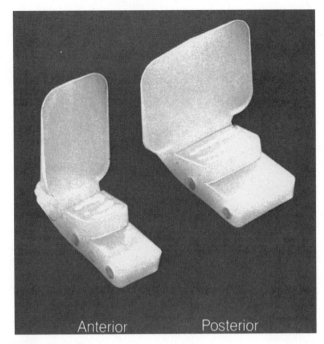

Figure 66-18 BAI bite blocks. (Courtesy of Rinn Corporation, Elgin, IL.)

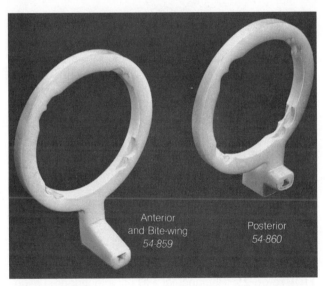

Figure 66-19 Rinn aiming rings. (Courtesy of Rinn Corporation, Elgin, IL.)

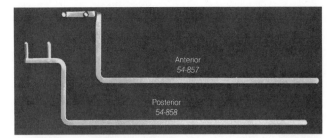

Figure 66-20 Rinn indicator rods (arms). (Courtesy of Rinn Corporation, Elgin, IL.)

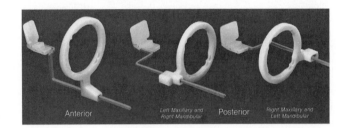

Figure 66-21 Rinn BAI components properly assembled. (Courtesy of Rinn Corporation, Elgin, IL.)

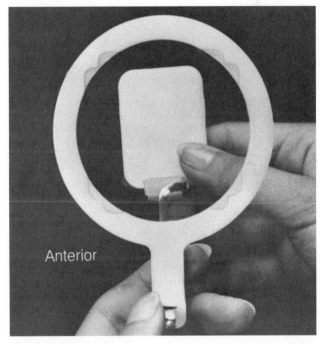

Figure 66-22 Anterior instrument is correctly assembled with film on target.

the assembled components. Position the prongs in the right side of the bite block for right maxillary and left mandibular projections. Assembled components must be inverted.

The angled portion of the indicator rod must be positioned away from the biting surfaces of the bite block:

1. Two prongs of the indicator rod are inserted into holes in the bite block.
2. Indicator rod is inserted into aiming ring slot.

3. Backing plate of bite block is fixed to open film slot for easy insertion of film packet, ensuring the film packet is inserted completely into the slot, with the dot in the slot.

4. Instrument is correctly assembled when film can be seen through aiming ring "on target" (Figures 66–22 and 66–23).

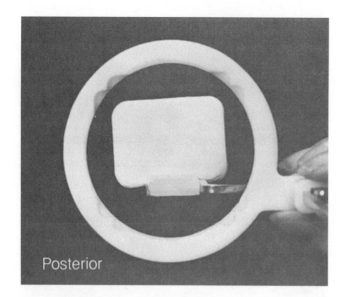

Figure 66-23 Posterior instrument is correctly assembled with film on target.

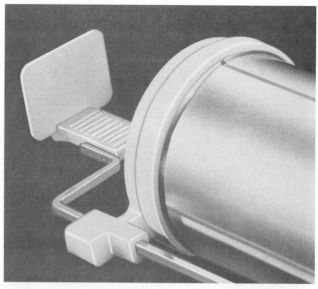

Figure 66-24 Round PIDs are set flush with and centered on the aiming ring. Shown with XCP bite block. (Courtesy of Rinn Corporation, Elgin, IL.)

5. The PID is placed. When using the round PID, it is set flush and centered on the aiming ring. The arm of the indicator rod should run parallel with the PID (Figure 66-24). The rectangular PID fits into indented guides on the aiming ring for anterior and posterior films. These guides are provided for vertical and horizontal placement (Figure 66-25).

Instrument Placement Instructions

See Table 66–1.

Anterior Region (General Instructions)

1. Assemble anterior instrument (see Figures 66–21 and 66–22) and insert film packet vertically into anterior bite block, pushing film packet all the way into slot. Plain side of film packet should be positioned away from backing plate toward the aiming ring. Narrow #1 film is used. When using #2 films, slightly soften the corners of film packet to facilitate positioning.

2. *For maxillary anterior teeth.* With bite block placed on incisal edges of maxillary teeth to be radiographed and film positioned as close as possible to the lingual surfaces of teeth, instruct patient to protrude lower jaw and close slowly, but firmly, to retain position of film packet. A cotton roll may be placed between mandibular teeth and bite block for patient comfort (Figure 66-26).

For mandibular anterior teeth. With bite block placed on incisal edges of mandibular teeth and film positioned as close as possible to the lingual surfaces

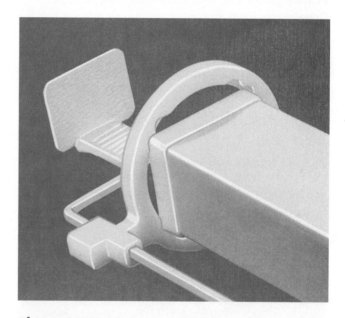

Figure 66-25 Rectangular PIDs fit into indented alignment guides on the anterior and posterior aiming rings. Shown with XCP bite block. (Courtesy of Rinn Corporation, Elgin, IL.)

of teeth, instruct patient to close slowly, but firmly, to retain position of film packet. A cotton roll may be placed between maxillary teeth and bite block for patient comfort (Figure 66-27).

3. Slide aiming ring down the indicator rod to skin surface, and center the PID of the x-ray unit in close approximation to aiming ring.

4. Press x-ray machine activating button and make exposure.

Table 66-1 Periapical Film Placement Technique

Teeth to be Radiographed	Placement of Film	Film Should Include the Following Teeth
Maxillary central and laterals	Center # 1 film on central and lateral.	Central, lateral, portion of cuspid and opposing central
Maxillary cuspid	Center #1 film on cuspid.	Cuspid in center, lateral, and first bicuspid
Maxillary bicuspids	Place anterior of #2 film to include the cuspid.	Cuspid, first and second bicuspids, first and second molars
Maxillary molars	Place anterior of #2 film to include distal of second bicuspid.	Distal of second bicuspid, first, second, and third molars
Mandibular central and laterals	Center #1 film on central and lateral.	Central, lateral, cuspid, and opposing central
Mandibular cuspid	Center #1 film on cuspid.	Cuspid in center, lateral and first bicuspid
Mandibular bicuspids	Place anterior of #2 film to include distal of mandibular cuspid.	Distal of cuspid, first and second bicuspids, first, second molars
Mandibular molars	Place anterior of #2 film to include distal of mandibular second bicuspid.	Distal of second bicuspid, first, second, and third molars

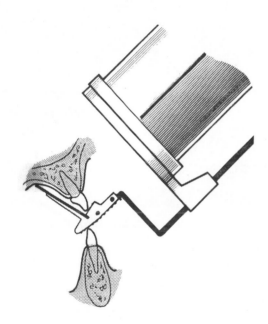

Figure 66-26 Maxillary anterior teeth. (Courtesy of Rinn Corporation, Elgin, IL.)

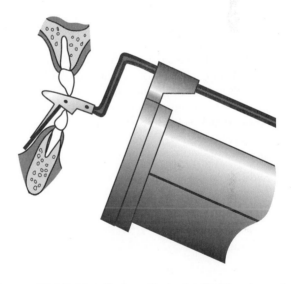

Figure 66-27 Mandibular anterior teeth. (Courtesy of Rinn Corporation, Elgin, IL.)

Posterior Region (General Instructions)

1. Assemble posterior instrument (see Figures 66-21 and 66-23) and insert #2 film packet horizontally into posterior bite block, pushing film packet all the way into slot. Plain side of film packet should be positioned away from backing plate toward the aim-

ing ring. Slightly roll upper anterior corner of film packet to facilitate positioning.

2. *For maxillary posterior teeth.* With bite block positioned on the occlusal surfaces of the maxillary teeth to be radiographed, position film as close as possible to lingual surfaces of teeth and instruct patient to close slowly, but firmly, to retain position of film packet. A cotton roll may be placed between mandibular teeth and bite block for patient comfort (Figure 66-28).

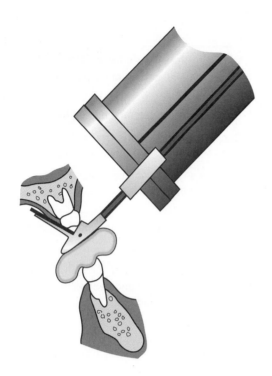

Figure 66-28 Maxillary posterior teeth. (Courtesy of Rinn Corporation, Elgin, IL.)

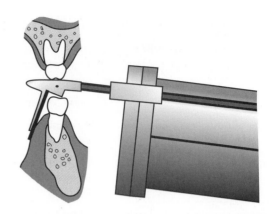

Figure 66-29 Mandibular posterior teeth. (Courtesy of Rinn Corporation, Elgin, IL.)

For mandibular posterior teeth. With bite block placed on occlusal surfaces of mandibular teeth to be radiographed, position film as close as possible to lingual surfaces of teeth and instruct patient to close slowly, but firmly, to retain position of film. A cotton roll may be placed between maxillary teeth and bite block for patient comfort (Figure 66-29).

3. Slide aiming ring down the indicator rod to skin surface and center the PID of the x-ray unit in close approximation to aiming ring.

4. Press x-ray machine activating button and make exposure.

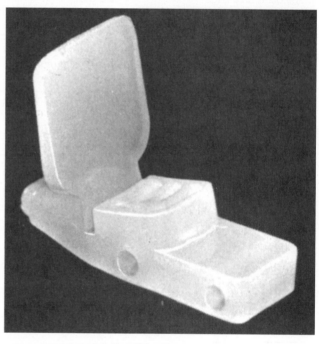

Figure 66-30 BAI anterior bite block (child). (Courtesy of Rinn Corporation, Elgin, IL.)

Radiographic Techique for the Child Patient (BAI)

The full-mouth survey for children is possible with a maximum of six to eight films. As with the adult patient, exposure should be kept to a minimum, under strict adherence to the ALARA (as low as reasonably achievable) concept (Chapter 61).

A #0 film is placed in the child's mouth with a plastic holder. The anterior bite block is reduced in size from that used for adults to accommodate a vertically positioned film. The backing plate is cut down to a level slightly lower than the height of the film. The length of the bite block biting surface remains the same as that used in the conventional technique, as do the aiming rings and indicator rods (arms).

Anterior Region

1. The anterior instrument is assembled (see Figures 66–21 and 66–22) and a #0 film packet inserted vertically into anterior bite block (Figure 66-30).

2. Steps 1–4 of the incisor region and conventional BAI technique are followed.

3. The exposure chart is checked before activating the exposure button. A child's tissue is less dense, and thus the exposure time will be less than for an adult.

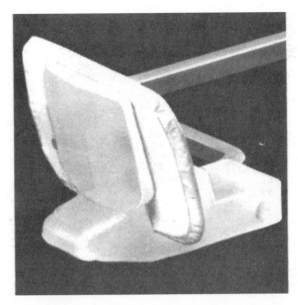

Figure 66-31 Posterior bite block (child). (Courtesy of Rinn Corporation, Elgin, IL.)

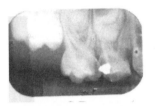 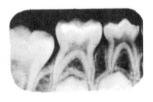

Figure 66-33 Posterior films (child). (Courtesy of Rinn Corporation, Elgin, IL.)

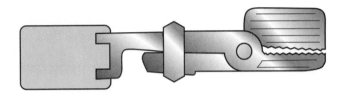

Figure 66-34 Film in position in Eezee-grip holder for anterior areas. (Courtesy of Rinn Corporation, Elgin, IL.)

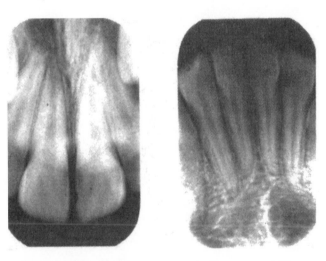

Figure 66-32 Incisor films (child). (Courtesy of Rinn Corporation, Elgin, IL.)

Rinn Eezee-Grip (Snap-A-Ray) Film Holder

Use of a film holder will help to place and stabilize the dental film as it is placed in the mouth. The Rinn Eezee-Grip (Snap-A-Ray), a bisecting-angle technique, can be used if you prefer to do your own angle bisecting. It is often used for selected single exposures.

The horizontal angulation is determined by directing the central ray at right angles to the tooth and film. The x-ray beam must be aimed through the interproximal spaces to avoid overlapping of tooth structures.

Both angulations depend on specific head positioning of the patient and correct film placement for successful performance of this technique. The Rinn Eezee-Grip is rather versatile as long as the limitations of the procedure are understood.

Posterior Region

1. The posterior instrument is assembled (see Figures 66-21 and 66-23) and a #0 film is inserted horizontally into posterior bite block (Figure 66-31).

2. Steps 1–4 of the posterior region and BAI technique are followed.

3. Exposure time is checked. Activating button is pressed and exposure made.

Note: Typical exposures for children are shown in Figures 66–32 and 66–33.

Parts of the Holder

The Rinn Eezee-Grip holder has a pronged end, which is used for anterior maxillary and mandibular projections (Figure 66-34). On the opposite end is a biting surface with a narrow and a wide jaw and a sliding friction ring that serves to lock the film in position. These biting surfaces are used for maxillary and mandibular posterior projections (Figure 66-35). The narrow jaw is most generally used for mandibular posteriors. The wide jaw is generally used with maxillary posteriors.

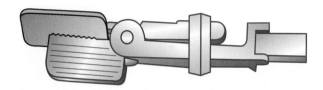

Figure 66-35 Film in position in Eezee-grip holder for most posterior areas. (Courtesy of Rinn Corporation, Elgin, IL.)

Preliminary Considerations

It is advisable to start with the maxillary incisor area, then proceed to the posteriors. The tubehead or PID for vertical and horizontal angulation should be adjusted, keeping the end of the collimator or PID and tubehead parallel with the film. The PID is placed close to but not touching the patient's face; this will ensure proper density and contrast for each film; refer to Chapter 69.

Head Positions for Proper Angulation. For maxillary periapical, interproximal, and maxillary occlusal examinations, the patient's head should be positioned in the headrest, so that the sagittal plane (the vertical line through the long axis of the body dividing it into right and left sides) is in a vertical position (Figure 66-36). An imaginary line from the tragus of the ear (the cartilaginous projection in front of the external auditory meatus) (external auditory meatus is the external opening of the ear) to the ala of the nose (the wing-like structure on the side of the nostril) should be horizontal (Figure 66-37). The plane of the occlusal surfaces of the maxillary teeth will then be approximately horizontal.

For the mandibular periapical examination, the headrest should be lowered until a line from the tragus to the corner of the mouth is horizontal (see Figure 66-37). The plane of the occlusal surfaces of the mandibular teeth will then be approximately horizontal when the mouth is open (as required during the exposure). In mandibular occlusal radiography, the head position is altered to suit the desired exposure.

In each instance, the horizontal, or occlusal, plane is considered to be at 0° angulation. Any line or plane intersecting the horizontal plane from above will be at a plus-degree angle to it; any line or plane intersecting it from below will be at a minus-degree angle to it. The angles for the beam of radiation in the procedures are designated as +° or -°.

Film Placement Using Rinn EEZEE-Grip Holder

Film Position for Anterior Exposures

a. Number 1 or 2 film is placed vertically in mouth.

b. The corners of the film are softened between thumb and forefinger. Film is placed in the pronged end of

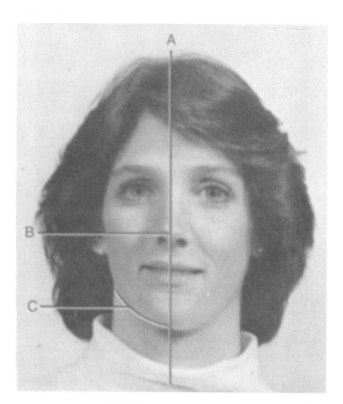

Figure 66-36 Planes for proper angulation: (A) sagittal plane; (B) tip of nose to tragus of ear; (C) one-fourth inch above mandible at apices of mandibular teeth.

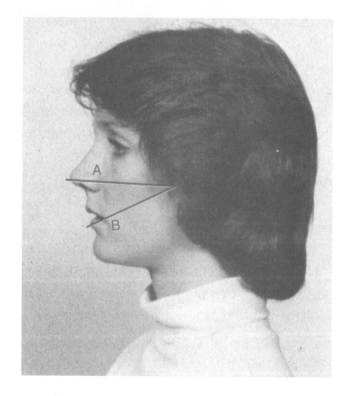

Figure 66-37 Planes for proper angulation: (A) ala of nose to tragus of ear; (B) corner of mouth to tragus of ear.

the holder, with dot of film in the slot, making sure not to crease the film.

c. The film is carried into place, not allowed to slide into position.

d. Patient is instructed to close firmly but gently to maintain the position of the film by resting teeth in grooves on opposite side of holder. Patient should retain the film holder with tips of fingers, and at the same time, push downward on the opposite end of the holder; the mandibular teeth will act as a fulcrum for the maxillary placement. The opposite retention would be used for the mandibular projections, Figure 66-38.

e. The PID placement and angulation chart is used for centrals or laterals and cuspids (Table 66–2).

Film Position for Posterior Exposures (Figures 66-39 and 66-40).

a. A #2 film is placed horizontally in mouth.

b. The corners of the film are softened between thumb and forefinger and placed in the jaw (biting surface)

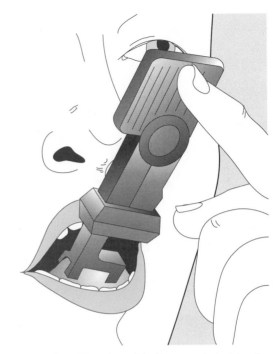

Figure 66-38 Film placed in Eezee-grip holder for mandibular central/lateral incisors.

Table 66-2	PID Placement and Angulation	
Area	**Cone Placement: Vertical and Horizontal "Ray"**	**Average Vertical Angulation**
Maxillary Arch		
Central/laterals	Center incisors on film Central ray directed between central/laterals Horizontal ray side of nose on ala/tragus line	+40°
Cuspids	Central cuspid on film Central ray directed at distal of cuspid Horizontal ray on ala/tragus line	+45°
Bicuspids (premolars)	Film placed to cover distal of maxillary cuspid Central ray directed below pupil of eye Horizontal ray on ala/tragus line	+30°
Molars	Film placed to cover distal of maxillary second bicuspid Central ray directed in a line with the outer canthus of eye Horizontal ray on ala/tragus line	+20°
Mandibular Arch		
Central/laterals	Center incisors on film Central ray directed between central/laterals Horizontal ray just above lower border of mandible	−15°
Cuspids	Central cuspid on film Central ray directed at distal of cuspid Horizontal ray along lower border or mandible	−20°
Bicuspids (premolars)	Film placed to cover distal of maxillary cuspid Central ray directed approximately at mesial of mandibular first molar Horizontal ray just above lower border or mandible	−10°
Molars	Film placed to cover distal of mandibular second bicuspid Central ray directed distal of second molar, approximately in a line with the outer canthus of eye. *Note:* For third molars, film may have to be placed further back in mouth in order to have full view of roots—PID will then have to be moved back also.	−5°

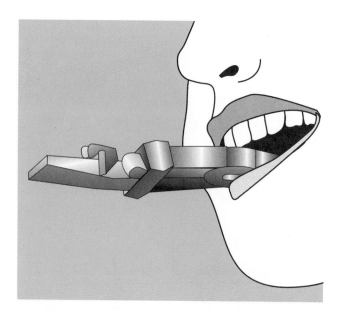

Figure 66-39 Film placed in Eezee-grip holder for maxillary posteriors.

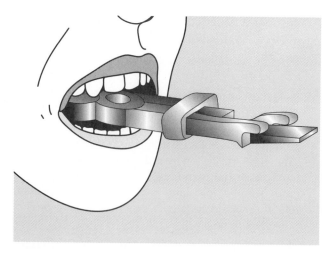

Figure 66-40 Film placed in Eezee-grip holder for mandibular posteriors.

of the holder with the dot in the slot (see Figure 66-35). The film should not be creased. The friction ring is slid into position, with just enough pressure to hold the film securely.

c. When using the wide biting surface of the holder for maxillary areas, the film can be positioned farther away from the lingual surface of the teeth by having the patient bite close to the outer edge. By so doing, the maxillary edge can be brought to the roof of the mouth and the lower edge away from the crowns of the teeth as far as the width of the Eezee-Grip jaw will permit. This will position the film almost, if not parallel, to most maxillary posterior teeth (see Figure 66-35). The mandibular posterior technique is the reverse of the maxillary area.

d. Use the PID placement and angulation for premolars and molars, given in Table 66-2.

Additional Retentive Methods/Holders

Placement and retention of the packets are the primary responsibility of the operator. **Digital retention** (the patient holds the film packet in place using the fingers and light pressure to prevent movement) should be avoided if possible. The operator should never hold the film. Disposable styrofoam blocks such as the Stabe bite blocks and plastic film holders are used as a matter of preference in most offices.

Supplementary views of teeth are often necessary to reveal some aspect of dental structure that may be

hidden when a standard placement and projection are used. In such instances, the horizontal angle, the vertical angle, and the method of placement may vary. In all cases, the important thing to remember is to avoid shaping the film to the arch; a flat film surface must be ensured regardless of the procedure used.

Paralleling Technique

Paralleling Technique Principles

Paralleling techniques require the use of a film-holding device. One of the most commonly used is the Rinn XCP instrument (extension cone paralleling).

Extension cone paralleling (XCP) is a practical technique for periapical radiography that minimizes dimensional distortion and presents the objects being radiographed in their true anatomical relationship and size. A film-holding device, very similar to that used for the bisected-angle technique, will direct the position of the film and PID to meet the principles of the paralleling technique. This systematic procedure is based on the following principles:

1. Paralleling the film with the longitudinal axes of the teeth to diminish dimensional distortion

2. Increasing the **anode-film (source) distance (AFD)** (the distance between the source of radiation to the film) to avoid image enlargement and **adumbration**; i.e., the images of the teeth are overshadowed by an object, as occurs with the superimposition of the malar bone over the apices of the teeth on a maxillary posterior film.

3. Directing alignment of the x-ray beam to assure correct vertical and horizontal angulation.

Advantages of the XCP Technique

1. *Simplicity.* Eliminates the need for predetermined angulation and positioning of the patient's head.

2. *Adaptability.* Can be used in most offices regardless of space limitations by rotating the chair or the patient's head.

3. *Reliability.* Anatomical accuracy of tooth size and length and size of canals is assured.

4. *Results.* Radiographs that reproduce anatomical structures in their normal size and relationship, free of distortion with minimal superimposition of the zygomatic shadow and exhibiting maximum detail and definition.

With the central ray directed perpendicularly to the two planes (the film and the teeth), a truer profile and relative registration of the shadow images are the result on the radiograph. This technique also employs a slightly increased **object-film distance** (the distance between the tooth and the film) and an increased AFD. Further advantages of this technique include:

● Sharpness of details

● Minimal enlargement and control of malar bone shadow

● Images of teeth nearly anatomically accurate from right-angle exposures and flat surfaces of film

● Alveolar crest in true relationship to the teeth

● Increased film clarity and contrast

Paralleling Technique

Along with the advantages of the paralleling technique, there are disadvantages. First, there is the problem of attaining parallel film placement in all areas of the oral cavity. Parallelism is rather easily established in the mandibular molar region, where the lingual alveolar process is relatively thin; therefore, the film can be placed closer to the teeth. In the maxillary molar and premolar (bicuspid) region, it is necessary to position the film at the midline of the palate and some distance from the teeth. In the maxillary anterior region, narrow films must be used, and as a result, often no more than one tooth is satisfactorily shown. The same problem holds for the mandibular anterior teeth.

The previous problems can be somewhat minimized by utilizing a styrofoam disposable bite block or plastic film holder. Both permit the film to be brought to the center of the vault, nearly parallel with the teeth, without discomfort to the patient. Of the several types of accessory devices for holding the film in position, experience has shown that they should be radiolucent (permitting the passage of x-rays), economical, easy to use, and capable of withstanding sterilization, or being disposable.

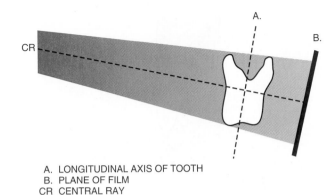

A. LONGITUDINAL AXIS OF TOOTH
B. PLANE OF FILM
CR CENTRAL RAY

Figure 66-41 Angulation of the central ray (Courtesy of Rinn Corporation, Elgin, IL.)

The paralleling technique for periapical radiography will minimize dimensional distortion and result in a more true anatomical relationship and size. It involves placing the plane of the film parallel with the long axes of the teeth. Basic to any technique is the principle that image sharpness is primarily affected by increased AFD, the size of the focal spot of the central ray, and motion (Figure 66-41). The paralleling technique favorably meets this criterion.

When a longer PID is used (and the AFD increased), the x-rays reaching the film tend to be more nearly parallel, and magnification of the image is decreased. Because magnification is less, it is possible to position the film farther away from the teeth in a plane parallel to the long axes. As with any technique, every effort must be made to eliminate motion of the patient or vibration of the tubehead during the exposure. Such motion increases the focal-spot size and results in a hazy or blurred image. When done properly, the paralleling technique will produce diagnostic intraoral radiographs with less distortion of the images (teeth and surrounding structures) than those produced with the bisected-angle technique (Figures 66-42 and 66-43). Certain essentials must be maintained for successful completion of this technique:

1. The film should be kept flat and an accessory device used.

2. Except in the mandibular molar area, the film is positioned lingually as far as possible to cover the apices of the teeth.

3. The film is positioned parallel with the long axes of the teeth.

4. The AFD is increased to minimize dimensional distortion.

5. The face of the open PID is kept parallel with the plane of the film and thus ensure that all of the film is covered by the x-ray beam.

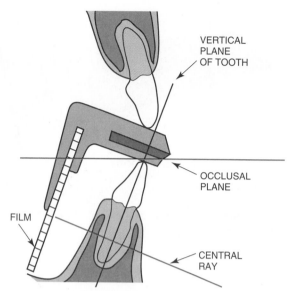

Figure 66-42 Film placed in disposable bite block for mandibular central or lateral exposure.

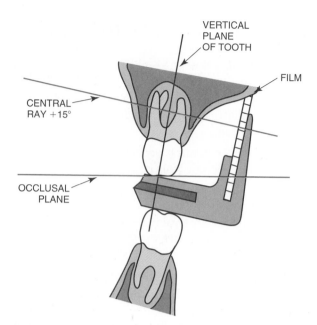

Figure 66-43 Film placed in disposable bite block for maxillary molar exposure.

For anterior maxillary and mandibular film exposures, #1 film is placed in a vertical position. For posterior maxillary and mandibular projections, #2 film is placed in a horizontal position.

Film Placement. It is important to remember that the position of the film must be more lingually placed for mandibular exposures and near the center of the vault for the maxillary:

1. The film is centered in the holder by sliding it along the backing support of the holder, with the dot in the slot. The film should be secured with the edge completely in the slot and with the plain side of the film away from the backing plate toward the aiming ring.

2. The lingual (palatal) corners of the film are softened between the thumb and forefinger.

3. The film and backing support are introduced in a slanted position, with the film parallel to the long axes of the teeth. The biting surface of the holder is seated on the biting edges of the teeth under survey.

4. The patient is asked to close the opposing teeth on the block to retain the film. *Note:* When using a disposable film holder or an XCP holder with an aiming ring, the biting portion that extends facially beyond the incisal or occlusal surfaces of the teeth will indicate the horizontal center of the film (see Figures 66-42 and 66-43).

5. The face of the open cone is positioned parallel to the plane of the film, which should then direct the central ray toward the center of the film and perpendicular to the film and object.

Paralleling (XCP) Instrument Components

Bite Blocks. Designed to achieve true parallelism of the longitudinal axes of the teeth and the plane of the film, XCP bite blocks have greater length to the grooved biting surface than those used for the bisected-angle technique. The backing plate for the anterior instrument is positioned at right angles to the biting surface. Anterior and posterior XCP bite blocks differ (Figure 66-44).

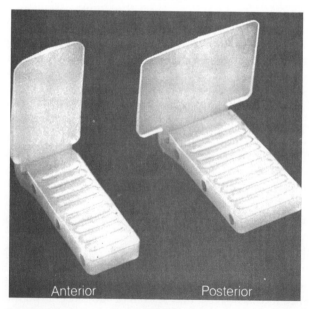

Figure 66-44 Rinn XCP bite blocks. (Courtesy of Rinn Corporation, Elgin, IL)

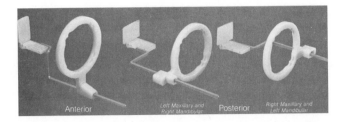

Figure 66-45 Rinn XCP instrument components properly assembled. (Courtesy of Rinn Corporation, Elgin, IL.)

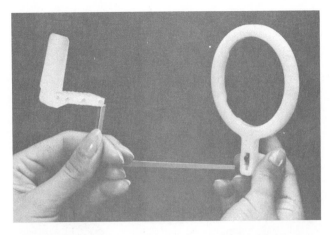

Figure 66-47 Insert indicator rod into the aiming ring slot.

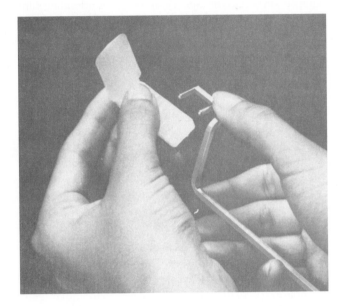

Figure 66-46 Insert the two prongs of the indicator rod into openings in the bite block as shown. On three-hole blocks, use the two forward holes (away from the backing plate). The third opening is for use when the bite block is shortened for pedo technique.

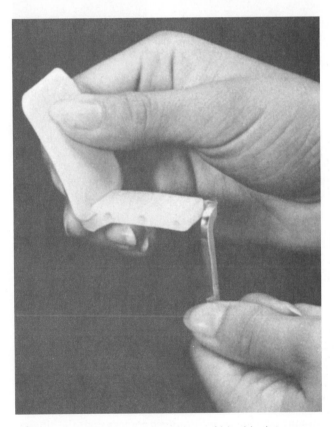

Figure 66-48 Flex backing plate of bite block to open film slot.

Aiming Rings. These plastic rings are used to bring the film "on target." The same rings are used for both BAIs and XCP. Aiming rings for anterior and posterior films differ.

Indicator Rods (Arms). The same rods are used for both BAI and XCP. Anterior and posterior rods (arms) differ.

Assembly Instructions

Figure 66-45 shows the properly assembled XCP instrument components. The angled portion of the indicator rod must be positioned away from the biting surfaces of the bite block.

1. Insert the two prongs of the indicator rod into the holes of the bite block. On anterior three-hole blocks, use the two forward holes (away from the backing plate). The third opening is for use when the bite block needs to be shortened for an extremely narrow arch (Figure 66-46).

2. Insert indicator rod into aiming slot (Figure 66-47).

3. Flex backing plate of bite block to open film slot for easy insertion of film packet. Make sure the film packet is inserted completely into the slot, with the dot in the slot (Figure 66-48).

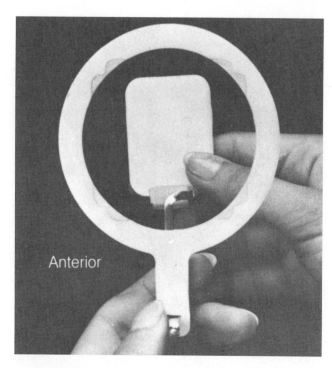

Figure 66-49 Anterior instrument is correctly assembled with film on target.

4. When assembling an anterior instrument, make sure that the film is "on target" (Figure 66-49).

Placing the Film Inside the Mouth

The instrument should be held by the paralleling rod and ring. For maxillary films, the top portion of the film is tilted toward the center of the mouth, making a V shape with the bite block. Keeping this angle, the bite block is guided up to contact the tooth of interest. This will avoid scraping the film across the intraoral tissues.

For mandibular films, the tongue is lifted with the index finger, and the lower border of the film packet is allowed to slide into place between the tongue and lingual side of the teeth. The film is kept approximately 1/4 inch away from the lingual side of the teeth. The film should not be placed in direct contact with the lingual surface of the teeth.

When instructing the patient to bring the teeth together on the bite block, the phrase, "Slowly, close, please" should be used. This will allow you to keep the film where it was placed and to remove your finger before the teeth close on it.

Maintaining Patient Cooperation

The film should be placed and exposed as quickly as possible. The film should be removed as soon as it has been exposed. At best, this procedure is not a comfort-able one for many patients. Keeping the film in the patient's mouth for as short a time as possible tends to increase patient cooperation.

The easiest films should be taken first, probably the maxillary anterior. With these successfully accomplished, the patient is likely to cooperate for the remaining exposures.

The dental assistant should be as quick and gentle as possible and be sure of herself or himself and learn as much of the procedure as possible by practicing it before actually exposing a full-mouth series of radiographs on a patient. See Table 66–1 for adequate film placement.

Maxillary Anterior Region (General instructions)

1. Assemble anterior instrument, and insert film packet vertically into anterior bite block, pushing film packet all the way into slot. Plain side of film packet should be positioned away from backing plate. Narrow #1 film is used. When using #2 film, slightly roll upper corners of film packet to facilitate positioning.

2. With the front edge of bite block placed on incisal edges of teeth to be radiographed, position film as posterior as possible and instruct patient to close slowly, but firmly, to retain position of film packet. A cotton roll may be placed between mandibular teeth and bite block for patient comfort (Figure 66-50).

3. Slide aiming ring down the indicator rod to skin surface, and align the PID of the x-ray unit in close approximation to aiming ring, centered and parallel to rod.

4. Press x-ray machine activating button and make exposure.

Maxillary Posterior Region (General Instructions)

1. Assemble posterior instrument and insert film packet horizontally into posterior bite block, pushing film packet all the way into slot. Plain side of film packet should be positioned away from backing plate. Slightly roll upper anterior or posterior corners of film packet to facilitate positioning.

2. With bite block placed on occlusal surfaces of teeth to be radiographed, entire horizontal length of bite block should be utilized to position film in mid-palatal area. Instruct patient to close slowly, but firmly, to retain position of film packet. A cotton roll may be placed between mandibular teeth and bite block for patient comfort (Figure 66-51).

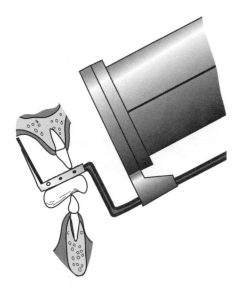

Figure 66-50 Maxillary anterior teeth. (Courtesy of Rinn Corporation, Elgin, IL.)

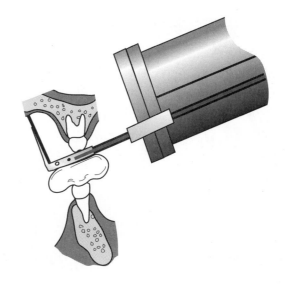

Figure 66-51 Maxillary posterior teeth. (Courtesy of Rinn Corporation, Elgin, IL.)

3. Slide aiming ring down the indicator rod to skin surface, and align the PID of the x-ray unit in close approximation to aiming ring, centered and parallel to rod.

4. Press x-ray machine activating button and make exposure.

Mandibular Anterior Region (General Instructions)

1. Assemble anterior instrument and insert film packet vertically into anterior bite block, pushing film packet all the way into slot. Plain side of film packet should be positioned away from backing plate. Narrow #1 film may be used.

2. With bite block placed on incisal edges of teeth to be radiographed, instruct patient to close slowly, but firmly, to retain position of film packet. A cotton roll may be placed between maxillary incisors and bite block for patient comfort (Figure 66-52).

3. Slide aiming ring down the indicator rod to skin surface and align the PID of the x-ray unit in close approximation to aiming ring, centered and parallel to rod.

4. Press x-ray machine activating button and make exposure.

Mandibular Posterior Region (General Instructions)

1. Assemble posterior instrument and insert film packet horizontally into posterior bite block, pushing

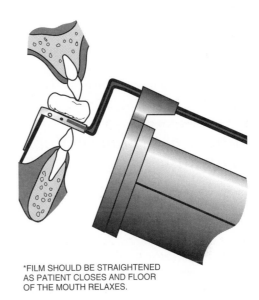

*FILM SHOULD BE STRAIGHTENED AS PATIENT CLOSES AND FLOOR OF THE MOUTH RELAXES.

Figure 66-52 Mandibular anterior teeth. (Courtesy of Rinn Corporation, Elgin, IL.)

film packet all the way into slot. Plain side of film packet should be positioned away from backing plate. Roll lower anterior corner of film packet slightly to facilitate positioning.

2. With bite block placed on occlusal surfaces of mandibular teeth to be radiographed, instruct patient to close slowly, but firmly, to retain position of film packet. A cotton roll may be placed between maxillary teeth and bite block for patient comfort (Figure 66-53).

3. Slide aiming ring down the indicator rod to skin surface and align the PID of the x-ray unit in close

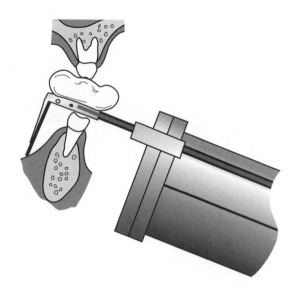

Figure 66-53 Mandibular posterior teeth. (Courtesy of Rinn Corporation, Elgin, IL.)

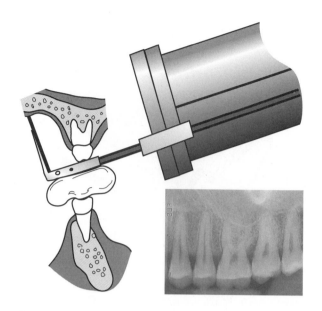

Figure 66-54 Variation problem: low palate. (Courtesy of Rinn Corporation, Elgin, IL.)

approximation to aiming ring, centered and parallel to rod.

4. Press x-ray machine activating button and make exposure.

Variations of the Conventional XCP Procedure

There are cases when the conventional XCP technique must be varied to achieve the desired results. Selected variations are added to this chapter.

Maxillary Posterior Region

Low Palates. Parallelism between the film and long axes of the teeth is difficult to accomplish in patients with low palatal vaults. If the discrepancy from parallelism does not exceed 15°, the resultant radiograph is usually acceptable (Figure 66-54). By using a two-cotton roll technique (one on each side of block), the film can be paralleled with the long axes, but the area of periapical coverage will be reduced (Figure 66-55). This may prove adequate in some instances, particularly if the teeth have short roots.

Increasing Periapical Coverage. Greater periapical coverage than can be obtained with the conventional technique may be desired in certain instances. This can be accomplished by increasing the vertical angulation 5°–15° more than the instrument indicates (Figure 66-56). Also, by altering the relationship of the film to the teeth on a horizontal plane, various aspects of multirooted teeth can be projected on the radiograph (Figure 66-57).

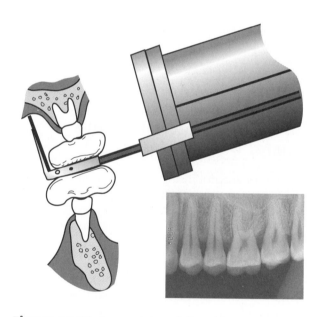

Figure 66-55 Low palate solution. (Courtesy of Rinn Corporation, Elgin, IL)

Mandibular Posterior Region: Overcoming Inadequate Periapical Coverage. With an excessive mandibular occlusal curve or in patients with long bicuspids, the conventional technique may result in inadequate coverage. Two methods are suggested to overcome this problem:

1. Projection of the bicuspid images higher on a conventionally positioned film can be accomplished by increasing the vertical angle negatively 5° to 15° more than the XCP instrument indicates (Figure 66-58).

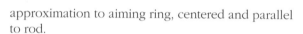

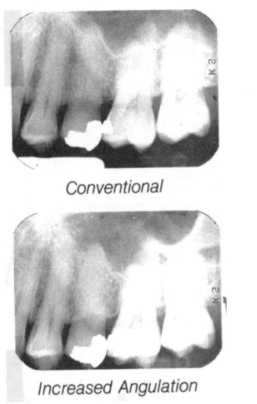

Conventional

Increased Angulation

Figure 66-56 Variation problem: increasing periapical coverage. (Courtesy of Rinn Corporation, Elgin, IL.)

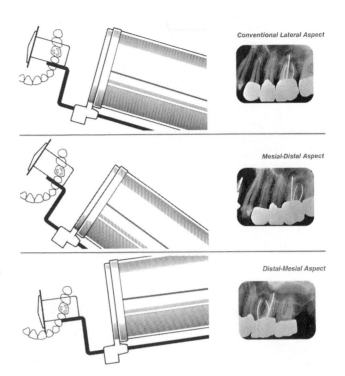

Conventional Lateral Aspect

Mesial-Distal Aspect

Distal-Mesial Aspect

Figure 66-57 Variation problem, showing various aspects of multirooted teeth. (Courtesy of Rinn Corporation, Elgin, IL.)

2. By placing the film vertically rather than horizontally in the posterior instrument and using a two-cotton roll technique (one on each side of the block), complete visualization of the bicuspid region will be accomplished. The purpose of the second cotton roll between the block and the mandibular bicuspids is to prevent unnecessary impingement of the film on the floor of the mouth (Figure 66-59).

Partially Edentulous Technique

The XCP instruments can be used in radiography of partially edentulous mouths by substituting a cotton roll or block of styrofoam (or a similar radiolucent material) for the space normally occupied by the crowns of the missing teeth and then following standard procedure (Figure 66-60). Care must be taken to angle the film at approximate parallelism to missing teeth.

Completely Edentulous Technique

When all the teeth are missing, cotton rolls, blocks of styrofoam, or a combination of both can be used with the XCP instruments, as illustrated. The thickness of the cotton rolls or styrofoam will determine the amount of film coverage of the edentulous ridges. The instrument

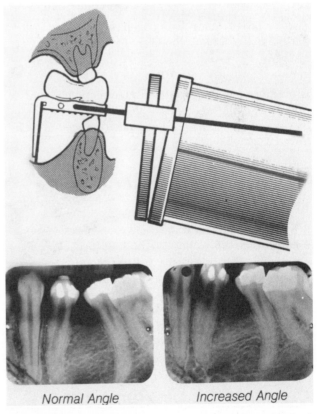

Normal Angle *Increased Angle*

Figure 66-58 Inadequate periapical coverage: Method 1. (Courtesy of Rinn Corporation, Elgin, IL.)

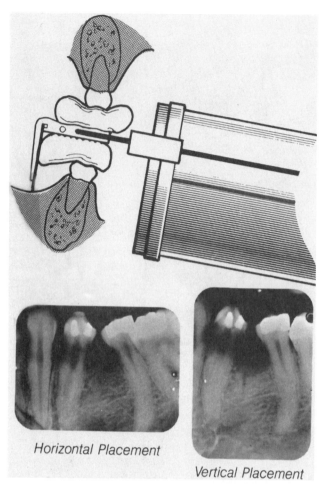

Horizontal Placement

Vertical Placement

Figure 66-59 Inadequate periapical coverage: Method 2 (Courtesy of Rinn Corporation, Elgin, IL.)

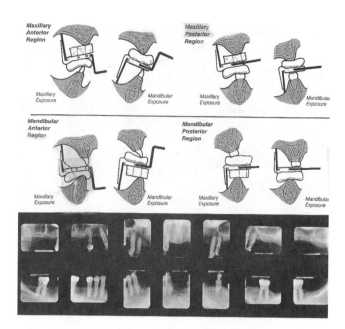

Figure 66-60 Partially edentulous technique. Exposure times should be reduced 25% from that of a standard technique. (Courtesy of Rinn Corporation, Elgin, IL.)

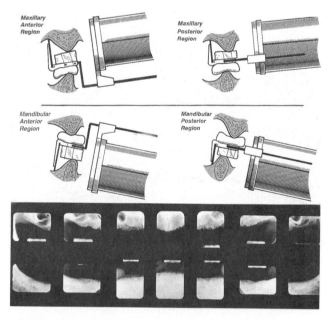

Figure 66-61 Completely edentulous technique. Exposure times should be reduced 25% from that of a standard technique. (Courtesy of Rinn Corporation, Elgin, IL.)

is positioned in the mouth with the film parallel to the ridge area being examined. The patient closes, holding the film in position, and the standard procedure is followed (Figure 66-61).

Technique for Limited Operatory Space (XCP Only)

It is well known that some x-ray procedures cannot be used in some offices because of limited space. Space is not a limiting factor with the XCP technique, because the patient no longer needs to be maintained in the standard dental radiographic posture. By rotating or tipping the patient's head or by adjusting the dental chair to a convenient position, it is always possible to align the extension tube (PID) with the XCP instrument regardless of space limitations or restricted mobility of the x-ray unit.

Occlusal Film Examination

The **occlusal film examination** is so-called because the film packet is placed in the occlusal plane for exposure.

Such exposures show sectional views of large dental areas on one film. In cases where periapical packets cannot be used, the occlusal packet is the logical substitute.

The image on the occlusal film discloses conditions that cannot be recorded conveniently on any other film.

Industrial and automobile accidents have greatly increased the incidence of jaw fractures. In an examination of such conditions, the dentist cannot always be satisfied with the information provided by extraoral radiographs. If the maxillae are involved, a few additional exposures may be necessary to detect obscure (not easily seen) and hairline fractures that would have an important influence on occlusion and the maxillary sinuses. Often, these added exposures must be made from several different angles.

Advantages

The occlusal film is particularly useful in revealing fractures of the palate and alveolar processes of the maxilla, as well as various portions of the mandible. Therefore, if the patient can open his or her mouth wide enough to insert the occlusal packet, valuable x-ray information may be secured. In cases where the patient suffers from **trismus** (lockjaw) or any severe form of mental affliction or disease that prevents the use of periapical or interproximal examination, occlusal packets can be slid between the teeth and radiographs made.

In addition, occlusal film has distinct applications in making rapid surveys of the teeth and jaws. It is of value in locating impacted teeth, foreign bodies, and calculi in the salivary ducts; in determining the extent of lesions, such as cysts, osteomyelitis, and some forms of malignancies; in recording changes in the size and shape of the dental arches; in showing the presence or absence of supernumerary teeth (particularly in the cuspid region); in observing the condition of the upper jaw following operations for closure of cleft palate; in revealing **odontomata** (an anomaly in tooth development, particularly of the hard tissues) that has blocked the eruption of teeth; in examining edentulous areas at the site of root fragments, cystic growths, necrotic areas, etc.; and in locating areas of destruction in malignancies of the palate.

Angulation

The position of the patient and the tubehead, the correct angle for projection, and the normal occlusal radiographs for the anterior and posterior areas of the maxilla and anterior areas of the mandible are illustrated in Figures 66-62 through 66-66.

Film Placement (Maxillary)

1. The patient is seated in an upright position in the dental chair. The maxillary occlusal plane must be parallel with the floor.
2. The smooth, or tube-side of the film packet is placed vertically toward the maxillary teeth, ideally allowing a 1/4 in. margin of film in front of the maxillary incisors with dot palced outside the oral cavity. The patient is instructed to close the teeth firmly on the packet to stabilize the film's position.

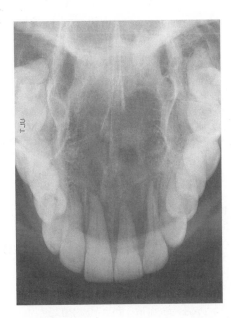

Figure 66-62 Maxillary occlusal radiograph, anterior view

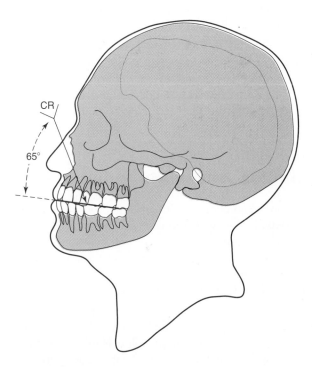

Figure 66-63 Angle for projection of central ray for maxillary occlusal radiograph, anterior view.

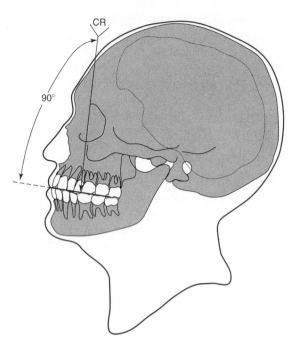

Figure 66-64 Angle for projection of central ray for maxillary occlusal radiograph, posterior view.

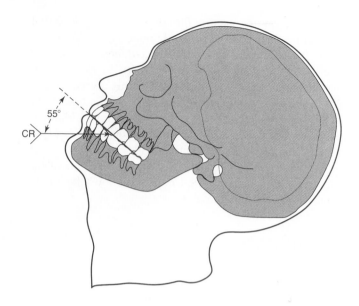

Figure 66-65 Angle for projection of central ray for mandibular occlusal radiograph, anterior view.

3. The film that extends beyond the biting surfaces is checked to make certain it remains parallel with the floor.

4. The patient is instructed to maintain this position and to close his or her eyes during the exposure of the film.

5. For the anterior view, the central ray is directed at the bridge of the nose and a +65° angulation is used (Figures 66-62 and 66-63). For the cross-section view, the central ray is directed above the forehead parallel to the film and a +90° angulation is used (Figure 66-64).

Film Placement (Mandibular)

1. For the anterior view, the patient is positioned in the dental chair with the occlusal plane at 55° to the floor (Figure 66-65). For the cross-section view, the patient's head is extended as far back as possible, positioning the inferior border of the mandible at a right angle, or 90°, to the floor (Figure 66-67).

2. The smooth, or tube-side of the film is placed vertically toward the mandibular teeth, allowing a 1/4 in. margin in front of the mandibular incisors with dot placed outside the oral cavity. The patient is instructed to close the teeth firmly on the film packet to stabilize its position.

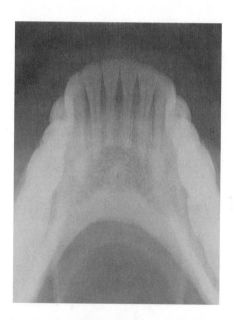

Figure 66-66 Mandibular occlusal radiography, anterior view.

3. For the anterior view, the PID is positioned at zero angulation and placed in close proximity, approximately 1/2 in. away from the chin, with the central ray directed at the midline of the chin. The angle of the PID and the plane of the film is bisected (Figures 66-65 and 66-66).

4. For the cross-section view, the PID is placed under the chin at zero angulation parallel to the film (Figure 66-67).

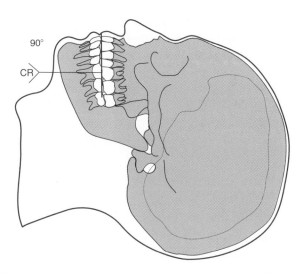

Figure 66-67 Angle for projection of central ray for posterior view.

SUGGESTED ACTIVITIES

● Watch a demonstration, then practice placing the film loop on four #2 periapical films. Observe the position of the raised dot. Review Figure 66-7.
  1. Use manikins to position each bite-wing film. Determine the correct vertical and horizontal angulation of the PID.
  2. Expose premolar and molar bite-wing films and process them.

● Using infection control procedures and a fellow student for your patient, seat the person in the dental chair, and make all preparations for a bite-wing radiographic survey. Check your procedures under the supervision of the instructor.
  1. Practice placement of the film and place angulation of the PID for both the bicuspid and molar bite-wing films. Have instructor check final film placement and PID alignment.

● Under the supervision of the instructor, prepare, place, and expose periapical films on a manikin or skull. Use the Rinn BAI and an 8- or 12-in. PID.

● Using the Eezee-Grip holder on a manikin or skull, practice exposing posterior periapical films.

● Demonstrate (to the class) by drawing and labeling the paralleling and the bisecting-angle techniques, indicating the x-ray tube with central ray, the object, the film, and bisecting plane where applicable.

● Under the supervision of the instructor, assemble the XCP instruments for anterior, right maxillary, and right mandibular posterior teeth.

● Using a fellow student and the XCP technique, practice placing film in half of the mouth, one maxillary quadrant and one mandibular quandrant, using instruments without exposure. Fellow students are most willing to give feedback on the comfort or discomfort of film placement.

● Practice placing, aligning, exposing, and processing the four occlusal x-ray films using an 8-inch or a 12-inch PID and appropriate angulations for each technique on a manikin. Be sure to check all procedures with your instructor.

REVIEW

1. The purposes for making interproximal surveys include checking for (1) the presence of interproximal caries, (2) overhanging restorations, (3) resorption of alveolar bone, and/or (4) gingival caries.
   a. 1, 2, 3
   b. 2, 3, 4
   c. 1, 2, 4
   d. 1, 3, 4

2. When making a bicuspid interproximal survey, the vertical angle of the PID is positioned at:
   a. 0° angulation
   b. +5° angulation
   c. +10° angulation
   d. -10° angulation

3. The principle of the bisected-angle technique states that the central ray is perpendicular to:
   a. The long axis of the tooth
   b. The imaginary line that bisects the long axis of the tooth and the film
   c. The film
   d. The backing plate of the film holder

4. When using the bisected angle technique and the central ray is directed at right angles to the long axis of the tooth, it will appear _____. If the ray is directed at right angles to the plane of the dental film, the image will appear _____.
   a. Elongated, foreshortened
   b. Foreshortened, elongated

5. Advantages of using the XCP technique include (1) reproducing anatomical structures in their normal size and relationship, (2) eliminating the need for predetermined angulation and position of patient's head, (3) closer object-to-film distance, and/or (4) ability to be used in areas of space limitations.
   a. 1, 2, 3
   b. 2, 3, 4
   c. 1, 2, 4
   d. 1, 3, 4

6. When placing the film for the maxillary posterior teeth using the XCP technique, the film is placed:
   a. As close to the teeth as possible
   b. As far away from the teeth as possible
   c. At half way between the teeth and the center of the mouth
   d. At the center of the mouth

7. XCP instruments may be used on edentulous patients by:
   a. Using digital retention
   b. Using cotton rolls
   c. Using styrofoam blocks
   d. Both b and c

8. Occlusal radiographs are made to:
   a. Reveal fractures of the palate and alveolar bone
   b. To detect calculi in the salivary ducts
   c. To detect unerupted teeth
   d. Both a and c
   e. All of the above

Extraoral Radiography

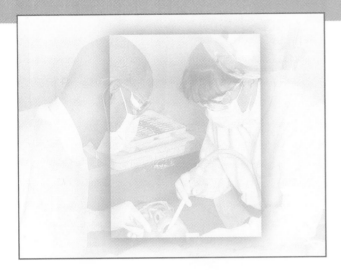

OBJECTIVES

After studying this chapter, the student will be able to:

- Describe the purpose for taking lateral jaw radiographs.
- Define panoramic radiography.
- Name advantages and give limitations of panoramic radiography in comparison to intraoral radiography.
- Identify equipment needed for panoramic radiography.
- Describe cassette-loading techniques.
- Describe patient preparation and positioning techniques.
- Describe the technique for preparation of the panoramic machine.
- Identify patient positioning errors and how they may be corrected.

Introduction

Extraoral x-ray films are exposed with the film positioned outside the mouth. They are valuable for examining the body and ramus of the mandible, the temporomandibular joint, the maxilla, and other areas of the face. They are not expressly used for the detection of caries.

It should be noted that the extraoral film carton *must* be opened and the film holder or **cassette** (film-holding device used during exposure) loaded in the darkroom. The methods of making some of the more frequently used extraoral radiographs of the head and its parts are shown in Figures 67-1 and 67-2.

Dental x-ray units are *not* designed for making radiographs of the torso or other extremities. When dental x-ray units are used for this purpose, the patient is subjected to greater radiation than he or she would be if proper equipment were used. Dental x-ray equipment should be used for this purpose *only in an emergency*.

Body of the Mandible (Lateral Oblique Jaw)

To visualize a large portion of the jaw, the lateral oblique jaw projection is used. The patient's head is positioned with the maxillary occlusal plane horizontal. The cassette or cardboard film holder is placed at the desired side of the head, between the headrest pad and the patient's head, with the front edge of the film held in the patient's hand. The longer dimension of the film is positioned horizontally, and the plane of the film is approximately vertical. The patient's head is rotated until the nose is 1/4 in. from the surface of the film holder. The chin is elevated moderately and the teeth held in normal occlusion. The sagittal plane of the patient's head

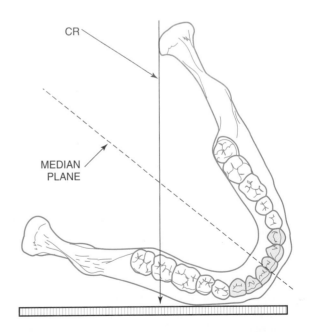

Figure 67-1 Angle for projection of central ray for body of the mandible—lateral oblique jaw.

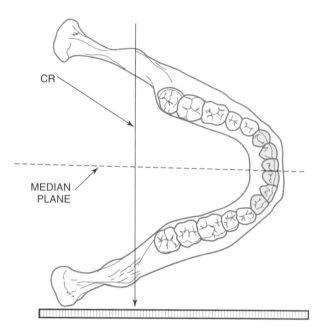

Figure 67-2 Angle for projection of central ray for condyle—lateral Jaw.

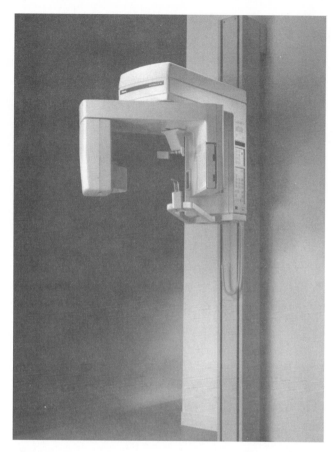

Figure 67-3 Panoramic machine. (Courtesy of GEN-DEX Corp.)

remains vertical at all times. The vertical angulation is tipped −17° upward. The point of entry for the central ray is 1/2 in. below and behind the angle of the undesired side of the jaw. The horizontal angulation is chosen so that the face or axis of the x-ray head parallels the top edge of the film holder. A paper clip fastened at the center of the lower edge of the tube side of the cardboard film holder is useful to identify the film that is used on the patient's right side. Refer to the manufacturer's instructions for exposure time.

Condyle (Lateral Jaw)

To visualize the condyle, the patient's head is positioned with the maxillary occlusal plane horizontally. The cassette or film holder is placed on the side of the head with its longer dimension vertical and centered over the desired condyle. It is held in this position by pressure exerted upon the back of the film by the palm of the patient's hand. The position-indicating device (PID) is removed from the x-ray machine. The vertical angulation setting is -5° upward. The point of entry for the central ray is at the mandibular foramen (not the mental foramen) on the undesired side of the jaw. The x-ray machine is placed in contact with the patient's cheek and the horizontal angulation determined so that the face or axis of the x-ray machine parallels the medial sagittal plane of the patient. Before the film is exposed, the patient is instructed to open his or her mouth to its fullest extent. Refer to manufacturer's instructions for exposure time (Figure 67-2).

Panoramic Radiography (Dental Pantomography)

Panoramic radiography is another type of extraoral radiography. Names used by manufacturers include Panorex, Panelipse, Panoral, or Orthopantomograph (Figure 67-3). This technique records both maxillary and mandibular dental arches on one film (Figure 67-4). It uses a principle called **tomography** (*tomo* = "section")—a radiographic technique used on a three-dimensional object that focuses on one plane (focal

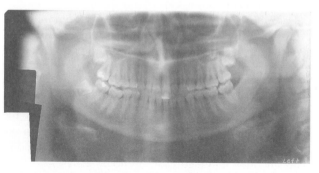

Figure 67-4 Panoramic radiograph.

trough) of the object while blurring out other surrounding structures located in different planes. Tomography is based on the principle whereby the x-ray tubehead and film are rotated about a pivot point that is located at the level of the selected plane of tissue to be exposed. The recording of the dental arches and their adjacent structures is achieved by moving the tubehead and the film through the x-ray beam with equal linear velocity.

Making a panoramic radiograph is similar to taking several photographs of a scenic valley in which the camera is moved to the right or left for each photograph. When all the pictures are developed, they can be pieced together and placed into one panoramic picture of the valley. Panoramic radiographs make it possible to take several pictures of the dental alveolar structures and have them laid out side by side automatically on one film.

Panoramic radiographs should not be considered to be the only diagnostic aid when assessing the patient's oral condition. They are very useful, however, in determining traumatic injuries, third molar positions, pathologic diseased areas, abnormal tooth eruption, and developmental anomalies. Some advantages and disadvantages are reviewed.

Advantages

- A principal advantage is its ability to cover a broad anatomic area using one film that not only shows the teeth and supporting structures but also includes the condyles laterally, a portion of the orbits of the eyes vertically, third molar impactions, and certain pathologic conditions that may not be visible on periapical radiographs.

- Patients who do not tolerate intraoral film placement or who are unable to open their mouths widely are more cooperative due to the simplicity of this technique.

- The time required to expose a panoramic radiographic film is very short by comparison with exposing a full-mouth series of intraoral films.

- There is a low dose of radiation exposure to the patient. One panoramic exposure may be comparable to four bite wings.

Disadvantages

- It is not a replacement for intraoral radiography due to its inability to detect anatomic detail; therefore, it is not useful in diagnosing incipient decay, periapical disease lesions, or periodontal disease. When using panoramic radiographs, it is advisable to include a set of bite-wing radiographs to aid in making proper diagnosis.

- Magnification, distortion, and overlapping teeth, especially in the premolar area, are prevalent. Areas that are not within the focal trough will be distorted or poorly visible.

- The cost involved in purchasing a panoramic x-ray machine is double or more than that of an intraoral x-ray machine. There are also added costs in purchasing processing racks, a darkroom safelight, and film.

Focal Trough

To understand how the image of the dentition will appear clearly on the radiograph, one needs to consider that having the teeth within the **focal trough** (an imaginary three-dimensional area formed in the shape of the dental arches or a "horseshoe" used to position the patient's jaws within its confines while making panoramic radiographs) will produce acceptable panoramic radiographs. Understanding this concept will aid the operator in patient positioning. If the teeth are not within the focal trough, they will be magnified, reduced, blurred, and out of focus. The focal trough, also called the image layer, is a three-dimensional region resembling the form of a horseshoe that is wider, at least 2 cm, or 3/4 in., in the posterior area, where the margin of error is less. The anterior area, being narrower, at least 6 mm, or 1/4 in., may create more distortion (Figure 67-5). The operator needs to be able to determine if the dental structures will be in the central area of the focal trough to produce sharper images.

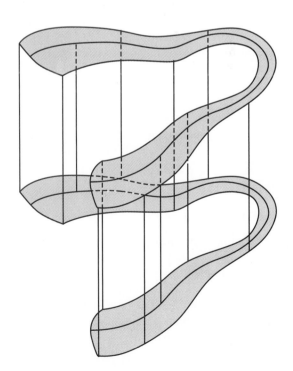

Figure 67-5 Focal trough.

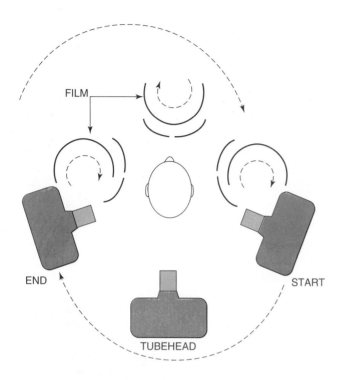

Figure 67-6 Tubehead rotation in panoramic radiography. Film cassette drum and tubehead move in opposite directions around the patient.

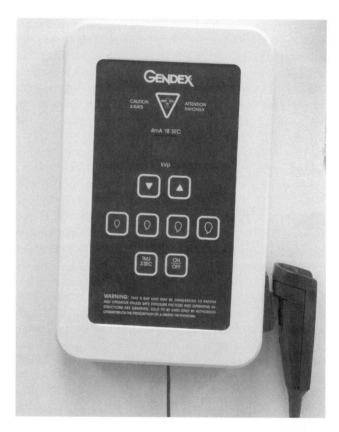

Figure 67-7 Panoramic machine control panel.

Tubehead Rotation

Manufacturers of panoramic machines determine the manner in which the tubehead rotates around the patient's head. Some have a double center rotation, having two centers of rotation, one for the right side and one for the left side of the patient's jaws. With this type of rotation, the machine will automatically shift to the second center of rotation. Others have a triple center rotation, or three centers of rotation moving in an automatic uninterrupted motion. Another type of rotation is called the continual moving center, which also moves, in an automatic uninterrupted motion (Figure 67–6).

Equipment

Control Panel

Most panoramic machines have preset timing factors on the control panel that are determined by the manufacturer. For example, it may have four settings to choose from, the first one being for a child, the second one for a small adult, the third for a medium-sized adult, and the last one for a large adult. This is to guide the operator in selecting the proper exposure setting, kilovolt peak (kVp), and milliamperes (mA); however, the operator can still make kVp and mA adjustments when necessary. The size of the patient will influence the setting of the machine. On some machines, there is a profile index meter located within the "head positioner" framework that takes a reading of the patient's head size. This reading is used in determining the proper setting for x-ray exposure (Figure 67-7).

The Tubehead

The tubehead is stationary and does not move vertically as does the intraoral x-ray tubehead. It slants upward slightly and rotates around the back of the patient's head when exposure is taking place. The collimator is in the shape of a slit, which allows the photons to exit in a narrow vertical rectangular beam, tall enough to affect the lower facial area up to the orbits of the eyes (Figure 67-8). The photons travel across the patient and affect the film through a vertical slit located on the drum or cassette. Because the x-ray beam is so narrow by comparison with the regular tubehead used for intraoral radiographs, the patient is exposed to less radiation. Even though the tubehead tilts upward and the patient receives less radiation, a lead apron without a thyroid collar is still used.

The Head Positioner

On each machine there is a place to position the patient's head. Within this framework, there will be the

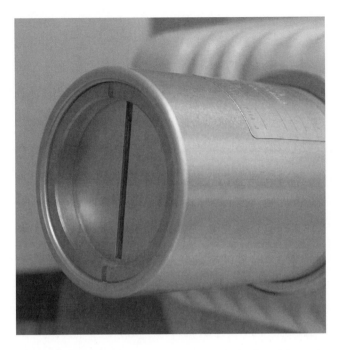

Figure 67-8 Collimator in tubehead is in the shape of a slit at the opening.

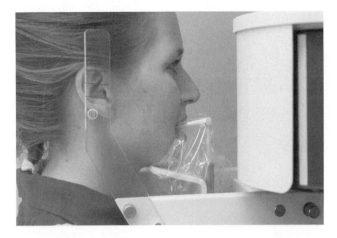

Figure 67-9 Head positioner and chin rest.

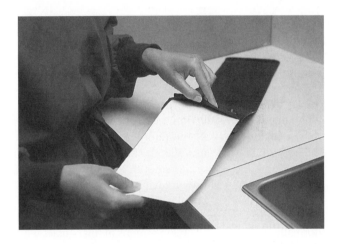

Figure 67-10 Film cassette that fits on the drum.

positioner guides, a bite block or rod, and a chin rest. These mechanisms aid the operator in positioning the patient accurately within the focal trough. It is of great importance that the patient be instructed to remain stationary, close the mouth, and place the tongue next to the palate. It should be noted that a knob controls the positioner guides where the operator is able to open or close in a horizontal direction to fit the patient's face. The bite block or rod is scored with grooves that serve to position the patient's maxillary and mandibular central teeth. The chin rest can be moved vertically to accommodate the patient (Figure 67-9).

Film Cassette and Intensifying Screen

The film cassette, which holds the intensifying screen and film, is located directly opposite the tubehead. On some machines the cassette is located in a "drum" and is flexible and rotates around the patient's head at the same speed as the tubehead. On other machines the cassette is rigid and moves slowly from side to side as opposed to rotating around the patient during the exposure (Figure 67-10).

Intensifying screens are composed of either rare earth or calcium tungstate phosphor. These materials glow or emit light when affected by x-ray photons, which in turn expose the film. Calcium tungstate was common

in previous years and emits blue light. The rare earth, which emits green light, is four times more efficient than calcium tungstate in converting x-ray energy into light and therefore uses less radiation. Because of the rapid reaction between these materials and x-ray photons, the patient receives less radiation (Figure 67-11).

Panoramic film is available in two sizes, 5 x 12 and 6 x 12 in., and is sensitive to blue light or green light for flexible or rigid cassettes. When ordering film, the size and type of film will dictate which one to purchase. If rare intensifying screen is used, the film sensitive to green light should be purchased; if calcium tungstate intensifying screen is used, the film sensitive to blue light should be purchased. "Panoramic" film should not be confused with "duplicating" film (Figure 67-12).

When inspecting the flexible cassette, it is always wise to look for smudges on the intensifying screen, as they will transfer onto the radiograph as dark spots. Smudges can be removed with a special screen cleaner.

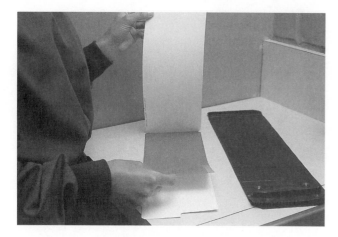

Figure 67-11 Intensifying screens.

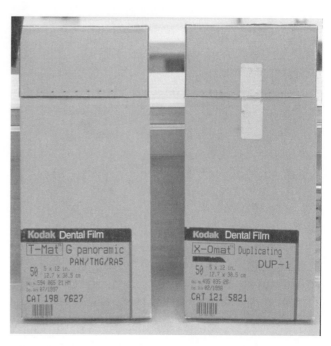

Figure 67-12 Panoramic film and duplicating film.

When loading the film in the darkroom under a special safelight and making certain it is shielded from white light, the film is inserted between two intensifying screen sheets, placing it as far as the film will go. One must observe that panoramic film is "extremely" sensitive to white light, and therefore, the darkroom must be white light safe. As the film is placed in the cassette, one must ensure that all of the film is making contact with the intensifying screens. With the flap of the cassette still open, one hand is used to smooth and remove any air pockets, as they will impair image formation.

Rigid cassettes are flat or curved, are constructed stronger, and wear longer. They are easier to load and will normally keep the intensifying screens in full contact with the film, and there is less chance of trapping air pockets.

Procedure

There are three areas of preparation to consider: preparation of the film, preparation of the x-ray machine, and preparation of the patient.

Preparation of the Film

The main areas of concern are to ensure that the proper film is positioned adequately between the intensifying screens inside the cassette and protection of film from white light. There are other critical considerations:

- Because panoramic film is so sensitive to light, loading of the film *must* take place in a darkroom where a proper safelight is used, such as the Kodak GBX-2.

- The intensifying screens have two sides. The inside portion should never be placed on the outward side as the phosphor will not affect the film in this position. Handling of the screens should be minimal due to the tendency of scratching them or allowing particles of foreign matter to adhere.

- The film should be handled with care, avoiding fingerprints or smudges, always holding it by the edges, as it is inserted into the intensifying screen as far as possible. Then it is placed into the cassette. The cassette should be checked for air pockets. Once film is loaded into the cassette and closed, it is mounted on the drum or cassette holder/carrier on the x-ray machine (Figure 67-13).

Preparation of the X-Ray Machine

- The film and cassette are loaded following specific manufacturer's instructions. It is necessary that the film be in the proper place. If mounted upside down,

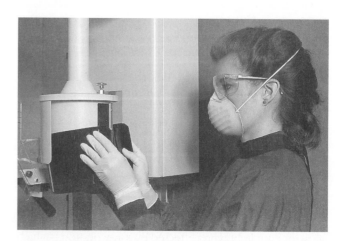

Figure 67-13 Cassette carrier or drum.

only half of the film will be exposed. Also, if the cassette is not placed at the starting point, the radiograph will be off center.

- The x-ray machine should be turned on and the appropriate setting selected.

- The tubehead should be in the starting position.

- The bite block/rod should be disinfected and covered with a plastic barrier.

Preparation of the Patient

- The procedure is explained to the patient.

- The patient is asked to remove all metallic and non-metallic objects from the head and neck area. These may include hairpins, hair clips, hats, hearing aids; all jewelry from ears, nose, neck, tongue, and lips; and dentures, removable bridges/partials, and retainers.

- The patient is draped with a lead apron protecting the patient on the front and back with no thyroid collar.

- The patient is instructed to sit or stand, extend the neck as straight and tall as possible, making sure the back is in a straight position, not "slouching."

- The patient's chin is positioned in the chin rest while guiding the anterior teeth to bite on the bite block, edge to edge. The teeth must be in contact with one of the grooves on the bite block, used to align the teeth in the focal trough.

- The positioner guide is adapted to the patient's face to establish the size of patient's frame.

- The patient's head is straight, ensuring that the **midsagittal plane** (an imaginary line that divides the body in right and left sides) is perpendicular to the floor and is evenly dividing the face in right and left sides.

- For the horizontal plane, the **Frankfort plane** (an imaginary line that is parallel to the floor and measured from the top of the ear canal to the inferior portion of the orbit of the eye) is used. Some x-ray machines use a light that illuminates the patient's Frankfort and midsagittal planes. Other machines use the ala-tragus line to match the lines on the positioner guide (Figure 67-14).

- The patient is instructed to swallow while placing his or her tongue at the roof of the mouth, close the lips, close the eyes, and not move while the x-ray tubehead is in motion. This process takes approximately 20 seconds or less (see Figure 67-9).

Processing

An identification tag with the date, patient's name, and dentist's name is made. This is used to label the film hanger (rack) when processing manually. A similar label is made and placed on the radiograph immediately after processing radiographs.

It is critical when unwrapping the film from the cassette that one does not cause static electricity to occur, as this will create an artifact of significant size. If loading a film hanger (rack) for manual processing, the film must be handled with caution, keeping in mind the nature of the film's sensitivity to light. The same processing time and temperature as that used with intraoral films is recommended. (Refer to Chapter 65 for processing techniques.)

Troubleshooting Errors

Errors are discussed and the correction given:

1. *Positioning the patient too far forward.* This will cause the anterior teeth to be outside of the focal trough; the anterior teeth will be out of focus or blurred and will look narrow. The premolars will be extremely overlapped. The spine will look superimposed on the area of the ramus.

   Correction: Ensure that the patient's anterior teeth are biting correctly on the bite block's grooves as indicated. If the patient has missing anterior teeth, the ridge should be placed slightly behind the groove (toward the tubehead). A cotton roll should be used to elevate the ridge to a more normal position.

2. *Positioning the patient too far back.* This will cause the anterior teeth to be outside the focal trough. The anterior teeth will be out of focus or blurred and will look wide. There may be ghosting of the mandible and spine (see #11).

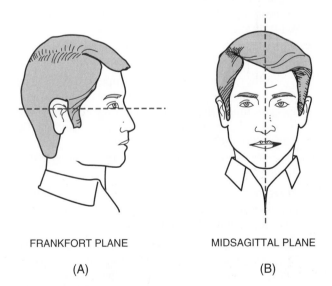

FRANKFORT PLANE

(A)

MIDSAGITTAL PLANE

(B)

Figure 67-14 (A) Midsagittal plane divides face in right and left sides. (B) Frankfort plane is an imaginary line from top of ear canal to the lower portion of the orbit that is parallel to the floor.

Correction: Ensure that the patient's anterior teeth are biting correctly in the grooves of the bite block as indicated. If the patient's anterior teeth are flared out, position the incisal edges further forward (away from tubehead), thus allowing the ridges (apices of anterior teeth) to be in the focal trough.

3. *Patient's head tilted too far down.* This will cause an exaggerated smile line to appear on the radiograph. The roots of the mandibular anterior teeth will be outside the focal trough. The hyoid bone will be superimposed on the mandibular anterior area. The premolars will be extremely overlapped. The condyles may be cut off.

   Correction: Ensure that the Frankfort plane is parallel to the floor when using a panoramic unit that has this guideline. On other panoramic units, the ala-tragus line is used to line up with the positioner guide.

4. *Patient's head tilted too far up.* This position will cause a reverse smile with the roots of the maxillary anterior teeth to be outside the focal trough. The maxillary anterior roots will be out of focus and the palate/floor of the nasal cavity will superimpose this area.

   Correction: Ensure that the Frankfort plane is parallel to the floor or that the ala-tragus line is lined up with the positioner guide.

5. *Patient's midsagittal plane is not perpendicular to the floor or the head is tilted to one side.* This position will appear to show one side of the mandible higher than the opposite side. One condyle will appear larger and its neck will look elongated.

   Correction: Ensure that the midsagittal plane is perpendicular to the floor. The operator may check the positioner guides to establish that the face is in central position.

6. *Patient's head is twisted.* The teeth on one side of the arch appear enlarged and overlapped; conversely, on the opposite side, teeth appear very narrow and not as overlapped. The ramus on one side appears much wider than the opposite side. The condyles differ in size. One side of the jaw will be malpositioned outside the focal trough and the opposite side of the jaw will be malpositioned inside the focal trough.

   Correction: Ensure that the patient's midsagittal plane is aligned with the center of the chin rest and that the patient is facing forward.

7. *Patient's tongue is not next to the palate.* A radiolucent or dark area will appear at the apices of maxillary teeth, preventing periapical diagnosis.

   Correction: Ensure that the patient understands to place the tongue next to the palate. Patient should be instructed to swallow and hold that position during the entire time of exposure.

8. *Patient's mouth is open.* A radiolucent or dark oval area will appear around the crowns of the incisors.

   Correction: Ensure that the patient understands to close the lips during the entire time of exposure.

9. *Patient moved during exposure.* One or more areas may be blurred due to patient movement during exposure. A small area of the panoramic radiograph will portray a blurred image, which results only while that increment was being exposed.

   Correction: Ensure that the patient understands that there is to be no movement during entire time of exposure.

10. *Patient's neck and back were not erect or straight but were "slouching."* This will cause the cervical spine to be prominent in the center of the film. The radiopaque area does not permit diagnosis in this area.

    Correction: Ensure that the patient understands to keep the spine erect and the neck stretched in an upward direction and to lower the shoulders.

11. *Radiopaque artifacts were present such as jewelry, partials, hearing aid, thyroid collar, etc., producing ghost images.* The real image of the object will appear in detailed form on the correct side; however, the **ghost image** will appear on the opposite side and it will be enlarged and slightly at a higher level than the real image.

    Correction: Ensure that the patient has removed all articles that will cause an artifact to appear on the radiograph. Do not use a thyroid collar or a neck chain.

12. *Irregular movement of the machine (tubehead).* This will appear as vertical dark lines spaced evenly on the radiograph, due to the machine's malfunction.

    Correction: Replace the worn part on the panoramic unit.

13. *Static electricity.* The appearance of smudges, "lightning-like" or "tree-like" radiolucent markings on the radiograph caused at the time of removing the exposed film from the cassette or due to low humidity or static producing materials.

    Correction: Avoid creating friction by quick removal of exposed film from cassette or unexposed film from its package. Use antistatic solutions to clean intensifying screens.

14. *Film placed incorrectly in the cassette.* A portion of the radiograph does not have an image. Film was not placed all the way into the fold of the intensifying screen.

    Correction: Ensure that the film is placed all the way into the "fold" of the intensifying screen.

15. *Intensifying screen was positioned inside out.* This will cause the radiograph to appear extremely light with very little image due to the film not being in

contact with the phosphor of the intensifying screen.

Correction: Ensure that the intensifying screen is not inside out while loading film into cassette. Look for the fold and observe that the tape that holds both sheets together is on the "outside" of the intensifying screen.

16. *Cassette not placed adequately into cassette carrier.* This will cause a partial image to appear on the radiograph. There will be a blank area on one side of the radiograph.

    Correction: Ensure that the cassette is positioned appropriately on the cassette carrier or drum according to manufacturer's instructions. It is important to know where the beginning of the film is located.

17. *Double exposure.* This will cause double images to appear on the radiograph and the radiograph will appear darker or have more density.

    Correction: Load the film in the cassette and place it in the cassette carrier yourself. Be assured that there is "new" film in the cassette.

SUGGESTED ACTIVITIES

● Practice loading a cassette according to instructions in the darkroom using the Kodak GBX-2 safelight.

● Practice positioning a fellow student for making a panoramic radiograph. Follow the step-by-step procedure in this chapter.

● Practice duplicating a panoramic radiograph (refer to Chapter 65) and process it.

REVIEW

1. Name the two major areas that would require a lateral jaw radiograph: (1) full head, (2) body of the mandible, (3) condyle, and/or (4) occlusal aspect.
   a. 1, 2   c. 3, 4
   b. 2, 3   d. 1, 4

2. Indicate what problems may occur if the patient's jaws are not in the focal trough: (1) magnification of structures, (2) reduction of structures, (3) blurred and out of focus, and/or (4) exaggerated smile.
   a. 1, 2, 3   c. 1, 2, 4
   b. 2, 3, 4   d. 1, 3, 4

3. What is the purpose of using intensifying screens in panoramic radiography?
   a. They reduce the amount of radiation the patient would otherwise receive.
   b. They protect the film from white light.
   c. They glow when affected by x-ray photons.
   d. They add to the rigidity of the cassette.
   e. Both a and c

4. Name the limitations of using panoramic radiography: (1) it produces slight magnification of images, (2) it produces overlapping images around the bicuspid area, (3) it produces too much radiation, and/or (4) the detail and definition are not as precise as intraoral radiographs.
   a. 1, 2, 3
   b. 2, 3, 4
   c. 1, 2, 4
   d. 1, 3, 4

5. Match the troubleshooting errors on the left with the radiographic appearance on the right:

   ___ a. Patient too far back

   ___ b. Patient too far forward

   ___ c. Patient's head tilted down

   ___ d. Patient's head tilted up

   ___ e. Patient's head twisted

   ___ f. Patient's tongue not at palate

   ___ g. Patient's mouth open

   ___ h. Patient slouching, not erect

   ___ i. Radiopaque artifacts on image

   ___ j. Intensifying screen inside out

   1. Teeth on one side are enlarged and overlapped and teeth on opposite side are narrow and not overlapped

   2. An exaggerated smile line

   3. Anterior teeth out of focus and look wide

   4. A radiolucent oval around crowns of incisors

   5. Jewelry, thyroid collar, or other objects appear radiopaque with a ghost image on opposite side of radiograph

   6. Cervical spine very prominent in center of radiograph

   7. Radiolucency at the apices of maxillary teeth

   8. Radiograph appears extremely light with little image

   9. Reverse smile with roots of maxillary teeth out of focus

   10. Anterior teeth out of focus and look narrow

Digital Imaging Systems in Oral Radiography

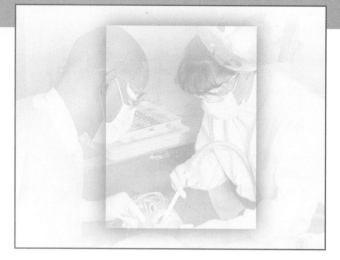

OBJECTIVES

After studying this chapter, the student will be able to:

- Identify component parts of a digital imaging system.
- Describe the purpose of electronic sensors.
- Discuss the advantages and disadvantages of using digital imaging.
- Discuss the principles of digital imaging.
- Identify how much reduction of radiation can be attained by using digital imaging.

Introduction

With the computer age upon us, radiography has adopted many changes. Several years ago the concept of using computer technology in radiology was considered to be a thing of the distant future. As electronics (having to do with electrons) have evolved in dentistry, **digital imaging** (an image comprised of computer pixel elements) has gained increased favor and is now being used in several universities and dental offices.

This chapter will focus on how the component parts of the digital imaging system work, how the image is acquired, and how the data are recorded. Examples of advantages and disadvantages will be discussed and an overview of the procedure of its use will be given.

What is Digital Imaging?

Digital imaging radiography is a method by which an image is processed into a digital format that can be displayed for viewing and electronically stored by means of a computer. Capturing the image can be done using either indirect or direct methods.

Indirect Method

The *indirect method* involves the digitizing of a traditional dental radiograph by using a video camera on a scanner device. Some newer methods use a special dig-

itizing plate in place of dental film. After exposure, the plate is placed in a scanner that converts the image information into the digital format for the computer.

Direct Method

The *direct method* uses a sensor directly in the mouth. These are called **charged coupled-devices (CCDs)**. The image is directly captured by the sensors and converted to the digital format for immediate viewing on the computer monitor.

Digital imaging radiography offers several features that potentially promote the quality of diagnosis: the use of color, the ability of magnification, and the ability to alter degrees of density to the image on the screen, known as contrast enhancement.

A digital image (an image that has been recorded with a nonfilm receptor) requires less ionized radiation, in some cases by as much as 90% reduction of exposure, as compared to radiographs. It makes use of intraoral **electronic sensors** (filmless portion of the digital imaging system) instead of film and uses a computer (an electronic device that has the ability to retain entered data in its memory) and a printer (output mechanism that converts data into printed form) instead of using a viewing screen (Figure 68-1). It records data, which are stored in the memory of the computer. These data can be viewed on the monitor screen and printed out as hard copy (printed copy) to be kept in the patient's file or sent to an insurance company or to another dentist.

How It Works

Digital imaging is based on the premise that the information is acquired by using a computer as the main

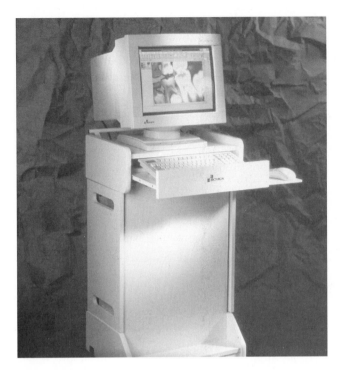

Figure 68-1 Full digital imaging system. (Courtesy of Schick Technologies, Inc.)

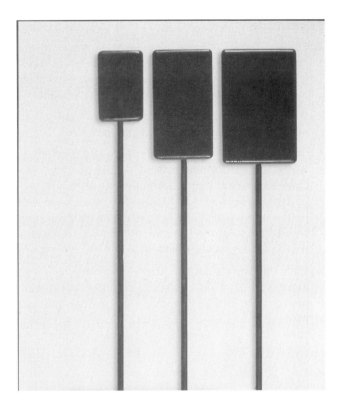

Figure 68-2 Electronic sensors. (Courtesy of Schick Technologies, Inc.)

component of the digital system. The newer systems offer a set of electronic sensors, used in place of film. A remote module contains the support circuitry for the sensors and for data transmission to the computer. The keyboard allows the operator to input data. The computer has the ability to retain entered data in its memory. The monitor can display the image in color or black and white. The printer can make a hard copy (printed copy). One must keep in mind that the x-ray machine, though not part of the system, is also a key element because it produces the x-ray photons that affect the electrons within the sensors to produce a latent image. The latent image is transmitted and stored on the computer and displayed on the monitor.

Other systems use **digital image receptors (DIRs)** comparable to the electronic sensors. These receptors form a digital image in the following manner. Within the DIR is the CCD array, which is a silicon chip containing an active area that connects to a computer electronically. This chip, being sensitive to either x-ray photons or visible light, is limited in size depending on the size of the receptor. When the image is made, it can be stored in the computer memory for image processing or displayed on the monitor. With these models, the exposure to radiation for the patient is reduced by approximately 50% when compared to using D-speed film and x-ray photons to produce a radiograph.

Electronic Sensors. It is important to discuss the electronic sensors in more detail as they are the filmless por-

tion of the digital imaging system and are the key to producing images. They consist of an integrated circuit with a large array of photodetectors. Sensors come in different sizes, similar to the same sizes of film, and may be attached to a flexible cord. For example, one company makes three sizes, 0, 1, and 2, comparable to film sizes of 0, 1, and 2, the most frequently used of these would be sizes 1 and 2 (Figure 68-2). At this time other companies have sizes that are similar in width but not always in length. When the length is shorter, the full images of the teeth may not always be seen. They may not include the apical portion or may include the apical portion but not a portion of the crown. Therefore, numerous exposures would be made to compensate for the size of the sensor.

Infection Control. When using the sensors, it is imperative to know how to barrier them to establish infection control. Sensors cannot be sterilized in an autoclave due to their delicate nature, and placing them in a chemical sterilizer would be out of the question due to the time factor. The use of a plastic barrier is recommended with additional spraying of a disinfectant prior to using it on the next patient. Purchasing extra sensors for the sole purpose of preventing transmission of diseases is not economical.

Advantages

- The reduction of ionized radiation exposure to the patient by as much as 90% is a key factor in considering this method of recording radiographic data. This is possibly the greatest advantage to the consumer.

- Images can be viewed immediately as opposed to processing of films, which may require up to 15 or 20 minutes.

- Patient education where there is little need to convince the patient that a restorative procedure is necessary in promoting oral health. The patient is able to understand what is taking place by visually inspecting the problem area on the monitor and able to participate in making oral care decisions.

- With the elimination of film and processing films, there would be no need to purchase radiographic film or processing chemicals, thus saving time and money.

Disadvantages

- The high cost of the system.

- Resolutions of sensors and screen monitors are not as defined as the traditional film.

- Positioning of electronic sensors in the oral cavity, keeping in mind that a cord is attached to the sensor, makes it more difficult for the operator to handle the procedure.

- When using digital imaging systems that use smaller electronic sensors, the operator would be required to make more exposures for a complete set of images of all teeth.

- The problem of infection control is still an issue for the operator as the sensors are not able to withstand the heat generated in autoclaves. It is also possible but not wise, logistically, to use chemical sterilization by immersion for 10 hours.

Digital Imaging Procedure. The procedure in producing an image is as follows:

- The x-ray machine and computer are turned on. The patient's name is entered into the computer. A computer-designed template for a full-mouth set consisting of 18 to 20 windows or less is selected.

- The patient is draped with a lead apron and thyroid collar.

- Instructions are given the patient and the procedure is explained.

- The sensor with a plastic barrier is placed in the patient's mouth. Some companies provide holders similar to Rinn holders, which will fit their sensors.

- The x-ray tubehead is directed to the area of interest where the sensor is already in place.

- The exposure is made using up to 90% less radiation exposure than when using regular "D-speed" film. The sensor reacts to x-ray **emissions** (discharge of electrons), and the **electrons** (negatively charged particles of an atom) that register the latent image are transferred to the computer where they are changed into digital data and displayed as an image on the monitor.

- Once it is registered on the monitor, the dentist may enlarge and reposition the image on the screen, using a mouse. Certain areas can be highlighted in color, if desired. Arrows can be added for clarification or to point out areas of special concern. The picture can be changed into a reverse image where the light areas become dark and vice-versa (Figure 68-3).

- Transmitting a copy of the image to another dentist or to an insurance company can be done immediately by using a phone line, provided that the receiver has a compatible computer. This is similar to sending a facsimile (FAX). A hard copy (printed copy) can be made by printing out the information seen on the monitor screen. The patient's name would already be recorded. This feature could avoid labeling errors.

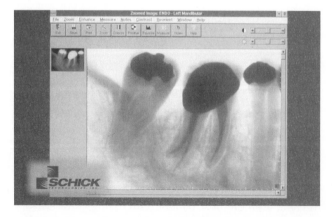 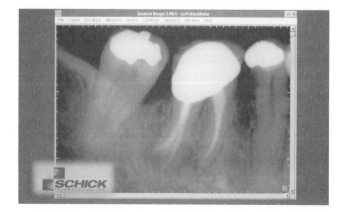

Figure 68-3 Changes in images for contrast, color, and depth. (Courtesy of Schick Technologies, Inc.)

SUGGESTED ACTIVITY

● Using a manikin and an intraoral CCD sensor, make an exposure using the lowest setting on the x-ray machine. Using the image on the monitor screen, try to enhance it by adding more contrast until the desired effect is reached.

REVIEW

1. Digital imaging system component parts include which of the following: (1) an x-ray machine, (2) electronic sensors, (3) a computer, and/or (4) a monitor.
   a. 1, 2, 3
   b. 2, 3, 4
   c. 1, 2, 4
   d. 1, 3, 4

2. What is an electronic sensor?
   a. The filmless portion of the digital imaging system
   b. A film converted into a digitized sensor
   c. An integrated circuit with a large array of photodetectors
   d. All of the above
   e. Both a and c

3. Indicate what are some advantages of the digital imaging system: (1) reasonable cost of equipment, (2) reduces ionized radiation exposure to the patient by as much as 90%, (3) images are viewed immediately on the monitor, and/or (4) processing solutions are not needed.
   a. 1, 2, 3
   b. 2, 3, 4
   c. 1, 2, 4
   d. 1, 3, 4

4. Indicate some disadvantages of the digital imaging system: (1) resolution of sensors and screen monitors are not as good as a radiograph, (2) positioning of electronic sensors with a cord attached into the oral cavity, (3) more difficult to do patient education using the monitor, and/or (4) more difficult to achieve infection control.
   a. 1, 2, 3
   b. 2, 3, 4
   c. 1, 2, 4
   d. 1, 3, 4

5. Once the digital image is registered on the monitor, the operator is able to:
   a. Change the image by highlighting desired areas in color
   b. Add arrows to point out areas of special concern
   c. Transmit a copy to another office or insurance company via the phone line
   d. All of the above
   e. Both a and b

CHAPTER 69

Image Detail and Quality Analysis of Radiographs

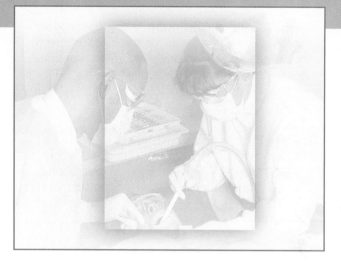

OBJECTIVES

After studying this chapter, the student will be able to:

● Distinguish between radiolucent and radiopaque and give an example of each.

● Explain why it is important to have a small anode target when producing photons.

● Describe how penumbra can be diminished.

● Explain how magnification can occur and how to diminish it.

● State three factors that influence the density on a radiograph.

● Explain why the inverse square law exists.

Introduction

As dental radiographs are now accepted as routine in dental practice and are generally accepted by the public, the operator of the dental x-ray equipment must not fail to exhibit "reasonable and ordinary skill" in this area of dental care. Radiographs must be on file with the patient's record for future use. They must be factual and provide evidence of the need for operative dental procedures and, on occasion, in court.

One must remember that, in a court of law, the best evidence is factual. However, mere introduction of radiographs in court is not assurance of their value if the films are inadequate because of poor placement, exposure, or processing.

The radiographs in Figure 69-1 show the basic selection of landmarks that may be visible on radiographs placed in the proper area for a complete periapical series, including bite wings.

It is the radiographer's duty to determine if radiographs have proper diagnostic qualities. There are many factors that influence these qualities. For example, when a radiograph appears too dark or too light and the image appears blurry and out of focus, one could determine that something went wrong. These problems should be considered and repeated mistakes avoided. It is important for the radiographer to be able to determine what the problem was and correct it.

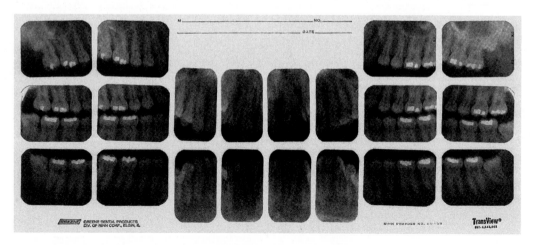

Figure 69-1 Complete radiographic series. (Courtesy of Rinn Corporation, Elgin, IL.)

The Radiographic Image

Radiolucent and radiopaque are terms used to describe the darkness and lightness of images on radiographs. The image on a radiograph depicts many shades of gray, including some black and white areas.

Radiolucent

The dark areas are known as **radiolucent** because x-ray photons were able to penetrate through open spaces or soft tissue reaching the film, creating dark shadows. Examples are soft tissues and sinuses.

Radiopaque

The light areas are known as **radiopaque** because x-ray photons are blocked by dense structures such as bone, enamel, dentin, and metallic restorations that absorb or block some or all photons from reaching the film.

The Visual Image

The visual image is a graphic representation of the internal structures of an object placed in the path of the x-ray beam. The primary objective is to obtain maximum differentiation of tissues on the film. This differentiation is realized only when the film has four visual qualities: radiographic density, radiographic contrast, radiographic distortion (or lack of it), and radiographic detail. Although the quality of the x-ray beam depends on certain factors concerned with the production of the beam, the visual (diagnostic) quality of the radiograph depends on radiographic density and contrast.

Radiographic Density. *Density* is described as the degree of darkness on a radiograph and is influenced by the following:

- *Varying the milliampere (mA) setting.* By increasing the mA, more x-ray photons will be produced that affect the film and the radiograph will appear darker or it will be more dense. The operator should remember that the mA controls the *quantity* or number of photons produced. Fifteen milliamperes produces a larger quantity of photons than 10 mA does (Figure 69-2).

- *Varying the kilovoltage peak (kVp) setting.* The density of the radiograph can also be controlled by the kVp. The higher the kVp, the higher the energy of the x-ray photons, and a larger number of high energy photons will affect the film (Figure 69-3).

- *Varying the exposure time.* An increase in exposure time also allows a longer time frame for photons to affect the film, thereby increasing the density of the radiograph (Figure 69-4).

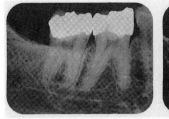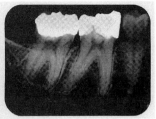

Figure 69-2 Varying mA's—controls density by producing the number of electrons.

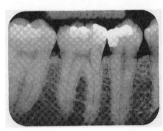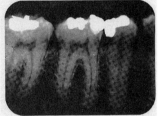

Figure 69-3 Varying kVp's—higher or lower contrast.

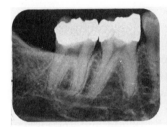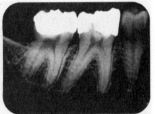

Figure 69-4 Varying exposure time—light and dark radiographs.

Radiographic Contrast. **Contrast** is described as the number of shades of gray seen on a radiograph. The higher the contrast, the fewer shades of gray will be evident. When lower than 70 kVp is used, it will produce a **short scale** or high contrast. This means that it will be hard to define the shades of gray because they will be either too dark or too light with not many grays in between (Figure 69-5A). The opposite is true when higher than 85 kVp is used, it will produce a **long scale** or low contrast with more visible shades of gray (Figure 69-5B). A step wedge is used to determine how many different shades of gray on a radiograph can be produced (Figure 69-6). It is made of aluminum containing several steps of layered thicknesses used to test the x-ray machine's effectiveness in producing varying degrees of contrast.

Other influencing factors affecting the contrast of the radiograph are known as "object contrast" and are listed here:

- Object density (how compact the object is)
- Object thickness
- X-ray beam quality (how penetrating it is)
- Amount of scatter radiation affecting the film

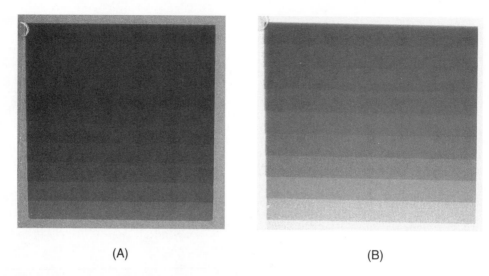

(A)   (B)

Figure 69-5 Short scale vs. long scale. Compare radiographs taken at 40 kVp, where they have short scale or high contrast, with radiographs taken at 100 kVp, where they have many shades of gray or long scale and low contrast.

Radiographs should be of diagnostic quality; otherwise they are useless. The radiographer needs to determine, in advance, if the machine has proper kVp, mA, and exposure time settings for each individual. Generally, these settings are adjustable, which allows the operator to make changes as deemed necessary for object density and thickness. For example, if a child was the patient, the settings should be lowered to compensate for the child's small frame. If a large obese adult is to follow the child, the settings on the same machine need to be increased to allow the beam to penetrate more tissue and to compensate for the focal-film distance. If the same setting was used for both of these patients, the radiographs on the child would be very dark in comparison to the large adult's radiographs, which would be very light.

Film Fog Affecting Contrast. Film fog is known as the undesirable film exposure to light, radiation, or chemicals that affect the quality of a radiograph by increasing overall darkness. These occurrences can take place in the following manner:

- *Light fog.* Any time the film is exposed to white light whether it happened before or during processing where the darkroom is not light safe (Figure 69-7).

- *Exposure to radiation.* This could take place when stored film is unprotected from radiation while the patient is being exposed.

- *Processing techniques.* This may take place when the film is chemically fogged by processing it in the developer for an extended length of time or the temperature of the solutions is elevated.

Figure 69-6 Step wedge scale.

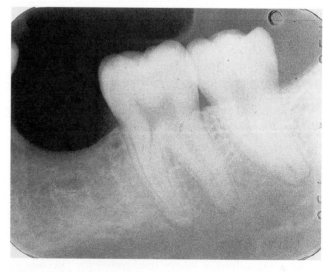

Figure 69-7 Film fog.

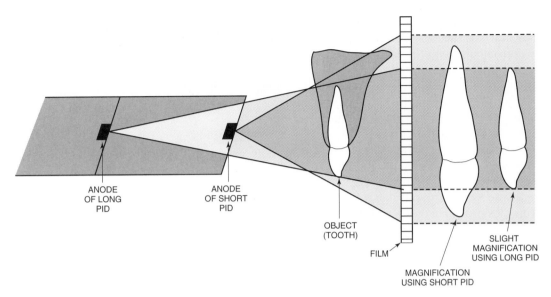

Figure 69-8 Short vs. long PID. The shorter the PID, the more magnification of the object.

Radiographic Distortion

Distance from Source to Object and Film. The distance from the anode to the object and film affects the film in the following ways: causes lack of sharpness, (definition), magnification, and distortion.

Definition. The definition of a radiograph pertains to the overall sharpness of the image of the object. When the object appears fuzzy, it exhibits **penumbra**, meaning that it does not have a sharp or clear image. If the object appears to have a shadow, it exhibits **umbra**. Factors causing poor definition are as follows:

- *Movement of the patient, film, or tubehead* will cause the radiograph to appear blurred, exhibiting poor definition in which the dentist cannot see the image clearly. This situation can be compared to photographs that appear blurred when the subject moved or when the photographer moved the camera.

- The *anode focal spot size* will control the image detail on the radiograph. The focal spot is made smaller than the actual focal spot area by inclining the anode at 20°. The smaller the focal spot, the smaller the area of effective focus. This means that the source of x-ray photons would come from one small area or point, about 1 mm in size. If this happens, less distortion or penumbra will occur on the image because all photons would be generated in the same spot, as opposed to having a large focal spot where photons would be coming from a large area, creating increased penumbra.

- *Focal-film distance (FFD)* refers to the distance from the source of photons or the anode focal spot to the film. If the distance is shorter, as when an 8-in. position-indicating device (PID) is used, it will magnify

(enlarge) the image. However, if the distance is longer, as when a 16-in. PID is used, the image will conform more precisely to the size of the object (Figure 69-8).

- *Object-film distance (OFD)* refers to the distance created from the object (tooth) to the film. It is more desirable to have the film as close to the object as possible in a parallel position; otherwise, magnification (enlargement) of the object will take place.

- *Size of silver halide crystals in film emulsion.* The type of film affects the definition of the radiograph. E-speed film is composed of larger silver halide crystals that contributes to the "grainy" appearance on the radiograph, in comparison to D-speed film that produces sharper definition.

Magnification

There are two factors that affect magnification:

- Focal-film distance—using a short PID instead of a long one

- Object-film distance—placing the film away from the object (teeth)

Distortion. Distortion means that the size or shape of the object is not accurate. There are some factors that can cause distortion:

- *PID angulation.* When excessive angulation occurs, it causes the image to appear foreshortened (shorter than the real object). Ideally, the PID should be perpendicular to the object and film, and the object and film should be as parallel to one another as possible. If the angulation of the PID is less than the prescribed angulation, the opposite distortion occurs. The image appears *elongated* (longer than the real object).

• *Film not being parallel to the object.* When using the parallel technique, in which the PID is perpendicular to the object and film, and the object and film are parallel to one other, distortion is minimized. However, when using the bisecting-angle technique, where only the crown portions of the teeth are in close proximity to the film and where the PID is directed at the bisection of the angle formed by the long axis of the teeth and the film, distortion takes place. This is due to the alignment of the object in relation to the film. Foreshortening or elongation of the object may be viewed. Another cause for distortion is due to arching of the film (not being parallel to the teeth) as in digital retention. As a result, the entire film is bent, resulting in elongation or a stretched-out look to take place (Figure 69-9).

Inverse Square Law

The **inverse square law** states that the intensity of the beam is inversely proportional with the square of the distance from the source. The intensity of the x-ray beam diminishes more and more as it travels further away from the anode. It has been mentioned that the operator should be at least 6–8 feet away from the path of the primary beam to not be affected by its rays. Therefore, it stands to reason that the effect of the rays or its penetrating power dissipates as the distance from the anode increases. By using a long PID as opposed to a short PID, the operator needs to realize that there has to be an adjustment made in the exposure time. To be able to compensate for the extended distance, the exposure time needs to be increased by a factor of 4. To do this, a formula has been established using the FFD in relation to the exposure time. Suppose that the FFD was changed from 8 to 16 in., now being twice as long as it was before. The word "twice" refers to the number 2. This is squared, giving a total of 4. It would be reasonable to take the exposure time allotted for an 8-in. PID and "quadruple" it, or multiply by 4. when using the 16-in. PID. In other words, supposing that 2/10 was the timing used with an 8-in. PID, now 2/10 would be multiplied by 4 and the new exposure time using a 16-in. PID would be 8/10. It would take this much more timing (8/10) using a 16-in. PID to achieve the same intensity that 2/10 timing did for the 8-in. PID.

The inverse square law formula is summarized as follows.

Baseline:	Timing
PID size = 8 in.	2/10

Increase to:
PID size = 16 in. (twice as long),
2 x 2 = 4
4 x 2/10 (old timing) = 8/10

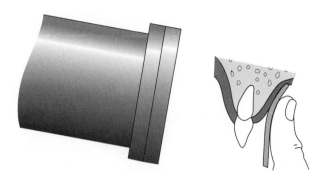

Figure 69-9 Film not parallel to object.

To bring this theory into perspective, the use of squares will demonstrate how the intensity of the beam becomes weaker as it travels further. Figure 69-10 shows that at 8 in., the intensity of the beam affected 4 squares, but at 16 in. it affected 16 squares; however, the intensity was much weaker. To achieve the same intensity as at 8 in., the exposure time would have to be increased.

Film Inadequacies

Several factors contribute to inadequate radiographic images and render them useless for proper diagnosis, as seen in Table 69-1. Some common inadequacies and their causative factors are listed. Care must be taken to avoid such results when making and handling radiographs.

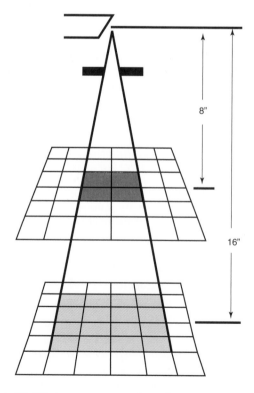

Figure 69-10 Inverse square law diagram.

Table 69-1 Radiographic Inadequacies and Causative Factors

Inadequacy	Causative Factor	Inadequacy	Causative Factor
Elongation 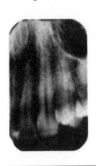	Insufficient vertical angulation	Density—too light 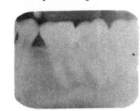	Insufficient exposure Insufficient develpoment Excessive fixation Solutions too cold Use of aged, contaminated, or poorly mixed solutions Outdated films Wrong side if film placed toward tube (leaded side of packet toward teeth)
Foreshortening 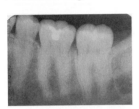 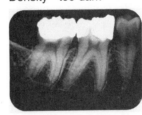	Excessive vertical angulation	Density—too dark 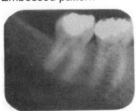	Excessive exposure Excessive development Too warm temperature of developer Unsafe safelight Exposure to overhead light (may be black after processing
		Embossed pattern 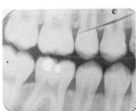	Foil side of film placed next to teeth
Partial image 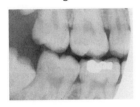	Cone-cut (either incorrect direction of central ray or incorrect film placement) Incompletely immersed in processing solutions Film touched other film or side of tank during processing	Dark lines 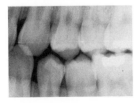	Moon-shaped mark left by fingernail Film bent or creased Wrapper sticking to film when opened due to excess patient's saliva (not drying film surface after exposure) Static electricity (film removed with force prior to processing)
Overlapping	Incorrect horizontal angulation (central ray not directed through interproximal)	Stains and spots 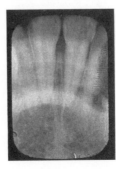	Finger marks Unclean hanger and/or clips Developer, fixer, water, or dust splatter Splattering dry films with solutions or water Air bells adhering to film surface (insufficient agitation of films) Insufficient rinsing after developing before fixing Overlapping of films in tanks or on drying racks Paper wrapper stuck to film during processing
No Image	Machine not functioning properly Machine not turned on during exposure Film placed in fixer before developer		

(Continued)

Table 69-1 Radiographic Inadequacies and causative Factors (Continued)

Inadequacy	Causative Factor	Inadequacy	Causative Factor
Blurred image	Movement of film, patient, or tube during exposure Film exposed a second time	Light fog	Exposure to light (either prior to or during processing Unsafe safelight Darkroom leak
Stretched appearance of teeth or supporting tissues)	Film plane was bent, not flat, overcontoured	Reticulation	Sudden temperature changes between processing solutions and wash water
		Latent film	Incomplete processing and/or rinsing
Fog Chemical fog	Deterioration of processing solutions Imbalance of chemicals in solutions		
Radiation fog	Improper storage of film (both unused and exposed prior to processing)	Discoloration	Too warm a storage place Stored too close to chemicals

SUGGESTED ACTIVITIES

- Using a step wedge, expose films at varying mA, kVp, and exposure time and make a comparison of density of each radiograph. Which one demonstrated the highest density? Which one demonstrated the lowest density? Which one demonstrated higher contrast? Which one demonstrated lower contrast?

- Expose first film at 15 mA, 90 kVp, and average exposure time.

- Expose second film at 10 mA, 80 kVp, and average exposure time.

- Expose third film at 10 mA, 65 kVp, and less than average exposure time

REVIEW

1. The quantity of photons produced is controlled by the:
   a. mA
   b. kVp
   c. exposure time
   d. Both a and b

2. The contrast of a radiograph is controlled by the:
   a. mA
   b. kVp
   c. exposure time
   d. Both b and c

3. Indicate how fog can occur on a radiograph: (1) overexposure to radiation, (2) leaving the film in the fixer for an extended period of time, (3) exposing film to white light during processing, and/or (4) leaving unexposed film on the counter top while x-rays are being made.

    a. 1, 2, 3

    b. 2, 3, 4

    c. 1, 2, 4

    d. 1, 3, 4

4. What factor(s) can cause radiographic magnification?

    a. focal-film distance

    b. object-film distance

    c. focal-object distance

    d. Both a and b

    e. Both b and c

5. Indicate in what ways image distortion can occur on a radiograph: (1) bending the film, (2) excessive PID angulation, (3) film not being parallel to object, and/or (4) processing in the developer too long.

    a. 1, 2, 3

    b. 2, 3, 4

    c. 1, 2, 4

    d. 1, 3, 4

CHAPTER 70

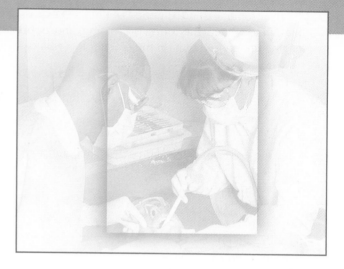

OBJECTIVES

After studying this chapter, the student will be able to:

● List five factors to consider when reviewing radiographs.

● Explain the difference between radiopaque and radiolucent.

● Describe the appearance of various tooth structures on a radiograph.

● Identify the anatomical landmarks of the maxilla and mandible on radiographs.

Introduction

A thorough knowledge of radiographic anatomy is a prerequisite in evaluating normal radiographic images. The operator must have a thorough knowledge of the anatomy of the head and all the landmarks of the skull. *Note:* Refer frequently to Figures 70-1A, B, and C as the structure of the head is discussed.

As already described in previous chapters, radiopaque and radiolucent are terms used to describe the darkness or lightness of images in radiographs. Radiopaque refers to anatomical areas that appear lighter in radiographs. This results from more x-rays being absorbed by the object. Radiolucent areas are those that appear darker, such as the periodontal ligament. This results from more x-rays passing through the area to expose the film. Table 70-1 summarizes maxillary and mandibular radiolucent and radiopaque structures.

Density of Tooth Structures

Enamel, Dentin, and Cementum (Radiopaque)

Because tooth substance is the densest component of the human body, it absorbs more x-rays than any other tissue of comparable size and thickness. The normal tooth has an outer covering called enamel, a middle layer called dentin, and cementum that covers the root. Dentin and cementum have nearly the same capacity to absorb x-rays; therefore, radiographic evidence does not differentiate between the two. Both present a uniform gray or white radiographic shadow with no evidence of particular structure or shape.

The coronal portion of the tooth covered by a thin layer of enamel is revealed in radiographs as a homogeneous cap that has greater whiteness than that of the dentin. The line of demarcation between enamel and dentin is sharp and clearly defined. In normal teeth the enamel is of uniform density except in depressions, which are situated chiefly on the mesial and distal aspects of the crown. Because the enamel is thinner, less radiation is absorbed and the darkness of that particular portion of the radiograph increases.

The Pulp Chamber and Root Canals (Radiolucent)

The pulp chamber and root canals are continuous cavities within the teeth. They contain soft tissue that absorbs fewer x-rays than the surrounding dentin does; therefore, a dark shadow is produced within the shadow of the tooth itself. The shape of the pulp chamber is, on the whole, fairly constant, and there is a general pattern for each of the various types of teeth. It is common for some teeth to show an elongation or an increase in the size of one or more of the *cornua* (projections). This may be of great importance in the preparation for restorations. In children of normal health and development, the size of the pulp chamber is rather large. As they grow older, most persons reveal considerable reduction in the size of the pulp chamber. The change may be seen in both the coronal portion and the root canals.

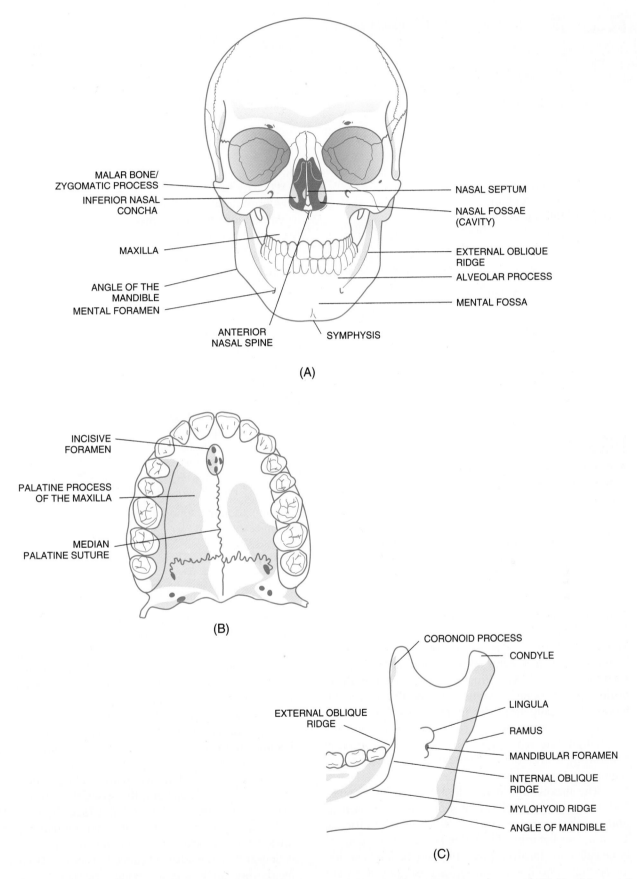

Figure 70-1 Anatomical landmarks of the skull showing (A) facial bones, (B) palatine process, and (C) lingual aspect of mandible.

Table 70-1 A Summary of Radiographic Landmarks

Maxillary Arch	
Anterior Area	**Posterior Area**
Radiolucent	
Median palatine suture	Maxillary sinus
Incisive foramen	
Nasal cavity/fossa	
Maxillary sinus (anterior portion)	
Radiopaque	
Anterior nasal spine	Maxillary tuberosity
Nasal septum	Floor of nasal cavity/palatine process
Inferior turbinate bones	Malar bone (zygomatic process)
Lower border of the nasal cavity	Floor or maxillary sinus
Wall of maxillary sinus	Coronoid process (seen on maxillary radiograph)

Mandibular Arch	
Anterior Area	**Posterior Area**
Radiolucent	
Lingual foramen	Mental foramen
	Mandibular canal
Radiopaque	
Genial tubercles	Mental process (ridge)
	Mylohyoid ridge
	External oblique ridge
	Internal oblique ridge
	Walls of mandibular canal

Other Landmarks	
Radiolucent	**Radiopaque**
Pulp chamber and pulpal canals	Enamel, dentin, cementum
Periodontal ligament	Lamina dura
Medullary spaces	Cortical plate
Nutrient canals	Trabeculae

The Alveolar Process (Radiopaque)

The alveolar process is a part of the maxilla (and mandible) and forms the investing and supporting tissues for the teeth. As a structural material, **cancellous bone** (spongy bone) is homogeneous, although it differs mechanically from **compact bone** (hard dense bone) in that it possesses less strength. Cancellous bone is usually found where the chief function of the bony structure is to transmit tensile and compressive strains (Figure 70-2A).

The maxilla and mandible are made up of outer and inner alveolar plates of bone, termed **cortical plates**, which serve as cortices of the alveolar process. The tooth socket is lined by a thin layer of dense cortical bone called the **lamina dura**. Beyond the lamina dura, the spongy cancellous bone serves to support the teeth and to anchor them to the mandible or maxilla. On the lingual and labial surfaces of the spongy bone are covering plates of dense bone named alveolar plates. The alveolar plates, spongy bone, and lamina dura are termed the alveolar process. The radiolucent parts of spongy bone when viewed on a radiograph are called **medullary spaces**; the thin radiopaque lines separating them are called **trabeculae** (Figure 70-2B).

Adjacent to the lamina dura lies the periodontal ligament. This is delicate, thin, vascular tissue of a density insufficient to absorb any appreciable amount of x-rays. On the other side of the ligament lies the lamina dura, which does cast a shadow. With a dense structure on either side of the ligament, the space that the ligament occupies appears as a thin dark line (see Figure 70-2A).

The bone adjacent to the periodontal ligament lines the tooth socket. In common with cortical bone, it is denser than the adjacent cancellous bone. Because of its density, this layer of bone (the lamina dura) is revealed in radiographs as a thin white line. This line is of utmost importance in radiographic interpretation. If

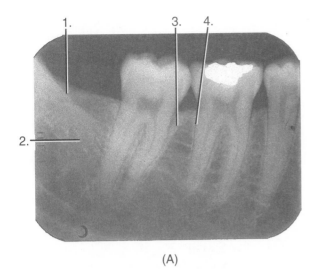

(A)

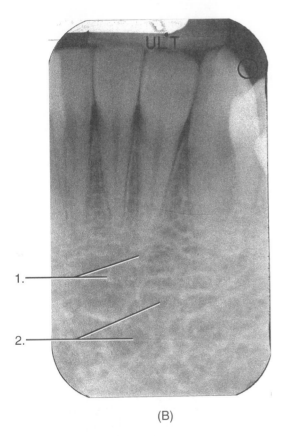

(B)

Figure 70-2 (A) Alveolar process with (1) compact bone, (2) cancellous bone, (3) lamina dura, and (4) periodontal ligament. (B) Alveolar process with (1) trabeculae and (2) medullary spaces.

one bears in mind the great variety of shapes of the roots of teeth and the physical factors that enter into the production of the shadow of the lamina dura, it is easy to understand why there must be great radiographic differences in the lamina dura. Differences in thickness, density, shape, and the number of shadows would be expected merely from the study of cross sections of sockets as seen in dried skulls. All these differences in

the radiographic appearance of lamina dura have no clinical significance as long as the lamina dura is continuous throughout its extent. Any deviation from this, slight deficiency, or discontinuity is highly suggestive and probably indicative of an abnormal condition.

The Maxilla and Mandible

It is important to note that no radiographic differentiation is possible between the cancellous bone of the alveolar process and the cortical plates that cover the lingual and buccal aspects of those processes. In the maxilla, the whole of the supporting bone, extending from the alveolar crest to the floor of the antrum and the nasal fossa, commonly presents a finer network of trabecular pattern and a uniform appearance. The mandible, however, usually does not present a uniform trabecular pattern and is more open (Figure 70-2B).

Landmarks of the Maxilla

There are two maxillary processes that, together, form the upper jaw. Each bone, consisting of four processes, also contains a large air-filled cavity within it called the maxillary sinus.

The Nasal Cavity (Radiolucent)

The **nasal fossae** or cavities often appear in the radiograph as dark shadows, at least in some part, because they contain air. Since the lower portions of the **inferior turbinate** (osseus) **bone** occupy some part of the nasal fossae, the dark area is not of uniform density. The **nasal septum**, which presents a gray or white dividing shadow of variable width, separates the fossae (Figures 70-1A and 70-3A).

The nasal fossae are roughly pear shaped when seen in the large extraoral radiographs made in the posterior and anterior projection. In the intraoral radiographs, only portions of the fossa are seen. These shadows, resembling the letter W, have rounded inferior margins denoting the **lower border of the nasal cavity**, with the nasal septum forming the central portion of the letter (Figures 70-1A and 70-3A).

The nasal septum commonly presents a wide radiopaque shadow that divides the right from the left nasal cavity or fossae, and it usually deviates slightly from the midline. A hazy gray shadow may be seen arising from the lateral wall of both fossae, which may extend to the septum or may fall short by a considerable distance. This shadow represents the anterior portions of the inferior turbinate bones. In the midline, at the inferior aspect of the nasal fossa, there usually is a small white inverted V that represents the **anterior nasal spine** (Figures 70-1A and 70-3A).

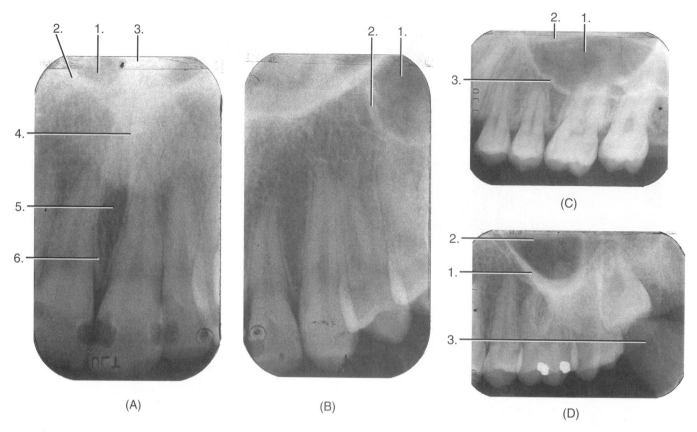

Figure 70-3 Maxillary radiographs: (A) 1, nasal fossae; 2, lower border of the nasal cavity; 3, nasal septum; 4, anterior nasal spine; 5, incisive foramen; 6, median palatine suture. (B) 1, maxillary sinus; 2, wall of maxillary sinus. (C) 1, maxillary sinus; 2, floor of nasal cavity; 3, floor of maxillary sinus. (D) 1, malar bone; 2, floor of nasal cavity; 3, coronoid process..

Incisive Foramen (Radiolucent)

In the palate, superimposed between the roots of the two central incisors, is the **incisive foramen** (Figures 70-1B and 70-3A). It varies widely in shape from a mere slit to a round, oval, or heart-, diamond-, or pear-shaped structure. This foramen transmits the nasal palatine nerves and vessels. The radiographic interpretation of this structure is important, because it is often mistaken for a pathologic process and is sometimes the site of a cyst.

Median Palatine Suture (Radiolucent)

In radiographs of the maxillary central incisor region, a radiolucent line extends from the alveolar crest to the posterior aspect of the palate. Sometimes, a short funnel-shaped widening appears in the anterior, which may be mistaken for an abnormality. This is the **median palatine suture**. The margins of the suture are lined by cortical bone; therefore, there is a radiopaque border along the edge of each maxilla (Figures 70-1B and 70-3A).

Maxillary Sinus (Radiolucent)

The **maxillary sinus**, a cavity and bone which contains air, is revealed in radiographs as a dark shadow (Figure 70-3C). As in all normal cavities and bone, the margins of the cavity consist of a thin layer of dense bone, the cortex, which appears as a thin white line in radiographs. These lines are termed the **floor of maxillary sinus** (horizontal aspect) (Figure 70-3C) and **wall of maxillary sinus** (vertical aspect) (Figure 70-3B). Because there are differences in the thickness of the walls and the width of the sinus, the dark shadow of the antrum is not uniformly dense throughout.

The relationship of the sinus to the teeth is not a constant one. The width of bone between the roots of the teeth and the floor of the sinus varies in thickness. The bone is thin; the roots of the teeth may form elevations on the floor of the sinus, and these elevations form recesses. *Septa* may also divide the sinus into two or more cavities.

The maxillary sinus is seen as a dark shadow with a thin white cortical border. The radiographic characteristics of this cortical line are important because they often serve to differentiate a normal antrum from a

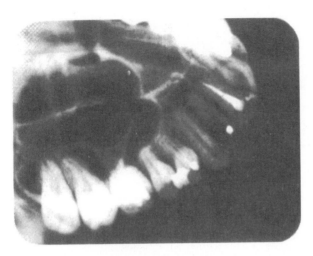

Figure 70-4 Maxillary cuspid-molar region.

pathologic lesion closely resembling the antral shadow. Although the cortex of the sinus is always continuous, there are appearances that suggest small interruptions in the line; these are only a simulation of interruptions. In intraoral radiographs, the sinus cavity is usually seen to extend from the bicuspid area to the tuberosity (Figure 70-4). The anterior aspect of the sinus meets the floor of the nasal fossa, and an inverted Y-shaped shadow appears, the diverging limbs of which represent the sinus wall in the cortex of the nasal fossa that curves anteriorly. The leg of the letter, or the long line, represents the lateral cortex of the nasal fossa passing backward to the pharyngeal end (Figure 70-3B). This Y-shaped shadow is of value in differentiating some cysts in this region, for it tends to be obliterated in such conditions. In some cases of doubt, the persistence of the shadow may be evidence against the presence of a lesion.

The Malar Bone (Radiopaque)

The prominence of the cheek is produced by the **malar bone** or zygomatic process (Figures 70-1A and 70-3C, D). Only the inferior portion of the zygomatic process appears in intraoral radiographs. A gray or white shadow, depending on the thickness of the bone and the proportion of dense bone, is seen. The extent of the inferior border varies, beginning over the second bicuspid or first molar area and extending backward, usually beyond the limits of the film. The lowest part of the bone may be situated above the first molar or, less often, the second molar from which it passes backward and upward with varying degrees of sharpness. Depending on anatomical and technical factors, the relation of the shadow of the malar bone to the shadow of the roots of the teeth is variable.

Intraoral radiographs of the malar bone give this relationship a U appearance that overlies the larger shadow of the antrum as a whole. Since the limbs of the U are made up of dense cortical bone, they present a white shadow that is accentuated by the dark background of the antrum or sinus.

Palatine Process (Radiopaque)

The superior surface of the **palatine process** forms a part of the **floor of the nasal cavity**; the inferior surface of the palatine process forms the roof of the mouth (Figures 70-3C, D).

The Coronoid Process (Radiopaque)

Numerous anatomical structures appear in radiographs of the maxillary third molars. One of these structures is the **coronoid process**, which may be mistaken for a retained root or an unerupted tooth. The coronoid process, a component part of the mandible, usually appears as a cone-shaped shadow with the apex, which may be blunt or relatively pointed, directed upward and forward (Figures 70-1C and 70-3D).

Landmarks of the Mandible

At birth, the mandible is in two pieces, joined at the midline by soft tissue only. Within a year after birth, the suture is usually closed.

Mental Process or Ridge (Radiopaque)

The anterior and inferior aspect of the chin is usually thickened by the presence of a triangle of smooth and shiny denser bone, which stands out above the surface of the adjacent bone. This dense ridge of bone extends from the symphysis of the mandible to the region of the bicuspid. It is called a **mental process** or mental ridge and varies in different persons (Figure 70-5A). It is more visibly pronounced on a person with heavy bones than one with light bones, thus showing corresponding differences on radiographs. In conventional intraoral radiographs the apex of the triangle may or may not be apparent, depending on the actual depth of the mandible at this side. When the apex is present, it appears to be formed by two dense lines that converge toward the midline. On some occasions, the density of the whole triangle is so great that it interferes with the clear view of the apices of the incisors.

Genial Tubercles (Radiopaque)

In the midline of the lingual surface of the mandible, there frequently may be seen an elevation situated well below the roots of the incisors representing the **genial tubercles** (Figure 70-5B). In periapical radiographs, they appear as a localized area of increased density with a small, dark radiolucent spot, the **lingual foramen**, in

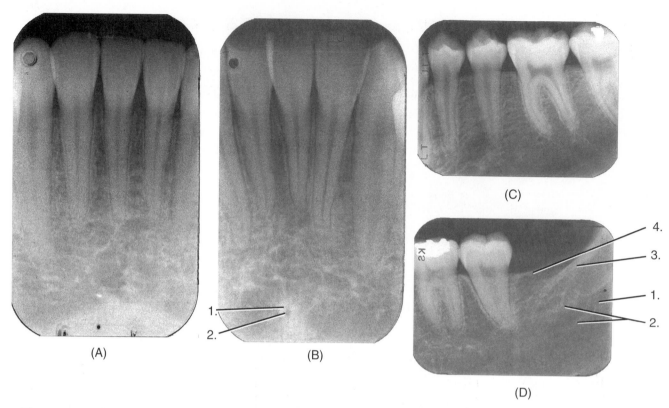

Figure 70-5 Mandibular radiographs: (A) Mental ridge. (B) 1, genial tubercles; 2, lingual foramen. (C) Mental foramen. (D) 1, mandibular canal; 2, walls of the mandibular canal; 3, external oblique ridge; 4, internal oblique ridge.

the center (Figure 70-5B). In occlusal radiographs showing the floor of the mouth, these tubercles protrude, sometimes quite extensively, from the surface of the bone, suggesting to the inexperienced observer that an abnormality is present.

The Mental Foramen (Radiolucent)

The position of the **mental foramen** is variable, common sites being at or just below the apex of the second bicuspid or a little medial to and below the apex (Figure 70-5C). The mental foramen appears on the radiograph as an area of radiolucency. The shadow may be oval, round, oblong, or any regular shape or there may be no shadow at all. When present, it varies in size from a few millimeters to a centimeter.

Poor angulation sometimes results in a radiolucent area, the mental foramen appearing at the apex of a mandibular bicuspid. In this position, it may be mistaken for a pathologic condition as an abscess; therefore, it is very important to observe that the superimposition of the shadows of the root and foramen are not associated with any discontinuity of the lamina dura. Teeth have been needlessly removed because the superimposition of the mental foramen and root was misinterpreted as disease.

The Mandibular Canal (Radiolucent)

The **mandibular canal** commences at the mandibular foramen in the ascending ramus. It passes downward until it arrives at the body of the mandible where it turns forward to pass into the anterior portion of the bone. The mandibular foramen varies greatly in its radiographic manifestations. Usually it appears as a funnel-shaped area of increased radiolucency with wide variation in the width, length, and depth of the funnel (Figure 70-5D).

The mandibular canal, being a space in bone, appears as a dark shadow in radiographs. Because it is a normal anatomical space, it is lined by a cortical layer of bone, termed **walls of the mandibular canal** (Figure 70-5D). Although such shadows are observed, there is no one typical radiographic image because of the wide variations in the appearance of the canal. In most people, the canal appears as a dark, narrow ribbon between two white radiopaque lines (walls). However, in others, it is not even apparent but is seen as two faint, more or less parallel, white lines without any intermediate alteration in bone density.

Nutrient Canals (Radiolucent)

Blood vessels lying in channels or grooves traverse the maxilla and mandible to supply the teeth and gingival tissues. These are known as **nutrient canals**. Except for the mandibular canal, these vascular channels usually do not appear on radiographs. However, occasionally it is possible to see them. Radiographs may reveal vascular markings on the walls of the maxillary sinus; or they may be seen in the mandible, most frequently in the incisive region. These channels appear as dark linear shadows situated between the roots of adjacent teeth and more or less parallel with them. The canals fall short of the gingival crest and disappear at various distances below the level of the root apices.

External Oblique Ridge (Radiopaque)

On the external surface of the mandible is a ridge that descends along the ramus of the mandible and passes downward and outward to become the **external oblique ridge** (Figures 70-1A and C and 70-5D).

If this ridge continues past the third molar, it proceeds downward and forward on the outer part of the body of the mandible, terminating at or above the lower border. This structure may appear on the radiograph as a radiopaque line traversing the mandibular third molar region.

Internal Oblique Ridge and Mylohyoid Ridge (Radiopaque)

On the internal aspect of the ramus of the mandible is a prominent ridge that passes downward and forward from the ramus to the third molar. This is called the **internal oblique ridge** (Figures 70-1C and 70-5D). On a radiograph it may show as a thin white line and is usually inferior to the external oblique ridge but not as dense. The **mylohyoid ridge**, or line, is a ridge formed from the attachment of the mylohyoid muscle (Figure 70-1C). It may appear to be in the same alignment as the internal oblique as if it were a continuation of that ridge. However, the mylohyoid is more horizontal along the inside of the mandible and below the posterior or molar region.

Coronoid Process

The coronoid process of the ascending ramus varies markedly in different persons. The process is usually cone shaped. The appearance of the coronoid process was covered in an earlier section on landmarks of the maxilla.

- Using a full-mouth series of radiographs, locate as many of the landmarks of the maxilla as you can. List each one and indicate which of the radiographs showed those with normal radiographic appearance. List those with variations within the normal, and indicate which radiograph you viewed to detect it.

- Locate as many landmarks as you can while viewing radiographs of the maxilla and mandible. On a sheet of paper divide it in half lengthwise and list all the radiopaque radiographic landmarks on one side and all the radiolucent on the other and determine which ones pertain to the maxilla and which ones pertain to the mandible.

- Locate landmarks that you may expect to find in a panoramic radiograph based on location as seen in this chapter.

REVIEW

1. Indicate which radiolucent landmarks may be found on the maxillary arch: (1) nasal cavity, (2) nasal septum, (3) maxillary sinus, and/or (4) median palatine suture.
   a. 1, 2, 3   c. 1, 2, 4
   b. 2, 3, 4   d. 1, 3, 4

2. Indicate which radiopaque landmarks may be found on the maxillary arch: (1) incisive foramen, (2) floor of the nasal cavity, (3) malar bone, and/or (4) wall of the maxillary sinus.
   a. 1, 2, 3   c. 1, 2, 4
   b. 2, 3, 4   d. 1, 3, 4

3. Indicate which radiolucent landmarks may be found on the mandibular arch: (1) lingual foramen, (2) mental foramen, (3) mandibular canal, and/or, (4) genial tubercles.
   a. 1, 2, 3   c. 1, 2, 4
   b. 2, 3, 4   d. 1, 3, 4

4. Indicate which radiopaque landmarks may be found on the mandibular arch: (1) external oblique ridge, (2) walls of the mandibular canal, (3) floor of the nasal cavity, and/or (4) internal oblique ridge.
   a. 1, 2, 3   c. 1, 2, 4
   b. 2, 3, 4   d. 1, 3, 4

5. Thin radiopaque lines separating the medullary spaces are called:
   a. Trabeculae
   b. Cancellous bone
   c. Cortical bone
   d. Lamina dura

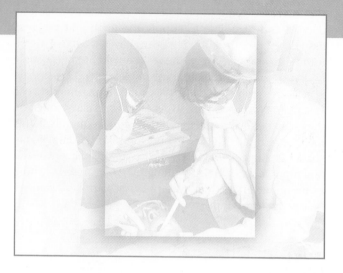

OBJECTIVES

After studying this chapter, the student will be able to:

- Differentiate between interpretation and diagnosis.
- Explain who may interpret radiographs.
- Explain who may make a diagnosis.
- Describe the type of radiographs utilized to document interproximal caries.
- Discuss each type of interproximal caries and how each one is interpreted.
- Explain how the healthy alveolar crest should look in the posterior and anterior areas.
- Describe vertical and horizontal bone loss.
- Explain which conditions exhibit radiolucent characteristics.
- Explain which conditions exhibit radiopaque characteristics.

Introduction

Radiographic interpretation is used to determine healthy from diseased tissues and normal from abnormal structures. The dental health care professional should be familiar with and understand these differences when viewing radiographs.

Clarification regarding interpretation and diagnosis is made. Radiographic **interpretation** is the recognition and description of the images on a radiograph. **Diagnosis** is the determination of which one of several diseases or conditions may be producing the symptoms.

Radiographic interpretation can be accomplished by any of the dental health care professionals, provided they have had previous instruction. A diagnosis is determined only by the dentist, after a clinical and radiographic evaluation.

The terms radiolucent (dark) and radiopaque (light or white) have been discussed in Chapter 70.

Interpretation of Carious Lesions

Carious lesions are the most common reasons for making dental radiographs. As carious lesions occur, tooth structure is destroyed. Radiographically, the carious lesion is visible as a radiolucency due to the decreased density in the tooth structure which allows penetration of x-ray photons (Figure 71-1).

The dentist performs a clinical examination to detect carious lesions. However, due to the fact that it is virtually impossible to detect **interproximal** (between two teeth) caries on posterior teeth, radiographs are useful as a diagnostic tool for a complete diagnosis.

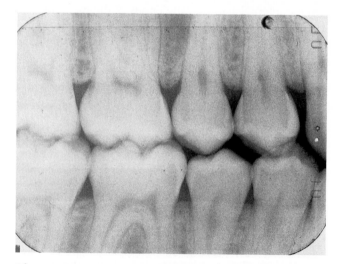

Figure 71-1 Carious lesions between maxillary bicuspid, distal of maxillary second bicuspid, and mesial of mandibular first molar.

Use of Bite-Wing Radiographs

The use of bite-wing radiographs taken at a parallel, or 90°, angle with open interproximals greatly aids in the diagnosis. Periapical radiographs taken at a greater vertical angle lose pertinent information and are not as useful in the diagnosis of carious lesions.

Recognizing Incipient Interproximal Carious Lesions

It is usually not difficult to recognize large carious lesions radiographically, but small interproximal incipient carious lesions are difficult to locate. It may be helpful to realize that these usually exist at or just below the contact area between two teeth. The carious lesion appears as a small radiolucent triangular formation on only the enamel portion of the tooth. It extends from the edge of the enamel to less than halfway into the enamel.

Recognizing Moderate Interproximal Carious Lesions

The moderate interproximal carious lesion is still located only on the enamel and extends close to the **dentinoenamel junction (DEJ)** (the line where the enamel and dentin meet) but does not affect the DEJ or the dentin. It appears as a wedge-shaped radiolucency on the enamel portion.

Recognizing Advanced Interproximal Carious Lesions

As the carious lesion advances through the enamel past the DEJ, it affects the dentin, causing a small portion to appear radiolucent. The lesion extends to a halfway point between the DEJ and the pulp.

Recognizing Severe Interproximal Carious Lesions

Severe interproximal caries involve the enamel past the DEJ and extend past the halfway point between the DEJ and the pulp. Radiographically, they appear as small wedges at the enamel, but when the dentin is involved, there is significant destruction that reaches close to the pulp.

Recognizing Occlusal, Buccal/ Lingual, and Root Carious Lesions

Occlusal carious lesions are a little more difficult to recognize. The dentist or dental hygienist usually discovers these lesions with an explorer. Radiographically, incipient occlusal caries are not seen, but moderate and severe occlusal caries are visible because they extend into the dentin. The moderate occlusal is barely seen just below the DEJ in the dentin, whereas the severe occlusal carious lesions are clearly into the dentin and appear quite large (Figure 71-2).

Buccal/lingual carious lesions appear as a radiolucent dot if they are large enough; otherwise, they are recognized clinically with an explorer.

Root carious lesions are recognized when radiolucencies appear below the **cementoenamel junction (CEJ)** (line where the enamel and cementum meet).

Other Carious Lesions

Other carious lesions are located under a restoration and are known as **recurrent caries**. These appear radiolucent under a restoration, and a person with **rampant caries** appears to have carious lesions on almost every tooth in the oral cavity (Figure 71-3).

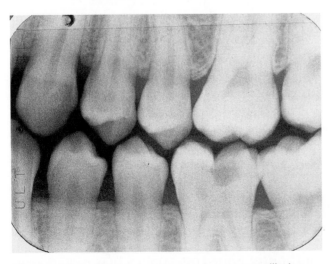

Figure 71-2 Occlusal carious lesion on mandibular first molar.

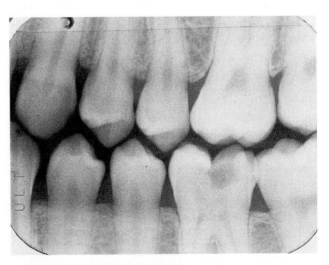

Figure 71-3 Rampant carious lesions.

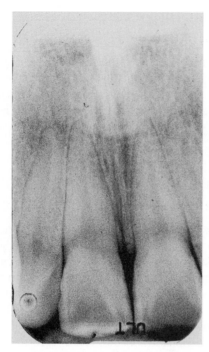

Figure 71-4 Cervical burnout on maxillary central incisors.

Cervical Burnout

Cervical burnout is a term used to point out a radiolucent area at the cervical portion of the tooth that is not diseased or defective. Although not a carious lesion, it may be easily confused for one. Cervical burnout appears as a wedge-shaped radiolucency near the CEJ on the mesial or distal portions of the tooth (Figure 71-4).

Interpretation of Periodontal Conditions

Three structures should always be evaluated radiographically: the alveolar crest, lamina dura, and periodontal ligament.

The Alveolar Crest

To detect bone loss and other destructive conditions, the alveolar crest is evaluated. In a healthy mouth the alveolar crest for the posterior teeth should possess a smooth flat surface; for the anterior teeth it should be defined and pointed and the height should be at 1.5 to 2 mm below the CEJ. Radiographs that show a truer alveolar crest height use the parallel technique as opposed to the bisecting-angle technique. Horizontal and vertical bite wings are also used. Bite-wing radiographs are made not only of posterior teeth but also of anterior teeth. Vertical bite wings are made of the anterior area.

If bone destruction of the alveolar crest exists, the height will diminish vertically or horizontally. There will

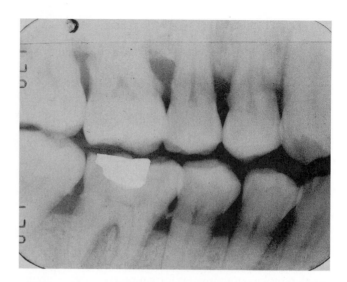

Figure 71-5 Vertical bone loss on mesial of maxillary first molar.

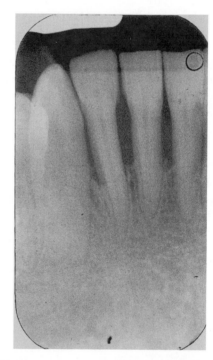

Figure 71-6 Horizontal bone loss on mandibular anterior teeth.

be **localized bone loss** in a few teeth or **generalized bone loss** throughout the maxillary or mandibular arches.

Vertical Bone Loss. Vertical bone loss occurs and is identified when the bone level between two adjacent teeth measures differently from the CEJ (Figure 71-5).

Horizontal Bone Loss. Horizontal bone loss occurs when the bone level of adjacent teeth is at the same distance from the CEJ (Figure 71-6).

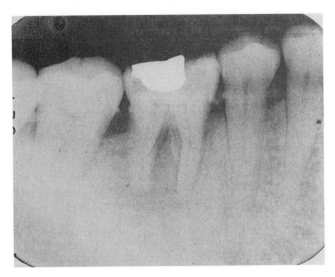

Figure 71-7 Furcation involvement on mandibular first molar.

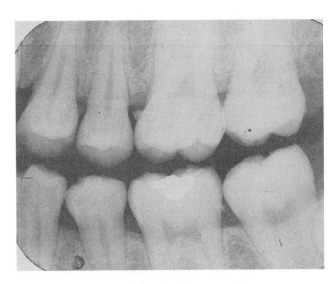

Figure 71-8 Calculus deposits.

Furcation Involvement. When bone loss occurs past the furcation (the area between the roots of a multirooted tooth), it is said to have furcation involvement (Figure 71-7).

Lamina Dura

Lamina dura is the compact bone that lines the tooth socket. When viewed radiographically, it appears as a white radiopaque line beside the periodontal ligament. It should be intact and unbroken.

Periodontal Ligament

The periodontal ligament should be well defined around the root of the tooth. When viewed radiographically, it appears dark or radiolucent. Should it become thickened, it may be diseased.

Causes for Bone Loss

Calculus is a local irritant and a major contributor to periodontal disease, which in turn causes bone loss. The appearance of calculus on radiographs is radiopaque. Supragingival calculus may appear as spiny interproximal projections close to the CEJ (Figure 71-8), whereas subgingival calculus may be more difficult to see radiographically.

Overhanging restorations are considerably irritating to the soft tissues and also contribute to periodontal disease.If the overhanging restoration is such that it prevents effective flossing, deterioration of tissues usually occurs; therefore, bone loss is likely to result (Figure 71–9).

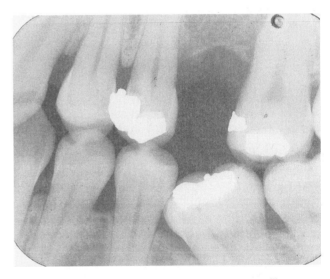

Figure 71-9 Overhanging restoration on maxillary second bicuspid.

Interproximal open contacts allow food and bacteria to be trapped, causing irritation and ultimately contribute to bone loss.

Radiolucent Conditions

- A *radicular cyst* or *periapical abscess* may form at the apex of an endodontically involved tooth and is viewed radiographically as a round saclike radiolucency (Figure 71-10).

- *Fractures* occur in the crowns or roots of teeth. Crown fractures are clinically visible; however, root fractures are only visible radiographically where they exhibit a radiolucent irregular line. Fractures may

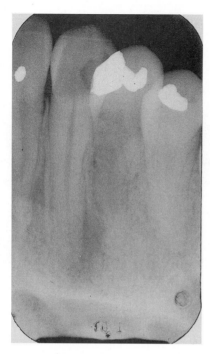

Figure 71-10 Periapical abscess at apex of maxillary cuspid.

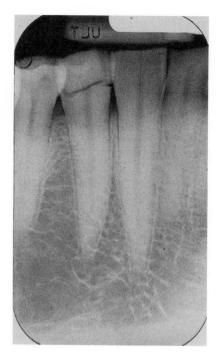

Figure 71-11 Fractured tooth on mandibular first bicuspid.

occur in bone, exhibiting a radiolucent irregular line (Figure 71-11).

- *Widened periodontal ligament* suggests there is periapical disease involvement.

- *Root resorption* may be external or internal.

- *External root resorption* becomes evident when an outside force causes osteoclastic activity to destroy the root apex. This can be observed in orthodontic cases where tooth movement was excessive, causing the roots to appear blunted and shortened. External root resorption also occurs when an unerupted tooth places lateral forces on the root of an erupted tooth, as with a horizontally impacted third molar positioned adjacent to the root of a second molar.

- *Internal resorption* is visible within the pulpal canals or the pulp chamber. The space of the pulpal canal appears to have an enlarged section that is continuous with the pulpal canal, and resorption in the pulp chamber appears round and overextends into the surrounding dentin.

- *Avulsion* is the complete displacement of a tooth from its alveolus, generally caused by a traumatic accident. When viewed radiographically, the socket appears radiolucent due to the absence of the tooth. However, the alveolus may have splintered bone fragments which appear as radiopaque particles.

Radiopaque Conditions

- *Hypercementosis* indicates increased formation of cementum around the root of the tooth. The root appears bulbous, presenting difficulty in recognizing the periodontal membrane.

- *Condensing osteitis* affects mandibular nonvital teeth more than maxillary teeth and most often occurs on the mandibular first molars. It is seen as an opaque area just below the root of the tooth or surrounding the root and may be due to chronic pulpitis or inflammation.

- *Sclerotic bone* or osteosclerosis is a radiopaque diffuse and well-defined composite of bone seen below vital teeth. It is not associated with diseased or pathologic lesions (Figure 71-12).

- *Pulp stones* appear as opaque calcifications within the pulp chamber or pulp canals. They do not cause a problem, unless the tooth is treated endodontically; otherwise they are harmless (Figure 71-13).

- *Pulpal obliteration* means that the pulp of the tooth no longer exists but rather is filled with dentin material, rendering the tooth nonvital.

- *Pulp sclerosis* is usually connected with the aging population. The pulp chamber and canal decrease in size.

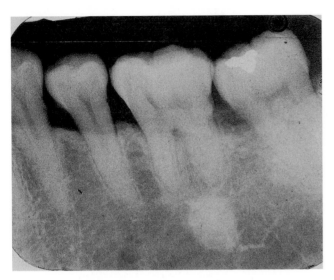

Figure 71-12 Sclerotic bone/osteosclerosis below mandibular first molar.

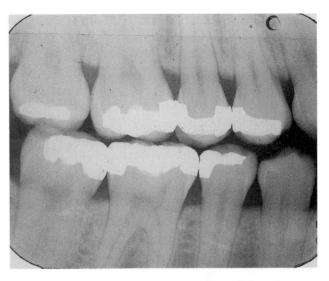

Figure 71-13 Pulp stones on maxillary first and second molars.

Anomalies and Unusual Conditions

● *Luxation* is the abnormal displacement of teeth. It may be recognized as intrusion or extrusion. *Intrusion* means that a tooth was driven into its socket or bone, appearing shorter than adjacent teeth or missing altogether, indicating the tooth was driven deep into its socket, very likely due to trauma. *Extrusion* means that a tooth has grown out of its socket, appearing longer than adjacent teeth due to nonexistent teeth on the opposite arch where the tooth normally would occlude.

● *Torus mandibularis* or *torus palatinus* is the excess bony outgrowth on the lingual side of the bicuspid area of the mandible or center of maxilla. When observed radiographically, it appears as radiopaque nodules (Figure 71-14).

● *Dens in dente* means "tooth within a tooth," primarily affecting maxillary lateral incisors. It is a defect prone to decay due to a deep lingual pit on the tooth and is recognized radiographically as a small inverted teardrop at the cingulum.

● *Supernumerary teeth* are extra teeth located in various areas. Typically, areas of the mandibular premolars, maxillary third molars, and sometimes maxillary laterals are affected. Their positions when unerupted are seen radiographically as tooth-shaped radiopacities (Figure 71-15).

● *Mesiodens* is considered to be a supernumerary tooth located between the maxillary centrals. Sometimes it does erupt between the two maxillary centrals and is usually underdeveloped.

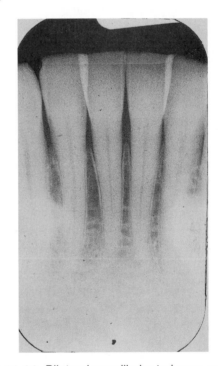

Figure 71-14 Bilateral mandibular tori seen as two radiopaque spots on either side of radiograph.

● *Taurodontism* is the unusual shape of a tooth whereby it exhibits an elongated pulp chamber and small stubby roots and is identified only radiographically (Figure 71-16).

● *Dilacerated roots* are roots that have unusual bends, sometimes at a near 90° angle. The unusual bending is attributed to difficulties encountered during eruption. These teeth become very difficult to extract or treat endodontically.

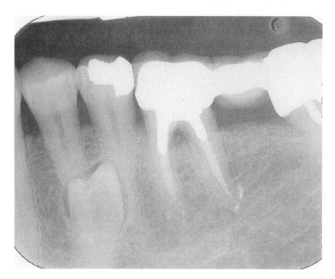

Figure 71-15 Supernumerary tooth below first and second mandibular bicuspids.

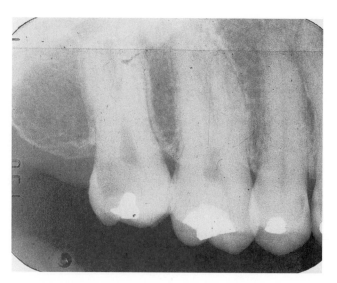

Figure 71-16 Taurodontism exhibiting elongated pulp and small stubby roots on maxillary second molar.

● *Supernumerary roots* are found in teeth that have an extra root. For example, mandibular bicuspids that typically have one root but, through root bifurcation, acquire an extra root.

● *Root tips* are viewed radiographically as radiopaque root tip fragments in the alveolus. Root tips are severed when the tooth is extracted.

● *Gemination* is the incomplete formation of two teeth that occurred when a single tooth germ attempted to divide. Clinically and radiographically, it exhibits two crowns on one root.

Restorations

There are many restorative materials currently in use that should be identified radiographically by dental health care professionals. Restorative materials range from metallic to acrylic, composite, and porcelain. Generally, metallic restorations are radiopaque and acrylic, composite, and porcelain may vary from radiolucent to slightly radiopaque.

Metallic Restorations

Amalgam restoration is the most widely used restorative material in dentistry. It is used predominantly on posterior teeth. Amalgam is also used in other areas besides posterior teeth: on maxillary anterior linguals at the cingulum where pits tend to develop (Figure 71-17), on gingival one-third class V cavities, and at the apex of an apicoectomy where it is retrofilled. Amalgam appears very radiopaque on radiographs because x-ray photons are unable to penetrate this material. They are stopped and absorbed by the amalgam material, thus producing a white radiopaque image.

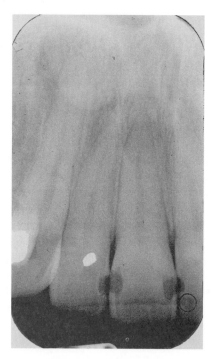

Figure 71-17 Amalgam restoration on maxillary anterior tooth at the cingulum

To identify amalgam restorations, it should be understood that they do not have very smooth margins but rather tend to be uneven and irregular. They are commonly seen as mesiocclusal (MO), distocclusal (DO), mesiocclusodistal (MOD), buccal, and lingual restorations. There are some problems associated when using amalgam material. Amalgam is in a plastic state when restoring the tooth. When a two- or three-surface restoration is being placed, a matrix band is used to support the material and hold it in place. Thus, there is a

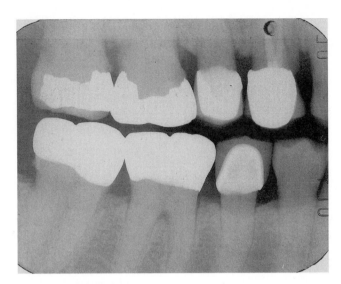

Figure 71-18 Gold crowns on mandibular first and second molars.

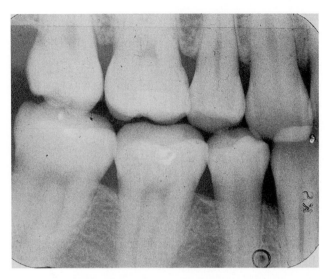

Figure 71-19 Composite restoration on maxillary and mandibular first molar occlusals.

possibility of creating overhanging margins when a wedge is omitted that would seal the gingival margin at the base of the matrix band, preventing this problem. As noted previously, overhanging restorations are contributors to periodontal disease (see Figure 71-9). Amalgam material may become permanently embedded in the gingiva during the process of restoring the tooth. When this occurs, it causes an *amalgam tattoo.*

Gold restorations are just as radiopaque as amalgam restorations except they have smooth margins as opposed to amalgams with irregular margins (Figure 71-18). Gold restorations are used where strength is required and where there is insufficient tooth structure to retain a restoration. Crowns, inlays, onlays, and bridges are constructed of gold alloy.

Stainless steel crowns cover the full crown portion of the tooth. They are generally used as temporary crowns, and their margins do not follow the contour of the tooth as does a full gold crown. Radiographically they appear somewhat transparent because they are not as dense as gold or amalgam.

Nonmetallic Restorations

Porcelain restorations are not as radiopaque as gold or amalgam restorations. The density is similar to dentin and therefore just as radiopaque. When porcelain is combined with a metal in fabricating a crown or bridge, the metal portion of the restoration is placed in the center, which covers the prepared tooth. The portion of the restoration that replaces the facial surface and cusps is made of porcelain and appears radiopaque on the radiograph.

Composite and acrylic restorations appear less dense than metallic restorations. Composite material has

fillers to give it a radiopaque appearance (Figure 71-19), while acrylic restorations that lack fillers will appear radiolucent and may be difficult to distinguish from a carious lesion. One way to distinguish these materials is to analyze the form of the radiolucent cavity. If it has a definite form, whether square or round, it is obvious that a cavity preparation was made and restored, whereas a carious lesion will have no definite form.

Cements are used as temporary restorations, bases under deep restorations, and luting agents when cementing crowns. Cement that is used as a base will appear as radiopaque material, more dense than dentin but less than metal. A metallic restoration that is very radiopaque is usually placed over it and the density of the two materials is distinguishable.

SUGGESTED ACTIVITIES

- Review radiographs with several types of restorations. Identify amalgam, gold, composite, and cement base.
- Select radiographs in this text that identify anomalies and unusual conditions.

REVIEW

1. The following are causes for bone loss, except:
   a. Interproximal open contacts
   b. Calculus
   c. Pulp stones
   d. Overhanging restorations

2. For the following conditions mark those that appear radiolucent with a 1 and those that appear radiopaque with a 2:

___ a. Internal resorption

___ b. Pulp stones

___ c. Pulpal obliteration

___ d. Fractures

___ e. Condensing osteitis

___ f. Hypercementosis

___ g. Periapical abscess

3. Match the conditions on the left with their descriptions on the right:

___ a. Dens in dente   1. Extra teeth

___ b. Gemination   2. Roots that have unusual bends

___ c. Torus   3. Abnormal displacement of teeth

___ d. Mesiodens   4. Incomplete formation of two teeth that share one root

___ e. Supernumerary teeth   5. Teeth that have extra root(s)

___ f. Dilacerated root   6. A supernumerary tooth located between maxillary centrals

___ g. Luxation   7. Excess bony outgrowth

___ h. Supernumerary roots   8. Tooth within a tooth

4. Identify the restorations on the left as seen radiographically with the definitions on the right:

___ a. Gold restoration   1. A full crown that appears somewhat transparent, whose margins do not contour the tooth

___ b. Porcelain restoration   2. A radiopaque restoration with smooth margins

___ c. Stainless steel crown   3. A radiopaque restoration predominantly used on posterior teeth whose margins are irregular

___ d. Amalgam restoration   4. A radiopaque restoration used in crowns and bridges, not as dense as metallic restorations, similar to dentin in density

Mounting, Labeling, and Filing Dental Radiographs

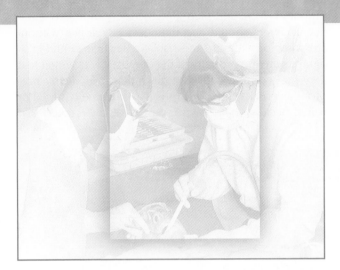

OBJECTIVES

After studying this chapter, the student will be able to:

- Name two desirable qualities for dental mounts.
- Differentiate between a bite-wing mount and a peri-apical mount.
- State the advantages and disadvantages for various types of dental mounts.
- State the method of determining the right and left sides of the dental arch on a radiograph.
- Demonstrate the proper procedure for mounting bite-wing radiographs.
- Name three reasons for keeping dental radiographs.
- Determine proper storage.
- State the proper labeling and filing procedures for dental radiographs.

Introduction

Dental mounts should be stiff and have a sufficiently glazed surface to promote permanent filing of radiographs. Their construction should ensure that the radiographs remain rigid and securely in place.

Mounts come in various sizes and with 1, 2, 4, 7, 14, 16, 18, 20, and 28 windows. Bite-wing mounts have either 2 or 4 windows. The most commonly used peri-apical mounts have 16–20 windows.

Types of Mounts

Clear Plastic Mounts

Advantages

- Reasonable price
- Little storage problem
- Water repellent
- Reusable
- Easy to handle

Disadvantages

- Subject to scratches
- Crack, split (cannot be reused)
- Glare of surrounding films inhibits diagnosis

Plastic Mounts

Advantages

- Same as for clear plastic
- Frosted quality cuts out light glare

Disadvantages

- Same as for clear plastic

Cardboard Mounts

Advantages

- Blocks out view of any object detracting from radiographs
- Less cost than plastic

Disadvantages

- Soil easily
- Absorb water
- Film is not held tightly
- Bend and break easily
- Difficult to mount radiographs
- Seldom reusable
- Bulky

Mounting

When bite-wing radiographs are mounted, the operator must keep in mind that the center of the mount is the median line and that the distal portion of the area appears along the right margin of the radiograph and is, therefore, the left side of the dental arch. If it appears along the left margin, the right side is indicated. This view of the radiographs when mounted represents the facial aspect to the operator.

Labeling and Filing

All radiographic films of a patient should be kept in the same envelope and filed alphabetically in a steel cabinet. Drawers should accommodate envelopes without crowding or without excess space. Because dental radiographs are the property of the dentist, it is essential that they be kept in a cool, dry place that is as nearly fireproof as possible. Radiographs may become crimped or soiled because of moisture. Care should be taken that

Procedure 78 Mounting Radiographs

Materials Needed

2- or 4-window mount for bite wing and 16-, 18-, or 20-window mounts for full mouth
Radiographs
Rubber finger cot or white cotton gloves

Radiographic Characteristics

- The process of mounting a full-mouth set of radiographs requires the operator to recognize radiographic characteristics that will be helpful in this process; for example:

- The "smile line" or curve of spee is seen on posterior radiographs.

- Sizes of anterior teeth in the maxillary arch are larger than those of the mandibular arch.

- Maxillary molars have three roots while mandibular molars have two distinct roots.

- The pulp chambers on maxillary molars appear triangular or circular and are not as distinct as those of the mandibular molars.

- The trabecular pattern on the mandibular arch is more noticeable.

- Roots tend to drift distally.

- Anatomical landmarks such as the maxillary sinus and nasal cavity are usually visible on the maxillary arch.

Instructions

1. Cover the index finger with the rubber finger cot. Hold the film edgewise with the thumb and forefinger to avoid leaving finger marks on the radiograph. If gloves are used, make certain they are clean and free of lint

2. Separate anterior from posterior radiographs

3. Determine the right side of the radiograph

   a. Convex dot is toward the operator.

   b. Molars appear along distal margin of the radiograph, bicuspids along the mesial margin of the radiograph.

   c. Occlusal or "smile line" curves slightly upward from mesial to distal.

4. Posterior radiographs are mounted horizontally and anterior radiographs vertically.

5. Hold radiograph with the convex side of the dot *toward* the operator. The dot should be placed toward the occlusal or incisal edge.

6. Hold mount in one hand and place radiograph in mount with the other hand.

7. Start by mounting the bite-wing radiographs and place them toward the center of the mount.

8. Continue with the posterior bicuspid and molar radiographs, matching them to bite-wings for visible restorations.

9. Finish mounting the anterior radiographs following stated guidelines (trabecular pattern and sizes of teeth and anatomical landmarks).

Procedure 79 Labeling and Filing Radiographs

Materials Needed

Steel cabinet
manila envelope (size needed for radiographic mount)
Mounted radiographs

Instructions

Film Mount

1. Write patient's full name in full on the top line:

   M _____

   (Example: Mrs. Janet W. Smith)

2. Write date radiographs were taken on the second line:

   DATE _____

3. Fill in the number according to the patient file system:

   NO. _____

   NUMBER OF FILMS: _____

4. Fill in the dentist's name and who referred the patient:

   DR. _____

   REFERRED BY _____

Radiograph Envelopes

1. Write patient's full name in the upper left corner of envelope:
   - Last name, title, first name, and middle initial.
   - Example: Smith, Mr. James Lowell

2. Place envelope in the indexed section of file indicated by the first letter of the last name.
   - Alphabetize according to first three letters of last name and initials of first name.
   - Example: James, Mrs. Susan R.

     Jamison, Mr. Robert T.

     Jorgensen, Miss Sarah L.

     Jorgensen, Mr. Thomas D.

     Juergens, Mrs. Lillian M.

3. Never seal envelopes.

the radiographs are not bent, scratched, or otherwise damaged as this impairs their diagnostic value.

All files should be kept for at least a period of five years as a means of comparing progress of dental treatment; as a legal protection in case of malpractice suits; to indicate the necessity of operation and the results obtained; and for identification of deceased persons after ordinary characteristics of identification no longer exist.

SUGGESTED ACTIVITIES

- Practice labeling a mount and corresponding envelope.
- Practice mounting bite-wing radiographs and periapical radiographs by using ones that are kept on file.
- When you have mounted one set and viewed it for accuracy, evaluate to see where the identification dots were placed and whether they are all convex or concave.
- Practice mounting rapidly and without error until it can be accomplished in 5 minutes or less.

REVIEW

1. How can one determine the right from the left side when mounting radiographs?
   a. View the mounted radiographs as though the patient's facial aspect were facing the operator.
   b. View the mounted radiographs as though the operator were inside the patient's mouth.
   c. Convex dot is toward operator.
   d. Concave dot is toward operator.
   e. a, c
   f. b, d

2. Indicate which helpful guidelines are used in the mounting process: (1) maxillary molars have two roots and are more distinct, (2) the "smile line" is used with posterior radiographs, (3) maxillary anterior teeth are larger than mandibular anterior teeth, and/or (4) sinus cavity is seen on the maxillary posterior teeth.
   a. 1, 2, 3
   b. 2, 3, 4
   c. 1, 2, 4
   d. 1, 3, 4

3. Where should the identification dot be located on periapical radiographs?
   a. Toward the apical areas
   b. Toward the mesial side
   c. Toward the distal side
   d. Toward the occlusal and incisal areas

4. Indicate how anterior and posterior radiographs are mounted: (1) posteriors horizontally, (2) posteriors vertically, (3) anteriors horizontally, and/or (4) anteriors vertically.
   a. 1, 3
   b. 2, 4
   c. 1, 4
   d. 2, 3

5. Indicate the method(s) of labeling the mount and envelope: (1) placing the patient's last name then first name on the mount, (2) placing the patient's first name then last name on the mount, (3) placing the patient's last name then first name on the envelope, and/or (4) placing the patient's first name then last name on the envelope.
   a. 1, 3
   b. 2, 4
   c. 1, 4
   d. 2, 3

Abandonment Wrongful cessation of provision of care to a patient who is still under treatment.

Abraded Scraping of the skin as a result of injury or mechanical means.

Abrasion The process of wearing away.

Abrasive agents Pertains to hard particles with sharp or rounded edges that produce scratches when applied to a surface.

Abscess Pus formation at a localized area, such as at the apex (root tip) of a tooth or on periodontal tissue.

Absorbed dose The amount of x-radiation absorbed by matter (tissue).

Abutment An anchor tooth, root, or implant used for the support or retention of a fixed or removable prosthesis.

Accelerator A substance that speeds up a reaction.

Accepted Dental Therapeutics A publication of the American Dental Association that publishes information on drugs mainly used by dentists.

Acquired pellicle A thin bacteria-free, translucent film that forms initially on the teeth.

Acute In radiology, it refers to exposure to a large dose of radiation in a short time.

Acute necrotizing ulcerative gingivitis (ANUG) Also known as Vincent's infection and trench mouth, an acute, severe, and rapidly progressive gingival inflammation that destroys the periodontium and tends to become chronic; characterized by a feeling of illness, bad breath, and appearance of ulcers in the mouth.

Addiction Physiologic or psychological dependence to continue the use of a substance, especially alcohol or drugs with a tendency to increase the dosage to get the original effect.

Admixed A combination of the low-copper lathe-cut alloy and high-copper spherical alloy particles.

Adsorption Adhesion of a virus to the outer surface of a host cell.

Adumbration The images of the teeth are overshadowed by an object.

Aerobic The ability of an organism to use oxygen in metabolism and grow in its presence.

Aerosolization Infecting the atmosphere with airborne pathogens.

Agar-agar A colloid material extracted from a certain type of seaweed.

AIDS (acquired immunodeficiency syndrome) One of the most serious health problems caused by a virus and considered to be a worldwide epidemic.

ALARA "As Low As Reasonably Achievable" The term used in conjunction with radiation protection to keep exposures to a minimum.

Algae Small eucaryotic cells that live primarily in water and are important in photosynthesis.

Alginic acid Crystalline compounds that are typically water-soluble and are extracted from seaweed.

Aligned Arranged in a line.

Alimentary canal The digestive tube from the mouth to anus.

Alkali A substance that can neutralize acids. In radiography, sodium carbonate is used in the developer to promote developing action.

Allergen A foreign substance to the body system that causes a reaction or sensitivity.

Allergy Reaction to a drug that may be life threatening.

Alloy Composed of two or more metals.

Alopecia Hair loss.

Alveolectomy The process of reshaping the alveolar ridge by removing and smoothing bone.

Alveolitis Inflammation in the tooth socket due to loss of clot formation.

Alveolus (alveoli) Sockets for the teeth, also called alveolar process.

Amalgamation The actual chemical reaction that occurs between the alloy and mercury to form the silver amalgam.

Amalgamator A specially designed machine used to triturate (mix) a dental alloy with mercury to produce a silver amalgam restorative material.

Amalgam carrier A device used to carry dental amalgam to the prepared tooth.

Amalgam dust Minute particles of alloy and mercury.

Ambulatory When a person is able to walk.

Ameloblasts Specialized cells that form enamel.

Amelogenesis Beginning of enamel formation.

American Dental Assistants Association (ADAA) A national professional organization that represents dental assistants in legislative, educational, and career concerns.

American Dental Association (ADA) A national professional organization that deals with issues within the profession of dentistry. It possesses several branches, one of which is the Commission on Dental Accreditation, has direct authority on the accreditation of all schools of dentistry, dental hygiene, and some voluntary ADA-approved dental assisting and laboratory technology schools.

American Dental Hygienists Association (ADHA) A national professional organization that represents dental hygienists in legislative, educational, and career concerns.

American National Standards Institute (ANSI) Occupational and Educational Eye and Face Protection Standard (Z87.1-1989) A standard used when manufacturing eyewear and face protection.

Amide A chemical compound whereby a substitution of an ammonia atom for an acid radical takes place.

Amine An organic compound containing nitrogen.

Amylon Greek word for starch.

Anaerobic The ability to survive and grow in the absence of oxygen.

Anaphylaxis An allergic hypersensitivity reaction by the body to a foreign substance or drug that causes a fall in blood pressure, asthma, and swelling of the larynx.

Anatomic crown That part of the tooth crown covered with enamel.

Anatomic root That part of the tooth root covered with cementum.

Anatomy Study of structures and parts of the body.

Anchor tooth A tooth that receives the dental dam clamp.

Aneroid A type of manometer that utilizes atmospheric pressure instead of a liquid such as mercury.

Anesthesia Temporary loss of feeling or sensation by means of depressing the central nervous system or local interruption of nerve impulses to a specific area.

Angina pectoris Chest pain resulting from decreased blood supply to the heart muscle.

Angulation Alignment of the central ray in either direction, horizontally or vertically.

Ankyloglossia "Tongue tied" or short lingual frenum attachment between the tongue and the floor of the mouth.

Anode A positive electrode that attracts negative ions. In the dental x-ray tube, it incorporates the tungsten target.

Anode-film (source) distance (AFD) The distance between the source of radiation to the film.

Anomalies Any deviation from the normal.

Antagonist Drugs that counteract the action of another drug, decreasing or concealing the effect of the other.

Antecubital fossa A fossa located anteriorly at the bend of the elbow.

Anterior nasal spine A radiopaque pointed projection found anterior to the nasal fossae.

Antibody A specific substance produced by the body in response to a specific antigen.

Antigen A foreign substance, usually a protein, which when it enters the body incites the body to produce antibodies specific to that antigen.

Antigenically Pertaining to antibody production.

Antihistamine Drugs that counteract the action of another drug or allergen, decreasing or concealing the effect of the other.

Anti-inflammatory An agent that counteracts inflammation and its effects.

Antimicrobial Controls or destroys microorganisms.

Antipyretic An agent that reduces elevated temperatures.

Apex The pointed, anatomical area at the end of the tooth root.

Apexification Complete removal of pulpal tissues of a necrotic primary tooth with anticipated results of forming a calcified plug to seal the apex.

Apexogenesis Partial removal of a vital pulp that lies within the crown of a tooth, leaving the root portion intact.

Apical foramen Pertaining to the opening at the apex of the tooth root.

Apposition The body's process of laying down new bone. Also the deposition of the matrix for the hard dental structures.

Aqueous Containing water.

Arch wire Shaped in the form of the dental arch that fits into the buccal tubes and is attached to the brackets to provide movement to the teeth.

Arrhythmia Irregular heart rate.

Arterioles The smallest of arteries which join with capillaries in the circulatory system.

Articulator A mechanical hinge that acts as the temporomandibular joint.

Artifact In radiography, any image that appears on a radiograph but was not intended to be there.

Aseptic technique Methods used to prevent infection.

Asymmetry Right and left sides are not the same size.

Asymptomatic Without symptoms.

Atomization To separate into atoms.

Atrium The upper chambers of each half of the heart.

Atrophic Pertaining to wasting away or reduction in size.

Attenuation The process of absorption of the x-ray beam as it passes through matter and thus becomes weaker.

Attrition Loss of tooth structure due to wear.

Atypical Not typical.

Aura A sensory awareness preceding an epileptic seizure.

Auscultate Listening for abnormal sounds while performing an examination.

Autograft Graft taken from one part of the body and placed in another part.

Automix A device that mixes the material.

Autonomic Working independently.

Autopolymerization The process of polymerization when two materials are mixed together.

Autotransformer A device that is used to make small electrical adjustments in the dental machine, due to fluctuations in electrical current.

Avulsed A tooth that is forcibly knocked out or torn from its socket.

Axial Any surface of the tooth that is parallel to the long axis of the tooth.

Bacillus A cylindrical bacterium; also called a rod.

Backup A copy made of a file usually on a diskette or tape cartridge in the event the original is lost or damaged.

Bacteria Single-celled organisms that are the simplest cells; also called procaryotes.

Bacterial filtration efficiency (BFE) A standard of filtration used when manufacturing face masks.

Band A fixed orthodontic appliance consisting of a metallic ring that is cemented on the tooth.

Base The portion of the denture made of acrylic resin that seats and makes contact with the tissue underneath. A metallic mesh embedded within the acrylic resin adds strength. The layer of cement that acts as an insulator and protective barrier under a restoration.

Baseline Ratio of nitrous oxygen to oxygen that produces the desired level of sedation.

Baseplate A preformed semirigid acrylic resin material that temporarily represents the base of the denture.

Behavior The manner in which a person conducts him- or herself under specified circumstances.

Bell stage When the enamel organ assumes the shape of a bell during tooth development.

Benign Doing little or no harm. Not malignant.

Beta particles High speed electrons.

Bevel A slanting of the enamel margins of a tooth preparation.

Bicuspid/premolar A posterior tooth with points and cusps for grasping, tearing, and chewing.

Bifurcation The anterior area where roots divide in a two-rooted tooth.

Bilateral Pertaining to both sides.

Bioburden Visible organic materials such as blood, saliva, and debris.

Biocompatible Compatible with oral tissues.

Biohazard material Biological, hazardous, or potentially infectious material.

Bisect To cut in half.

Bisected angle Based on the principle of projecting the x-ray beam at right angles to an imaginary line which bisects the angle formed by the longitudinal axis of the tooth and the plane of the film packet.

Bite wing Interproximal radiographs generally of the bicuspids and molars.

Black paper envelope Black paper sheath that protects the film from light.

Bloodborne pathogens Pertains to disease-causing microorganisms that are present in human blood.

Bloodborne Pathogen Standard (by OSHA) Standards developed by OSHA for the protection of health care workers.

Blood vessels Pertaining to the arteries, veins, and capillaries.

Bodily movement When a tooth is moved in its entirety.

Bone allograft A bone graft obtained from another person.

Brachial artery The main artery located at the inside of the arm.

Bracket An attachment to the band or directly to the tooth that provides a means for the arch wire to be secured to the bands or teeth.

Bremsstrahlung radiation X-radiation produced by speeding electrons that interact with tungsten atoms at their nucleus or nearby, causing abrupt stopping or deflection of entering electrons.

Bruxism Involuntary grinding or clenching of teeth.

Buccal Pertaining to the cheek or a surface closest to the cheek.

Buccal groove A groove that develops on the occlusal surface and continues over to the buccal surface, usually found on mandibular molars.

Buccal mucosa Inside the cheek area.

Buccal ridge A ridge on the buccal surface which extends from the tip of the cusp to the cervical margin found on maxillary bicuspids.

Buccal tube Where the ends of the arch wire are secured.

Bud stage First stage of tooth development.

Calcification The process by which organic tissue becomes hardened by the deposit of calcium and other mineral salts.

Calcination When gypsum is heated, some of the water is driven off and forms plaster or stone.

Calcining The process of heating the gypsum particles so that some of the water molecules are driven off in the form of steam.

Calculus Mineralized layers of plaque attached to the teeth.

Cancellous (bone) Spongy, having a latticelike structure.

Canine/cuspid An anterior tooth with a long thick root.

Canthus of the eye Anatomical area where the upper eyelid meets the lower eyelid.

Capillaries The smallest blood vessels in the body that connect with arterioles and venules.

Capsid The geometric protein case that is formed around viruses.

Cap stage When the enamel organ assumes the shape of a cap during tooth development.

Capsule Plastic or metal, screw-type or friction-fit small container used to mix amalgam in the amalgamator.

Carcinoma A malignant epithelial neoplasm that tends to invade surrounding tissue and to metastasize to distant regions of the body.

Cardiac muscle Heart muscle (myocardium).

Cardiac sphincter The sphincter located between the esophagus and the stomach that allows food to enter the stomach and prevents reflux to the esophagus.

Caries Bacterial disease of the calcified dental tissue.

Carious Decayed.

Carrier An individual who harbors disease organisms without being ill with the disease.

Caruncle A small fleshy elevation in close proximity to the opening of Wharton's duct.

Cassette A device used to hold film and intensifying screens during exposure of extraoral radiographs.

Cast Replica of the teeth or dental arch that is used as a working model.

Catalyst A substance capable of promoting or altering the speed of a chemical reaction, but that does not take part in the reaction.

Cathode A negative electrode that attracts positive ions. In the dental x-ray tube, it incorporates the tungsten filament.

Cavitation The implosion of billions of microscopic bubbles that collapse into themselves within the ultrasonic cleaner.

Cavosurface The junction of the cavity and the exterior tooth surface.

Cell A unit of structure, of development, and of function, both normal and abnormal.

Cell membrane The thin sheet of fats and protein that is the primary covering of a cell involved in transport and metabolism.

Cell wall A thick, rigid support structure that surrounds the cell membrane of algae, fungi, and bacteria and prevents them from bursting.

Cement line The layer of cement formed around the margin of the restoration.

Cementoblasts Cells that form cementum.

Cementoclasts Cementum-destroying cells.

Cementocytes Cementum-forming cells.

Cementoenamel junction (CEJ) The line of union of the cementum and enamel of the tooth.

Cementogenesis Beginning of cementum formation.

Cementum The substance covering the root surface of the tooth.

Central groove A groove found on the occlusal surface that separates the buccal from the lingual cusp.

Central processing unit (CPU) Comprised of the chips where all the computing takes place, or the "brain" of the computer.

Centric occlusion The relationship of maxillary and mandibular teeth when the jaws are closed, the teeth are in maximum contact, and the heads of the condyles are in the most retruded, unstrained position in the glenoid fossa.

Cephalometric radiograph An extraoral radiograph of the lateral view of the head and facial structures.

Cerebral edema Fluid in the brain.

Cerebrovascular accident Also known as stroke, where a cerebral blood vessel is blocked or ruptured, preventing blood flow to that part of the brain.

Certified Dental Assistant (CDA) A person who has earned a Certified Dental Assistant credential by meeting the eligibility requirements to take and pass the certification exam in chairside duties, radiation health and safety, and infection control given by the Dental Assisting National Board (DANB).

Certified Dental Laboratory (CDL) A dental laboratory that has met certain standards imposed by the National Board for Certification (NBC).

Certified Dental Technician (CDT) A person who has earned a Certified Dental Technician credential by meeting the eligibility requirements to take and pass the certification exam in dental laboratory procedures given by the National Board for Certification (NBC).

Cervical loop When the outer and inner enamel epithelium merge at the site of the cervix of the tooth during tooth development.

Cervix Necklike structure.

Charged-coupled device (CCD) The portion of the electronic sensor that is considered to be the electronic connector to the computer.

Chelation A chemical reaction between two substances that join together to form an adhesive bond.

Chemotherapy Application of chemical agents that are toxic to the fast growing cells or microorganisms but not harmful to the patient.

Cholesterol A substance pertaining to fat that circulates in the bloodstream.

Chromogenic Producing color or pigment.

Chromosome The condensed molecule of DNA that carries the hereditary information for most organisms. There are a total of 46, or 23 pairs, of different shapes and sizes.

Chronic In radiology, it refers to small doses of radiation over a long period of time.

Chronology Accepted order of past events.

Chuck A small metal cylinder located inside the head of the handpiece used to hold the shank portion of the rotary instrument.

Ciezynski's rule of isometry The normal ray is directed perpendicularly to a plane which lies midway between the plane of the teeth desired and the plane of the film.

Ciliary body Muscle attached to the lens of the eye that helps to focus the eye.

Cingulum A bulge or prominence of enamel found on the cervical third of the lingual surface of an anterior tooth.

Civil Law A law that deals with a situation between two persons where there was damage or injury or where there was a binding agreement.

Clasp/retainer The semicircular metallic projection that surrounds the abutment tooth, providing retention to the prosthesis.

Cleft An opening or crevice.

Cleft lip A congenital malformation caused by complete or partial failure of the lips to unite during fetal development.

Cleft palate A congenital malformation caused by complete or partial failure of the palate to unite during fetal development.

Clinical crown The crown portion of a tooth that is visible in the oral cavity.

CNS Central nervous system.

Coalesce To grow together.

Coccus A spherical, ball-shaped bacterial cell. When grouped in chains, they are called streptococci and in clusters they are staphylococci.

Code of ethics Standard of moral principles and practices that a profession closely follows.

Coenzymes A nonprotein organic substance that works with enzymes as an enzyme activator.

Collagen A vital crystalline, protein substance present in all connective tissue.

Collimator A disc made of radiopaque material, usually lead, with a round or rectangular aperture that restricts the size of the x-ray beam.

Colloid Gelatinous substances with large inorganic molecules that remain suspended and do not diffuse or spread once the chemical change occurs.

Colonies Clusters of bacteria.

Colony A clinging mass of cells that is the main body form of fungi and bacteria. It is created when a parent cell goes through hundreds of divisions.

Commissure Angle of the mouth.

Communication An exchange of information, ideas, views, meanings, and understanding.

Compact bone Hard dense bone.

Composite restoration A tooth-colored resin restorative material.

Concave Having an inward curvature, almost spoonlike in appearance.

Cone cut Improper positioning of the PID rendering a radiograph with an unexposed area.

Condense The process of packing the amalgam into the prepared tooth.

Conditioner A substance such as acid etchant that prepares the tooth to receive a sealant.

Confidentiality The nondisclosure of certain patient information except to another authorized person.

Conjunctiva Mucous membrane that lines the eyelids.

Connector A term used to describe one of the bars that connects the framework from right to left sides or from the framework to the acrylic saddle of a partial denture.

Consciousness Protective reflexes are intact, including ability to maintain airway and capability of rational responses to question or command.

Consent An adult who willingly gives authorization for proposed treatment.

Constrict Narrowing of a blood vessel.

Contact dermatitis Skin irritation or allergy due to making contact with an agent that produces an inflammatory reaction.

Contiguous Touching along a boundary or at a point.

Contralateral tooth A comparable tooth located on the opposite side of the same arch.

Contrast The number of shades of gray seen on a radiograph.

Convex Having an outward curvature.

Core The portion of the endodontic pin that receives the cast restoration.

Cornea The clear transparent portion of the eyeball.

Coronal Pertaining to the crown portion of the head.

Coronal surface The surface on the crown portion of the tooth.

Coronoid process One of two prominences of the superior part of the mandible located on the anterior of the ramus.

Corpuscles "Little bodies," or small rounded bodies pertaining to blood cells.

Corrosion A chemical reaction of a nonmetallic substance with a metal.

Corrosive Destructive materials that are either above or below 7.0 pH, as are alkalies or strong acids, and are reactive when the two combine.

Cortical plate The compact bone that covers cancellous bone, located on the facial and lingual surfaces of the maxillary and mandibular jaws.

Cosmic radiation Coming from the sun and stars.

Coulomb/kilogram (c/kg) An SI unit of measurement of ion pairs in 1 kilogram of air; 1 C/kg equals 3880 R.

Cranial nerves Twelve pairs of nerves that have their origin in the brain.

Cranium Composed of eight bones that contain and protect the brain.

Crepitus Grinding sounds coming from a joint.

Criminal law A law that deals with a person who has committed an act or crime that threatens society and may be subject to punitive action.

Crossbite When maxillary anterior incisals and/or posterior buccal cusps are in linguoversion position and do not overlap mandibular teeth.

Crozat appliance A palatal spreading appliance consisting of a split plastic palate with a screw in its center that opens or closes the space.

Curettage Scraping and cleaning out the diseased and infected tissues with a dental surgical curette.

Crypt A space within the alveolar bone that holds the unerupted tooth.

Cumulative Repeated exposure to ionized radiation producing effects in the body.

Cumulative effect Drugs not excreted quickly from the body that tend to accumulate, causing an increased effect.

Cusp Pertaining to a pointed or rounded elevation on the working surface of a cuspid, bicuspid, or molar.

Cuspidor A bowl with circulating water, used by the patient for spitting or emptying the mouth.

Cutaneous pain Located near the surface of the skin, which interprets pain as sudden and sharp.

Cyanotic When oxygen level is low, there is reduced hemoglobin in the blood, causing a bluish appearance on the skin.

Cyst The dormant survival stage a protozoan enters during hostile conditions; encapsulated sac containing fluid, semifluid, or solid material.

Cytoplasm The semiliquid substance that makes up the primary content of the interior of a cell.

Data Information.

Database A collection of stored data dealing with one subject that can be retrieved and manipulated to produce information.

Debridement Removal of foreign matter or dead tissue.

Decalcification The loss of calcium salts from the enamel in the first step of the decay process.

Decomposition The process of decay.

Decontamination The removal or destruction of bloodborne pathogens by the use of physical or chemical means.

Deglutition The act of swallowing.

Delinquent accounts Accounts that have an outstanding unpaid balance.

Delirium tremens Disorientation with visual and hearing hallucinations due to the habitual and excessive use of alcohol.

Dementia Loss of thought processes and memory.

Demineralization Removal of mineral elements from mineralized tissues.

Density (1) As applied to radiographs, refers to the degree of blackening of the film and the amount of light transmitted through the film. (2) Object density refers to the object's resistance to x-ray passing through it. (3) Thickness and bulk of a substance such as bone.

Dental assistant An unlicensed or noncertified person employed in a dental office who performs basic supportive dental assisting procedures under the supervision of a licensed dentist.

Dental Assisting National Board, Inc. (DANB) A governing board recognized by the American Dental Association that deals with various dental assistant certifying examinations such as CDA, CDPMA, and COA.

Dental health care worker (DHCW) Any member of the dental health team.

Dental laboratory technician (DLT) A member of the dental health team who performs supportive dental laboratory tasks.

Dental lamina Thin layer of tooth-producing cells.

Dental papillae Originating as connective tissue within the cap that proliferates to form the dental pulp and dentin.

Dental sac Dense band of connective tissue that surrounds the enamel organ and the dental papilla.

Dentifrice Another term for toothpaste.

Dentin The material forming the main inner portion of the tooth structure.

Dentinal tubules The shape that dentin takes simulating small tubes.

Dentinoclasts Dentin-destroying cells.

Dentinoenamel junction (DEJ) The line of union of the dentin and enamel within the tooth.

Dentinogenesis Beginning of dentin formation.

Dentist A licensed person having earned a Doctor of Dental Surgery (DDS) or Doctor of Medical Dentistry (DMD) who provides dental care to patients.

Dentofacial Pertaining to the teeth and face.

Deposition The body's process of activating osteoblasts to develop new bone.

Depression Diminished functional activity.

Desensitization Making it less sensitive.

Dessicated Thoroughly dried up.

Developer A processing solution that is comprised of several chemicals and is responsible for making the latent image visible on the film.

Developmental groove A shallow groove or line on the surface of a tooth.

Diabetic coma Loss of consciousness due to excessive amounts of blood sugar and little or no insulin in the system.

Diagnosis The recognition of a disease or condition and distinguishing it from another, based on its signs and symptoms.

Diastolic pressure Occurs when the heart is at rest and the surge of blood within the arteries is at the lowest arterial pressure.

Die A replica of a single tooth or several teeth on which a restoration is fabricated.

Differentiation A series of changes whereby the cells acquire completely different individual characteristics.

Diffusion The capability of cell membranes to selectively allow substances to pass in or out of the cell.

Diffusion hypoxia Lack of adequate amount of breathed oxygen, causing a person to develop a headache, nausea, and lethargy.

Digital image An image that is made up of pixels.

Digital image receptors (DIR) Another name for electronic sensors.

Digital retention The patient holds the film packet in place, using his or her fingers and light pressure to prevent movement.

Digitize The process of recording an image using a computer.

Dilacerated The root(s) of the tooth is (are) bent or curved.

Dilate Expansion of an orifice or vessel.

Dimensional distortion Changes that continue to take place whereby the dimensions are altered due to the relaxation of internal stresses.

Direct supervision Performance of clinical duties by an auxiliary while the dentist is physically present in the dental office and who will evaluate the procedure upon completion.

Disclosing solution/tablet A special dye used to detect plaque in the oral cavity.

Disease The pattern of response of a living organism to some form of injury.

Disinfection The process of using chemicals, ultraviolet light, or ionizing radiation as a means to kill bacteria with the exception of spores and resistant micoorganisms.

Dissipated Driven off.

Distal Pertaining to a surface away from the midline.

Distal fossa A fossa located on the distal side of the occlusal surface.

Distocclusion The mesiobuccal cusp of the maxillary first molar is aligned between the mandibular second bicuspid and first molar.

Distolingual groove A groove located only on the distal fossa of maxillary molars that continues onto the lingual surface ending at the middle third of the crown of the tooth.

Divergent Slightly narrowed at the pulpal floor.

Dorsum The upper surface (of the tongue).

Dose-response curve Refers to the direct correlation between radiation dose and the response (damage) of tissues.

Double-ended instrument Having two working ends using the same handle.

Dry strength The dry strength may be two or more times the wet strength.

Duct A canal or passage for fluids.

Dura mater The outermost membrane of the brain.

Duty of care The ethical responsibility owed by one individual to another, such as the dentist to the patient.

Dysphagia Difficulty in swallowing.

Ecto Pertaining to the outer layer.

Ectoderm The outer embryonic tissue layer.

Edema When body tissues retain an excessive amount of fluid, causing localized swelling.

Edentulous Without teeth.

Elastic hook A hook that serves to attach elastic bands for additional orthodontic force.

Electrode The point from which a discharge of current takes place.

Electrolyte A substance that undergoes chemical change to form ions in solution.

Electronic mail (e-mail) Distribution of messages in soft copy form.

Electronic sensors Filmless portion of the digital imaging system, used in place of film.

Electrons Negatively charged particles within the atom.

Electrostatic energy The binding force that keeps the negative electrons in their orbits by the positive nucleus.

Elongation Images of teeth appear longer than the actual teeth due to insufficient vertical angulation.

Embrasure A V-shaped space in a gingival direction between the proximal surfaces to two adjoining teeth in contact.

Embryo A young organism up to the end of the second month of intrauterine life.

Emergency Medical Service (EMS) Emergency care made available to persons who are experiencing life-threatening conditions.

Emetic A substance that induces vomiting.

Emissions The discharge of a substance or, in radiology, electrons.

Enamel The hard tissue that covers the anatomic crown of the tooth.

Enamel matrix A layer of cells that gives form to the crown of the tooth.

Enamel organ Originates as the tooth bud that subsequently develops the enamel of the tooth.

Enamel rods/prisms Many-sided columns of enamel.

Endo Pertaining to the layer within.

Endocardium The inner lining of the heart cavity.

Endodontic Pertaining to a tooth treated with a root canal.

Endospore The dormant, highly resistant cell that is formed by some bacteria to survive adverse conditions in the environment.

Endotracheal Within the trachea.

Engineering controls Pertaining to controls that isolate or remove the bloodborne pathogens hazard from the workplace.

Enteral Drugs placed directly into the gastrointestinal tract where absorption of the drug takes place in the small intestine.

Envelope The membrane that surrounds certain viruses (hepatitis B and AIDS) and is used to invade a host cell.

Enzyme A secretion of living cells, usually a protein, capable of causing or accelerating a chemical reaction.

Epidemic A contagious disease that spreads rapidly and extensively among many individuals in a geographic area.

Epidemiology The study of the cause, occurrence, and transmission of disease.

Epilepsy A central nervous system disorder caused by abnormal electrical discharges within the brain, resulting in abnormal muscular movements and loss of consciousness.

Epithelial nests Remnant cells of the enamel organ present in the periodontal ligament.

Epithelium The covering of the internal and external surfaces of the body.

Ergonomic Concerned with the design and structure of machines and facilities that contribute to the well-being of an individual's body.

Erosion Disintegration of tooth surfaces other than those used in mastication.

Erythema Redness of the skin caused by dilation of capillaries; sometimes results from radiation.

Erythematous Reddish appearance of the skin or mucosa.

Ester A chemical compound formed by combining an organic acid with alcohol.

Ethics The part of philosophy that deals with moral conduct, judgment, and being able to apply these capacities.

Etiology The cause of disease.

Eucaryotic A more complex type of cell found in animals, plants, fungi, and algae that contains a nucleus and organelles for performing various specific functions.

Euphoria A sense of well-being.

Excretory Elimination of waste products from the body such as urine, feces, and sweat.

Excursion Lateral or protrusive movement of the lower jaw.

Exfoliation The process of shedding primary teeth.

Exostosis Excessive bony outgrowth generally occurring bilaterally on the mandibular lingual premolar region, termed torus (on one side) or tori (on both sides) mandibularis or on the maxillary along the palatine suture, termed torus palatinus.

Exothermic reaction Chemical reaction whereby heat is released.

Expectorate The act of ejecting or spitting out.

Extended functions dental assistant (EFDA) A licensed dental assistant who performs additional clinical duties beyond those performed by the dental assistant under the supervision of a licensed dentist.

Extension cone paralleling (XCP) A practical technique for periapical radiography that minimizes dimensional distortion and presents the objects being radiographed in their true anatomical relationship and size.

External oblique ridge A ridge that descends along the ramus of the mandible and passes downward and outward.

Extirpation Complete removal or eradication of soft tissue.

Extraoral Outside of the oral cavity.

Extrusion A tooth that is partially displaced outwardly from its socket due to injury or tooth loss from the opposing arch.

Exudate Leakage of fluid (pus or tissue fluid) from a cavity.

Facial Pertaining to a surface facing the cheek and collectively to the labial and buccal surfaces.

Fermentation The process of decomposition of complex substances through the action of enzymes, produced by bacteria, molds, and yeasts.

Fetal period From the third month of gestation to full term.

Fiberoptic A light system that uses special glass fibers called optical bundles to carry a source of light to a dental handpiece or mirror.

Fibroblasts Cells that form fibrous tissues.

Fibrous Containing fibers.

Fibrous capsule A tough protective capsule that surrounds the synovial fluid and attaches onto the bones.

Fibrous sheath Also known as the dental sac in which the development of a tooth occurs.

Filament A coil made of tungsten, also called wolfram wire, located in the cathode of an x-ray tube, that when heated, produces electrons.

Filings Alloy particles.

Filliform papillae Cone-shaped papillae on the tongue.

Film thickness Thickness of cement.

Final set Occurs after the plaster or stone has completed its crystallization and all the heat has been driven off.

Finger rest A pivot point that allows the hand to turn and move the instrument.

Fissure A natural groove found on enamel or bone, commonly the result of the imperfect fusion of the enamel.

Fixed maintainer A space maintainer cemented in place.

Fixer A processing solution comprised of several chemicals responsible for removing the silver halide crystals and clear the film.

Flammable An agent that is capable of producing flames.

Flange The extension of the acrylic portion of the saddle or base that reaches the border of the prosthesis.

Flash Excess restorative material that goes beyond the cavosurface or gingival margins.

Floor of maxillary sinus A thin, horizontal radiopaque line located below the maxillary sinus.

Floor of nasal cavity A thin, horizontal radiopaque line appearing above the maxillary sinus on a posterior periapical radiograph. Located on the superior surface of the palatine process.

Floppy disk Portable unit for storing computer information.

Fluorosis A condition of the teeth due to excessive ingestion of fluoride that causes teeth to have brown stains.

Focal spot Also known as the "tungsten target," located at the anode of the x-ray tube, where high-speed electrons hit to produce x-ray photons and heat.

Focal trough An imaginary three-dimensional area formed in the shape of the dental arches or a "horseshoe" used to position the patient's jaws within its confines while taking panoramic radiographs.

Focusing cup A concave reflector cup of molybdenum that focuses the electrons emitted by the filament into a narrow beam to the tungsten target at the anode.

Food and Drug Administration (FDA) A U.S. office that controls and inspects manufacture of drugs for public safety.

Fordyces granules Sebaceous glands located on the buccal mucosa and inner lips.

Foreshortening Images of teeth appear shorter than the actual teeth due to excessive vertical angulation.

Formative phase The development of an enamel matrix during tooth formation.

Foramen (foramina) A natural opening in the bone.

Fossa A hollow, grooved, or depressed area in a bone or tooth.

Framework The metallic portion of the removable denture that provides strength. It contains the base connector, lingual or palatal bar/major connector, clasps/retainers, and rests.

Frankfort plane An imaginary line that is formed starting at the top of the auditory meatus and extending through the lower border of the orbit of the eye.

Free gingival groove The line that separates the free gingiva from the attached gingiva.

Free radicals Produced during ionization of water within tissues. They are capable of forming hydrogen peroxide, a toxin, or poison to tissues.

Frena (frenum, singular) Folds of mucous membrane which connect the inner surface of the lip to the midline of the gingiva.

Frenectomy A surgical procedure to remove, reposition, or incise the frenum to give added mobility to the lip or tongue.

Fulcrum A point of rest and support that provides stability.

Fungi A kingdom of eucaryotic organisms including mushrooms, yeasts, and molds.

Fungiform papillae Mushroom-shaped papillae on the tongue.

Furcation Pertaining to the space between two roots in a multirooted tooth.

Gait The manner in which the patient carries him- or herself.

Gamma A particular arrangement of atoms.

Ganglion A mass of nerves found outside the brain or spinal cord.

Gastrointestinal tract Pertaining to the stomach and intestines of the digestive tract.

Gel The semi-solid state of a hydrocolloid.

Gelation The process of changing from a sol to a gel.

Gelation temperature The temperature at which the change from the sol state to a semi-solid material occurs.

Generalized bone loss Involving bone loss throughout the maxillary or mandibular arches.

General supervision Performance of clinical duties by an auxiliary with the dentist's permission but without the physical presence of the dentist.

Genes Units of heredity.

Genetic effects Radiation effects that are passed on to future generations.

Genial tubercles Two small radiopaque processes of bone located below the roots of the incisors in the midline of the lingual surface of the mandible.

Geriatric Elderly patients.

Ghost images A radiopaque artifact created by an object such as jewelry that is projected to the opposite side and on a higher plane of the radiograph as an out-of-focus magnified image.

Gingival crest The edge, or tip, of the free gingiva.

Gingival hyperplasia Overgrowth of the gingiva.

Gingival recession Changes that occur in both the composition make-up of the gingiva and the relation of the gingiva to the tooth where the gingiva recedes rootward, possibly due to advancing age, improper oral hygiene, malocclusion, and physiologic or pahtologic disturbances.

Gingival sulcus The shallow furrow formed where the gingival tip meets the tooth enamel.

Gingivectomy Surgical removal of the inflamed and diseased gingiva and of deep suprabony pockets.

Gingivitis Inflammation limited to the gingiva.

Gingivoplasty Surgical removal of gingival deformities to create normal and functional form.

Gland A cell or a group of cells that have the ability to draw specific substances from the blood and alter them for later release.

Glenoid Shallow or slightly cupped depression in a bone.

Glossopalatine arch Also known as anterior tonsilar pillar arch, located within the palatine velum anterior to palatal tonsils.

Glucose Sugar in the bloodstream.

Glycerol A sugar alcohol present in chemical combination of all fats.

Glycol An alcohol derived from a carbohydrate that is used in alginate to make it dustless.

Gnarled enamel A variation in the direction of enamel rods in which they become intertwined, increasing the strength of enamel.

Golden rule "Do unto others as you would have them do unto you."

Gomphosis Principal fibers of the periodontal ligament that support the gingival tissue and suspend the tooth in the socket.

Gram negative Bacteria that stain with a red dye in the gram stain.

Gram positive Bacteria that stain with a purple dye in the gram stain.

Grand mal Epileptic seizure usually involving convulsions and loss of consciousness.

Granulation tissue Tissue that appears granular due to new fleshy projections formed in an area where healing is not taking place.

Granuloma Collection of granular tissue at the apex of a tooth due to inflammation.

Gray (Gy) An SI unit for absorbed dose. Used in place of the rad; 1 Gy equals 100 rad.

Grit Particle size of the abrasive that controls the cutting action.

Gypsum powder Plaster of Paris.

Half-life Time required by the body to metabolize or inactivate half the amount of a substance taken in.

Half-value layer (HVL) The reduction of the intensity of the x-ray beam by 50% after aluminum filtration is added.

Hamulus A spiny projection that protrudes from the medial wing of the pterygoid process.

Hard copy The printed page of data generated by the computer.

Hard disk A storage device composed of magnetically treated rigid platters that is able to store much more information than diskettes.

Hard radiation A term used to describe shorter, high-frequency wavelengths of radiation.

Hardware The physical electronic and mechanical components of a computer system.

Harelip Imperfect fusion of the upper lip.

Headgear An extraoral orthodontic device used to control orthopedic growth and tooth movement.

Headgear tube Where the inner bow of the orthodontic headgear is secured.

Heatless Creating less heat.

Hemoglobin Oxygen-carrying red blood cells.

Hemostasis Less flow of blood to the injection site causing less bleeding.

Hepatitis Inflammation of the liver.

Hepatitis A (HAV) Known as "infectious" hepatitis. Occurs usually in children and young adults and is transmitted by oral-fecal route.

Hepatitis B (HBV) Known as "serum" hepatitis and transmitted by infected blood, sexual contact, infected needle puncture, and mother to fetus/infant.

Hepatitis C (HCV) Chronic liver disease transmitted through blood transfusions, contaminated sharps, infected needle puncture, sexual body fluids, and childbirth.

Hepatitis D (HDV) Occurring simultaneously with hepatitis B, immunization against HBV will provide protection against HDV. Transmitted by contaminated sharps, sexual body fluids, and childbirth.

Hepatitis E (HEV) Similar to hepatitis A and transmitted by contaminated water and fecal-oral route.

Hepatitis G (HGV) Occurs worldwide and is transmitted by infected blood.

Herpes simplex A highly infectious viral disease that produces vesicular lesions that burst, ulcerate, and scab within 5–10 days.

High-voltage transformer Also known as the "step-up transformer" located within the tubehead to increase voltage from 110 or 220 volts to 65,000 up to 100,000 volts.

Histamine Substance released by the body in the presence of a foreign substance (allergen).

Histodifferentiation The development stage where cells differentiate and become specialized.

HIV (human immunodeficiency virus) A disease that invades the body and generally develops into AIDS.

Horizontal angulation Alignment of the central ray using a horizontal movement to position the PID at a mesial or distal angulation; establishes open or closed interproximals.

Hormones Chemical messengers produced by cells of the body and transported by the bloodstream.

Host The organism that serves as the habitat and source of nutrition for a parasite; it is usually harmed by the association.

Humidity Amount of water in the air.

Hydration Addition of water to the powder.

Hydrogenated oils A process whereby hydrogen atoms are added to the oil to change it into a solid state, such as margarine.

Hydrophillic Capable of taking up water.

Hyperemia The first stage of inflammation where excessive blood is present.

Hyperreactive The response from a person who has low tolerance to pain.

Hypersensitivity (Allergy) The state of being abnormally sensitive or susceptible to a drug or chemical.

Hypo A component chemical found in the fixer, also known as sodium thiosulfate or hyposulfite of soda that removes unexposed silver halide crystals not affected by the developer. Fixer is also known as hypo.

Hypoallergenic (Hypo = "below") Below the level to cause an allergic reaction.

Hypocalcification A condition of diminished calcium from excessive fluoride intake (over 2 ppm) during tooth development.

Hyporeactive The response from a person who has a high tolerance to pain.

Iatrosedation Does not require the administration of drugs but instead uses stress reduction behavior and patient management techniques such as acupressure, hypnosis, or the manner of communication whereby the patient develops trust and confidence in the doctor.

Identification dot A small raised dot placed on intraoral film to identify the right from the left side.

Idiosyncrasy An unexpected effect following administration of a drug.

Imbibition The process of taking on additional water, causing a swelling of the material.

Impaction Pertaining to an embedded tooth which has been unable to erupt in the oral cavity.

Impervious Material resistant to moisture, light, and penetration of microorganisms.

Implied consent Verbal authorization given by an adult who agrees to proposed treatment.

Implosion The formation of minute bubbles that collapse into themselves in the special solution by the action of the ultrasonic cleaner.

Incisal Pertaining to the biting edge of an anterior tooth.

Incisive foramen A radiolucent opening on the anterior portion of the palate located at the midline between the central incisor roots.

Incisors Pertaining to the central and lateral teeth that incise to divide or cut.

Increment Small amounts of material.

Incontinence Loss of urinary bladder control.

Incubation period The time between the infection of the individual by a microroganism and the first manifestation of the disease.

Indirect vision Using a mouth mirror to view an area within the mouth.

Inert substance Pertaining to a substance that is not active and remains idle.

Infectious disease Illness that is due to a microorganism growing in the body and causing damage to the tissue and organs.

Infectious wastes Also referred to as biohazardous waste. Examples are contaminated sharps, blood-soaked items, and extracted teeth.

Inferior turbinate bones A hazy gray radiopaque shadow located on the lateral wall of the nasal fossa.

Informed consent Written authorization given by an adult who agrees to proposed treatment.

Infra Inferior or below.

Ingot Metal cast into a bar.

Initiation The beginning development of a tooth.

Initial set The time between the spatulation and the time the mixture loses its gloss and becomes firm or solid enough to handle but is still moist and slightly pliable.

Innocuous Harmless or benign.

Inoculation The process by which microorganisms enter the body.

Insertion The point of muscle attachment that is movable.

Insoluble Incapable of dissolving.

Insomnia Sleeplessness or unable to sleep.

Insulin shock Diabetic condition resulting from an overdose of insulin, resulting in hypoglycemia.

Intensifying screen A white plastic-like film holder composed of rare earth or calcium tungstate that emits light or glows when struck by radiation, which in turn exposes film.

Intercostal paralysis Paralysis of muscles between the ribs.

Interdental papilla Triangular folds of gingival tissue between the teeth.

Internal oblique ridge A radiopaque line located on the internal aspect of the ramus of the mandible that passes downward and forward from the ramus to the third molar.

International System A charting system designed to be used with the computer that uses a two-digit number to identify each tooth, The numbering for permanent teeth start with 1–4, and for primary teeth the numbering starts with 5–8, depending on the quadrant.

Internet Large computer network.

Interpretation The explanation of what is viewed on a radiograph.

Interprismatic substance The calcified substance that separates each enamel rod or prism.

Interproximal Between the proximal surfaces of adjacent teeth.

Interseptal/septum The portion of the dam located interproximally between two dental dam holes.

Intraligamentary Within the (periodontal) ligament.

Intrauterine Within the uterus, pertaining to embryonic life.

Intrusion A tooth that is partially driven into its socket and does not meet occlusion with the opposing arch.

Invasive To allow infective microorganisms to gain entry into the body.

Inverse square law A principle that states that the intensity of the beam is inversely proportional with the square of the distance from the source of radiation.

Invert/invaginate The process of "tucking" or folding the raw edges of the dental dam holes that surround the isolated teeth to prevent moisture contamination.

Ionization The process by which a balanced atom becomes an unbalanced atom, or particle, with an electrical charge of positive or negative.

Iris Pigmented membrane surrounding the pupil.

Irradiation The application of radiation for therapeutic purposes.

Irreversible colloids Have the ability to change from a liquid state to a semi-solid state but not vice-versa.

Jaundice Yellow appearance over all the skin, including the sclera or white portion of eyes.

Keratotic Pertaining to the formation of horny growth.

Labial Pertaining to the lips or a surface closest to the lips.

Labial lamina A thin layer of tissue that forms the lips in histodifferentiation.

Labial ridge A ridge on the labial surface that extends from the cusp tip to the cervical line, found on maxillary cuspids.

Labiodental Pertaining to the areas of the lips and teeth.

Lacrimal Pertaining to tears.

Lactobacillus One of the microorganisms that forms inside a carious lesion.

Lamina dura/Alveolar process proper Dense bone that lines the root sockets of the teeth.

Laminae Thin layer or plates.

Laryngoscope A viewing instrument inserted into the larynx.

Latent Refers to a virus going into a dormant, inactive phase in its host cell.

Latent image The invisible radiographic representation of dental structures on an exposed but not processed film.

Latent period The time period that elapses between the time or radiation exposure and the time when observable signs are manifested.

Lay terms Adjusting technical terms into ones that will be understood by the average person.

Lead foil A thin sheet of embossed lead foil located on the back side within the film packet for protection of scattered radiation.

Lesion Disease-related or external injury-induced tissue damage or discoloration.

Leukoplakia Precancerous condition exhibiting white patchy lesions.

Ligature tie Made of thin wire or elastomeric material and utilized to tie the arch wire to the orthodontic brackets on the bands or teeth.

Light tight When the darkroom is free of white light.

Linea alba buccalis A white line demarcation on inside cheek where maxillary and mandibular teeth occlude.

Line angle Formed by the junction of any two surfaces of a tooth crown, and its name is derived by combining the names of the two surfaces.

Lines of Retzius Contour incremental lines observed in enamel, caused by brief pauses in its development where diminished calcification occurs.

Lines of Schreger/enamel lamellae Narrow cracks in enamel that become filled with organic material during formation.

Lingual Pertaining to the tongue or a surface nearest the tongue.

Lingual foramen A radiolucent small dark spot located above the genial tubercles, radiographically appearing in the center of the genial tubercles.

Lingual groove A groove that develops on the occlusal surface of mandibular molars and second bicuspids and continues over to the lingual surface dividing the mesiolingual cusp from the distolingual cusp.

Lingual ridge A ridge on the lingual surface that extends from the tip of the cusp toward the cervical line, found on maxillary cuspids.

Linguoversion Turned toward the lingual side.

Lobes A developmental segment of a tooth.

Localized bone loss Bone loss involving a few teeth.

Localized exposure Refers to ionized radiation exposure to a small part of the body.

Long axis Vertical length of tooth.

Longitudinal Lengthwise.

Long-scale contrast Low contrast, depicting many shades of gray on a radiograph; has a result of using higher kilovoltage.

Long-term effect Effects of radiation manifested years later due to chronic exposure to radiation.

Lower border of nasal cavity Radiopaque rounded inferior margins of the nasal cavity.

Lumen The space within a tube, such as a blood vessel or needle.

Luting Cementation.

Luxation Displacement of organs or dislocation of a joint.

Lysis Refers to a virus continuing into the phase of multiplication in its host cell, which results in the destruction of the host cell.

Macroscopic Visible with the naked eye.

Mainframe A large system that places computers in many locations within a building allowing them to input and retrieve information from a central unit.

Malaise A feeling of illness or depression.

Malaligned Pertaining to teeth that are out of alignment in the dental arch.

Malar bone (zygomatic process) The inferior portion of the cheek bone that appears as a radiopaque U overlying the maxillary sinus.

Malaria A prominent and severe protozoan infection spread by the bite of certain mosquitoes.

Malignant Tending to become progressively worse and to result in death.

Malocclusion Any deviation from normal occlusion.

Malpractice An act of professional negligence that causes injury or harm to a patient.

Mamelon A rounded eminence on the incisal edge of a newly erupted incisor.

Mandate Something imposed by an administrative board as a moral obligation.

Mandibular canal A radiolucent space between two white radiopaque (white) lines in the mandibular bone located below molar and bicuspid roots.

Man-made/artificial radiation Produced by man, i.e., nuclear, dental, and medical x-rays.

Manometer A device used in measuring gaseous or liquid pressure (blood pressure).

Marginal ridge The rounded borders of the enamel that form the margins of the occlusal surfaces of the bicuspids and molars mesially and distally.

Master cone The selected gutta percha point that fits adequately whereby it fills and seals the canal up to 1 mm from the apex.

Mastication Masticate, or grind with the teeth; the act of chewing and grinding.

Materia alba White curds of matter composed of dead cells, food, and other components of the dental plaque.

Material Safety Data Sheets (MSDS) Data collected on hazardous agents that may be found in materials used in a dental office.

Matrix band A contoured, thin strip of stainless steel used to form the missing wall(s) of the prepared tooth.

Maturation phase When the enamel matrix undergoes calcification during tooth formation.

Maxillary sinus (antrum) A radiolucent cavity and bone which contains air located above the maxillary bicuspid and molar roots; also known as antrum of Highmore.

Maximum permissible dose (MPD) The maximum dose that an occupational person may receive within a prescribed time.

Media The nutrient material that is used to culture or grow microorganisms in the laboratory.

Median line An imaginary line dividing the two central incisors.

Median palatine suture A radiolucent line located at the maxillary central incisor region extending from the alveolar crest to the posterior of the palate.

Median sulcus (tongue) The middle line that divides the tongue in symmetrical halves.

Medullary spaces The radiolucent bone marrow portions of the spongy bone.

Meniscus (Interarticular disc) A fibrous cartilage within a joint.

Mental Pertaining to the chin.

Mental foramen A radiolucent oval, round, or oblong space located around the mandibular bicuspid apices.

Mental process (ridge) The anterior and inferior aspect of the chin that appears radiopaque in a triangular shape below the apices of the mandibular incisors.

Mercury A metal that is liquid at room temperature.

Mercury vapor Undetectable mercury molecules present in the air.

Mesenchyme The meshwork of embryonic connective tissue in the mesoderm from which are formed the connective tissues of the body and also the blood and lymphatic vessels.

Mesial Toward the midline.

Mesial fossa A fossa located on the mesial side of the occlusal surface.

Mesiocclusion The mesiobuccal cusp of the maxillary first molar is aligned between the mandibular first and second molars.

Meso Pertaining to the middle layer.

Mesoderm The middle embryonic tissue layer.

Mesognathic profile Pertaining to a straight profile.

Metabolic Pertaining to metabolism whereby the sum of all physical and chemical changes take place within an organism.

Metastasis (plural metastases) The distant spread of the tumor cells from the site of origin.

Microbiology The study of living things that are too small to be observed with the naked eye and that require magnification with a microscope.

Microcomputer Also known as the personal computer, consisting of one system.

Microleakage A space between the tooth and the restoration.

Microorganism Any tiny cell or group of cells that cannot be adequately seen or studied without the aid of a microscope, including viruses, bacteria, algae, protozoa, yeasts, and molds. Also called microbe.

Microscopic Referring to a property of cells or other structures that cannot be viewed readily without magnification.

Midsagittal plane An imaginary line that divides the body in right and left sides evenly.

Milliampere (mA) 1/1000th of an ampere. The strength of a unit of electrical current.

Millimicrometer One-millionth of a millimeter or one-thousandth of a micrometer.

Mineralization Placement of minerals in a mineralized tissue.

Minicomputer A computer system that has a central unit with monitors and keyboards placed in other rooms that can input data.

Mitosis A process of division in eucaryotic cells in which the chromosomes divide evenly between the two new cells that are formed.

Mixed dentition When loss of deciduous teeth takes place and permanent teeth start to take their positions.

Mixed nerves Nerves possessing both sensory and motor fibers.

Modified pen grasp A method of grasping an instrument, handpiece, or oral vacuum when performing operative dentistry.

Molar A posterior tooth with a broad occlusal surface for chewing.

Molecules The smallest units of a compound.

Monomer Molecule with one mer—*mono* means "one."

Monosaturated fats Refers to those fats that neither raise nor lower serum cholesterol, such as olive oil.

Morphodifferentiation The stage of development at which the basic form and relative size of the tooth are determined.

Morphology The science of organic form and structure.

Motor or efferent nerves Nerves that stimulate movement of muscles by carrying impulses from the brain to the muscles in response to pain.

Mottled enamel Teeth severely affected by fluorosis exhibiting cracking and pitting.

Mottling Enamel surfaces that become pitted as a result of fluorosis.

Mould Shape of artificial teeth.

Mucous (Mucin) A slimy gluelike secretion.

Mull Additional trituration given whereby the mixture is brought together after the pestle is removed.

Mycoses Infections of living tissue by a fungus (mold or yeast).

Mylohyoid ridge A prominent radiopaque ridge located horizontally along the inside of the mandible and below the posterior or molar area.

Myocardial infarction Also known as a heart attack, where the coronary artery becomes occluded, preventing blood flow to the myocardium (heart muscle).

Myocardium Heart muscle.

Narcolepsy Sleeping sickness.

Nares Another term for nostrils.

Nasal fossae (cavities) A radiolucent cavity situated above the apices of the maxillary central incisors.

Nasal septum A wide radiopaque shadow that divides the right from the left nasal cavity or fossae.

Nasmyth's membrane The enamel cuticle partially remaining on a tooth surface after tooth eruption.

Nasociliary Pertaining to nerves of the nose.

Nasopharyngeal A tube inserted through the nose to provide ventilation to the patient.

National Board for Certification (NBC) A governing board recognized by the American Dental Association (ADA) that deals with certification of dental laboratory technicians.

Natural/terrestrial radiation Coming from natural sources and part of human environment.

Necrosis Condition in which dead cells or tissues are in contact with living cells.

Negligence An act that a reasonable person would not do under the same or similar circumstance (act of commission) or failure to do an act that a reasonable person would do under the same or similar circumstance.

Neoplasm A tumor that may be benign or malignant.

Neutrocclusion The mesiobuccal cusp of the maxillary first molar is aligned with the buccal groove of the mandibular first molar.

Nib The working end of an instrument such as the condenser.

Nonverbal communication A mode of communication involving actions, attitudes, and gestures.

Nucleated Containing a nucleus.

Nucleus The control center of the cell that influences growth, repair, and reproduction of the cell.

Nutrient canals Blood vessels that supply the teeth and gingival tissues and appear as radiolucent linear shadows between the roots of adjacent teeth.

Object-film distance The distance between the tooth and the film.

Obligate parasite A pathogenic microorganism that must live inside its host cell to carry out its full life cycle.

Oblique On a slant, neither perpendicular nor horizontal.

Oblique ridge A ridge that runs diagonally across the occlusal surface of maxillary molars.

Obtundent A medicament that provides soothing relief to the patient.

Obturate To fill the root canal(s) of a tooth with a restorative material.

Obturator Portion of a prosthesis used to close a congenital opening or cleft of the palate.

Occiput Back part of the head.

Occlude When the biting surfaces of maxillary and mandibular teeth meet.

Occlusal The chewing surface of the posterior teeth.

Occlusal edge Also known as occlusal margin. The tip of the buccal cusp of a bicuspid is located in the center of the biting edge.

Occlusal film examination A radiographic examination that employs one film to inspect large areas of the maxilla or mandible.

Occupational exposure When an employee is exposed to HBV, HCV, HIV, or OPIM while performing duties in the work place.

Odontoblastic process/Tomes' dentinal fibrils Collagenous tissue retained within the dentinal tubules during tooth formation.

Odontoblasts Specialized cells that form dentin.

Odontomata An anomaly in tooth development, particularly of the hard tissues.

Odontology A study of the external form and relationship of the teeth.

Oncology Study of tumors.

Open bay Where several dental chairs are positioned in one large treatment room.

Openbite When there is no overlap but rather an open space between the incisal edges of the maxillary and the mandibular incisors while the posterior teeth are in occlusion.

Operating system Software that directly controls the hardware.

Ophthalmic Pertaining to the eyes.

Organelle A tiny package inside a cell that has a membrane covering and performs a particular function for the cell, such as metabolism or transport.

Orifice An opening to a cavity.

Origin The point of attachment at one end of the muscle which is more or less stationary.

Oropharyngeal A tube inserted into the pharynx through the mouth to provide ventilation to the patient

Orthodontics The dental specialty concerned with the study and supervision of growth and development of dentition and related anatomical structures from birth to maturity.

Orthostatic or postural hypotension Decrease in blood pressure when the patient is returned to a sitting position after reclining.

Osseointegration A process whereby the bone grows around the implant and attaches itself.

Osseous Bony material.

Ossification Conversion into bone.

Osteoblasts The cells responsible for bone formation.

Osteoclasts Specialized bone-destroying cells.

Osteoplasty The surgical reshaping of the alveolar bone.

Osteoradionecrosis Destruction of the bone due to radiation exposure.

OTC Over the counter, not needing a prescription.

Other potentially infectious materials (OPIM) Any human body fluid that may or may not be contaminated by blood, i.e., semen, vaginal secretions, cerebrospinal fluid, synovial fluid, pleural fluid, pericardial fluid, peritoneal fluid, amniotic fluid, saliva, and any other body fluid visibly contaminated with blood such as saliva or vomitus.

Otic Pertaining to the ear.

Outer wrapping A plastic or waterproof paper that protects the film from moisture and light.

Ovale Egg shaped.

Overbite When there is a greater than normal vertical overlap between the incisal edges of the maxillary central incisors and the mandibular central incisors.

Overjet A horizontal distance that exists due to the protrusion of the most anterior maxillary incisor to the facial aspect of the most anterior mandibular incisors.

Ovum Fertilized egg from the mother.

Oxidation When solutions combine with oxygen, causing them to break down.

Palatal Area involving the palate, or roof of the mouth.

Palatine process The superior surface forms a part of the floor of the nasal cavity; the inferior surface forms the roof of the mouth.

Palatine tonsils Two prominent masses, consisting of lymphoid tissue, located on either side of the oral cavity between the glossopalatine and pharyngopalatine arches.

Palatine uvula A small conical extension at the midline of the soft palate free edge.

Palatine velum A curtainlike partition of the soft palate.

Palmer System A charting system that uses quadrants with numbers or letters. Numbers 1–8 are used to identify permanent teeth and letters A–E to identify primary teeth.

Palpation Process of examination for detection by the use of hands or fingers on the external surfaces of the body.

Papillae Projections located over the dorsum of the tongue.

Papule Small elevated solid lesion, less than 5 mm.

Parasite Any organism that lives on or in the body of another organism, called its host.

Parasitic worm An animal such as a fluke or roundworm that invades and grows in a host.

Parenteral Drugs that bypass the gastrointestinal tract and are absorbed in a different manner.

Parietal Forming walls of a cavity (skull).

Particulate radiation Small particles of matter such as electrons, protons, neutrons, alpha particles and beta particles that travel at high speeds in a straight line.

Password A meaningful number of characters used to identify a specific computer user.

Pathogen Microbe capable of causing disease.

Pathogenic Capable of causing infection and disease.

Penumbra An indistinct fuzzy outline of the object on the image of a radiograph.

Periapical film Pertaining to a film that captures the apex of the roots of teeth and their surrounding areas.

Pericardium The fibrous sac in which the heart is enclosed.

Pericoronitis An inflammation or infection of the gingival tissues surrounding the crown of an erupting tooth.

Periodontal ligament The tissues that support and anchor the tooth in its socket.

Periodontal pocket Detachment of the gingiva leaving an extremely wide and deep space in the gingival crevice.

Periodontia The science of treating diseases of the supporting tissues of the teeth.

Periodontitis Inflammation involving the periodontal ligament and supporting structures.

Periodontium The tissues that surround and support the teeth such as the alveolar process, periodontal ligament, and gingiva.

Periosteum A fibrous sheath that covers the cortical plate.

Peristalsis Muscular contractions of the alimentary canal that aids in breaking up food into smaller particles and mixes them with digestive juices and continually moves the food mass through the canal.

Personal protective equipment (PPE) A term used in reference to protective clothing, eyewear, masks, and gloves for effective infection control for the health care worker's skin protection.

Pestle A mechanical rod used to break up the material within the capsule.

Petit mal Mild form of epileptic attack that does not include seizures.

Pharmacosedation Sedatives that calm and reduce anxiety by depressing the central nervous system without loss of consciousness.

Pharyngo Refers to the pharynx or throat.

Pharyngopalatine arch Also known as posterior tonsilar pillar, located at the most posterior arch dividing the oral cavity and pharynx.

Phase Denotes a change in structure.

Photoelectric effect One of the interactions produced by an x-ray photon with matter; the x-ray photon gives up all of its energy, ceasing to exist, when it ejects a tightly-bound electron from its shell which continues its journey as a photoelectron.

Photopolymerization The process of polymerization when a visible blue light is used.

Photosensitivity Reaction to light (sunlight) exposure.

Physiology Study of the functions of the body systems.

Pit A pinpoint depression on the surface of a tooth, usually located at the end of a groove or where two or more grooves join.

Plaque Accumulation of bacteria and products of saliva that clings to the teeth.

Plasma A faintly straw-colored fluid of the blood consisting of 90% water.

Plexus A network of veins.

Pneumocystis carinii **pneumonia (PCP)** A particular type of lung disease associated with AIDS.

Point angle Formed by the junction of three surfaces of a tooth; its name is derived by combining the names of the three surfaces.

Polygonal Having many sides.

Polymer A long chain of many mers or molecules of a compound capable of being chemically combined—*poly* means "many."

Polymerization A chemical reaction that occurs between the initiator (peroxide) and the activator (amine) or the use of visible blue light that causes the material to set up or harden.

Polyunsaturated fats Include the common vegetable oils having a lesser number of hydrogen atoms.

Pontic Suspended portion (tooth replacement) of a bridge; the part of the appliance that replaces a missing tooth or teeth.

Porte polisher A single-ended handle built with an adjustable loop that holds small wooden points used to manually polish teeth.

Porous Has more open spaces within the structure.

Positioner An appliance that will help maintain the teeth in their new positions after orthodontic treatment.

Position-indicating device (PID) Sometimes known as the cone; an open-ended cylindrical or rectangular device varying from 8 to 16 in. in length that fits over the aperture of the tubehead, used to direct and restrict the central beam toward the patient.

Post The metallic pin that is cemented within the endodontically treated pulpal canal to lend support to a fixed appliance.

Potentiation The potency generated from a combination of two drugs are greater than the sum of the independent effects of each drug.

Predentin An uncalcified layer of material located within the dentinal tubules which subsequently calcifies.

Premature Taking place earlier than anticipated.

Premedication Medication given in advance of the procedure.

Primary dentin Dentin formed in a newly developed tooth.

Primary radiation Also known as direct, useful, or central rays, projected from the target that reaches the object.

Primitive First in time, original.

Procaryotic A type of cell that is very small and simple in structure, lacking a nucleus and organelles.

Prognathic profile Profile that exhibits a prominent chin.

Proliferation Multiplication of cells.

Prosthesis The replacement for one or more teeth and associated tissues.

Protoplasm Pertaining to a combination of the cytoplasm and the substance in the nucleus of a cell; the essential constituent of a living cell.

Protozoa A type of single-celled microorganism that feeds by engulfment and usually has some form of locomotion.

Protuberance Rounded projection.

Proximal Nearest or adjacent to.

Psychotropic Any substance that acts on the mind.

Pterygoid Wing-shaped bone.

Pulp The vital tissues of the tooth consisting of nerves, blood vessels, and connective tissue.

Pulpalgia Severe constant pain in the pulp of a tooth.

Pulp canal/root canal Portion of the pulp confined to the root.

Pulp cavity The space within the central portion of the crown and root of the tooth, surrounded by dentin, normally filled with pulp tissue.

Pulp chamber The portion of the pulp found within the crown portion of the tooth.

Pulpectomy Involves the removal of pulpal tissues from the chamber and pulpal canals, treatment with zinc oxide-eugenol, and a permanent restoration.

Pulpitis, irreversible Inflammation and deterioration of the pulp requiring endodontic treatment.

Pulpitis, reversible Inflammation of the pulp where there is a chance for recovery without endodontic treatment.

Pulpotomy Involves the removal of pulpal tissue up to the pulpal canals, treatment with formocresol or calcium hydroxide, and restoration.

Punitive Punishment for negligence imposed on another. The amount charged usually exceeds the actual cost of damages.

Putrefaction Decomposition of proteins with the production of foul-smelling products.

Putty-wash A technique whereby a putty tray and impression material are used together to get a final impression.

Pyloric sphincter The sphincter located between the stomach and the small intestine that allows food to enter the intestine and prevents reflux to stomach.

Quadrant Half of a maxillary or mandibular arch or one-fourth of the teeth in the entire mouth.

Quality assurance (QA) Procedures established that promote the production of the highest quality diagnostic radiographs.

Quality factor (QF) As applied to ionizing radiation, the term refers to the penetrating power of the rays.

Radial artery The artery located at the inner wrist used to take a person's pulse.

Radiation-absorbed dose (rad) One unit of radiation absorbed by matter, equivalent to 1 roentgen (R) or 0.01 gray (Gy).

Radiation caries Rampant caries that develop in a person who was exposed to high doses of radiation.

Radiobiology The study of ionizing radiation effects on living tissue.

Radiograph A processed exposed film consisting of shadows of a three dimensional object on film that can be viewed and interpreted.

Radiography The art or science of making radiographs; the act of making a radiograph.

Radiolucent Those images on the film that appear darker; the darkness is related to the lack of density of the object, which allows more x-rays to go through it and expose the film. Some restorative materials, certain diseases, and soft tissues will appear radiolucent on a radiograph.

Radiolysis The destructive change that takes place in a cell under the influence of radiation.

Radionuclide Any atomic nucleus specified by its atomic number, atomic mass, and energy state.

Radiopaque Those images on the radiograph that appear whiter or lighter; the lightness is related to the density of the object being exposed (bone, enamel, dentin). Certain restorative materials of dense metallic structure will also appear radiopaque on a radiograph.

Radioresistant Cells such as bone, muscle, nerve, and enamel are more resistant to ionized radiation. They can absorb more radiation without much damage.

Radiosensitive Cells such as reproductive, blood-forming, and intestinal epithelium are less resistant to ionized radiation and are more subject to damage.

Rampant caries Carious lesions appearing on almost every tooth in the oral cavity.

Ramus (rami-plural) Pertaining to a branch.

Rapport The term applied to a pleasant relationship in which there is concern and understanding.

Reactor Causes a chemical change.

Recurrent caries Carious lesions located under existing restorations.

Reduction A term that describes the removal of the bromide from the metallic silver, which remains behind to form the image.

Reference radiograph A radiograph made previously under ideal conditions of exposure and processing, kept as a measuring device for subsequent radiograph assessment.

Reflux Another term for backflow.

Registered dental assistants (RDA) A licensed dental assistant who performs additional clinical duties beyond those performed by the dental assistant under the supervision of a licensed dentist.

Registered dental assistant in extended functions (RDAEF) A licensed person who performs additional clinical duties beyond those performed by the dental assistant and RDA under the supervision of a licensed dentist.

Registered dental hygienist (RDH) A licensed person who mainly performs clinical duties in preventive dental health and, in some states, may perform all of the functions of dental assistants and RDAs under the supervision of a licensed dentist.

Regulated wastes Wastes that are regulated by OSHA and defined as potentially infectious.

Relative biologic effectiveness (RBE) Similar to quality factor but used only in reference to laboratory investigations.

Remission When signs and symptoms become less severe or are no longer evident.

Remnant radiation Radiation that has passed through the object to expose the film and produce an image. It is the image-forming radiation.

Removable maintainer A maintainer that can be removed and replaced by the patient.

Resin tags The mechanical interlocking of the resin to the etched enamel surface.

Resorption Loss of substance and reduction of the volume and size of tissues by activating osteoclasts.

Rest A metallic projection that fits on the occlusal or lingual aspect of a tooth to prevent the prosthesis from seating too far gingivally.

Retainer Fixed or removable appliances used to hold teeth in place.

Reticular Netlike initial formation of dentin.

Reticulation A condition where the film was exposed to sudden temperature changes between solutions and water, causing the emulsion to swell and shrink.

Retract To hold back away from the area or operation.

Retrognathic profile Profile that exhibits a weak chin.

Retrograde restoration Tooth is filled at the root end.

Reversible hyhdrocolloid The capacity of the hydrocolloid to change from a liquid to a gel (semi-solid state) and vice versa under certain conditions.

Rheostat A device used to regulate an electric current without interrupting the circuit of flow.

Rhodium A reflective metal used on the surface of the glass of a mirror.

Ribosomes Tiny particles found in all cells that serve as the sites for synthesizing proteins.

Rickettsia Tiny bacteria carried by arthropods that are obligate intracellular parasites.

Ridge A linear elevation on the surface of a tooth that is named according to its location and form, such as buccal ridge, incisal ridge, and marginal ridge.

Roentgen equivalent (in) man (rem) Unit of dose equivalent, or the absorbed dose of any type of ionizing radiation that produces the same biologic effects as 1 rad; equivalent to 0.01 Sv or 10 mSv.

Roentgen unit (R) An international unit based on the ability of radiation to ionize air. The unit of exposure corresponding to ionization of air of one electrostatic unit in 0.001293 gram of dry air at standard temperature and pressure.

Rotation When a tooth faces the wrong side but its long axis is positioned correctly.

Rotundum Round shaped.

Router A device that bridges between the local-area network and the Internet.

Saddle/base The acrylic resin portion attached to the framework that holds the artificial teeth and contacts the tissue.

Safelight A low-intensity red-orange light that uses a filter to sufficiently illuminate a darkroom without exposing or fogging film.

Salivary calculus A hard mass containing lime salts and found in saliva.

Salivation Secretion of saliva.

Sarcoma A malignant neoplasm of the soft tissues arising from supportive and connective tissue such as bone.

Saturated fats Contain a greater number of hydrogen atoms and are usually solid at room temperature.

Scattered radiation Radiation that may be deflected from matter and travel in directions not planned by the procedure.

Scribe A line drawn on the temporary crown to indicate proper height.

Seating lug An attachment welded to the orthodontic band used to seat the band to the tooth.

Secondary dentin Dentin that forms adjacent to the pulp cavity after teeth have erupted.

Secondary radiation Rays that have passed through matter, or the primary radiation that has interacted with matter.

Secretion The biological expulsion of material that has been chemically modified by a cell to serve a purpose elsewhere in the body.

Sella turcica Central portion or cradlelike structure of the sphenoid bone where the pituitary gland is located.

Semipermeable membrane Created by a varnish in preventing the passage of acids from the cements along the dentinal tubules to the pulp.

Sensory or afferent nerves Carry impulses from one part of the body to the brain; concerned with sensation.

Separator Appliances used to open up a space interproximally between teeth that will be receiving orthodontic bands.

Septa A wall or partition that separates two chambers.

Serous Pertaining to serum, a clear liquid.

Sharps Classified by OSHA as contaminated items that cut or puncture the skin.

Sharps injury Any injury caused by a sharp, including, but not limited to, cuts, abrasions, or needlesticks.

Sharps injury log A written or electronic record of any sharps injury.

Shelf life The stability of a dental material when it is stored.

Short-scale contrast High contrast, depicting few shades of gray on a radiograph as a result of using lower kilovoltage.

Short-term effects Effects of radiation manifested within a short time due to acute exposure to radiation.

Sievert (Sv) An SI unit for dose equivalent. Used in place of the rem; 1 Sv equals 100 rem.

Silicosis A condition in the lungs due to inhaled silica.

Silver halide crystals A component part of the emulsion on a film; the crystals that are suspended in gelatin forming the latent image when affected by radiation.

Single-ended instrument Having one working end.

Sinus Large hollow spaces within the bone.

Sinusitis A bacterial infection or inflammation of the mucous membranes that line the sinuses.

Smear layer A microscopic layer of mineralized tooth and bacterial debris.

Smooth muscles Involuntary muscles that contract and relax, i.e., to move food or fluids.

Soft copy What the computer monitor displays.

Soft radiation A term used to describe longer, lower frequency wavelengths or radiation.

Software A set of instructions that tells the hardware which tasks to perform.

Sol The liquified colloidal solution.

Soluble Capable of being dissolved.

Somatic cells All body cells except reproductive.

Source individual A person whose blood or other potentially infectious materials may have infected the employee.

Spacer Wax that provides the necessary space needed for the elastomeric impression material when fabricating an acrylic tray.

Species The most specific classification level that refers to a single type or distinct kind of organism.

Sphenoid Wedge-shaped bone.

Spherical Round in shape.

Spicules Sharp bone fragments that are removed for alveolar bone contouring.

Spirilla A rigid bacterial shape that is coiled like a corkscrew.

Spirochete A flexible coiled bacterium with a snakelike movement.

Splint Custom appliances whose object is to retain the traumatized tooth (teeth) in approximately the same position in the dental arch as before the injury.

Spores Dense, thick-walled cells that are the reproductive structures of fungi.

Spreadsheet A special feature in software that creates tables or places information using columns.

Squamous cell Flat, scalelike epithelial cell.

Standard Universal Precautions The same infection control procedures must be used for all patients for any given dental procedure.

State Board of Dental Examiners An administrative body created by the Dental Practice Act to interpret and provide definite procedure to ensure that regulations are fulfilled.

State Dental Practice Act Contains the legal restrictions and controls on the dentist, the dental auxiliaries, and the practice of dentistry.

Statute Laws, rules, and regulations.

Step-down transformer Reduces voltage of incoming alternating current to 3–5 volts to control the required amount of heat at the tungsten filament within the cathode.

Step-up transformer Increases the voltage of incoming alternating current from 110–220 volts to the required 65,000–100,000 volts.

Sterile A condition of being completely free of living organisms or viruses.

Sterilization The process of destroying all microorganisms and their pathogenic products. It is accomplished by moist heat (steam) under pressure or by dry heat.

Sternocleidomastoid muscle A muscle that arises from the sternum and clavicle and attaches to the mastoid process of the skull.

Stethoscope Instrument used to hear sounds within the body.

Stippled To have the appearance of an orange peel.

Stomodeum A depression at the head end of the embryo that becomes the front part of the mouth.

Stone dies A replica of a single tooth or several teeth on which a restoration is fabricated.

Stray radiation Rays that flow from parts of the tube other than the target.

Streptococcus mutans The first type of microorganism that attaches itself to the acquired pellicle and multiplies in the presence of carbohydrates, especially sugars.

Striated muscles Voluntary muscles that possess striations (bands of light and dark) that move the skeletal bones. Also known as skeletal or striped.

Study cast A plaster replica of the patient's mouth.

Styloid Slender and pointed.

Subgingival Located below the gingiva.

Submandibular Below the mandibular area.

Submental Below the chin area.

Substernal Under the sternum (central bone on chest where ribs attach).

Succedaneous Permanent teeth that replace primary teeth.

Sulcus A groove or depression.

Superficial Situated on or near the surface.

Supine The position assumed by a person who is lying on the back facing upward.

Supra Over or above

Suprabony Above the bone.

Supragingival Located above the gingiva.

Suture Where two bones join each other.

Symphysis Line of fusion where two distinct bones join and blend together as one.

Synergy Substances working together to achieve an effect of which each is individually incapable.

Syneresis Loss of water by evaporation due to exposure to the air, resulting in shrinkage in dimension.

Synovia A thick, sticky fluid found in joints of bones.

Synthetic A man made material.

Synthesis A reaction, or series of reactions, in which a complex compound is created from elements and simple compounds.

Systeme Internationale (SI) Radiation measurements that use the metric system.

Systemic Pertaining to the whole body.

Systolic pressure Occurs when the heart contracts, sending a surge of blood within the arteries that causes the highest arterial pressure.

Tactile Pertaining to the sense of touch.

Tarnish Simple surface discoloration of a silver alloy.

Template A clear plastic device made in the shape of the alveolar ridge with open markings to locate the implant.

Tendons Fibrous cords that attach muscles to bone.

Tetracycline An antibiotic.

Thermal Pertaining to temperature.

Therapeutic Pertaining to the treatment or curing of disease.

Thermionic emission (electron cloud) Electrons produced by the heated tungsten filament at the cathode.

Thermoplastic Having the ability to transform from a glassy, brittle solid to a softened, moldable plastic by the use of heat.

Thiazide diuretic Lowers blood volume through renal excretion of water and sodium ions.

Thixotropic Ability of gel to turn into fluid by applied stress and return to a gel state.

Threshold dose The amount or dose of radiation that causes damage to tissues, and prior to that threshold, there was no response.

Thrombocytes Also known as platelets that aid with clotting of blood.

Thrombosis A blood clot that blocks the lumen of the artery where it forms.

Thrush Candidiasis of the oral mucosa characterized by white patches on a red, moist, inflamed surface.

Thumb-to-nose grasp A method of grasping the oral vacuum when performing operative dentistry on posterior teeth.

Tidal volume The amount of air inhaled and exhaled during rest.

Tipping When a tooth leans laterally, mesially, or distally and its long axis tips toward a horizontal plane.

Titer The quantity of a substance required to cause antibody formation.

Titration Small incremental amounts of drug is given until desired dosage is achieved.

Tolerance The body builds tolerance to drugs with prolonged use.

Tomes' dentinal fibril A protoplasmic extension of an odontoblast (dentin-forming cell), found within the dentinal tubules.

Tomes' dentinal tubules Hollow structures found in the dentin that extend from the surface of the pulp to the dentinoenamel junction.

Tomography A radiographic technique used on a three-dimensional object that focuses on one plane of the object while blurring out other surrounding structures located in different planes.

Tongue thrust A pattern of swallowing in which the tongue is placed between the incisor teeth or alveolar ridges that may result in an open bite, deformation of the jaws, and abnormal function.

Tonus A slight state of contraction called muscle tone.

Torque movement When a tooth is in a linguoversion or labioversion position to the arch.

Toxic Resembling or caused by poison; poisonous.

Trabeculae The pattern of the cancellous bone that separates the medullary spaces.

Transillumination Passing a light through the crown of the tooth.

Transthorax Across the chest.

Transverse Pertaining to projecting across the palate.

Transverse ridge A ridge formed by two triangular ridges that join and cross the occlusal surface of a posterior tooth.

Trendelenburg position A supine position that places a person's head at a lower point than the chest and knees.

Triangular ridge A ridge that descends from the tips of the cusps of bicuspids and molars toward the center part of the occlusal surface.

Tributaries Vessels that flow into the larger veins.

Trifurcation Division into three, as in a three-rooted tooth.

Trismus Contraction of the muscles of mastication causing lockjaw.

Triturate The mechanical means of combining the dental alloy with mercury.

Trophozoite The active feeding stage of a protozoan life cycle.

Tubercle A small, rounded elevation on a bone for attachment of a tendon.

Tuberosity A rounded prominence or projection located at the most distal portion of the maxillary dentition.

Tungsten filament A coiled tungsten wire located at the cathode of the x-ray tube that produces the electron cloud.

Tungsten target Located at the anode of the x-ray tube where the high-kinetic-energy electrons strike to produce x-ray photons.

Umbra Shadow of object exhibited on a radiograph.

Undercut Type of cavity design whereby the pulpal wall itself is slanted to lock in the restoration in place.

Unilateral Pertaining to one side.

Universal System A charting system that uses numbers 1–32 for permanent teeth and letters A–T for primary teeth, starting with the maxillary right last molar as 1 or A.

Urticaria A condition of the skin where elevations of pale wheals appear that may be due to an allergic reaction.

Utility gloves Protective puncture-resistant gloves used for operatory disinfection and instrument clean-up.

Vallate (Circumvallate) pallae Cup-shaped papillae.

Vaporize Particles of matter scatter and freely float in the air.

Vaso Pertaining to blood vessel.

Vasoconstrictor Drugs that constrict (narrow) the lumen of blood vessels.

Vasodilator Drugs that relax the muscles of blood vessel walls, increasing their lumen.

Vector An animal such as an insect that spreads infection to humans.

Venous sinuses Venous channels situated between two layers of the dura mater on the brain.

Ventricle The lower chambers of each half of the heart.

Venules The smallest of veins which unite with capillaries in the circulatory system.

Verbal communication A mode of communication that involves the spoken or written word.

Verrucous Wart-like appearance.

Vertical angulation Alignment of the central ray using an up and down motion to position the PID at a positive (+), directing the ray downward, or negative (-) angulation, directing the ray upward. This establishes elongation or foreshortening.

Vertical bone loss Occurs when bone level of two adjacent teeth is at different heights from the cementoenamel junction.

Vesicle Small thin-walled blister containing clear fluid, less than 1 cm.

Vestibule An opening forming an entrance to another cavity.

Viewbox A source of light that uses fluorescent tubes under a frosted window to examine radiographs.

Virulence Of sufficient strength to cause disease.

Virus A tiny infectious particle that takes over its host cell and multiplies inside it.

Visceral pain Located deep within the body such as muscles, organs, and cavities where pain is interpreted as dull and is less localized. Pertains to being alive.

Viscosity Thickness of a fluid that causes it not to flow.

Wall of maxillary sinus Thin layer of dense bone that lines the maxillary sinus vertically.

Walls of mandibular canal Thin cortical bone that lines the passage of the mandibular canal.

Washed-field technique The use of water as a coolant when cutting and shaping tooth tissues with a high-speed dental handpiece.

Wavelength The distance between one crest of a wave to the crest of an adjacent wave of electromagnetic energy. The shorter the wavelength, the stronger or more energetic it is.

Wax pattern A wax replica of the anatomy of the tooth that is being replaced by a cast restoration.

Web sites A collection of viewable documents located on a computer server.

Wedge A triangular shaped device made of wood or plastic used between two teeth to brace the matrix band and prevent overhangs of restorative material.

Wet strength The strength present when the water is in excess of that required to bring the gypsum back to its natural water content.

Wheals Pale elevations on the skin, white in the center with pale red borders, accompanied by itching.

Whole body exposure Refers to ionized radiation exposure to the whole body at one time.

Wicking Penetration of glove material through inherent defects.

Xerostomia Dryness of the mouth due to salivary gland secretion dysfunction.

X-rays A type of electromagnetic radiation with extremely short and high-frequency wavelengths, capable of penetrating matter.

Barton, R. E. (1988). *The dental assistant* (6th ed.). Philadelphia, PA: Lea & Febiger.

Brand, R. W. & Isselhard, D. E. (1994). *Anatomy of oro-facial structures* (5th ed.). St. Louis: Mosby.

California Department of Consumer Affairs. (1994). *Dental Practice Act with Rules and Regulations.* Sacramento, CA: Author.

Carranza, F. A. & Perry, D. A. (1986). *Clinical periodontology for the dental hygienist.* Philadelphia: Saunders.

Centers for Disease Control and Prevention. (1987). Handpiece sterilization procedures. *Dental Products Report, 21,* 47–51.

Clark M. S. & Brunick, A. L. (1999). *Handbook of nitrous oxide and oxygen sedation.* St. Louis: Mosby.

Computer Age Dentist. (1997). *Tomorrow's practice management solutions...Today* [Brochure]. Santa Monica, CA: Author.

Council on Dental Therapeutics of the American Dental Association. (1982). *Accepted dental therapeutics.* Chicago: Author.

Darby, M. L., & Walsh, M. M. (1995). *Dental hygiene theory and practice.* Philadelphia: Saunders.

Dentrix Dental Systems. (1997). [Brochure].

Donovan, T. E. (1995). *Restorative dental materials: A clinical approach.* Los Angeles: University of Southern California.

Dunn, S. M., & Kantor, M. L. (1993). Digital radiology facts and fictions. *JADA, 124,* 39–44.

Ehrlich, A. (1997). *Medical terminology for health professions* (3rd ed.). Albany: Delmar.

Ferracane, J. L. (1995). *Materials in dentistry: Principles and applications.* Philadelphia: Lippincott, Williams & Wilkins.

Ferretti, A. (1999). *Radiographic imaging for dental auxiliaries: Extraoral radiography* (3rd ed.) Philadelphia: Saunders.

Finkbeiner, B. L., & Finkbeiner, C. A. (1996). *Practice management for the dental team* (4th ed.). St. Louis: Mosby-Year Book.

Finkbeiner, B. L., & Johnson, C. S. (1999). *Mosby's comprehensive review of dental assisting.* St. Louis: Mosby.

Frommer, H. H. (1996). *Radiology for dental auxiliaries* (6th ed.). St. Louis: Mosby-Year Book.

Gage, T. W. & Picket, F. A. (1996). *Mosby's dental drug reference.* St. Louis: Mosby-Year Book.

Glass, B. J. (Ed.). (1996). *Successful panoramic radiography.* Rochester, NY: Eastman Kodak Co.

Gluck, G. M., & Morganstein, W. M. (1998). *Jong's community dental health* (4th ed.). St. Louis: Mosby-Year Book.

Goaz, P. W., & White, S. C. DDS. (1994). *Oral Radiology Principles of Interpretation* (3rd ed.). St. Louis: Mosby-Year Book.

Gould, B.E. (1997). *Pathophysiology for the health-related professions.* Philadelphia: Saunders.

Haring, J. I. & Lind, L. J. (1993). *Radiographic interpretation for the dental hygienist.* Philadelphia: Saunders.

Haring, J. I. & Lind, L. J. (1996). *Dental radiography: Principles and techniques.* Philadelphia: Saunders.

Ibsen, O. A., & Phelan, J. A. (1996). *Oral pathology for the dental hygienist* (2nd ed.). Philadelphia: Saunders.

Journal of the American Dental Assistants Association, Recommendations for follow-up of health-care workers after occupational exposure to hepatitis C virus, May/June 1998.

Malamed, S. F. (1995). *Sedation: A guide to patient management.* St. Louis: Mosby-Year Book.

Malamed, S. F. ((1997). *Handbook of local anesthesia* (4th ed.). St. Louis: Mosby Yearbook.

Malamed, S. F. (2000). *Medical emergencies in the dental office* (5th ed.). St Louis MO: Mosby.

Microbiotics. (1998). *Hepa filtration, a global problem that has remedies* [Brochure].

Miles, D. A., Van Dis, M. L., Jensen, C. W., & Ferretti, A. (1999). *Radiographic imaging for dental auxillaries* (3rd ed.). Philadelphia: Saunders.

Monahan, R. (1996). [Legal aspects of the doctor-patient relationship]. Unpublished handout.

Neville, B. W., Damm, D. D., & White, D. K. (1999). *Color atlas of clinical oral pathology* (2nd ed.). Philadelphia: Lippincott, Williams & Wilkins.

Office Safety & Asepsis Procedures (OSAP) Research Foundation. (1995). Infection control in dentistry guidelines. Booklet.

Office Safety & Asepsis Procedures (OSAP) Research Foundation. Monthly Focus #8. (1996a). Personal protective equipment. Annapolis MD.

Office Safety & Asepsis Procedures (OSAP) Research Foundation, Monthly Focus #12. (1996b). Vaccinations update. Annapolis MD.

Office Safety & Asepsis Procedures (OSAP) Research Foundation. (1997). "Chemical Agents for Surface Disinfecting Reference Chart." Author.

Office Safety & Asepsis Procedures (OSAP) Research Foundation. (1997). *Infection Control in Dentistry Guidelines*, "Radiographic Asepsis." Author.

Office Safety & Asepsis Procedures (OSAP) Research Foundation. Monthly Focus #4. (1997a). Criticality of instrument cleaning.

Office Safety & Asepsis Procedures (OSAP) Research Foundation, Monthly Focus #5. (1997b). The sterilization process.

Office Safety & Asepsis Procedures (OSAP) Research Foundation, Monthly Focus #2. (1998). The dental infection control program.

Office Safety & Asepsis Procedures (OSAP) Research Foundation, Monthly Focus #4. (1998). Latex-associated allergies & conditions.

O'Hehir, T. E. & Suvan, J. (1997). *Perio reports—compendium of current research*. Flagstaff, AZ: Modern Press.

OSHA. (Amended 1999). *Bloodborne pathogens standard #5193*.

Phillips, R. W. (1984). *Elements of dental materials for dental hygienists and assistants* (4th ed., pp. 101–109). Philadelphia: Saunders.

Preston, J. D. (1998). Digital tools for clinical dentistry. *California Dental Association Journal* 26, 915–922.

Product literature, VistaCam Video Imaging System, Air Techniques, Costa Mesa, CA.

Product literature, Capture-It Clinical Image Management Software, Densply New Image, Densply International, York, PA.

Product literature, UltraCam Intraoral Systems, UltraView 3.0, Carrollton, TX.

Product literature, TeliCam System II, Dental Medical Diagnostic Systems, Westlake Village, CA.

Requa, B. S. & Holroy, S. V. (1982). *Applied pharmacology for the dental hygienist*. St. Louis: Mosby.

Scott, A. & Fong, E. (1998). *Body structures & functions* (9th ed.). Albany: Delmar.

Talaro, K. P., & Talaro, A. (1999). *Foundations in microbiology* (3rd ed.). Dubuque IA: William C. Brown.

Thomas, C. L. (1997). *Taber's cyclopedic medical dictionary* (18th ed.). Philadelphia: F. A. Davis.

U.S. Department of Labor, Occupational Safety and Health Administration. (1991). *Occupational exposure to bloodborne pathogens standard* (29 CFR part 1910.1030). *Federal Register* (56.64004–64182).

Wilkins, E. M., (1999). *Clinical practice of the dental hygienist* (8th ed.). Philadelphia: Lippencott, Williams & Wilkins.

Woodrow, R. (1997). *Essentials of pharmacology for health occupations* (3rd ed.). Albany, NY: Delmar.

Yost, G. Independent Computer Consultant. (Feb. 1999). Interview.